FLUIDS AND ELECTROLYTES WITH CLINICAL APPLICATIONS

A PROGRAMMED APPROACH

FIFTH EDITION

JOYCE LeFEVER KEE, R.N., M.S.

Associate Professor Emerita
College of Nursing
University of Delaware
Newark, Delaware

BETTY J. PAULANKA, R.N., Ed.D.

Dean
College of Nursing
University of Delaware
Newark, Delaware

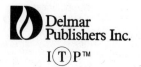

Delmar Publishers Inc.

I(T)P™

NOTICE TO THE READER

Cover design: Katie Hayden

Delmar staff:
Acquisitions Editor: Patricia E. Casey
Associate Editor: Elisabeth F. Williams
Project Editors: Melissa Conan/Christopher Chien
Production Coordinator: Mary Ellen Black
Art and Design Coordinator: Timothy J. Conners

For information, address

Delmar Publishers Inc.
3 Columbia Circle, Box 15015
Albany, NY 12203-5015

Printed in the United States of America
Published simultaneously in Canada
by Nelson Canada,
a division of The Thomson Corporation

1 2 3 4 5 6 7 8 9 10   XXX   00 99 98 97 96 95 94

Library of Congress Cataloging-in-Publication Data

Kee, Joyce LeFever.
    Fluids and electrolytes with clinical applications : a programmed
approach / Joyce LeFever Kee, Betty J. Paulanka. -- 5th ed.
        p.   cm.
    Includes bibliographical references and index.
    ISBN 0-8273-5134-8
    1. Body fluid disorders--Programmed instruction.   2. Water
-electrolyte imbalances--Programmed instruction.   3. Water
-electrolyte imbalances--Nursing--Programmed instruction.   4. Body
fluid disorders--Nursing--Programmed instruction.   5. Body fluid
disorders--Programmed instruction.   6. Water-electrolyte imbalances-
-Programmed instruction.   7. Body fluid disorders--Nursing-
-Programmed instruction.   8. Water-eletrolyte imbalances--Nursing-
-Programmed instruction.   I. Paulanka, Betty J.   II. Title.
RC630.K43 1994
616.3'9--dc20
                                                                                    93-46613
                                                                                    CIP

To
My Children—Eric, Katherine, and Wanda

Joyce LeFever Kee

To
My Children—Christie and Elaine

Betty J. Paulanka

Margaret R. Poppiti, R.N., M.S., C.N.N.
Dialysis Center
V.A. Medical Center
Wilmington, Delaware
  Renal Failure

Larry Purnell, R.N., Ph.D.
Assistant Professor
College of Nursing
University of Delaware
Newark, Delaware
  Gastrointestinal Surgery
  Increased Intracranial Pressure
  Burns and Burn Shock

Julie Waterhouse, R.N., M.S.
Assistant Professor
College of Nursing
University of Delaware
Newark, Delaware
  with
Marilyn Halstead
  Clinical Oncology

Consultants

Devasmita Choudhury, M.D.
Director, Dialysis Center
V.A. Medical Center
Wilmington, Delaware
  Renal Failure

Lucille Pulliam, R.N., Ph.D.
Associate Professor
College of Nursing
University of Delaware
Newark, Delaware
  Fluid Problems of Aging Adults

Larry Purnell, R.N., Ph.D.
Assistant Professor
College of Nursing
University of Delaware
Newark, Delaware
  Intravenous Therapy

Gail Wade, R.N., M.S.
Instructor
College of Nursing
University of Delaware
Newark, Delaware
  Fluid Problems of Infants and Children

Olga Ward, R.N.
Parenteral Therapist
Medical Center of Delaware
Wilmington, Delaware
  Intravenous Therapy

CONTENTS

Part I
Fluids, Electrolytes, and Acid-Base Balance and Imbalance

Chapter 1
BODY FLUID AND ITS FUNCTION

Chapter 2
FLUIDS AND THEIR INFLUENCE ON THE BODY

Chapter 3
ELECTROLYTES AND THEIR INFLUENCE ON THE BODY

Chapter 4
ACID-BASE BALANCE AND IMBALANCE

Part II
Clinical Situations

Chapter 6
FLUID PROBLEMS OF INFANTS AND CHILDREN

Chapter 7
FLUID PROBLEMS OF THE AGING ADULT

Chapter 8
GASTROINTESTINAL SURGERY

Chapter 12
INCREASED INTRACRANIAL PRESSURE

Chapter 13
CLINICAL ONCOLOGY

Chapter 17
CHRONIC OBSTRUCTIVE PULMONARY DISEASE

Nurses are involved continually in the assessment of fluid and electrolyte imbalance. Medical advances and new treatment modalities have increased the importance of a strong background in the physiologic concepts associated with these imbalances. Additionally, the expanded role of nurses requires them to function more autonomously in assisting clients to control fluid and electrolyte imbalances. Every seriously or chronically ill person is likely to develop one or more imbalances. Even those who are only moderately ill are at a high risk for these imbalances. Nurses are responsible for maintaining homeostasis of fluid and electrolyte balance when caring for clients. After completing this book, the participant should understand more fully the effects of fluid, electrolyte, and acid-base balance and imbalance on the body as they occur in many clinical health problems.

The fifth edition of this programmed text, *Fluids and Electrolytes with Clinical Applications*, has been completely revised to meet the current assessment, management, and nursing interventions recommended for fluid and electrolyte imbalances and related clinical health problems. The format of most chapters includes a chapter outline, behavioral objectives, pathophysiology, etiology, clinical manifestations, clinical management, clinical applications, case studies, and nursing diagnoses with nursing interventions and appropriate rationales. Many new charts containing specific information and rationale are included to clarify pertinent content related to selected topics. There are over 125 tables and diagrams, each followed by content frames to help participants gain a deeper understanding of the material and develop personal self-confidence in the nursing management of fluid and electrolyte imbalances. A new chapter entitled Increased Intracranial Pressure contains the fluid, electrolyte, and acid-base imbalances associated with increased intracranial pressure. Nursing assessment factors and nursing diagnoses with nursing interventions are included in the first four chapters regarding general concepts of fluid, electrolyte, and acid-base balance and imbalances and in each of the twelve specialty chapters.

Chapter 2 contains the four common fluid imbalances: extracellular fluid volume deficit, extracellular fluid volume excess, extracellular fluid shift, and intracellular fluid volume excess. Chapter 3 contains the six electrolytes: potassium, sodium, calcium, magnesium, phosphorus, and chloride. The fourth chapter discusses acid-base balance and imbalances, particularly metabolic acidosis and alkalosis and respiratory acidosis and alkalosis. The first four chapters follow the above stated format.

Chapter 5 has been revised to include updates on intravenous (IV) solutions and flow rates, expanded information on total parenteral nutrition (TPN), a new section on infusion devices, and nursing diagnoses and interventions for clients receiving intravenous infusions.

There are a total of twelve specialty chapters related to specific health problems in which fluid and electrolyte imbalance is a major concern. These chapters discuss fluid problems of infants and children; aging adults with fluid and electrolyte imbalances; gastrointestinal surgery; trauma and shock; congestive heart failure; renal failure; increased intracranial pressure; clinical oncology; diabetic ketoacidosis; burns and burn shock; cirrhosis of the liver; and chronic obstructive pulmonary disease (COPD). Case studies, nursing assessment factors, and nursing diagnoses with interventions are included in each chapter.

The content of this book has been geared to three levels of learning within the nursing profession. First, it is intended for beginning students who have had some background in the biological sciences or who have completed an anatomy and physiology course. Second, it is for students who have a sufficient background in the biological sciences, chemistry, and physics but who need to learn about intravenous therapy and specific clinical health problems that cause fluid and electrolyte imbalances. Many of these students might wish to review the entire text to reinforce their previous knowledge and/or practice their skills in handling clinical nursing assessments and interventions. Finally, this book is intended to aid graduate nurses to review and improve their knowledge of fluid and electrolyte changes in order to assess their clients' needs and enhance the quality of client care.

Each participant can work at his or her own pace while learning the principles, concepts, and applications of fluids and electrolytes as presented in this book. This self-instructional method of learning helps the instructor to use class time more efficiently, while enabling students to apply their knowledge to clinical situations in their clinical practicum.

Throughout, an asterisk (*) on an answer line indicates a multiple-word answer. The meanings for the following symbols are: ↑ increased, ↓ decreased, > greater than, < less than. A dagger (†) indicates the most common signs and symptoms. A glossary covers words and terms used throughout the text. It should be useful to the student who has minimal preparation in the biological sciences.

Joyce LeFever Kee, R.N., M.S.
Betty J. Paulanka, R.N., Ed.D.

ACKNOWLEDGMENTS

We would like to express our appreciation to the students who used this programmed text in its various forms before the first edition was published. By testing their acquired knowledge and ability to apply it after they read the manuscript, necessary changes were made to improve the text. We extend our thanks to the students and faculty who tested the revisions for the second edition and made valuable suggestions for additions to, omissions from, and clarification of the frames and material covered.

For the third and fourth editions, our deepest appreciation is extended to students in the College of Nursing and the following professors: Sally Marshall (renal failure section), Julie Waterhouse (cancer section), Elizabeth Jenkins (parenteral therapy chapter), Evelyn Hayes (electrolyte chapter), Carolyn Freed (congestive heart failure section), and Brent Thompson (fluid problems in children section).

For the fifth edition, we wish to extend our deepest appreciation to Larry Purnell, Julie Waterhouse, Margaret Poppiti, Devasmita Choudhury, Lucille Pulliam, Gail Wade, and Olga Ward for their contributions and assistance.

We especially wish to thank Don Passidomo, head librarian at the V.A. Medical Center, Wilmington, Delaware, for his valuable assistance and service and for the literature search on fluids and electrolytes.

We also offer our sincere thanks to Patricia E. Casey, Aquisitions Editor, Elisabeth F. Williams, Associate Editor, and Deborah L. Angell, Editorial Assistant, at Delmar Publishers Inc. for their helpful suggestions and assistance with this revision.

TO THE INSTRUCTOR

Class time is frequently spent on reviewing material or presenting new material that can easily be given through programmed (learning) instruction. This method of instruction enables the teacher to minimize the time spent in lecture on fluids and electrolytes, thus devoting more time to clinical discussions and seminar format to enhance the students' understanding of fluid and electrolyte imbalance by active class participation.

You may find it helpful to cover the material in this book by one of three ways: (1) assigning the students a chapter at a time; (2) assigning the students and first five chapters to be completed by a certain date and specialty chapters to be coordinated with clinical experiences; or (3) assigning the students a given length of time to complete the entire text and having them present material using their clinical experience.

TO THE STUDENTS

Many students believe that the subject of fluids and electrolytes is very difficult to comprehend. This programmed book provides you with important data on fluids and electrolytes from various points of view. If you apply this material to clinical problems and previous and present experiences, it is not so difficult to understand and retain.

By taking easy steps provided in this book, you can proceed through the chapters more quickly than you might expect. This book is written using a self-instruction format that allows you to proceed at your own speed. Each step is a learning process. A better quality of learning occurs when you either complete a chapter at a time or spend a minimum of two hours at one sitting. Never end the study period without at least completing all frames related to a single topic.

It is helpful to begin each study session with the final frames from the previous material; this enables you to check your retention of material that was presented previously. The case study reviews in each chapter give immediate reinforcement of the data learned. The nursing assessment factors and nursing diagnoses with interventions should be useful when applying fluid, electrolyte, and acid-base concepts in various clinical settings. A glossary is included to assist you with words and terms used throughout the text.

Study each diagram and table before proceeding to the frames. If you make mistakes in the program, you need not be concerned so long as you rectify the mistakes. This learning modality and the content in this book should increase your knowledge and understanding of fluids and electrolytes. This model of learning can be a great asset for applying this knowledge to your clinical practicum experiences.

Joyce LeFever Kee
Betty J. Paulanka

PART I

FLUIDS, ELECTROLYTES, AND ACID-BASE BALANCE AND IMBALANCE

CHAPTER 1

BODY FLUID AND ITS FUNCTION

Behavioral Objectives

Upon completion of this chapter, you will be prepared to:

- Compare the percentage of water found in the body of the average adult, newborn infant, and embryo.
- Identify the three compartments (spaces) where water is distributed in the body.
- Identify the two classifications of body fluid and their percentages.
- Describe five functions of body fluids.
- Define homeostasis in terms of its role in maintaining body fluid equilibrium.
- Describe how the body loses and maintains body fluid.
- Define the following homeostatic mechanisms: osmotic pressure, oncotic pressure, semipermeable membranes, selectively permeable membranes, osmol, and osmolality.
- Describe the effects of the above homeostatic mechanisms on the movement of body fluid.
- Describe four measurable pressures that determine the flow of fluid between the vessels and tissues in terms of their effects on the exchange of fluid.
- Describe the concept of a pressure gradient.
- Explain the significance in colloid osmotic (oncotic) and hydrostatic pressure gradients.
- Discuss the body's regulators of fluid balance.
- Describe isotonic (iso-osmolar), hypotonic (hypo-osmolar), and hypertonic (hyperosmolar) solutions in terms of their effects on body cells.
- Discuss the relationship between milligrams and milliequivalents and the significance of this relationship in the body.
- Describe the effects of selected fluid changes on the observable symptoms of patients in your clinical area.

Introduction

The human body is a complex machine that contains hundreds of bones and the most sophisticated interaction of systems of any structure on earth. Yet, the substance that is basic to the very existence of the body is the simplest substance known—water. In fact, it makes up almost two thirds of an adult's body weight.

The body is not static—it is alive and solid particles within its framework are able to move into and out of cells and systems, and even into and out of the body, only because there is water.

The basis of all fluids is water, and as long as the quantity and composition of body fluids are within the normal range, we just take it for granted and enjoy being healthy. But if the water content of the body for some reason departs from this range, the whole delicate balance of body systems is disrupted, and disease can find an easy target.

In this chapter, distribution of body fluids, fluid compartments, functions of body fluid, intake and output for homeostasis, definitions, fluid pressures, regulators of body fluid, and osmolality of body fluid and solutions are discussed. Also included are a case study review, nursing assessment factors, nursing diagnoses, and nursing interventions.

An asterisk (*) on an answer line indicates a multiple-word answer. The meanings for the following symbols are: ↑ increased, ↓ decreased, > greater than, < less than.

1   The greatest single constituent of the body is water, which represents about 60% of the total body weight in the average adult. In the early human embryo, 97% of body weight is water, and in a newborn infant, 77% of body weight is water.

Label the following drawings with the proper percentage of water to body weight.

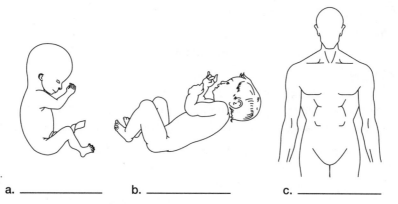

a. _____   b. _____   c. _____

a. 97%; b. 77%; c. 60%

2   In the average adult, the proportion of water to   *_____   is 60%.

body weight

3   Which has the highest percentage of water in relation to body weight (adult, newborn infant, embryo?)   _____ . Which has the lowest?   _____ .

embryo; adult

4 Speculate why the early human embryo and the infant have a higher proportion of water to body weight than the adult.

* _____

_____.

Many people think the extra water in infants acts as a protective mechanism. Since infants have larger body surface in relation to their weight, extra water acts as a cushion against injury.

■　　　　　　　■　　　　　　　■

5 Because body fat is essentially free of water, the leaner the individual, the greater the proportion of water in total body weight.

Who has more water as body weight—a person with more body fat or a person with less body fat?

* _____ .

a person with less body fat

■　　　　　　　■　　　　　　　■

FLUID COMPARTMENTS

6 Body water is distributed among three types of "compartments": cells, blood vessels, and tissue spaces between blood vessels and cells which are separated by membranes.

Label the three compartments where body water (fluid) is found.

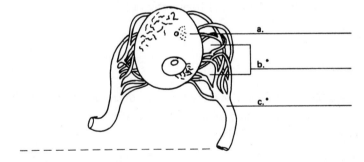

a. _____

b.* _____

c.* _____

a. *cell*
b. *tissue space*
c. *blood vessel*

■　　　　　　　■　　　　　　　■

7   The term for the water (fluid) in each type of "compartment" is as follows:

1. In the cell—*intracellular* fluid or *cellular* fluid.
2. In the blood vessels—*intravascular* fluid.
3. In tissue spaces between blood vessels and cells—*interstitial* fluid.

Label the diagram with the proper terms for body water in each of the three compartments.

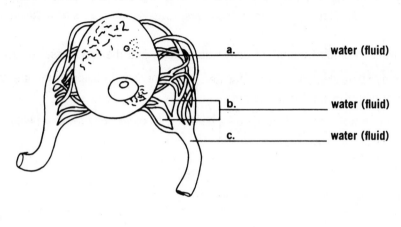

a. _____ water (fluid)

b. _____ water (fluid)

c. _____ water (fluid)

- - - - - - - - - - - - - - - - - -

a. *intracellular*
b. *interstitial*
c. *intravascular*

■   ■   ■

8   There are three prefixes that will be used frequently in this text:

inter-   between
intra-   within
extra-   outside of

The two major classes of body water or body fluid are described as intracellular fluid and extracellular fluid. The corresponding areas, or "compartments," that house this fluid are the intracellular space and the extracellular space.

The prefix *intra* means _____ . The prefix *extra* means _____

*_____ .

within; outside of

■   ■   ■

9 Fluid within the cell is classified as intracellular fluid, whereas intravascular fluid and interstitial fluid are classified as extracellular fluid.

The area within the cell is called the _____ space, whereas the tissue spaces between blood vessels and cells and the area within blood vessels are known as the _____ space.

intracellular; extracellular

■   ■   ■

10 Label the three "compartments" of body water (fluid) and the two classes of body water (fluid) represented in the diagram.

Compartments

a. _____

b. * _____

c. * _____

Classes

a. * _____

b. _____

Compartments

a. cell

b. tissue space

c. blood vessel

Classes

a. cellular or intracellular

b. extracellular

■   ■   ■

11 Approximately two thirds of the body fluid is contained in the intracellular compartment.

We have already said that the total body weight in the adult body is _____% water; therefore, intracellular fluid must represent _____ % of the total body weight, and extracellular fluid represents _____ % of the total body weight.

60; 40; 20

■   ■   ■

12 If one fourth of the extracellular fluid is intravascular fluid, then three fourths of extracellular fluid is * _____ .

interstitial fluid

■   ■   ■

13 Therefore, extracellular fluid represents _____ % of the total body weight, of which *_____ is interstitial fluid.

Interstitial fluid represents _____ % of total body weight. Intravascular fluid represents _____ % of total body weight.

20; three fourths; 15; 5

■   ■   ■

FUNCTIONS OF BODY WATER

14 The body is unable to maintain a healthy state without water.

Five main functions of body water are:

1. Transportation of nutrients, electrolytes, and oxygen to the cells
2. Excretion of waste products
3. Regulation of body temperature
4. Lubrication of joints and membranes
5. Medium for food digestion

Without water, the body would be (able/unable) _____ to maintain life.

unable

■   ■   ■

15 Name three of the five main functions of body water.

a. *_____

b. *_____

c. *_____

see Frame 14. Three of those functions should be selected.

■   ■   ■

INTAKE AND OUTPUT FOR HOMEOSTASIS

16 Since we already have learned that the percentage of body fluid varies with age and percentage of body fat, then the proportion of intracellular and extracellular fluid in a person with more body fat would be (greater/lesser) in proportion to body weight. _____ .

lesser

■   ■   ■

17 *Homeostasis* is a term used to describe the state of equilibrium of the internal environment. In relation to body fluids, homeostasis is the process of maintaining equilibrium or stability in relation to the physical and chemical properties of body fluid.

In a few words define the term *homeostasis*. *_____ . Explain the
relationship of homeostasis to body fluid. *_____

_____ .

state of equilibrium
It maintains equilibrium of the physical and chemical properties of body fluid.

■   ■   ■

18   The body normally maintains a state of equilibrium between the amount of water taken in and the amount of water lost.

If the body loses or gains water, it acts rapidly to compensate for this deficit or excess so that _____ will be maintained.

homeostasis or equilibrium

■   ■   ■

19   When body water is insufficient, urine volume diminishes and the individual becomes thirsty. Therefore, the patient drinks more water to correct the fluid (excess/deficit)

_____ .

deficit or loss

■   ■   ■

20   When we drink an excessive amount of water, our urinary output increases.

If you did not drink any fluids or if the body loses excessive water, the urinary volume would do which of the following:

( ) a. Increase
( ) b. Decrease

If there were an excess of water in the body, the urinary volume would adapt by which of the following:

( ) a. Increasing
( ) b. Decreasing

b. decrease; a. increasing

■   ■   ■

21   Refer to Figure 1-1. The three normal sources of body water intake are
_____ , _____ , and *_____ .

liquid, food, and oxidation of food

■   ■   ■

9

Figure 1-1. Normal pattern of water intake and loss.

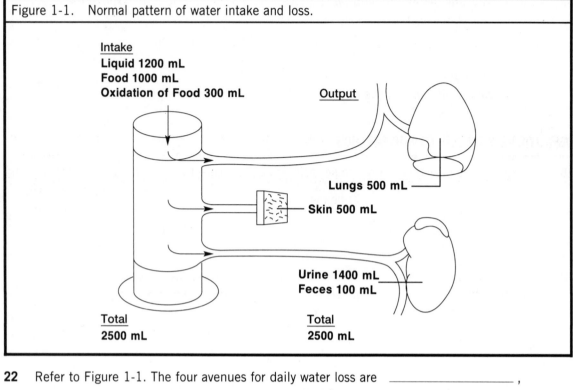

Intake
Liquid 1200 mL
Food 1000 mL
Oxidation of Food 300 mL

Output

Lungs 500 mL

Skin 500 mL

Urine 1400 mL
Feces 100 mL

Total
2500 mL

Total
2500 mL

22 Refer to Figure 1-1. The four avenues for daily water loss are _____ ,
_____ , _____ , and _____ .

lungs, skin, urine, and feces

■   ■   ■

23 If your water intake amounted to 2500 mL for the day and your water output was 2500 mL,
your body has maintained a state of _____ of body fluid.

equilibrium or homeostasis

■   ■   ■

24 The rate of water loss and gain is different in summer and winter. Describe why you think this
occurs. *_____

_____ .

*In the summer when the atmospheric temperature is high, water loss via skin and lungs
increases.*

■   ■   ■

25 Evaporation of water from the skin, as we perspire, is a protective mechanism against overheating the body.

Explain how evaporation of water acts as a protective mechanism. *_____
_____ .

It acts as a cooling system, keeping the body at a normal temperature.

■   ■   ■

DEFINITIONS RELATED TO BODY FLUIDS

26 Diffusion is the movement of molecules/solutes across a selectively permeable membrane along its own pathway, irrespective of all other molecules. Large molecules move *less* rapidly than small molecules. Molecules move faster from an area of higher concentration to an area of lower concentration.

Diffusion is the *_____
across a selectively permeable membrane. Small molecules move (faster than/slower than) large molecules. *_____ .

Molecules/solutes tend to move faster from *_____
_____ to *_____ .

movement of molecules/solutes; faster than
an area of higher concentration; an area of lower concentration

■   ■   ■

27 Body water loss by diffusion through the skin which is immeasurable and independent of sweat gland activity is called *insensible perspiration.*

When sweat gland activity occurs and water appears on the skin, this is called *sensible perspiration.*

In a relatively comfortable temperature would insensible perspiration or sensible perspiration occur? _____ . Why? *_____
_____ .

insensible
There is not enough heat to cause sweat gland activity, so only the normal loss occurs through insensible perspiration, with water diffusing through the skin and evaporating quickly.

■   ■   ■

28   Define the following terms:

Insensible perspiration. *_____.

Sensible perspiration. *_____.

immeasurable water loss by diffusion through the skin; water on the skin due to sweat gland activity

■   ■   ■

29   The volume of body water is primarily regulated by the kidneys. When water loss increases, e.g., through perspiration or diarrhea, the kidneys conserve water by (increasing/decreasing) the urinary output.

_____ .

decreasing

■   ■   ■

30   More definitions to know:

Membrane. A layer of tissue covering a surface or organ or separating spaces.

Osmosis. The passage of a solvent through a partition from a solution of lesser solute concentration to one of greater solute concentration.

   Note: Osmosis may be expressed in terms of water concentration instead of solute concentration. Then water molecules pass from an area of higher water concentration (fewer solutes) to an area of lower water concentration (more solutes).

Solvent.   A liquid with a substance in solution.

Solute.   A substance dissolved in a solution.

Permeability.   A capability of a substance, molecule, or ion to diffuse through a membrane.

Early literature described membranes of body cells as semipermeable. Today *semipermeable* refers to artificial membranes, i.e., cellophane membrane. *Selectively permeable membrane* refers to the permeability of the human membranes.

   Differentiate between:

Selectively permeable membrane. *_____.

Semipermeable membrane. *_____.

human membrane; artificial membrane

■   ■   ■

31 Explain the difference between a solvent and a solute.

Solvent. *_____ .

Solute. *_____ .

a liquid with a substance in solution; a substance dissolved in solution

■   ■   ■

32 In an effort to establish equilibrium, water in the body moves from a less concentrated solution (fewer solute particles per unit of solvent) to a more concentrated solution (more solute particles per unit of solvent) through a *_____ membrane.

selectively permeable or human

■   ■   ■

33 Osmotic pressure is the pressure or force that develops when two solutions of different strengths or concentrations are separated by a selectively permeable membrane.

To establish osmotic equilibrium, water moves from the (less/more) _____ concentrated solution into the (less/more) _____ concentrated solution.

The force that draws water across a selectively permeable membrane is called

*_____ .

less; more; osmotic pressure

■   ■   ■

34 In what direction does water flow? *_____

_____ . Why? *_____ .

from the lesser to the greater concentration; because more solute particles have a "pulling" effect which sets up a pressure gradient

■   ■   ■

35 Do you recall the meaning of *permeable*? If not, return to Frame 30.

A membrane is considered impermeable if an ion, substance, or molecule cannot diffuse freely across it.

Certain substances do not diffuse freely across the human membrane. When this happens, the membrane is considered _____ to that substance.

impermeable

■   ■   ■

FLUID PRESSURES (STARLING'S LAW)

36 Extracellular fluid (ECF) shifts between the intravascular space (blood vessels) and the interstitial space (tissues) to maintain a fluid balance within the ECF compartment.

Four fluid pressures regulate the flow of fluid between the intravascular and interstitial spaces in order to maintain fluid homeostasis or equilibrium.

ECF flows back and forth between the _____ space and the _____ space to maintain _____ .

intravascular; interstitial; homeostasis or equilibrium
■   ■   ■

37 E. H. Starling states that equilibrium exists at the capillary membrane when the fluid leaving circulation and the amount of fluid returning to circulation are exactly equal.

There are four measurable pressures that determine the flow of fluid between the intravascular and interstitial spaces. These are the colloid osmotic (oncotic) pressures and the hydrostatic pressures that are in both the vessels and the tissue spaces.

According to Starling, equilibrium exists at the *_____ .

capillary membrane
■   ■   ■

38 Three new terms to define:

Colloid: A nondiffusible substance; a solute suspended in solution.
Hydrostatic: A state of equilibrium of fluid pressures.
Oncotic pressure: osmotic pressure of a colloid (protein) in body fluid.

The osmotic pressure is *_____

_____

_____ .

the pressure that develops when two solutions of different strengths or concentrations are separated by a selectively permeable membrane OR the force that draws water (fluid) across a selectively permeable membrane
■   ■   ■

39 The measurable pressures influencing body fluid flow within the ECF compartment that are present in both the blood vessels and tissue fluid are *_____ and
*_____ .

the hydrostatic pressure and the colloid osmotic pressure (oncotic pressure)
■   ■   ■

40 Colloid means *_____ ; therefore, colloid osmotic pressure is the amount of pressure exerted from *_____ .

    Hydrostatic is the *_____ of fluid; therefore, hydrostatic pressure is the amount of pressure at _____ of fluid.

nondiffusible substances; nondiffusible substances
state of equilibrium; equilibrium

      ■   ■   ■

41 The colloid osmotic pressure and the hydrostatic pressure of the blood and tissues move fluid through the _____ membrane.

capillary

      ■   ■   ■

42 Do you know the meanings of the arterioles and venules? If not:

Arterioles. Minute arteries that lead into a capillary bed.
Venules. Minute veins that lead from the capillary bed.

    Which is larger, the arteriole or the artery? _____ . The venule or the vein? _____ .

artery; vein

      ■   ■   ■

43 Fluid exchange occurs only across the walls of capillaries and not across the walls of arterioles or venules. Therefore, fluid moves into the interstitial space at the arteriolar end of the capillary and out of the interstitial space into the capillary at the *_____ of the capillary.

venular end

      ■   ■   ■

44 Gases move from an area of higher concentration to an area of lower concentration. This is the opposite of the movement of fluid in osmosis, in which fluid moves from the (less/more) _____ concentrated solution into the (less/more) _____ concentrated solution.

    Since oxygen is in greater concentration in the capillaries, it moves into the interstitial fluid. Carbon dioxide passes in the opposite direction, from the higher concentration in the interstitial fluid to the *_____ in the capillaries.

less; more; lower concentration

      ■   ■   ■

45   In the capillaries, oxygen is in greater concentration and therefore moves

* _____ .

Carbon dioxide is in higher concentration in the interstitial fluid and therefore moves

* _____ .

into the interstitial fluid; into the capillaries

■   ■   ■

46   The capillary endothelium or capillary membrane acts as a selectively permeable membrane by permitting free passage of crystalloids. *Crystalloids* are diffusible substances which dissolve in solution. They are noncolloid substances.

Albumin, protein, and gelatin are colloids of what type of substance? _____ .

The amount of osmotic pressure that develops at a membrane depends mainly on the concentration of   *_____ .

Some examples of a nondiffusible substance are   *_____ .

nondiffusible; nondiffusible substances or colloids; albumin, protein, or gelatin

■   ■   ■

47   Blood contains blood cells and plasma. The red blood cell is normally bathed in plasma. Plasma and red blood cells have an equal quantity of nondiffusible solutes.

If the red blood cells were bathed in pure water, the presence of large quantities of nondiffusible substances inside the cell would cause the cells to (swell/shrink).

_____ .

swell

■   ■   ■

48   Fluid flows only when there is a difference in pressure at the two ends of the system. This difference in pressure between two points is known as the *pressure gradient*.

If the pressure at one end was 32 mm Hg and at the other end was 26 mm Hg, the pressure gradient is   *_____ .

6 mm Hg

■   ■   ■

49   The plasma in the capillaries has hydrostatic pressure and colloid osmotic pressure. The tissue fluids have hydrostatic pressure and colloid osmotic pressure.

The difference of pressure between the plasma colloid osmotic pressure and the tissue colloid osmotic pressure is known as the   *_____ .

The difference of pressure between the plasma hydrostatic pressure and the tissue hydrostatic pressure is known as the   * _____ .

It is this difference in pressure that makes the fluid flow between and among compartments.

colloid osmotic pressure gradient; hydrostatic pressure gradient

■   ■   ■

50   Refer to Figure 1-2. The plasma colloid osmotic pressure is 28 mm Hg (millimeters of mercury) and the tissue colloid osmotic pressure is 4 mm Hg.

The colloid osmotic pressure gradient would be   * _____ .

24 mm Hg

■   ■   ■

51   Refer to Figure 1-2. The hydrostatic fluid pressure is 18 mm Hg in the capillary, and the hydrostatic tissue pressure is −6 mm Hg; therefore, the hydrostatic pressure gradient is
* _____ .

24 mm Hg

■   ■   ■

52   The hydrostatic pressure gradient across the capillary membrane (24 mm Hg) is equal to the colloid osmotic pressure gradient across the membrane (24 mm Hg). Thus, the two pressures are _____ .

equal or same pressure

■   ■   ■

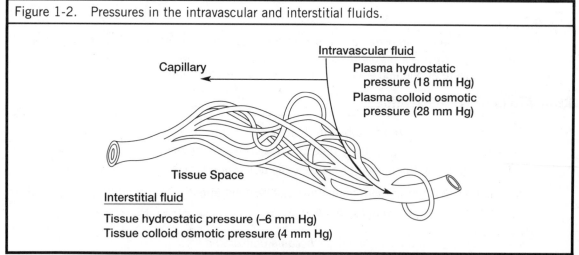

Figure 1-2.   Pressures in the intravascular and interstitial fluids.

Intravascular fluid
Capillary
Plasma hydrostatic pressure (18 mm Hg)
Plasma colloid osmotic pressure (28 mm Hg)

Tissue Space
Interstitial fluid
Tissue hydrostatic pressure (−6 mm Hg)
Tissue colloid osmotic pressure (4 mm Hg)

53   The plasma hydrostatic pressure gradient tends to move fluid out of the capillary. Why?   *_____

_____ .

Refer to Figure 1-2 if reply is unknown.

   The colloid osmotic pressure gradient tends to move fluid into the capillary. Why?   *_____

_____ .

The plasma hydrostatic pressure is higher than the tissue pressure.
Plasma osmotic pressure is higher than tissue pressure.

■   ■   ■

54   The balance between the two forces keeps the blood volume constant for circulation. In this way fluid does not accumulate in the intravascular or the interstitial compartments.

   Without the colloid osmotic forces, fluid (is/is not) _____ lost from circulation. Explain.   *_____

_____ .

   The blood volume is (sufficient/insufficient) _____ to maintain circulation.

is
Fluid stays in the tissues, causing accumulation and tissue swelling.
insufficient

■   ■   ■

55   Name the man who formulated the Law of Capillaries and define this law in your own words.

   Name.   _____ .

   Law.   *_____

_____ .

Starling
Plasma and tissue colloid osmotic and hydrostatic pressures regulate the flow of blood constituents between the interstitial and intravascular compartments.

■   ■   ■

REGULATORS OF FLUID BALANCE

56   Thirst, electrolytes, protein and albumin, hormones, lymphatics, skin, and kidneys are the major regulators that maintain body fluid balance. Thirst alerts the person that there is a fluid loss, thus stimulating the person to increase his or her oral intake.

   The thirst mechanism in the medulla may not respond effectively to fluid deficit in the older adult. Therefore, the older adult is more   *_____ .

prone to develop a fluid loss (deficit) or become dehydrated

■   ■   ■

57 When there is a body fluid deficit, what mechanism alerts the person that there is a fluid need? _____ .

thirst or thirst mechanism

■   ■   ■

A discussion regarding regulators of fluid balance follows Table 1-1. Study the actions of these substances or regulators.

Table 1-1. REGULATORS OF FLUID BALANCE	
Regulators	**Actions**
Thirst	An indicator of fluid need.
Electrolytes Sodium (Na)	Sodium promotes water retention. With a water deficit, more sodium is reabsorbed from the renal tubules.
Protein, albumin	Protein and albumin promote body fluid retention. These nondiffusible substances increase the colloid osmotic (oncotic) pressure.
Hormones Antidiuretic hormone (ADH)	ADH is produced by the hypothalamus and stored in the posterior pituitary gland (neurohypophysis). ADH is secreted when there is an ECF volume deficit. ADH promotes water reabsorption from the distal tubules of the kidneys.
Aldosterone	Aldosterone is secreted from the adrenal cortex. It promotes sodium reabsorption from the renal tubules.
Renin	Decreased renal blood flow increases the release of renin from the juxtaglomerular cells of the kidneys. Renin promotes peripheral vasoconstriction and the release of aldosterone (sodium and water retention).
Lymphatics	Plasma protein that shifts to the tissue spaces cannot be reabsorbed into the blood vessels. Thus, the lymphatic system promotes the return of water and protein from the interstitial spaces to the vascular spaces.
Skin	Skin excretes approximately 500 mL of water daily through normal perspiration
Lungs	Lungs excrete approximately 500 mL of water daily with normal breathing.
Kidneys	The kidneys excrete 1200–1500 mL of body water daily. The amount of water excretion may vary according to fluid intake and fluid loss.

58 The electrolyte sodium promotes the (retention/excretion) _____ of body water.

With a body fluid deficit, the reabsorption of sodium from the kidney tubules (increases/decreases) _____ .

retention; increases

■   ■   ■

59 Protein and albumin promote the (retention/excretion) _____ of body fluid (water). A decrease in protein can (increase/decrease) _____ the colloid osmotic pressure.

Another name for colloid osmotic pressure is *_____ .

retention; decrease; oncotic pressure

■   ■   ■

60 The three major hormones that influence fluid balance are _____ , _____ , and _____ .

ADH (antidiuretic hormone), aldosterone, and renin

■   ■   ■

61 The antidiuretic hormone, or ADH, increases the permeability of the cells of the kidney tubules to water, thus allowing more water to be reabsorbed. With a decrease in the production of ADH, what would occur? *_____

_____ .

an increased excretion of water from the kidney tubules

■   ■   ■

62 The posterior pituitary gland is influenced by the solute (sodium, protein, glucose) concentration of the plasma. If there is an increase in the amount of solute in the plasma, the posterior pituitary gland releases the hormone, ADH, which holds water in the body.

Explain how. *_____ .

For what reason should there be more water? *_____ .

It absorbs water from the kidney tubules.
to dilute the solute

■   ■   ■

63 A small increase of solute concentration in the plasma above the normal amount is sufficient to stimulate the posterior pituitary gland to release _____ .

Name two things that occur when there is less solute concentration in the plasma.

a. *_____

b. *_____

ADH
a. ADH would not be released.
b. More water would be excreted from the body.

■   ■   ■

64 When you drink a lot of fluids, what happens to the solute concentration of your plasma?
*_____ .

The posterior pituitary then (releases/retains) _____ ADH.

It becomes diluted.
retains

■   ■   ■

65 When the solute concentration increases, the thirst mechanism is stimulated and the individual ingests water.

Based on the above statement how can homeostasis be maintained? *_____

_____ .

by drinking water or other liquids when thirsty

■   ■   ■

66 Aldosterone promotes (water/sodium) _____ retention.

An increase in aldosterone release can be due to fluid volume (loss/excess) _____ and stress.

sodium; loss (deficit)

■   ■   ■

67 Sodium retention stimulates water retention in the *_____

_____ .

extracellular fluid (ECF) or vascular spaces

■   ■   ■

68 An ECF deficit causes the release of two (2) hormones called _____ and

_____ .

ADH and aldosterone

■   ■   ■

69   Increased renin secretion is a response to *_____
_____.

   How does renin affect fluid balance? *_____
_____.

   a decreased renal blood flow; it promotes aldosterone secretion
   ■   ■   ■

70   The response of the lymphatic system to the maintenance of fluid balance is *_____
_____.

   to promote the return of water and protein from the interstitial to the vascular spaces
   ■   ■   ■

71   If a person is febrile (increased body temperature) or there is an increase in humidity, diaphoresis may occur. This causes a fluid (loss/gain) _____ .

   Normally the amount of fluid lost through daily perspiration is _____ mL.

   loss; 500
   ■   ■   ■

72   Overbreathing or hyperventilation can (increase/decrease) _____ fluid loss through the _____ . The lungs normally cause a daily fluid loss of _____ mL.

   increase; lungs; 500
   ■   ■   ■

73   Kidneys conserve or excrete body water to maintain *_____.

   The amount of urine excreted per day is approximately _____ mL.

   fluid balance or homeostasis; 1200–1500
   ■   ■   ■

OSMOLALITY

74   Osmolality is determined by the number of dissolved particles (sodium, urea, and glucose) per kilogram of water. Sodium is the largest contributor of particles to osmolality. The other two major particle groups that contribute to osmolality are _____ and _____ .

   These dissolved particles exert an osmotic pull or pressure.

   urea and glucose
   ■   ■   ■

75 An *osmol* is a unit of osmotic pressure. The osmotic effects are expressed in terms of osmolality. A *milliosmol* (mOsm) is 1/1000th of an osmol and will determine the osmotic activity.

Six terms to know:

Osmolality. Osmotic pull exerted by all particles per unit of water, expressed as osmols or milliosmols per kilogram of water.

Osmolarity. Osmotic pull exerted by all particles per unit of solution, expressed as osmols or milliosmols per liter of solution.

Ion. A particle carrying a positive or negative charge. (A further explanation of ion will be found in Chapter 3.)

Dissociation. Separation, i.e., a compound separating or breaking down into many particles.

Serum. Consists of plasma minus fibrogen. It is obtained after coagulation of blood.

Plasma. Contains blood minus the blood cells. It is composed mainly of water.

What is larger, the osmol or the milliosmol? _____ . What is the relationship between ion and dissociation? *_____

_____ .

osmol; an ion is a positive or negative particle from dissociation (breakdown/separation) of a compound

■   ■   ■

76 According to Frame 75, 1 milliosmol is 1/1000th of an osmol. Then 1 osmol would equal _____ milliosmols.

Milliosmols determine the _____ activity of a solution.

1000; osmotic

■   ■   ■

77 The basic unit used to express the force exerted by the concentration of solute or dissolved particles is a(n) _____ .

The osmotic effect of a solute concentration in water is expressed as _____ , a property that depends on the number of osmols or milliosmols contained in a solution.

osmol; osmolality

■   ■   ■

78   Frequently the terms, serum and plasma, are used interchangeably. Plasma may be called blood plasma and serum may be called blood serum.

Serum and plasma are both found in what type of fluid?   *_____

_____ .

The difference between serum and plasma is that serum (does/does not) _____ contain fibrinogen. Serum is obtained after   *_____ in the blood specimen tube.

extracellular fluid (ECF) or vascular fluid; does not;
coagulation of blood

∎   ∎   ∎

79   Osmolality of fluid may be determined in serum and intravenous solutions. In serum, sodium, urea, and glucose are the most plentiful solutes and are the major contributors of serum osmolality. Sodium is most abundant in the (ECF/ICF) _____ and is available with most laboratory test results.

ECF

∎   ∎   ∎

80   The normal serum osmolality range is 280–295 mOsm/kg (milliosmols per kilogram). The serum osmolality may be measured by doubling the serum sodium level. For example, if the serum sodium is 142 mEq/L, the serum osmolality would be _____ mOsm/kg.

This provides a "rough estimate" of the serum osmolality.

Why is the serum sodium level used as an indicator of serum osmolality? _____

_____ .

284
Sodium is the most abundant solute/particle in the ECF.

∎   ∎   ∎

81   Another formula that may be used to determine the serum osmolality is:

$$2 \times \text{serum sodium} + \frac{\text{BUN}}{3} + \frac{\text{glucose}}{18} = \text{serum osmolality}$$

The two formulas that may be used to determine serum osmolality are:

a.   *_____

b.   *_____

a.   2 × serum sodium level = serum osmolality

b.   2 × serum sodium + $\dfrac{BUN}{3}$ + $\dfrac{glucose}{18}$ = serum osmolality

∎   ∎   ∎

82 Which of the two formulas (see Frame 81) would be the most accurate indicator of serum osmolality?

*_____ .

Why? *_____

_____ .

The formula that contains sodium, BUN, and glucose.
Using the three dissolved solutes in the vascular fluid is more accurate in determining the
serum osmolality than using only one solute.

■   ■   ■

83 Determine the serum osmolality from the following laboratory test results: serum sodium, 140 mEq/L; BUN, 12 mg/dL; serum glucose, 99 mg/dL.

Complete the following formula:

$$2 \times 140 + \frac{12}{3} + \frac{99}{18} = \underline{\hspace{3cm}} \text{ mOsm/kg}$$

289.5

■   ■   ■

84 If the serum osmolality is *not* within the normal range of _____ mOsm/kg, a fluid imbalance should be suspected.

There are three prefixes that are used for noting various types of osmolality. These are:

hypo = deficit or less than
iso = equal
hyper = excess or greater than

A serum osmolality of 288 mOsm/kg would be (hypo/iso/hyper) _____ osmolality.

280–295; iso-osmolality

■   ■   ■

85 Match the serum osmolality concentrations on the left with the type of osmolality:

_____	1. 299 mOsm/kg	a. Hypo-osmolality
_____	2. 292 mOsm/kg	b. Iso-osmolality
_____	3. 274 mOsm/kg	c. Hyperosmolality
_____	4. 305 mOsm/kg	
_____	5. 269 mOsm/kg	

1. c; 2. b; 3. a; 4. c; 5. a

■   ■   ■

86 The osmolality of an intravenous solution can be hypo-osmolar or hypotonic, iso-osmolar or isotonic, and hyperosmolar or hypertonic. The osmolality of the intravenous (IV) solution is determined by the average serum osmolality, which is 290 mOsm/L. The normal range for the osmolality of a solution is + 50 mOsm or −50 mOsm of 290 mOsm.

Early literature refers to the concentration of solutions as hypotonic, isotonic, and hypertonic. These terms are still in use; however, since the solute concentration is determined by the number of osmols or milliosmols in solution, hypo-osmolar, iso-osmolar, and hyperosmolar are the suggested terms.

The average osmolality of IV solution is 240 to _____ mOsm/L.

340

■   ■   ■

87 Plasma is considered to be a(n) (hypo-osmolar/iso-osmolar/hyperosmolar) _____ fluid.

The osmolality of solutions is compared to *_____ .

iso-osmolar; plasma osmolality or serum osmolality

■   ■   ■

88 Match the types of solutions on the left with their solute concentrations:

_____ 1. Iso-osmolar   a. Higher solute concentration than plasma

_____ 2. Hypo-osmolar   b. Same solute concentration as plasma

_____ 3. Hyperosmolar   c. Lower solute concentration than plasma

1. b; 2. c; 3. a

■   ■   ■

89 A solution having less than 240 mOsm is considered _____ , and a solution having more than 340 mOsm is considered _____ .

hypotonic (hypo-osmolar); hypertonic (hyperosmolar)

■   ■   ■

90 The following is a list of milliosmol values of IV fluids (solution). Classify them as iso-osmolar, hypo-osmolar, or hyperosmolar.

Milliosmol Values (mOsm)	Type of Osmolality
220	_____
75	_____
350	_____
310	_____
560	_____

hypo-osmolar; hypo-osmolar; hyperosmolar; iso-osmolar; hyperosmolar

■   ■   ■

91 Extracellular hyperosmolar fluid has a greater osmotic pressure than the cell; thus, intracellular water moves out of the cells and into the extracellular hypertonic (hyperosmolar) fluid by the process of _____ .

When cells lose water, what happens to their form and size?

* _____ .

osmosis
Cells shrink and become smaller in size.

■   ■   ■

92 A liter of 5% dextrose in water (D$_5$W) is 250 mOsm, and a liter of 0.9% sodium chloride or normal saline is 310 mOsm, having somewhat the same osmotic pressure as

_____ .

These solutions are (iso-osmolar/hypo-osmolar/hyperosmolar)

_____ .

plasma; iso-osmolar

■   ■   ■

93 The sum of 5% dextrose in normal saline equals _____ mOsm. This solution is a(n) _____ solution.

560; hyperosmolar

■   ■   ■

94 Name two common iso-osmolar intravenous (IV) solutions:

a. * _____

b. * _____

a. 5% dextrose (D$_5$W)
b. 0.9% sodium chloride or normal saline

■   ■   ■

95 In studying serum chemistry alterations and concentrations, one is concerned with how much the ions or chemical particles weigh. The weight of ions and chemical particles is measured in milligrams percent (mg%), which is the same as mg/100 mL or mg/dL. The number of electrically charged ions is measured in milliequivalents per liter (1000 mL), or mEq/L.

The term *milliequivalent* involves the chemical activity of elements, whereas milliosmol involves the _____ activity of the solution.

How do milligrams and milliequivalents differ? *_____

osmotic
Milligrams. The weight of ions.
Milliequivalents. The chemical activity of ions.

■   ■   ■

96 Milliequivalents provide a better method of measuring the concentration of ions in the serum than milligrams.

Milligrams measure the _____ of ions and give no information concerning the number of ions or the electrical charges of the ions.

weight

■   ■   ■

97 The following is a simple analogy to compare milligrams and milliequivalents.

If you were having a party and wanted to invite equal numbers of boys and girls, which would be more accurate—inviting 1500 pounds of girls and 1500 pounds of boys or inviting 15 girls and 15 boys? *_____ .

Why? *_____

_____ .

15 girls and 15 boys
Otherwise, you would have an unequal number of boys and girls, for not every child weighs exactly 100 pounds

■   ■   ■

98 From the example in Frame 97, which would be more accurate in determining the serum chemistry of chemical particles or ions in the body—milliequivalents or milligrams?

_____ .

You will find both measurements used in this book and in your clinical settings for determining changes in our serum chemistry. However, when referring to ions, milliequivalents will be used in this book.

milliequivalents

■   ■   ■

CLINICAL APPLICATIONS

99 There are several diseases that affect the plasma colloid osmotic pressure due to the loss of serum protein.

Memorize these five important definitions:

Protein. A nitrogenous compound, essential to all living organisms.
Plasma protein relates to albumin, globulin, and fibrinogen.
Serum protein relates to albumin and globulin.
Serum albumin is a simple protein that contains the main protein in the blood. It constitutes about 50% of the blood protein.
Serum globulin is a group of simple protein.

Clients with diagnoses of kidney and liver diseases or malnutrition lose serum protein. What are the two groups of simple proteins found in the serum?

_____ and _____ .

albumin and globulin
■   ■   ■

100 The main function of serum albumin is to maintain the colloid osmotic pressure of blood.

Without colloid osmotic pressure, what would happen to the fluid in the tissues? *_____

_____ .

Fluid would accumulate in the tissues and swelling would occur. This is known as edema.
■   ■   ■

101 Serum globulin is not fully understood, but one of its functions is to assist in maintaining the colloid osmotic pressure of the blood.

Gram for gram, the globulin molecule is larger than the albumin molecule; however, it is less effective in maintaining osmotic pressure. Name the diseases in which serum albumin leaks out of the capillaries. *_____ and *_____ .

When serum albumin leaks, the larger serum globulin molecule is retained and tries to compensate for the loss of albumin. As stated, globulin is not as effective as albumin in maintaining osmotic pressure; so what happens to the colloid osmotic pressure in the capillaries? *_____ .

What would happen to the fluid in the interstitial spaces? *_____ .

liver disease and kidney disease (also malnutrition)
Osmotic pressure would be lower (decrease).
Fluid accumulates in the tissue spaces and swelling occurs (edema).
■   ■   ■

102 Identify three possible nursing responsibilities you think are important when caring for clients with diseases that cause abnormal serum albumin and serum globulin levels.

    a.   *_____

    b.   *_____

    c.   *_____

Possible answers include:
a. report abnormal serum laboratory findings immediately
b. observe and report physical findings of swelling or edema
c. keep an accurate record of fluid intake and output

■   ■   ■

103 Edema, or swelling, occurs when there is fluid retention. Dehydration occurs with excess fluid removal or loss.

    If the osmolality of intravascular fluid is greater than the osmolality of intracellular fluid, would the cells (lose/gain) water? _____ .

    Would (edema/dehydration) occur to the cells? _____ .

lose; dehydration

■   ■   ■

104 With any vein obstruction, there is an increased venous hydrostatic pressure. This in turn inhibits the fluid moving out of the tissues, causing the tissues to   *_____

_____ .

retain/accumulate fluid and swell (edema)

■   ■   ■

105 Normal circulation of blood is dependent on differences in hydrostatic pressure in the arteries, capillaries, and veins.

    Increased hydrostatic pressure in the veins would   *_____

_____ .

cause a circulatory backup resulting in swelling of the tissues (edema)

■   ■   ■

CASE STUDY REVIEW

Mr. Kendall had been vomiting for several days. His urine output decreased. He was given 1 liter of 5% dextrose in water and then 1 liter of 5% dextrose in normal saline (0.9% NaCl).

1. In his adult stage, Mr. Kendall's body water represents _____ % of his total body weight. What percentage of his total body weight is in the intracellular compartment _____ % and what percent of water is in the extracellular compartment _____ %?

2. Explain why Mr. Kendall's urine output is decreased *_____

_____ .

3. The three primary sources for water intake are _____ , _____ , and *_____ .

   The four primary mechanisms for daily water loss (output) are _____ , _____ , _____ , and _____ .

4. Vomiting caused Mr. Kendall to lose body fluids and caused a decrease in urine output. The solute concentration was increased due to less circulating body fluid. As a result of an increased solute concentration, the posterior pituitary gland will release (more/less) _____ ADH.

5. Define osmolality and osmolarity.
   Osmolality. *_____ .
   Osmolarity. *_____ .

6. Mr. Kendall received 1 liter of 5% dextrose in water, which has a similar osmolality as plasma. A solution with osmolality similar to that of plasma is considered to be (iso-osmolar/hypo-osmolar/hyperosmolar) _____ .

7. The second liter he received was 5% dextrose in normal saline. This solution is a(n) _____ solution.

8. The osmolality of plasma is _____ mOsm. A solution with less than 240 mOsm is considered _____ .

9. One-half of normal saline (0.45% NaCl) solution has 155 mOsm. What is this type of solution? _____ .

Mr. Kendall developed edema of the lower extremities. Laboratory results documented a lower than normal serum protein.

10. Factors regulating the flow of body constituents between the interstitial and intravascular compartments are stated by *_____

_____ .

11. Define the following four terms.
    a. *Pressure gradient.* *_____
    b. *Crystalloids.* *_____ .
    c. *Colloids.* *_____ .
    d. *Albumin.* *_____ .

12. Pressure gradients are responsible for the exchange of fluid between the capillaries and the _____ .

13. The amount of colloid osmotic pressure that develops depends on the concentration of nondiffusible substances such as *_____ .

14. The direction of the movement of fluid depends on the results of the opposing forces.

    a. The hydrostatic pressure is greater than the colloid osmotic pressure at the arterial end of the capillary; thus the fluid moves out of the _____ and into the *_____ .

b. The osmotic pressure is greater than the hydrostatic pressure at the venous end of the capillary; thus the fluid moves out of the _____ and reenters the _____ .

15. Mr. Kendall's decrease in serum protein could account for his (edema/dehydration).
16. Mr. Kendall has a venous obstruction due to varicosities. This causes an increase in venous hydrostatic pressure, preventing fluid from moving out of tissues and into the circulation. Explain what happens to the fluid. *_____
_____ .

1. *60; 40; 20*
2. *Mr. Kendall is losing body fluid from vomiting and a lack of fluid intake.*
3. *liquid, food, and oxidation of food;*
   lungs, skin, urine, and feces
4. *more*
5. *Osmolality. Osmols or milliosmols per kilogram of water.*
   Osmolarity. Osmols or milliosmols per liter of solution.
6. *iso-osmolar*
7. *hyperosmolar*
8. *290; hypo-osmolar*
9. *hypo-osmolar*
10. *Starling's Law of Capillaries*
11. *a. Pressure gradient. Difference in pressure between two points in a fluid.*
    b. Crystalloids. Diffusible substances.
    c. Colloids. Nondiffusible substances.
    d. Albumin. Simple protein.
12. *tissues*
13. *protein or albumin*
14. *a. capillaries, surrounding tissues; b. tissues, capillary*
15. *edema*
16. *Fluid accumulates in the tissue, causing swelling (edema).*

NURSING ASSESSMENT FACTORS

- Assess the intake and output status of the client. Fluid intake and urine output are normally in proportion to each other.
- Recognize that infants and thin people have a higher proportion of body water than adults, older adults, and people with increased body fat.
- Assess excess fluid loss from the skin and lungs. Diaphoresis (excess sweating) and tachypnea (rapid breathing) cause excess body water loss through the skin and lungs.
- Obtain baseline vital signs. Baseline vital signs are used for comparison with future vital signs.
- Assess for fluid balance by checking the client's serum osmolality with the laboratory test results. The serum sodium, BUN, and glucose results are used in calculating the serum osmolality status of clients. If only the serum sodium value is available, double the sodium level for a rough estimate of the serum osmolality. A serum osmolality >295 mOsm/kg can indicate hemoconcentration due to fluid loss. A serum osmolality <280 mOsm/kg can indicate hemodilution due to fluid excess.

NURSING DIAGNOSIS

Fluid volume deficit and fluid volume excess, related to body fluid imbalance.

NURSING INTERVENTIONS AND RATIONALE

1. Monitor vital signs. Report abnormal vital signs or significant changes from baseline measurements.
2. Monitor intake and output. Report urine output of less than 600 mL per day and less than 25 mL per hour or more than 1500 mL per 24 hours.
3. Check the daily osmolality of IV solutions. Know that IV solutions with osmolality between 240 and 340 mOsm/L are iso-osmolar and are similar to plasma. Remember that a solution of 5% dextrose in water is 250 mOsm and a normal saline solution (0.9% sodium chloride) is 310 mOsm; both are iso-osmolar solutions. Continuous use of hypo-osmolar (0.45% sodium chloride) and hyper-osmolar [10% dextrose in water ([$D_{10}W$])] IV solutions may cause a fluid imbalance.
4. Monitor the fluid status of the client: check laboratory studies to determine the serum osmolality. Serum sodium, BUN, and glucose levels should be used to assess the serum osmolality.
5. Monitor the serum albumin and serum protein levels of clients with malnutrition, liver disease such as cirrhosis of the liver, and kidney disease. Low serum albumin and serum protein levels decrease the colloid osmotic (oncotic) pressure; thus fluid remains in the tissue spaces (edema). While diuretics are helpful in decreasing edema, they can also markedly decrease the circulating fluid volume.

CHAPTER 2

FLUIDS AND THEIR INFLUENCE ON THE BODY

Behavioral Objectives

Upon completion of this chapter, you will be prepared to:

- Describe the physiologic factors leading to extracellular fluid volume deficits or dehydration.
- State the difference between a hyperosmolar fluid deficit and an iso-osmolar fluid deficit.
- Describe the physiologic factors leading to extracellular fluid volume excess or edema.
- Compare the extracellular fluid volume shift in hypovolemia with the extracellular fluid volume shift in hypervolemia, or overhydration.
- Describe the physiologic factors leading to intracellular fluid volume shift or water intoxication.
- Identify nursing assessment associated with dehydration, edema, and water intoxication.
- Develop selected nursing diagnoses appropriate for clients with clinical manifestations of extracellular fluid volume deficits and excess and intracellular fluid volume excess.
- Identify selected nursing interventions to alleviate the symptoms of dehydration, edema, and water intoxication.

Introduction

Many disease entities have some degree of fluid and electrolyte imbalance. Much of the imbalance is the result of fluid loss, fluid excess, and/or fluid volume shift. Four major fluid imbalances—extracellular fluid volume deficit (ECFVD), extracellular fluid volume excess (ECFVE), extracellular fluid volume shift (ECFVS), and intracellular fluid volume excess (ICFVE)—are discussed in regard to pathophysiology, etiology, clinical manifestations (signs and symptoms), clinical applications, and clinical management. Nursing assessment factors, nursing diagnoses, and nursing interventions are listed for ECFVD, ECFVE, and ICFVE. Three case reviews related to clients with fluid imbalances are presented.

The physician computes and orders fluid replacement; however, the nurse should understand reasons for various types of fluid imbalances and should assess physical changes that may occur before and during clinical management.

An asterisk (*) on an answer line indicates a multiple word answer. The meanings for the following symbols are: ↑ increased, ↓ decreased, > greater than, and < less than.

EXTRACELLULAR FLUID VOLUME DEFICIT: DEHYDRATION

INTRODUCTION

Extracellular fluid volume deficit (ECFVD) is a loss of body fluid from the interstitial (tissue) and intravascular (vascular-vessel) spaces. With severe ECF loss, there may be an intracellular (cellular-cells) fluid loss.

1   Extracellular fluid loss results primarily from the loss of body fluid in the _____ and _____ spaces.

interstitial and intravascular

 ■   ■   ■

2   Severe loss of ECF may also result in _____ fluid loss.

intracellular or cellular

 ■   ■   ■

3   Dehydration is another name used to describe   *_____

_____ .

loss of water (extracellular fluid volume deficit or ECFVD)

 ■   ■   ■

PATHOPHYSIOLOGY

4   The concentration of body fluids (plasma/serum osmolality) is determined by the number of particles or solutes in relation to the volume of body water (refer to Chapter 1 for a description of osmolality).

The normal range of plasma/serum osmolality is   *_____

_____ .

280–295 mOsm/kg (milliosmols per kilogram)

 ■   ■   ■

5   If the serum osmolality is less than 280 mOsm/kg, there are (more/less) _____ solutes/particles in proportion to the volume of body water. This body fluid is described as (hypo-osmolar/iso-osmolar/hyperosmolar) _____ .

less; hypo-osmolar or hypotonic

 ■   ■   ■

6   If the serum osmolality is greater than 295 mOsm/kg, there are (more/less) _____ solutes in proportion to body water; the fluid imbalance is known as _____ .

more; hyperosmolar or hypertonic
                    ▪   ▪   ▪

7   A loss of the electrolyte sodium is usually accompanied by a simultaneous fluid loss. Sodium is one of the regulators of fluid balance (refer to Chapters 1 and 3). With a loss of sodium, body fluid is usually decreased or moves from ECF to ICF.

When fluid and sodium are lost in equal amounts, the type of fluid deficit that usually occurs is (iso-osmolar/hyperosmolar) _____ fluid volume deficit.

iso-osmolar or isotonic
                    ▪   ▪   ▪

8   When the amount of water lost is in excess of the amount of sodium lost, the serum sodium level is (elevated/decreased) _____ .

This type of fluid deficit is called   *_____ .

elevated; hyperosmolar fluid volume deficit
                    ▪   ▪   ▪

9   Plasma/serum osmolality increases with the retention of sodium, causing water to be drawn from the cells. With the elevation of serum sodium, the extracellular fluid becomes (hyperosmolar/hypo-osmolar) _____ , resulting in a(an) (increase/decrease) _____ in plasma/serum osmolality, which causes a withdrawal of fluid from the   *_____ .

hyperosmolar; increase; cells or intracellular compartment
                    ▪   ▪   ▪

10 A hyperosmolar fluid volume (hyperosmolar extracellular fluid) causes which of the following:

( ) a. Intracellular dehydration
( ) b. Intracellular hydration

Explain.   *_____ .

a. intracellular dehydration
The hyperosmolar extracellular fluid will pull intracellular fluid from the cells by osmosis.
                    ▪   ▪   ▪

11   With an iso-osmolar fluid volume loss, the plasma/serum osmolality is
      (increased/decreased/unchanged) _____ .

      unchanged

      ■   ■   ■

12   An iso-osmolar fluid volume loss is not classified as dehydration, although it is frequently
      considered a form of dehydration. This can occur when fluid and electrolyte losses are severe.

          A hyperosmolar fluid volume loss is referred to as _____ . Explain.
      *_____ .

      dehydration
      Moderate to severe fluid volume losses can cause symptoms of dehydration.

      ■   ■   ■

13   Compensatory mechanisms attempt to maintain fluid volume necessary for vital organs to
      receive adequate perfusion.

          When more than one third of the body fluid is lost, what might occur?   *_____
      _____ .

      vascular collapse or shock or inadequate organ perfusion

      ■   ■   ■

Etiology

   The causes of hyperosmolar and iso-osmolar fluid volume deficits differ somewhat. Both types of
fluid volume deficits may be caused by vomiting and diarrhea; however, the severity of vomiting and
diarrhea indicates which type of ECFVD results.

14   Usually with severe vomiting and diarrhea, the loss of water is greater than the loss of sodium.
      This type of fluid loss causes   *_____ .

      hyperosmolar fluid volume deficit

      ■   ■   ■

15   Common causes of ECFVD are vomiting and diarrhea. Vomiting and diarrhea can cause
      *_____ .

      Severe vomiting and diarrhea may cause
      *_____ .

      iso-osmolar fluid volume deficit; hyperosmolar fluid volume deficit

      ■   ■   ■

Table 2-1 lists the causes of hyperosmolar and iso-osmolar fluid volume deficits. Rationale is provided for each type of fluid volume deficit. Study the table carefully and refer to it as needed.

Table 2-1. CAUSES OF EXTRACELLULAR FLUID VOLUME DEFICITS	
Types and Causes	**Rationale**
Hyperosmolar Fluid Volume Deficit	
Inadequate fluid intake	A decrease in water intake can result in an increase in the numbers of solutes in body fluid. The body fluid becomes hyperosmolar.
Increased solute intake (salt, sugar, protein)	An increase in solute intake may increase the solute concentration in body fluid; the body fluids can become hyperosmolar with a normal or decreased fluid intake.
Severe vomiting and diarrhea	They can cause a loss of body water greater than the loss of solutes, such as electrolytes resulting in hyperosmolar body fluid.
Diabetes ketoacidosis	An increase in glucose and ketone bodies can result in body fluids becoming more hyperosmolar, thus causing diuresis. The resulting fluid loss is greater than the solute loss (sugar and ketones).
Sweating	Water loss is usually greater than sodium loss.
Iso-osmolar Fluid Volume Deficit	
Vomiting and diarrhea	Usually results in fluid losses that are in proportion to electrolytes (sodium, potassium, chloride, bicarbonate) losses *unless* the vomiting and diarrhea become severe.
Gastrointestinal (GI) fistula or draining abscess and GI suctioning	The GI tract is rich in electrolytes. With a loss of GI secretions, fluid and electrolytes are lost in somewhat equal proportion.
Fever, environmental temperature, and profused diaphoresis	With these causes, fluid and sodium are lost through the skin. With profused sweating, the sodium is usually lost in proportions equal to water losses.
	Depending upon the severity of the sweating and fever, symptoms of mild, moderate, or marked fluid loss may be observed.

Table 2-1. (Continued)

Types and Causes	Rationale
Hemorrhage	Excess blood loss increases fluid and solute loss from the vascular fluid. If hemorrhage occurs rapidly, fluid shift to compensate for blood losses can be inadequate.
Burns	Burns cause body fluid with solutes to shift from the vascular fluid to the burned site and surrounding interstitial space (tissues). This may result in an inadequate circulating fluid volume.
Ascites	Fluid and solutes (protein, electrolytes, etc.) shift to the peritoneal space, causing ascites (third-space fluid). A decrease in circulating fluid volume may result.
Intestinal obstruction	Fluid accumulates at the intestinal obstruction site (third-space fluid), thus decreasing the vascular fluid volume.

16 Match the type of ECFVD with its possible cause.

   a. IFVD (iso-osmolar fluid volume deficit)
   b. HFVD (hyperosmolar fluid volume deficit)

_____ 1. Hemorrhage
_____ 2. Diabetic ketoacidosis
_____ 3. Increased salt and protein intake
_____ 4. Burns
_____ 5. GI suctioning
_____ 6. Inadequate fluid intake
_____ 7. Profused diaphoresis and/or fever

1. a; 2. b; 3. b; 4. a; 5. a; 6. b; 7. a
■   ■   ■

17   Indicate which situations are representative of iso-osmolar and hyperosmolar fluid volume deficits.

   a. Iso-osmolar
   b. Hyperosmolar

   _____ 1. There is a proportional loss of both body fluids and solutes.
   _____ 2. The loss of body fluids is greater than the loss of solutes.
   _____ 3. A serum osmolality of 281 mOsm/kg occurring with ECFVD may indicate which type of fluid loss?
   _____ 4. A serum osmolality of 305 mOsm/kg occurring with ECFVD may indicate which type of fluid loss?

   1. a; 2. b; 3. a; 4. b

      ▪   ▪   ▪

CLINICAL MANIFESTATIONS

   The clinical manifestations (signs and symptoms) of ECFVD, both iso-osmolar and hyperosmolar, are listed in Table 2-2. The table describes the degrees of ECF loss (dehydration), percentage of body weight loss, symptoms, and body water deficit by liter for a man weighing 150 pounds.
   Study this table carefully; be able to name the degrees of dehydration, their symptoms, the percentage of body weight loss, and an estimation of body fluid loss in liters. Hopefully, you will be able to recognize and identify degrees of dehydration that can occur to your clients during your clinical experience. Refer back to this table as you find necessary.

18   Thirst is a symptom that occurs with mild, marked, and severe fluid loss. Lack of water intake is usually the contributing cause of mild dehydration.

   How can mild dehydration be corrected?   *_____ .

   increase water (fluid) intake

      ▪   ▪   ▪

19   With mild dehydration, the percentage of body weight loss is _____ %, which is equivalent to _____ liter(s) of body fluid loss.

   2; 1–2

      ▪   ▪   ▪

20   In the elderly, the thirst mechanism in the medulla does not alert the older person that there is a water deficit. Therefore, the older person may become *_____ without experiencing the symptom of thirst.

   dehydrated or mildly dehydrated

      ▪   ▪   ▪

Table 2-2. DEGREES OF DEHYDRATION

Degrees of Dehydration	Percentage of Body Weight Loss (%)	Symptoms	Body Water Deficit by Liter
Mild dehydration	2	1. Thirst	1–2
Marked dehydration	5	1. Marked thirst 2. Dry mucous membranes 3. Dryness and wrinkling of skin—poor skin turgor 4. Acid-base equilibrium toward greater acidity 5. Temperature—low-grade elevation, e.g., 99°F (37.2°C) 6. Tachycardia (pulse greater than 100) as blood volume drops 7. Respiration 28 and ↑ 8. Systolic BP 10–15 mm Hg ↓ in standing position 9. Hand veins: slow filling with hand lowered 10. Urine volume: <25 mL/h and highly concentrated 11. Specific gravity: >1.030 12. Body weight loss 13. Hct ↑, Hgb ↑, BUN ↑	3–5
Severe dehydration	8	1. Same symptoms as marked dehydration, plus: 2. Skin becomes flushed 3. Systolic BP 60 or ↓ 4. Behavioral changes, e.g., restlessness, irritability, disorientation, and delirium	5–10
Fatal dehydration	22–30 total body water loss can prove fatal	1. Anuria 2. Coma leading to death	

Abbreviations: BP, blood pressure; Hct, hematocrit; Hgb, hemoglobin; BUN, blood urea nitrogen.

21 Common symptoms of marked ECF loss include: decreased skin turgor, dry mucous membranes, increased pulse rate, weight loss, and decreased urine output.

What percentage of weight loss is associated with marked dehydration? _____ . This weight loss is equivalent to _____ liter(s) of body water loss.

5%; 3–5

■   ■   ■

22 The percentage of body weight loss is a guide for *_____ therapy.

replacement fluid or intravenous (IV) fluid

■   ■   ■

23 With marked and severe body fluid loss, the hematocrit, hemoglobin, and blood urea nitrogen (BUN) are (increased/decreased) _____ . Why? *_____

_____ .

increased; because of the increased number of solutes such as blood urea nitrogen and red blood cells or hemoconcentration

■   ■   ■

24 The red blood cell count, hemoglobin, hematocrit, and plasma/serum protein are elevated as a result of hemoconcentration (increased blood cells and decreased vascular fluid).

Hemoconcentration occurs with dehydration. Why? *_____

_____ .

With body fluid loss, red blood cell count is increased, along with other solutes.

■   ■   ■

25 With marked dehydration, increased urine concentration usually results. The specific gravity (SG) may be (increased/decreased) _____ such as SG (<1.008/>1.025) _____ . The urine output is (increased/decreased) _____ .

increased; >1.025; decreased

■   ■   ■

26 Indicate which symptoms are associated with *severe* dehydration.

( ) a. Bradycardia
( ) b. Tachycardia as blood volume drops
( ) c. Temperature 99.6°F
( ) d. Urine volume is increased
( ) e. Specific gravity of urine of 1.035 and higher
( ) f. Skin flushed
( ) g. Irritability
( ) h. Restlessness and disorientation
( ) i. Specific gravity of urine lower than 1.020
( ) j. Marked thirst

What percentage loss is associated with severe dehydration? _____ .

a. —; b. X; c. X; d. —; e. X; f. X; g. X; h. X; i. —; j. X
8%

■   ■   ■

CLINICAL APPLICATIONS

27 In early dehydration, the fluid is lost in equal quantities from both the extracellular and intracellular fluid spaces.

As dehydration continues, fluid is lost in greater quantities from the extracellular than from the intracellular fluid space, thus resulting in an ECF (excess/deficit) _____ .

deficit

■   ■   ■

28 When dehydration is severe, cellular dehydration from the intracellular fluid space occurs.

A severe ECF deficit can lead to an ICF (excess/deficit) _____ .

deficit

■   ■   ■

29 When there is a marked or severe fluid volume loss, hypovolemia occurs. Hypovolemia may be a new term to you. The prefix *hypo* indicates _____ . Volemia comes from the Latin word *volumen,* meaning "volume."

Hypovolemia is a diminished volume of circulating blood or vascular fluid. It is frequently referred to as a decrease in blood volume.

loss, less, deficit, or diminished

■   ■   ■

30   The nurse can make a quick assessment of dehydration, or hypovolemia, by checking the peripheral veins in the hand. First hold the hand above heart level for a short time and then lower the hand below heart level. The peripheral veins in the hand below heart level should be engorged within 5–10 seconds with a normal blood volume and circulating blood flow.

If the peripheral veins do not engorge in 10 seconds, this may be indicative of _____ _____.

dehydration or hypovolemia (low blood volume)

■   ■   ■

31   Body weight is an important tool for assessing fluid imbalance. Two and one-half pounds (2½) of body weight loss is equivalent to 1 liter of water loss.

Intake and output give the approximate amount of body fluid intake and output; however, *_____ gives the more accurate assessment of fluid balance.

body weight

■   ■   ■

32   Vital signs comprise another tool for assessing dehydration, or hypovolemia. With dehydration what would the following be?

Temperature   *_____.

Pulse   *_____.

Respirations   *_____.

Blood pressure   *_____.

Urine volume   *_____.

temperature: low-grade elevation
pulse: tachycardia (rate over 100)
respirations: increased
systolic blood pressure: ↓ 10–15 mm Hg (standing position)
urine volume: decreased or small amount and highly concentrated
(Kidney damage can occur if the systolic blood pressure is less than 60 for several hours.)

■   ■   ■

CLINICAL MANAGEMENT

In replacing body water loss, the total fluid deficit is estimated according to the percentage of body weight loss. The physician computes the fluid replacement for his or her client. The following is only an example. Many physicians use this method for replacement of fluid loss.

Mr. Smith, who was admitted to the hospital, had a weight loss of 10 pounds due to dehydration. His weight had originally been 154 pounds, or 70 kg (kilograms). To determine the percentage of body weight loss, divide the weight loss by the original weight; therefore, 10 ÷ 154 = 0.06, or 6%.

To determine the total fluid loss, multiply the percentage of body weight loss by kilograms of body weight; therefore, 0.06×70 kg $= 4.2$ liters.

33 Clinically, Mr. Smith has which of the following:

( ) a. Mild dehydration
( ) b. Marked dehydration
( ) c. Severe dehydration

b. marked dehydration

■   ■   ■

34 To determine the percentage of body weight loss, one *_____

_____ .

To determine the total fluid loss, one *_____

_____ .

divides the weight loss by the original weight
multiplies the percentage of body weight loss by kilograms of body weight

■   ■   ■

35 One third of body water deficit is from ECF (extracellular fluid), and two thirds of body water deficit is from ICF (intracellular fluid) (Chapter 1). To determine replacement therapy for the first day, you would multiply:

(a) $\frac{1}{3} \times 4.2$ L $= 1.4$ L (ECF replacement)
Replacement fluid needed for ECF is _____ liter(s), or
_____ mL.
(b) $\frac{2}{3} \times 4.2$ L $= 2.8$ L (ICF replacement)
Replacement fluid needed for ICF is _____ liter(s), or
_____ mL.
(c) 2.5 L, or 2500 mL, is added to replace the current day's losses (constant daily amount)

The total fluid replacement for the first day is _____ liter(s), or
_____ mL (sum of ECF and ICF and current day's losses).

a. 1.4; 1400
b. 2.8; 2800
c. 6.7; 6700

■   ■   ■

36 One third of the water deficit is from the *_____ , and two thirds of the water deficit is from the *_____ .

extracellular fluid; intracellular (cellular) fluid

■   ■   ■

37 The sodium (Na) deficit is the amount contained in the extracellular fluid loss of 1.4 liters. Explain the rationale for the sodium deficit.   *_____

_____ .

The potassium (K) deficit is the amount contained in the intracellular fluid loss of 2.8 liters. Explain the rationale for the potassium deficit.   *_____

_____ .

Sodium (Na) is the main cation of ECF, so with ECF loss, there is a loss of sodium. However, the serum sodium level may be elevated if the fluid loss is greater than Na loss.
Potassium (K) is the main cation of ICF, so with ICF loss, there is a loss of potassium. However, the serum potassium level may be elevated because the K leaves the cells and may accumulate in the ECF. If diuresis occurs, the serum potassium may be low.
■   ■   ■

38 In severe dehydration, cellular breakdown usually occurs, and acid metabolites, such as lactic acid, are released from the cells; thus, metabolic acidosis results. The serum CO_2 and the arterial bicarbonate (HCO_3) levels are decreased.

Bicarbonate is usually added to a liter or two of IV fluids. Constant use of saline (NaCl) is not indicated. Explain why.   *_____

_____ .

A low HCO_3 or serum CO_2 indicates a lack of HCO_3 ions, which are needed to neutralize the body's acidotic state. If Cl^- was administered, it would combine with H^+ and increase acidosis
■   ■   ■

39 The following suggested solution replacement is needed to correct the dehydration:

Lactated Ringer's, 1500 mL, to replace ECF losses.
Normal saline solution (0.9% NaCl solution), 500 mL.
Five percent dextrose in water (D_5W), 4700 mL, to replace the water deficit and increase urinary output.
Potassium chloride, 40–80 mEq, may be divided into the 3 liters to replace potassium loss, which is dependent upon the serum potassium level.

When potassium is restored in the cells, the intracellular fluid is (increased/decreased)

_____ .

Explain why you think this might happen.   *_____

_____ .

When potassium is being administered in the form of KCl (potassium chloride), explain your assessment concern and the appropriate rationale related to the client's urinary output.

*_____

_____ .

increased
Fluid flows into the cells as potassium returns to the cells. Cellular function is restored. Eighty to ninety percent of potassium is excreted via kidneys. Poor urinary output leads to potassium excess, so urine output should be 250 mL per 8 hours.

■   ■   ■

40 In correcting dehydration, two goals are to *_____

and *_____ .

replace fluid volume and reduce osmolality

■   ■   ■

41 Select all true statements.
Lactated Ringer's solution is helpful in treating dehydration because:

( ) a. It resembles the electrolytic structure of normal blood serum.
( ) b. It replaces the extracellular fluid volume.
( ) c. It replaces all of the electrolyte loss.
( ) d. It replaces potassium loss.

M/6 sodium lactate is helpful in treating dehydration because:

( ) a. It replaces the sodium loss.
( ) b. It aids in decreasing the CO_2 combining power of the plasma.
( ) c. It aids in increasing the CO_2 combining power of the plasma.
( ) d. It is helpful in the correction of metabolic acidosis.
( ) e. It is helpful in the correction of metabolic alkalosis.

Dextrose 5% in water is helpful in treating dehydration because:

( ) a. It replaces water deficit.
( ) b. It aids in increasing urine output.
( ) c. It aids in decreasing urine output.
( ) d. It replaces the sodium deficit.

a. X; b. X; c. —; d. —
a. X; b. —; c. X; d. X; e. —
a. X; b. X; c. —; d. —

■   ■   ■

42   Mild dehydration is frequently treated with dextrose, water, and small amounts of electrolytes.

Dextrose 5% in water (D_5W) is frequently given first followed by a solution of low electrolyte content such as   *_____

_____ . (These solutions could be given in reverse, according to the client's condition and physician's choice).

When administering D_5W, dextrose is metabolized quickly, leaving _____ .

lactated Ringer's solution or $D_5/\frac{1}{2}$ NSS (5% dextrose in 0.45% normal saline solution); water

■   ■   ■

CASE STUDY REVIEW

Mr. Cooper, age 55, has been vomiting persistently for 3 days. On admission, he weighed 153 pounds. His original weight was 165 pounds (75 kg). The nurse assessed his fluid state and noted that his mucous membranes and skin were dry. His temperature was 99.4°F (37.5°C), pulse 112, respirations 32, blood pressure 110/88, and urine output in 8 hours 125 mL with a specific gravity of 1.036. Electrolyte findings were serum K, 3.5 mEq/L; Na, 154 mEq/L; and Cl, 102 mEq/L. His hematocrit and BUN were elevated.

1. Name the type of Mr. Cooper's dehydration (fluid volume loss)   *_____ . Explain the rationale for your selection.   *_____
_____ .

2. Another name for dehydration is   *_____
_____ .

3. The nurse assesses Mr. Cooper's body fluid state. Name four of his symptoms and laboratory findings that are suggestive of the fluid imbalance (dehydration).

    a. *_____
    b. *_____
    c. *_____
    d. *_____

4. Determine the percentage of Mr. Cooper's body weight loss.   *_____
_____ .

5. Clinically, Mr. Cooper has which of the following:
    ( ) a. Mild dehydration
    ( ) b. Marked dehydration
    ( ) c. Severe dehydration

6. Mr. Cooper's total fluid loss is   *_____ .
    (Work space is provided.)

7. a. Calculate the replacement fluid needed for ECF loss.   *_____ .
    b. Calculate the replacement fluid needed for ICF loss.   *_____ .
    c. Calculate the replacement fluid needed for current day's losses.   *_____ .
    (constant daily amount)

8. What two laboratory results were indicative of dehydration other than the electrolytes?
    *_____ and _____ .

9. Hypernatremia frequently results from *_____ .
10. Mr. Cooper's serum potassium level of 3.5 mEq/L is considered low average. Do you think his cellular potassium is (increased/decreased)? Explain rationale. *_____
_____ .

11. If Mr. Cooper is hydrated without potassium added, the nurse should expect his serum potassium to be (increased/decreased). _____ .
Why? *_____
_____ .

12. What intravenous solution resembles the electrolyte structure of plasma?
*_____ .

1. *Hyperosmolar dehydration. Serum sodium is elevated with the fluid loss.*
2. *extracellular fluid volume deficit, or hypovolemia*
3. *a. dry mucous membrane and dry skin*
   b. vital signs—temperature slightly elevated, tachycardia, respiration increased, systolic blood pressure ↓
   c. elevated sodium level
   d. Hct and BUN increased
   Others—weight loss, urinary output ↓
4. *$12 \div 165 = 0.07 \times 100 = 7\%$*
5. *b. marked dehydration*
6. *$75 \text{ kg} \times 0.07 = 5.25 \text{ L loss}$*
7. *a. $\frac{1}{3} \times 5.25 \text{ L} = 1.75 \text{ L or } 1750 \text{ mL}$*
   b. $\frac{2}{3} \times 5.25 \text{ L} = 3.5 \text{ L or } 3500 \text{ mL}$
   c. 2.5 L or 2500 mL
8. *elevated Hct and BUN*
9. *water depletion*
10. *Decreased. With dehydration, K leaves cells.*
11. *Decreased. With hydration, K moves from the ECF back into cells; thus, serum K is lowered.*
12. *lactated Ringer's*

NURSING ASSESSMENT FACTORS

- Complete a client history identifying factors that may cause a fluid volume deficit (ECFVD), such as vomiting, diarrhea, lack of fluid intake, diabetes mellitus or insipidus, large draining wound, or use of diuretics.
- Assess the skin for: poor skin turgor by pinching the skin (pinched skin that remains pinched or returns slowly to its normal skin surface is indicative of poor skin turgor), dry mucous membranes, and/or dry cracked lips or tongue.
- Check vital signs: pulse rate, respiration, and blood pressure. When the blood volume decreases, the heart compensates for the fluid loss by increasing the heart rate. When the fluid volume continues to decrease, the systolic blood pressure begins to fall. Check the blood pressure, first, while the client is sitting and, then, while the client is standing (a fall of 10–15 mm Hg in systolic pressure could indicate marked dehydration). A narrow pulse pressure of less than 20 mm Hg could indicate severe hypovolemia.
- Check the urine output for volume and concentration. A decrease in urine output may be due to a lack of fluid intake or excess body fluid loss.

- Assess hand and/or neck vein filling. A decrease in venous filling (in the vessels of the hand) when the hand is below the heart level and in the jugular vein when the client is in a low Fowler's position may suggest a fluid volume deficit.
- Check laboratory findings such as BUN, hematocrit, and hemoglobin. Record and report abnormal findings.

NURSING DIAGNOSIS 1

Fluid volume deficit: dehydration related to inadequate fluid intake, vomiting, diarrhea, hemorrhage, or third-space fluid loss (burns or ascites).

NURSING INTERVENTIONS AND RATIONALE

1. Monitor vital signs every 4 hours depending upon the severity of the fluid loss. Compare the vital signs to the client's baseline vital signs. Check the blood pressure in lying, sitting, and standing positions.
2. Provide fluid intake hourly, using fluids client prefers, and those indicated by electrolyte deficits. If intravenous (IV) method is used for fluid replacement, monitor IV flow rate. Guard against overhydration and infiltration of the IV fluids.
3. Monitor skin turgor, mucous membranes, and lips and tongue for changes: improvement or deterioration.
4. Routinely check body weight. Remember 2.2 pounds (1 kg) loss is equivalent to 1 liter (1000 mL) of fluid loss.

NURSING DIAGNOSIS 2

High risk for impaired skin integrity, related to a fluid deficit in body tissues.

NURSING INTERVENTIONS AND RATIONALE

1. Utilize preventive measures to preserve skin and mucous membrane integrity. The client's position should be changed on a regular schedule.
2. Apply lotion to increase circulation to the bony prominents.
3. Check skin turgor. Note skin color and temperature.

NURSING DIAGNOSIS 3

Oral mucous membranes: altered, related to dehydration.

NURSING INTERVENTIONS AND RATIONALE

1. Provide oral hygiene several times a day. Inspect mouth for sores, lesions, or bleeding. Avoid use of drying agents such as lemon and glycerine swabs or certain mouth washes. Use half-strength hydrogen peroxide (H_2O_2) to remove dry debris from the mouth.
2. Apply water-soluble lubricant to the lips to prevent cracking and promote healing.
3. Promote adequate fluid replacement.
4. Avoid irritants (foods, fluids, temperature, etc).

NURSING DIAGNOSIS 4

Tissue perfusion, renal: altered, related to decreased renal blood flow and poor urine output secondary to ECFVD, or hypovolemia.

NURSING INTERVENTIONS AND RATIONALE

1. Monitor urinary output. Report if urine output is less than 30 mL per hour or 250 mL per 8 hours. Absence of urine output for 5–12 hours may indicate renal insufficiency due to decreased renal blood perfusion.
2. Note presence of pain on urination.
3. Monitor; report abnormal laboratory findings such as elevated BUN and elevated serum creatinine. Measure the specific gravity of urine every shift.
4. Weigh client daily, at the same time in the morning.

EXTRACELLULAR FLUID VOLUME EXCESS: EDEMA

INTRODUCTION

Extracellular fluid volume excess (ECFVE) is increased fluid in the interstitial (tissues) and intravascular (vascular or vessel) spaces. Usually it relates to the excess fluid in tissues of the extremities (peripheral edema) or lung tissues (pulmonary edema).

43 Hypervolemia and overhydration are interchangeable terms for ECFVE and edema.
Hypervolemia means *_____ .
Hypervolemia and overhydration contribute to fluid excess in tissue spaces, or edema.

Fluid overload is another term for overhydration and hypervolemia.

excess fluid volume in circulating blood volume
■   ■   ■

44 Edema is the abnormal retention of fluid in the interstitial spaces of the extracellular fluid compartment or in serous cavities. Frequently, edema results from sodium retention in the body, causing a retention of water and an increase in extracellular fluid volume. Three terms used for extracellular fluid volume excess are _____ ,
_____ , and _____ .

hypervolemia, overhydration, and edema
■   ■   ■

45 Edema is the abnormal retention of fluid in the *_____
_____ .

interstitial spaces of the ECF compartment or in serous cavities
■   ■   ■

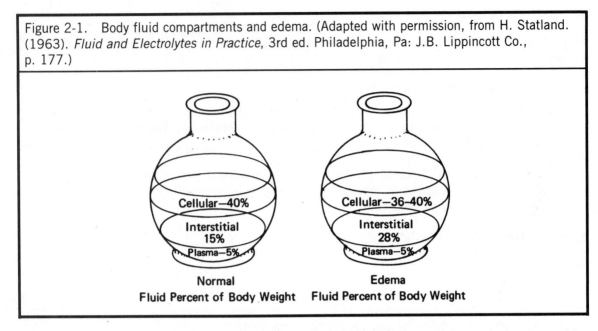

Figure 2-1.   Body fluid compartments and edema. (Adapted with permission, from H. Statland. (1963). *Fluid and Electrolytes in Practice*, 3rd ed. Philadelphia, Pa: J.B. Lippincott Co., p. 177.)

Figure 2-1 demonstrates the makeup of normal body fluid versus abnormal body fluid, such as with edema. As you recall from Chapter 1, 60% of the adult body weight is water; 40% of that is intracellular or cellular water, and 20% is extracellular water. Of the extracellular fluid, 15% is interstitial fluid and 5% is intravascular fluid or plasma. Note that with edema there is an increase of fluid in the interstitial space, which is between tissues and cells. The intracellular fluid may be decreased in extreme cases. Refer to the figure as needed.

PATHOPHYSIOLOGY

46   When sodium and water are retained in the same proportion, the fluid is referred to as iso-osmolar fluid volume excess. Actually the sodium level is increased even though the serum sodium level may be within the normal range. This is most likely due to (hemoconcentration/hemodilution) _____ .

hemodilution

■   ■   ■

47   Normally there is an exchange of fluid between the intravascular and interstitial spaces to maintain fluid balance in the extracellular fluid compartment.

The hydrostatic pressure in the arteries pushes fluid into the tissue spaces, and oncotic pressure in the arteries, which are made up of protein and albumin, holds fluid in the vessels. When there is fluid volume excess, the fluid pressure is greater than the oncotic pressure; therefore, (more/less) _____ fluid is pushed into the tissue spaces.

Excess fluid in the lower extremities due to fluid overload is known as (peripheral/pulmonary) _____ edema, and excess fluid that crosses the alveolar-capillary membrane of the lungs is known as (peripheral/pulmonary) _____ edema.

more; peripheral; pulmonary

 ■   ■   ■

48 Edema in the extremities (peripheral edema) occurs when there is a dysfunction of the heart, kidney, and/or liver. The fluid pressure in the vessels is increased and the fluid is pushed into the tissue spaces, primarily in the extremities.

If the kidneys cannot excrete excess vascular fluid, what might happen? *_____
_____ .

peripheral edema, or fluid is pushed into the tissue spaces

 ■   ■   ■

49 Excess vascular fluid may lead to (peripheral edema/pulmonary edema/eventually both)
*_____ .

peripheral and pulmonary edema (both)

 ■   ■   ■

ETIOLOGY

Physiologic factors leading to edema may be caused by various clinical conditions such as congestive heart failure (CHF), kidney failure, cirrhosis of the liver, steroid excess, and allergic reaction. Table 2-3 lists the physiologic factors for edema, the rationale, and the clinical conditions associated with each physiologic factor.

Study this table carefully; note whether there is an increase or decrease in the physiologic factors that can serve as an indication of edema. Be able to explain how edema occurs in the various clinical situations. Refer to this table as you find necessary.

50 Place I for increased and D for decreased beside the physiologic factors as they occur in edema:

____ a. Capillary permeability
____ b. Sodium retention
____ c. Lymphatic drainage
____ d. Plasma colloid osmotic pressure
____ e. Plasma hydrostatic pressure in the capillaries

a. I; b. I; c. D; d. D; e. I

 ■   ■   ■

Physiologic Factors	Rationale	Clinical Conditions
Plasma hydrostatic pressure in the capillaries	↑ Increased — Blood dammed in the venous system will cause "back" pressure in capillaries, thus raising capillary pressure. Increased capillary pressure will force more fluid into tissue areas, thus producing edema.	1. Congestive heart failure from increased venous pressure. 2. Kidney failure due to sodium and water retention. 3. Venous obstruction leading to varicose veins. 4. Pressure on veins because of swelling, constricting bandages, or casts.
Plasma colloid osmotic pressure	↓ Decreased — Decreased plasma colloid osmotic pressure results from diminished plasma protein concentration. Decreased protein content will cause water to flow from plasma into tissue spaces, thus causing edema.	1. Malnutrition due to lack of protein in diet. 2. Chronic diarrhea resulting in loss of protein. 3. Burns leading to loss of fluid containing protein through denuded skin. 4. Kidney disease, particularly nephrosis. 5. Cirrhosis of liver due to lack of protein. 6. Loss of plasma proteins through urine.
Capillary permeability	↑ Increased — Increased permeability of capillary membrane will allow plasma proteins to leak out of capillaries into interstitial space more rapidly than lymphatics can return them to circulation. Increased capillary permeability is predisposing factor to edema.	1. Bacterial inflammation causes increased porosity. 2. Allergic reactions. 3. Burns causing damage to capillaries. 4. Acute kidney disease, e.g., nephritis.

Table 2-3. PHYSIOLOGIC FACTORS LEADING TO EDEMA

51 Blood backed up in the venous system increases the capillary pressure, forcing more fluid into

*_____ .

The clinical conditions in which edema may occur as a result of an increase of plasma hydrostatic pressure are:

Table 2-3. (Continued)		
Physiologic Factors	**Rationale**	**Clinical Conditions**
Sodium retention	↑ Increased	Kidneys regulate level of sodium ions in extracellular fluid. Kidney function will depend on adequate blood flow. Inadequate blood flow, presence of excess aldosterone, or diseased kidneys, are predisposing factors to edema since they cause sodium retention.	1. Congestive heart failure causing inadequate circulation of blood. 2. Renal failure—inadequate circulation of blood through kidneys. 3. Increased production of adrenal cortical hormones—aldosterone, cortisone, and hydrocortisone—will cause retention of sodium. 4. Cirrhosis of liver. Diseased liver cannot destroy excess production of aldosterone. 5. Trauma resulting from fractures, burns, and surgery.
Lymphatic drainage	↓ Decreased	Blockage of lymphatics will prevent return of proteins to circulation. Obstructed lymph flow is said to be high in protein content. With inadequate return of proteins to circulation, plasma colloid osmotic pressure will be decreased, thus causing edema.	1. Lymphatic obstruction, e.g., cancer of lymphatic system. 2. Surgical removal of lymph nodes. 3. Elephantiasis, which is parasitic invasion of lymph channels, resulting in fibrous tissue growing in nodes, obstructing lymph flow. 4. Obesity because of inadequate supporting structures for lymphatics in lower extremities. Muscles are considered the supporting structures.

a. * _____

b. * _____

c. * _____

d. * _____

the tissue spaces (interstitial spaces)
a. CHF (congestive heart failure)
b. kidney failure
c. venous obstruction
d. pressure on the veins, e.g., from casts or bandages

■   ■   ■

52   A decrease in plasma protein results in a(n) (increase/decrease) _____ in the plasma colloid osmotic (oncotic) pressure. This causes water to flow from the vessels into the *_____ .

Name at least four clinical conditions in which edema occurs as a result of decreased plasma/serum colloid osmotic (oncotic) pressure. _____ , _____ , *_____ , and *_____ .

decrease; tissue spaces
malnutrition, burns, kidney disease, and liver disease
(all clinical conditions due to loss or lack of protein intake)

■   ■   ■

53   An increase in the capillary membrane permeability will permit plasma proteins to escape from _____ , causing more water to flow into *_____ .

Name at least three situations in which edema occurs as a result of increased capillary permeability. *_____ , *_____ , and *_____ .

capillaries; the tissue spaces (interstitial spaces)
bacterial inflammation, allergic reactions, acute kidney disease (e.g., nephritis), and burns

■   ■   ■

54   The kidneys regulate the level of _____ ions in the extracellular fluid. An inadequate blood flow, the presence of excess aldosterone, or diseased kidneys results in sodium (excretion/retention) _____ .

Name at least three clinical conditions that can cause sodium retention. _____ , *_____ , and *_____ .

sodium; retention
CHF (congestive heart failure), renal failure, adrenal cortical hormones (e.g., cortisone), cirrhosis of the liver, and trauma

■   ■   ■

55 Obstruction of the lymph flow prevents the return of proteins to the circulation. The obstructed lymph fluid is high in _____ content.

A decrease in protein content in the plasma causes the water to flow from
* _____ into * _____ .

Name at least three clinical conditions that cause a decrease in lymphatic drainage.
* _____ , * _____ , and _____ .

protein; the intravascular space; the tissue spaces
cancer of the lymphatic system, removal of the lymph nodes, obesity, and elephantiasis

■   ■   ■

56 Edema of the lungs, often called *pulmonary edema*, can occur in clients with limited cardiac or renal reserve. When the heart is not able to function adequately and the kidneys cannot excrete a sufficient amount of urine, the fluid backs up into the pulmonary circulatory system.

When the hydrostatic pressure of the blood in the pulmonary capillaries rises to equal or exceed the plasma colloid osmotic pressure, the water flows from vessels into the
* _____ , leading to pulmonary edema.

lung tissues

■   ■   ■

57 Giving excessive amounts of intravenous infusions to a person with pulmonary edema causes the blood volume to increase. This increased blood volume is called _____ .

Intravenous infusions should be regulated so that the rate of flow is not in excess of the urinary _____ .

hypervolemia; output

■   ■   ■

CLINICAL MANIFESTATIONS

There are numerous clinical manifestations of ECFVE as they relate to pulmonary edema and peripheral edema.

58 When the fluid volume excess (overhydration/hypervolemia) causes a "backup" of fluid that seeps into the lung tissue, * _____ results.

pulmonary edema

■   ■   ■

59 An early symptom of ECFVE is a constant, irritated cough. This is a sign of *_____

_____ .

overhydration or hypervolemia or fluid volume excess or early pulmonary edema
             ■   ■   ■

Table 2-4 lists the clinical signs and symptoms of ECFVE related to pulmonary and peripheral edema. Laboratory test results influenced by ECFVE are included. Rationale for each sign and symptom and potential abnormal laboratory results are listed.

Study the table carefully. As a nurse, you will frequently observe signs and symptoms of overhydration or hypervolemia. Be sure you recognize the signs and symptoms of edema and the related abnormal laboratory test results. Refer to the table as needed.

60 One of the first clinical symptoms of ECFV excess, or hypervolemia or overhydration, is

*_____ .

constant, irritating cough
             ■   ■   ■

Table 2-4. CLINICAL MANIFESTATIONS OF ECFVE—HYPERVOLEMIA, OVERHYDRATION, EDEMA

Signs and Symptoms	Rationale
Pulmonary Edema Constant, irritated cough	An irritated cough is frequently the first clinical symptom of hypervolemia. It is caused by fluid "backed up" into the lungs (lung congestion).
Dyspnea (difficulty in breathing)	Breathing is labored and difficult due to fluid congestion in lungs.
Neck vein engorgement	Jugular vein remains engorged when the patient is in semi-Fowler's or sitting position.
Sublingual vein engorgement	Engorged veins under the tongue may indicate hypervolemia.
Hand vein engorgement	Peripheral veins in the hand remain engorged with hand elevated above heart level for 10 seconds.
Moist rales in lung	Lungs are congested with fluid. Moist rales in lung can be heard with the stethoscope.
Bounding pulse	A full, bounding pulse is present with hypervolemia. The pulse rate may increase.

Table 2-4. (Continued)

Signs and Symptoms	Rationale
Cyanosis	Can be a late symptom of pulmonary edema as a result of the inadequate heart and kidney function.
Peripheral Edema Pitting edema in extremities	Peripheral edema present in the morning may result from inadequate heart, liver, or kidney function. A positive test of pitting edema is a finger indentation on the edematous area.
Tight, smooth, shiny skin over edematous area	Excess fluid in the peripheral tissues may cause the skin to be tight, smooth, and shiny.
Pallor, cool skin at edematous area	Excess fluid causes a decrease in circulation. The skin becomes pale, shiny, and cool.
Puffy eyelids	Swollen eyelids occur with generalized edema.
Weight gain	A gain of 2.2 to 2.5 pounds is equivalent to a gain of 1 liter of body water.
Laboratory Tests Decreased serum osmolality	Excess fluid dilutes solute concentration; thus serum osmolality is below 275 mOsm/kg.
Decreased serum protein and albumin, BUN, Hgb, Hct	Serum protein, albumin, BUN, and Hgb and Hct levels can be decreased due to excess fluid volume (hemodilution).
Increased CVP (central venous pressure)	An increase in CVP measurement of more than 12–15 cm H_2O is indicative of hypervolemia, evidenced as an increase in the fluid pressure.

61   Identify which of the following are signs and symptoms of pulmonary edema.

____ a. Dyspnea
____ b. Neck vein engorgement
____ c. Hand vein engorgement
____ d. Pitting edema in the extremities
____ e. Tight, smooth, shiny skin over edematous site
____ f. Moist rales in lung

a. X; b. X; c. X; d. —; e. —; f. X

■   ■   ■

62 In pulmonary edema, the alveoli (air sacs) are filled with fluid. Explain the effect this fluid throughout the lung tissue has on ventilation. *_____

_____ .

Pulmonary edema causes poor or inadequate ventilation.

■   ■   ■

63 When the jugular vein remains engorged after a person is put in a semi-Fowler's position (45° elevated), what type of fluid imbalance might this indicate? *_____

_____ .

extracellular fluid volume excess or hypervolemia

■   ■   ■

64 A quick assessment for hypervolemia, or overhydration, can be done by checking the peripheral veins in the hand. Instruct the client to hold a hand above the heart level. If the peripheral veins of the hand remain engorged after 10 seconds, this can be an indication of

_____ .

Explain how peripheral vein assessment for hypervolemia differs from peripheral vein assessment for hypovolemia. *_____

_____ .

hypervolemia
Hypervolemia is assessed with the hand above the heart level for vein engorgement, and hypovolemia is assessed with the hand below the heart level for flat vein or no engorgement.

■   ■   ■

65 The nurse can assess the lungs for evidence of hypervolemia by listening for
*_____ with a stethoscope.

moist rales

■   ■   ■

66 Cyanosis is a(n) (early/late) _____ symptom of pulmonary edema due to hypervolemia.

late

■   ■   ■

67 The influence of gravity has an effect on the distribution of fluid in the edematous person. In a lying position, there is a more equal distribution of edema, whereas in an upright position the edema is more prevalent in the lower extremities. This is called *dependent edema.*

The eyelids of a person with generalized edema may be swollen in the morning, but by afternoon, with increased activity, the swelling is (more/less) _____ marked.

less

■   ■   ■

68 With clients who are up and about, the peripheral edema is frequently found in the (ankles and feet/sacrum and buttocks) *_____ . For those who are bedridden, edema fluid is most likely be found in the *_____ .

ankles and feet
eyes or sacrum and buttocks, or more equally distributed

■   ■   ■

69 The type of edema associated with gravity and the person's body position is called
*_____ .

dependent edema

■   ■   ■

70 Explain why a nurse should assess for edema in the ankles and feet early in the morning.
*_____

_____

_____ .

Dependent edema should not be present after the client has been in a prone or supine position for the night. If edema is present in the morning, it is most likely due to cardiac, renal, or liver disease and can be called nondependent edema *(to differentiate between edema due to gravity versus edema due to cardiac, renal, or liver dysfunction; it can also be called* refractory edema *when edema does not respond to diuretics).*

■   ■   ■

71 Another tool for assessing edema and hypervolemia is body weight.

If the client has edema and has gained 2.2 pounds, this weight gain is equivalent to _____ liter(s) of water.

1

■   ■   ■

72 When hemoglobin and hematocrit measurements have been in a normal range and suddenly decrease, there is a fluid imbalance. This change is indicative of _____ .

If the hemoglobin and hematocrit increase, the fluid imbalance might be indicative of

_____ .

hypervolemia; hypovolemia or dehydration
■   ■   ■

CLINICAL APPLICATIONS

73 Many edematous persons are malnourished due to a loss of proteins or electrolytes. Unless contraindicated, the nurse should encourage the edematous client to eat foods high in _____ . Why? *_____

_____ .

protein
It increases plasma colloid osmotic pressure and thus pulls fluid out of the tissues.
■   ■   ■

74 Edematous persons often suffer from dehydration. Explain why? *_____

_____ .

The edema fluid is trapped in the interstitial space (tissue) and is not circulating, e.g., ascites and peripheral edema.
■   ■   ■

75 The tissues of an edematous person are said to be more vulnerable to injury, resulting in tissue breakdown.

A bedfast person with edema of the sacrum and buttocks is apt to develop _____ due to *_____

_____ .

decubiti (bedsores); tissue breakdown or constant pressure on the edematous tissues
■   ■   ■

76 Identify a nursing intervention to prevent decubiti in the edematous person. *_____

_____ .

frequent change of body position
■   ■   ■

77 Generalized edema is called *anasarca*. The following terms are used to describe fluid in various body cavities:

Peritoneal cavity, *ascites*
Pleural cavity, *hydrothorax*
Pericardial sac, *hydropericardium*
Anasarca means   *_____ .

   Identify the specific name used when fluid collects in the following body cavities:

Peritoneal cavity.   _____
Pleural cavity.   _____
Pericardial sac.   _____

generalized edema
ascites; hydrothorax; hydropericardium
      ■   ■   ■

CLINICAL MANAGEMENT

78 When edema is present, salt and water intake often increases the fluid retention.
   Water intake alone probably (will/will not)   _____   increase the edema.
Why?   *_____
_____ .

will not
Salt (sodium) has a water-retaining effect and without the sodium the water would not increase the edema. However, caution should be taken with giving excess amounts of water.
      ■   ■   ■

79 Thiazide diuretics such as hydrochlorothiazine (HydroDiuril) and loop or high ceiling diuretics such as furosemide (Lasix) assist in decreasing fluid volume excess by promoting sodium and water excretion.

   Decreasing fluid pressure in the vascular system assists fluid in flowing back from the tissue spaces into the vessels in order to be excreted.

   Diuretics aid in the excretion of body sodium and   _____ .

water
      ■   ■   ■

80 In cardiac insufficiency, the digitalis preparation digoxin may be needed to improve heart function and circulation.

The three Ds are frequently prescribed for the clinical management of ECFVE. They are: _____ , _____ , and _____ .

diuretics, digoxin (digitalis preparation), and diet (low sodium)

■　　　　　　　　　　■　　　　　　　　　　■

81 In nephrotic edema, cirrhosis of the liver with ascites, or any other marked hypoproteinemic state the administration of albumin, which is (hypo-osmolar/hyperosmolar) _____ , (increases/decreases) _____ the plasma colloid osmotic pressure; this causes the fluid to flow from the *_____ into the _____ .

hyperosmolar; increases; tissue space; plasma

■　　　　　　　　　　■　　　　　　　　　　■

82 Increasing protein intake in a malnourished person should (increase/decrease) _____ the oncotic pressure in the vessels, thus pulling water out of the tissues.

increase

■　　　　　　　　　　■　　　　　　　　　　■

CASE STUDY REVIEW

Mrs. Shea, age 72, was admitted to the hospital with complaints of shortness of breath, coughing, and swollen ankles and feet. Her blood pressure was 190/110, pulse 96, and respirations 28 and labored. Her hemoglobin and hematocrit were slightly low. She has a history of a "heart condition" and hypertension.

1. The nurse assesses Mrs. Shea's physical state. Her shortness of breath, coughing, and swollen ankles and feet may be indicative of *_____ . Other names for extracellular fluid volume excess include _____ , _____ , and _____ .

2. An early symptom of extracellular fluid volume excess or hypervolemia is *_____ _____ .

3. The five main physiologic factors leading to edema are *_____ , *_____ , *_____ , *_____ , and *_____ .

4. The two physiologic factors that may have caused Mrs. Shea's edema are *_____ and *_____ .

5. The nurse assesses Mrs. Shea's ankles and feet in the morning to differentiate between dependent and nondependent edema. If Mrs. Shea's ankles and feet remain swollen before she arises in the morning, the edema is described as _____ edema. The cause of this type of edema is *_____ .

6. The nurse assesses Mrs. Shea's peripheral veins. Her veins are still engorged after holding her hand above the heart level for 30 seconds. This can be indicative of *_____
_____ .

7. Mrs. Shea's shortness of breath or dyspnea and coughing may be due to _____ edema. Identify two assessment factors to assist the nurse in determining the type of edema present. *_____ and *_____
_____ .

8. Identify two causes of pulmonary edema. *_____ and _____ .

9. Mrs. Shea gained 5 pounds in 2 days. This weight gain would be equivalent to _____ liter(s) of body water gain, which is equal to _____ mL of body water.

10. Mrs. Shea's hemoglobin and hematocrit have been normal. At present, they are decreased, which may indicate _____ .
    Why? *_____
    _____ .

11. If Mrs. Shea developed generalized edema and was bedfast, what skin complication might result? _____

    Identify a nursing intervention that can be taken to prevent this complication? *_____
    _____ .

12. Identify the name for generalized edema. _____ .

1. extracellular fluid volume excess or edema
   edema, hypervolemia, and overhydration
2. constant, irritating cough
3. increased hydrostatic pressure, decreased colloidal osmotic pressure, increased capillary permeability, increased sodium retention, and decreased lymphatic drainage
4. Increased hydrostatic pressure and increased sodium retention
5. nondependent; inadequate heart, kidney, or liver function
6. extracellular fluid volume excess, or hypervolemia
7. pulmonary
   observe the jugular veins for engorgement when Mrs. Shea is in semi-Fowler's position and assess chest sounds for moist rales
8. inadequate heart and kidney function
9. 2; 2000
10. hypervolemia; dilution of red blood cells (RBCs) with a decrease in RBCs and an increase in water
11. decubiti; changing body position
12. anasarca

NURSING ASSESSMENT FACTORS

- Complete a client history to identify health problems that may contribute to the development of ECFVE. Examples of such health problems may include: reoccurring heart problem such as CHF, kidney or liver disease, infection, and malnutrition. Ask if there has been a recent weight gain.

- Obtain a dietary history that emphasizes sodium, protein, and water intake.
- Assess vital signs. Obtain baseline data that can be compared with past and future vital signs. Assess for a bounding pulse.
- Assess for signs and symptoms of hypervolemia (overhydration) such as constant and irritated cough, difficulty in breathing, neck and hand vein engorgement, chest rales, and abnormal laboratory results such as a decreased hematocrit and hemoglobin level that had previously been normal. Serum sodium levels may or may not be elevated.
- Make a quick assessment of hypervolemia by checking the peripheral veins in the hand: first lowering the hand and then raising the hand above the heart level. Overhydration is present if the peripheral veins remain engorged after 10 seconds.
- Assess extremities for peripheral edema. Check for pitting edema in the lower extremities in the morning before the client arises. Nondependent edema or refractory edema may be due to cardiac, renal, or liver dysfunction. Dependent edema (edema caused by gravity) is usually not present in the morning.
- Assess urine output. Decreased urinary output may be a sign of body fluid retention and/or renal dysfunction.
- Assess pulmonary status. Observe for the presence of pulmonary congestion or changes in respiratory status.

NURSING DIAGNOSIS 1

Fluid volume excess: edema, related to body fluid overload secondary to heart, renal, or liver dysfunction.

NURSING INTERVENTIONS AND RATIONALE

1. Monitor vital signs. Report elevated blood pressure and bounding pulse.
2. Monitor weight daily. Check weight every morning before breakfast. A weight gain of 2.2 pounds (1 kg) is equivalent to 1 liter or quart of water (1000 mL). Usually edema does not occur unless there is 3 or more liters of excess body fluids. Restrict fluids as necessary. Teach the client to monitor intake, output, and weight.
3. Observe for the presence of edema daily. Check for pitting edema in the extremities every morning. Press one or two fingers on the edematous area, and if indentation is present for 15 seconds or more, the degree of pitting edema should be recorded according to the length of time it takes for the indentation to disappear (+1 to +4). Monitor all IV fluids carefully.
4. Monitor diet. Teach appropriate food selections. Instruct the client to avoid using excess salt on foods [salt (sodium) holds water and increases the edematous condition]. Teach the client to avoid over-the-counter drugs without first checking with a nurse or physician.
5. Encourage the client with a liver disorder such as cirrhosis of the liver to eat foods rich in protein. Protein increases the plasma/serum oncotic (colloid osmotic) pressure, thus pulling fluids from the tissue spaces and decreasing edema.
6. Encourage rest periods to support diuresis.

NURSING DIAGNOSIS 2

Breathing patterns: ineffective, related to increased capillary permeability causing fluid overload in the lung tissue (pulmonary edema).

NURSING INTERVENTIONS AND RATIONALE

1. Monitor breathing patterns. Assess rate and depth of respiration. Check chest sounds and chest excursion. Note changes and location of adventitious sounds.
2. Observe for changes in skin color and nasal flaring. Note any coughing. Report any progression of symptoms to physician.
3. Use semi-Fowler's position for those with dyspnea or orthopnea.

NURSING DIAGNOSIS 3

Skin integrity: altered, related to edematous tissues (peripheral edema).

NURSING INTERVENTIONS AND RATIONALE

1. Monitor client's mobility. Turn edematous clients frequently to prevent decubiti. Edematous persons are prone to tissue breakdown.
2. Identify and record changes in skin surfaces regarding color, temperature, and skin turgor.
3. Ambulate the client to improve circulation and enhance fluid reabsorption from the tissue spaces to the vascular space.
4. Monitor laboratory results pertinent to electrolyte status and fluid balance. Report changes.

NURSING DIAGNOSIS 4

Tissue perfusion: decreased, related to hypervolemia as manifested by peripheral (tissue) edema.

NURSING INTERVENTIONS AND RATIONALE

1. Monitor fluid intake. Water and sodium restrictions may be necessary.
2. Monitor urine output. Urine output should be >30 mL per hour or >250 mL per 8 hours. Large amounts of urine output can indicate a decrease in urine retention.
3. Administer diuretics as ordered. Assess fluid balance.
4. Check serum electrolyte values while client is receiving diuretics. The more potent diuretics excrete not only sodium, but the important electrolyte potassium. Encourage foods high in potassium; potassium supplements may be necessary. Urine output should be closely monitored when potassium is given.

EXTRACELLULAR FLUID VOLUME SHIFT

INTRODUCTION

In the extracellular fluid compartment, fluid volume with electrolytes and protein shifts from the intravascular to the interstitial spaces. This fluid is referred to as *third-space fluid*. The fluid is nonfunctional and is considered to be physiologically useless. Later, third-space fluid shifts back from the interstitial space to the intravascular space.

83 Extracellular fluid is constantly shifting between the intravascular and interstitial spaces for the purpose of maintaining fluid balance.

When abnormal amounts of fluid shift into the tissue spaces and remain there, it is called

* _____ .

third-space fluid

∎   ∎   ∎

84 Excess fluid in the tissue spaces, or third-space fluid, is nonfunctional and is considered

*_____ .

physiologically useless fluid
　　　　　　　■　　　　　　　■　　　　　　　■

ETIOLOGY

85 Clinical causes could be as simple as a blister or sprain or as serious as massive injuries, burns, ascites, abdominal surgery, a perforated peptic ulcer, and intestinal obstruction.

When massive amounts of fluid shift to the tissues and remain there, what happens to the state of vascular fluids?　*_____

_____ .

Hypovolemia or fluid loss from the vascular space. If severe, shock can develop.
　　　　　　　■　　　　　　　■　　　　　　　■

86 Minor causes of third-space fluid may be _____ and

_____ .

Identify three severe health problems that can cause third-space fluid:

_____ , _____ , and _____ .

blisters and sprains
burns, trauma (massive injuries), and ascites (severe liver disease) (also, abdominal surgery, intestinal obstruction, or perforated ulcer)
　　　　　　　■　　　　　　　■　　　　　　　■

87 Burns and abdominal surgery are common causes of third-space fluid. With these two conditions, there are two phases of fluid shift.

In the first phase fluid is shifting from the intravascular space to the interstitial space. With burns, fluid remains at the burned site and surrounding tissues for 3–5 days.

In the second phase, the fluid shifts from the　*_____ to the

*_____ .

interstitial space (tissue and injured area); intravascular space
　　　　　　　■　　　　　　　■　　　　　　　■

CLINICAL MANIFESTATIONS

In a fluid shift due to tissue injury, it takes approximately 24–48 hours for the fluid to leave the blood vessels and accumulate in the injured tissue spaces. Edema may or may not be visible.

88 When fluid shifts out of the vessels, changes in the vital signs occur which are similar to shocklike symptoms. These vital signs are similar to those of marked dehydration. Indicate whether the following vital signs increase or decrease in such fluid shifts.

*_____ Pulse rate
*_____ Respiration
*_____ Systolic blood pressure

increased pulse rate; increased respiration; decreased systolic blood pressure (depends on the severity of fluid loss to the injured site)

■   ■   ■

89 Three to 5 days after an injury causing tissue destruction, fluid shifts from the injured site to

*_____ .

blood vessels or intravascular space

■   ■   ■

90 If the kidneys cannot excrete the excess fluid from the vascular space (blood vessels) that resulted from the fluid shift, what type of fluid imbalance might occur? _____

_____ .

hypervolemia or overhydration or ECFVE

■   ■   ■

91 Name three clinical signs and symptoms of hypervolemia/overhydration.
*_____ , _____ , and *_____

_____ .

constant, irritated cough, dyspnea, and moist chest rales (also hand and neck vein engorgement and full bounding pulse)

■   ■   ■

CLINICAL MANAGEMENT

92 An assessment must be completed in order to determine the cause of the third-space fluid. In the case of burns when severe tissue destruction results, the fluid shift may be so severe that (hypervolemia/hypovolemia) _____ occurs.

hypovolemia

■   ■   ■

93 During the first phase of a fluid shift to the burn tissue site, intravenous infusion in the amount of two to three times the urine output may be necessary to maintain the circulating fluid volume.

   During the second phase of fluid shift, (more/less) _____ IV fluids would be needed. Why? *_____

_____ .

less
Large quantities of fluid shift back into the vascular space and too much intravenous fluid may cause a fluid overload.

   ■   ■   ■

94 During the second phase of the fluid shift, the urine output (increases/decreases)

_____ .

Explain. *_____ .

increases
Urine excretion increases, with sufficient kidney function, to prevent fluid overload.

   ■   ■   ■

INTRACELLULAR FLUID VOLUME EXCESS: WATER INTOXICATION

INTRODUCTION

95 Intracellular fluid volume excess (ICFVE) results from an excess of water or decrease in solutes in the intravascular system. Fluid in the blood vessels is (hypo-osmolar/iso-osmolar/hyperosmolar) _____ when there is an ICFVE.

hypo-osmolar

   ■   ■   ■

96 Another name for ICFVE is *_____ . As a result of this fluid imbalance, the serum osmolality is (increased/decreased) _____ .

water intoxication; decreased

   ■   ■   ■

PATHOPHYSIOLOGY

   Hypo-osmolar fluid (decreased concentration in the circulating vascular fluid) moves by the process of osmosis from the areas of lesser concentration to the areas of greater concentration. The intracellular fluid (cells) is iso-osmolar, so the hypo-osmolar fluid from the vascular space flows into the cells, thus causing the cells to swell.

97 Fluid shifts from the areas of lesser concentration to the areas of greater concentration due to the process of (diffusion/osmosis) _____ .

osmosis

■   ■   ■

98 Excess fluid that may accumulate in the cells can cause *_____

_____ .

(intra)cellular fluid overload or cellular edema

■   ■   ■

99 In an ICFVE, the cerebral cells are usually the first cells involved in the fluid shift from the vascular to the cellular space.

What might happen if there are large amounts of fluid shifting into the cerebral cells?

*_____ .

cerebral edema or cellular fluid overload

■   ■   ■

100 An excess secretion of the antidiuretic hormone (ADH) causes fluid to be reabsorbed from the renal tubules. This can result in what type of vascular fluid? _____ .

hypo-osmolar

■   ■   ■

101 Edema may result from an excess of _____ , whereas water intoxication results from an excess of _____ .

With edema, there is excessive fluid in the *_____ compartment, whereas with water intoxication there is excess fluid in the *_____ compartment.

sodium; water; extracellular fluid; intracellular fluid

■   ■   ■

102 Water intoxication (is/is not) _____ the same as edema. Generally, edema is the accumulation of fluid in the interstitial spaces. With water intoxication, the excess hypo-osmolar fluid (increases/lowers) _____ serum osmolality.

As the result of the hypo-osmolar fluid in the vascular space, water moves into the cells, causing the cells to (shrink/swell) _____ .

is not; lowers; swell

■   ■   ■

ETIOLOGY

Intracellular fluid volume excess is not as common as ECFVD and ECFVE, but if untreated, it can cause serious health problems.

Common causes of water intoxication are the intake of water-free solutes and the administration of hypo-osmolar intravenous fluids such as 0.45% sodium chloride ($\frac{1}{2}$ normal saline solution) and 5% dextrose in water (D_5W). Dextrose 5% in water is an iso-osmolar IV solution; however, the dextrose is metabolized quickly, leaving water or a hypo-osmolar solution.

103 The two most common types of fluid imbalance are _____ and _____ . The initials ICFVE stand for *_____ .

ECFVD and ECFVE; intracellular fluid volume excess
      ■   ■   ■

104 There are four major conditions that may cause ICFVE:

    a. Excessive nonsolute water intake
    b. Solute deficit (electrolytes and protein)
    c. Increased secretion of antidiuretic hormone (ADH)
    d. Kidney dysfunction (inability to excrete excess water)

    These conditions may cause an increase in (hypo-osmolar/hyperosmolar) _____ fluid in the vascular space (vessels).

hypo-osmolar
      ■   ■   ■

Table 2-5 lists four major conditions and laboratory tests to assess for ICFVE, their causes, and rationale. Study the table carefully and refer to it as needed.

105 Name four major conditions that might cause water intoxication. *_____ , *_____ , *_____ , and *_____ .

excess nonsolute water intake, solute deficit or lack of electrolytes and protein, increased secretion of inappropriate ADH (SIADH), and kidney dysfunction or renal impairment
      ■   ■   ■

106 The iso-osmolar IV solution D_5W becomes a hypo-osmolar solution when *_____

_____ .

dextrose is metabolized rapidly, leaving water solution. When D_5W is used continuously without other solutes, hypo-osmolar fluid results, causing ICFVE or water intoxication.
      ■   ■   ■

Table 2-5. CAUSES OF INTRACELLULAR FLUID VOLUME EXCESS: WATER INTOXICATION		
Conditions	**Causes**	**Rationale**
Excessive water intake	Excessive plain water intake	Water intake with few or no solutes dilutes the vascular fluid.
	Continuous use of IV hypo-osmolar solutions (0.45% saline, D_5W)	Overuse of hypo-osmolar solutions can cause hypo-osmolar vascular fluid. Dextrose is metabolized rapidly, leaving water.
	Brain injury or tumor	Cerebral cell injury may increase ADH production, causing excessive water reabsorption.
	Psychogenic polydipsia	Compulsive drinking of plain water almost continuously can result in water intoxication.
Solute deficit	Diet low in electrolytes and protein	Decrease in electrolytes and protein may cause hypo-osmolar vascular fluids.
	Irrigation of nasogastric tube with water (not saline)	GI tract is rich in electrolytes. Plain water can wash out the electrolytes
Excess ADH secretion	Stress, surgery, drugs (narcotics, anesthesia), pain, and tumors (brain, lung)	Overproduction of ADH is known as secretion (syndrome) of inappropriate antidiuretic hormone (SIADH), which causes mass amounts of water reabsorption by the kidneys and results in hypo-osmolar fluids.
Kidney dysfunction	Renal impairment	Kidney dysfunction can decrease water excretion.
Abnormal laboratory tests	Decreased serum sodium level and decreased serum osmolality	Because of hemodilution, the solutes in the vascular fluid are decreased in proportion to water.

107 Overproduction of ADH or SIADH causes (more/less) _____ water reabsorption from the tubules of the kidneys.

Two causes of excess secretion of ADH are _____ and

_____ .

more; stress and surgery [also drugs (narcotics) and pain]
■   ■   ■

108 If the circulation through the kidneys is impaired and there is an excessive amount of plain water intake, the fluid imbalance most likely to occur is *_____ .

Impairment of the renal circulation can occur due to arteriosclerosis. If the kidneys do not receive sufficient blood circulation, kidney (function/dysfunction) _____ can result.

water intoxication from water taken without solutes; dysfunction
■   ■   ■

109 As the result of ICFVE, the serum osmolality is most likely *_____ , and the serum sodium level is most likely _____ .

low or decreased or <280 mOsm/kg; decreased
■   ■   ■

CLINICAL APPLICATIONS

110 It is difficult for a person to drink himself into water intoxication unless the renal mechanisms for elimination fail.

If excessive water has been given and the kidneys are not functioning properly, what is most likely to occur? *_____ .

water retention or water intoxication
■   ■   ■

111 The most common occurrence of water intoxication is seen in postoperative clients when oral and intravenous fluids have been forced without compensatory amounts of salt. In these situations, the amount of water taken in exceeds that which the kidneys can excrete.

A postoperative client receiving several liters of 5% dextrose in water (D_5W) with ice and sips of water PO (by mouth) can develop a fluid imbalance called *_____

_____ .

water intoxication or ICFVE (due to intake of copious amounts of hypo-osmolar fluids)
■   ■   ■

112 Also, after surgery, an overproduction of the antidiuretic hormone (ADH), known as the syndrome of inappropriate ADH secretions (SIADH), can occur due to trauma, anesthesia, pain, and narcotics. Because of the overproduction of ADH, water excretion (increases/decreases) _____ , causing the urine volume to (rise/drop) _____ and the vascular (intravascular) fluid volume to (rise/drop) _____ .

decreases; drop; rise

■   ■   ■

CLINICAL MANIFESTATIONS

The clinical signs and symptoms and rationale of water intoxication or intracellular fluid volume excess are explained in Table 2–6. Study the table and be cognizant of the signs and symptoms. Refer to the table as necessary.

Table 2-6.   CLINICAL SIGNS AND SYMPTOMS OF INTRACELLULAR FLUID VOLUME EXCESS—WATER INTOXICATION

Type of Symptoms	Signs and Symptoms	Rationale
Early	Headache Nausea and vomiting Excessive perspiration Acute weight gain	Cerebral cells absorb hypo-osmolar fluid more quickly than other cells.
Progressive Central nervous system (CNS)	Behavioral changes: Progressive apprehension Irritability Disorientation Confusion Drowsiness Incoordination Blurred vision Elevated intracranial pressure (ICP)	Hypo-osmolar body fluids pass into cerebral cells first. Swollen cerebral cells can cause behavioral changes and elevate ICP.
Vital signs (VSs)	Blood pressure ↑ Bradycardia (slow pulse rate) Respiration ↑	Vital signs are the opposite of shock. VS are similar to those in increased ICP.
Later (CNS)	Neuroexcitability (muscle twitching) Projectile vomiting Papilledema Delirium Convulsions, then coma	Severe CNS changes occur when water intoxication is not corrected.
Skin	Warm, moist, and flushed	

113 Identify four early symptoms of water intoxication. _____ ,
* _____ , * _____ , and * _____ .

headache, nausea and vomiting, excessive perspiration, and weight gain

           ■   ■   ■

114 Central nervous system symptoms are (least/most) _____ prominent with water intoxication. Explain why? * _____

_____ .

most
Hypo-osmolar body fluids pass into cerebral cells; swollen cerebral cells cause behavioral changes

           ■   ■   ■

115 Name three behavioral changes that occur with progressive symptoms of water intoxication.
_____ , _____ , and _____ .

apprehension, irritability, disorientation, and confusion

           ■   ■   ■

116 The intracranial pressure is (increased/decreased) _____ with water intoxication.

increased

           ■   ■   ■

117 With progressive intracellular fluid volume excess, the vital sign measurements reflect:

    a. Blood pressure _____
    b. Pulse rate *_____
    c. Respiration _____

    a. increased
    b. decreased, or bradycardia
    c. increased

           ■   ■   ■

118 Name five later symptoms of water intoxication or intracellular fluid volume excess.
* _____ , * _____ , _____ ,
_____ , and _____ .

muscle twitching, projectile vomiting, papilledema, delirium, and convulsions

           ■   ■   ■

119 The skin in the later stages of water intoxication is *_____

_____ .

warm, moist, and flushed

■   ■   ■

CLINICAL MANAGEMENT

Overall Objective: To reduce excess water in the body.
   Two ways to reduce water in water intoxication are:

1. Reduce water intake
2. Promote water excretion

120 In *less* severe cases of water intoxication, water restriction may be sufficient, or an extracellular replacement solution such as lactated Ringer's or normal saline solution may be given to increase the osmolality of the extracellular fluid.

   The overall objective in the clinical management of water intoxication is *_____

_____ .

   Name two ways in which this objective is accomplished. *_____ and
*_____ .

to reduce excess water in the body; reduce water intake and promote water excretion.

■   ■   ■

121 Concentrated saline may be given in severe cases of water intoxication to raise extracellular electrolyte concentration in hope of drawing water out of the (intracellular space/interstitial space) *_____ and (increasing/decreasing) _____ urinary output.

intracellular space; increasing

■   ■   ■

122 However, administration of additional salt to a person who already has too much water can result in expansion of the interstitial fluid and blood volume, and the development of (water intoxication/edema) _____ .

   An osmotic diuretic, e.g., mannitol, includes diuresis and a loss of retained fluid, especially from the cerebral cells.

edema

■   ■   ■

123 Identify three methods for promoting water excretion.

a. *_____

b. *_____

c. *_____

a. *water restriction*
b. *extracellular replacement solution, e.g., lactated Ringer's or normal saline solution (0.9% NaCl)*
c. *concentrated saline solution, and also*
d. *osmotic diuretics, e.g., mannitol*

■   ■   ■

124 For less severe cases of water intoxication, the clinical management includes
*_____ and/or *_____.

For more severe cases of water intoxication, identify two possible clinical management interventions. *_____
and/or *_____.

water restriction; extracellular replacement solution
intravenous concentrated saline solution; osmotic diuretics

■   ■   ■

125 An osmotic diuretic induces *_____
_____.

diuresis and a loss of retained fluid, especially from cerebral cells

■   ■   ■

CASE STUDY REVIEW

Ms. Cline, age 19, returned from having an appendectomy performed. She received 1 liter of 5% dextrose in water during the procedure and another liter postoperatively. She was allowed to have crushed ice and sips of water. That evening she became nauseated, and the third liter of 5% dextrose in water was added. The following day she received 2 more liters of 5% dextrose in water. Ms. Cline took several glasses of crushed ice. Her first day postoperatively she complained of a headache. Later she was drowsy, disoriented, and confused. Her blood pressure evidenced a slight increase, and a drop in her pulse rate was noted.

1. The nurse assessed Ms. Cline's fluid state. From the history and her symptoms, the nurse assessed a fluid imbalance was present indicative of *_____
_____.

2. Excessive amounts of 5% dextrose in water along with glasses of crushed ice without any other solute intake can cause *_____ .

   Explain why. *_____

   _____ .

3. Name Ms. Cline's early symptoms of intracellular fluid volume excess. *_____ .
4. As the fluid imbalance progressed, name three symptoms that indicated water intoxication or intracellular fluid volume excess. _____ , _____ , and

   _____ .

5. Her vital signs were similar to those of *_____

   _____ .

6. Can an overproduction of ADH increase her water intoxication? _____ Explain how. *_____

   _____ .

7. Name the type of intravenous solution to be administered to correct severe cases of water intoxication. *_____ .

8. Identify how this fluid imbalance could have been prevented. *_____

   _____ .

1. water intoxication or intracellular fluid volume excess
2. Water intoxication. With 5% dextrose in water, the dextrose is metabolized by the body, leaving water. The intravenous solution and crushed ice cause the plasma to become hypo-osmolar.
3. Headache. If your answer was nausea—possibly; however, early nausea is most likely the result of the surgery and anesthesia.
4. drowsiness, disorientation, and confusion
5. increased intracranial pressure
6. Yes. After surgery, there can be an increased secretion of ADH, due to trauma, anesthesia, pain, and narcotics. This increases water retention and, with the hypo-osmolar fluids she received, could increase the state of water intoxication.
7. concentrated saline solution, e.g., 3% saline, hyperosmolar solution to "pull" water out of the cells
8. Ms. Cline should have received intravenous fluids containing saline (solute) together with dextrose.

NURSING ASSESSMENT FACTORS

- Complete a history to identify possible causes of intracellular fluid volume excess (ICFVE) such as excessive administration of hypo-osmolar solutions [continuous use of D₅W without solutes (saline)], oral fluid without solutes, major surgical procedure that might cause SIADH, and kidney dysfunction in which urine output is decreased.
- Assess vital signs. Obtain baseline data that can be compared with past and future vital signs. Note if the systolic blood pressure increases even slightly, pulse rate decreases, and respirations increase. These signs are indicative of an accumulation of cerebral fluid (cerebral edema).

- Assess for behavioral changes, such as confusion, irritability, and disorientation. Headache is an early symptom of ICFVE. These symptoms can result when hypo-osmolar fluid in the vascular space shifts to the cells, increasing cellular fluid. Cerebral cells are usually the first cells affected.
- Assess for weight changes. With ICFVE or water intoxication, there is normally an acute weight gain. With peripheral edema, the weight gain occurs more slowly.

NURSING DIAGNOSIS 1

Fluid volume excess: water intoxication, related to excessive ingestion and infusion of hypo-osmolar fluids and solutions, major surgical procedure causing SIADH.

NURSING INTERVENTIONS AND RATIONALE

1. Monitor fluid replacement. Assess osmolality of fluid replacement and consult with the physician for appropriate replacement balance. Report if the client is receiving only 5% dextrose in water continuously. Dextrose is metabolized rapidly by the body, leaving water, a hypo-osmolar solution.
2. Offer fluids that contain solutes, such as broth and juices, to the postoperative client. Giving plain water and ice chips increases the hypo-osmolar state. Immediately postoperatively and for 24–48 hours, there may be an overproduction of ADH [SIADH, or secretion (syndrome) of inappropriate antidiuretic hormone], causing an increase in water reabsorption.
3. Monitor fluid balance. The urine output after surgery and trauma can be compromised. The SIADH is frequently seen following surgery and trauma, which causes more water to be reabsorbed from the kidney tubules and dilution of the vascular fluid. Urine output is decreased due to water reabsorption.

NURSING DIAGNOSIS 2

Injury, high risk for, related to cerebral edema secondary to ICFVE.

NURSING INTERVENTIONS AND RATIONALE

1. Monitor vital signs and observe for behavioral changes. Assess the client for progressive signs and symptoms of water intoxication such as headache, behavioral changes (irritability, drowsiness, confusion, disorientation, delirium), changes in the vital signs ($\uparrow$ BP, $\downarrow$ P, $\uparrow$ R), and warm, moist, flushed skin.
2. Protect the client from injury during periods of confusion and disorientation. Keep bed rails up, assist the client with ambulation, assist the client with meals, and frequently reorient to place and time.
3. Observe for signs of seizure activity. Convulsions usually occur with severe ICFVE.

CHAPTER 3

ELECTROLYTES AND THEIR INFLUENCE ON THE BODY

Behavioral Objectives

Upon completion of this chapter, you will be prepared to:

- Describe the relationship of nonelectrolytes, electrolytes, and ions in body fluids.
- Name the principal cation and anion of the extracellular and intracellular fluids.
- Describe the physiologic functions of potassium, sodium, calcium, magnesium, phosphorus, and chloride.
- List the normal ranges of serum and urine potassium, sodium, calcium, magnesium, phosphorus, and chloride.
- Identify the various clinical causes (etiology) of potassium, sodium, calcium, magnesium, phosphorus, and chloride deficits or excesses.
- List the signs and symptoms of hypo-hyperkalemia, hypo-hypernatremia, hypo-hypercalcemia, hypo-hypermagnesemia, hypo-hyperphosphatemia, and hypo-hyperchloremia.
- Relate the electrolyte imbalances to drug action and interaction.
- Describe methods commonly utilized in electrolyte replacement therapy.
- Explain the nursing interventions to selected clinical situations (clinical applications).
- List foods that are rich in potassium, sodium, calcium, magnesium, phosphorus, and chloride.

Introduction

Chemical compounds may react in one of two ways when placed in solution. In one way, their molecules may remain intact as in urea, dextrose, and creatinine in the body fluid. These molecules do not produce an electrical charge and are considered nonelectrolytes.

In the other reaction, the compound develops a tiny electrical charge when dissolved in water. The compound breaks up into separate particles known as ions; this process is referred to as ionization, and the compounds are known as electrolytes. Some electrolytes develop a positive charge (cations) when placed in water; others develop a negative charge (anions).

The chemical composition of seawater and human body fluid is very similar. The principal cations of seawater are sodium, potassium, magnesium, and calcium, and so it is with the body fluid. The seawater contains as principal anions chloride, phosphate, and sulfate, the same as body fluid.

In this chapter six electrolytes [potassium, sodium, calcium, magnesium, phosphorus (phosphate), and chloride] are discussed in relation to human body needs (functions), pathophysiology, etiology, clinical manifestations, and clinical management. Normal serum and urine levels, drug-laboratory test interactions, and foods rich in these electrolytes are presented. Clinical applications and case studies are discussed using the nursing process (nursing assessment, nursing diagnoses, and interventions).

An asterisk (*) on an answer line indicates a multiple-word answer.

The meanings for the following symbols are: ↑ increased, ↓ decreased, > greater than, < less than.

ELECTROLYTES: CATION AND ANION

1   *Electrolytes* are compounds that, when placed in solution, conduct an electric current.

   Pure water does not conduct electricity, but if a pinch of salt, which contains sodium and chloride, is dropped into it, what do you think happens to the water?   *_____

_____ .

   Salt would produce an electrical charge. The water would conduct electricity.

   ■   ■   ■

2   *Ions* are dissociated particles of electrolytes that carry either a positive charge called a *cation* or a negative charge called an *anion*.

   Dissociated particles of electrolytes are called _____ .

   The particles which carry a positive charge are called _____ and those which carry a negative charge are called _____ .

   ions; cations; anions

      ■   ■   ■

3   What is the difference between a cation and an anion?   *_____

_____ .

   a cation carries a positive charge and an anion a negative charge

   ■   ■   ■

   Table 3-1 gives the principal cations and anions in human body fluid. Since we will be referring to these elements and their symbols throughout the program, take a few minutes now to memorize them. Be sure to note the + and − symbols. There will not be a separate section on bicarbonate

Table 3-1. CATIONS AND ANIONS			
Cations		**Anions**	
Na^+	(Sodium)	Cl^-	(Chloride)
K^+	(Potassium)	HCO_3^-	(Bicarbonate)
Ca^{++}	(Calcium)	HPO_4^{--}	(Phosphate)
Mg^{++}	(Magnesium)		

and phosphate in this chapter; however, they will be covered in the chapter on acid-base, so be sure to remember them. When you think you are ready, go ahead to the frames that follow. Refer back to the table as necessary.

4   Place a C in front of the cations and an A in front of anions.

     ___ a. K   ___ e. Na

     ___ b. Mg   ___ f. Ca

     ___ c. Cl   ___ g. HPO_4

     ___ d. HCO_3

a. C; b. C; c. A; d. A; e. C; f. C; g. A

          ■   ■   ■

5   If you have had chemistry, these ions and their symbols should be familiar to you. Complete the following chart using proper names and/or symbols.

Names of Ions	Symbols
Sodium	___
___	K
Calcium	___
___	Cl
Bicarbonate	___
___	HPO_4
___	Mg

Names	Symbols
Potassium	Na
Chloride	Ca
Phosphate	HCO_3
Magnesium	

          ■   ■   ■

6   For electrical balance, the quantities of cations and anions in a solution, expressed in milliequivalents (mEq) always equal each other.

     Electrolytes differ in their chemical activity, for sodium has one positive charge and calcium has *_____ .

two positive charges

          ■   ■   ■

7   The term *milliequivalents* is used to express the number of ionic charges of each electrolyte on an equal basis. It measures the _____ activity of ions or elements. Refer to Chapter 1 if needed to explain milliequivalents.

  The total cations in milliequivalents must equal the total _____ in milliequivalents.

chemical; anions

    ■   ■   ■

8   Milliequivalents consider electrolytes in terms of their *_____ rather than their weight.

chemical activity

    ■   ■   ■

9   Electrolytes have different weights but are considered during therapy in terms of their chemical activity, which is expressed as (milliequivalents/milligrams) _____ .

milliequivalents

    ■   ■   ■

Table 3-2 gives the weights and equivalences of five ions. Note how the weights of the named ions differ, but the equivalences remain the same according to their ionic charge. You are not expected to memorize the weights of these ions.

Table 3-2. ELECTROLYTE EQUIVALENTS		
Kind of Ion	**Weight (mg)**	**Equivalence (mEq)**
Sodium$^+$	23	1
Potassium$^+$	39	1
Chloride$^-$	35	1
Calcium^{++}	40	2
Magnesium^{++}	24	2

10   An ion with two charges has the same equivalence as *_____ .

another ion with two charges

    ■   ■   ■

11 Name a cation and an anion with the same equivalence but different weights.   *_____

_____ .

Sodium and chloride or potassium and chloride

        ■   ■   ■

12 The electrolyte composition of fluid differs within the two main classes of body fluid.

The two main classes of body water are _____ and

_____ fluid. Describe the extracellular fluid. *_____

_____ .

intracellular and extracellular. The extracellular fluid consists of intravascular and interstitial fluid.

        ■   ■   ■

Table 3-3 gives the ion concentrations of the intravascular fluid (which is frequently referred to as plasma), interstitial fluid, and intracellular fluid. Take a few minutes to memorize the fluids and their greatest concentration of ions. Memorizing the numbers is not necessary. Refer back to the table when necessary.

Table 3-3. ELECTROLYTE COMPOSITION OF BODY FLUID (mEq/L)		
	Extracellular	
Ions	**Intravascular or Plasma**	**Interstitial**	**Intracellular**
---	---	---	---
Na^+	142	145	10
K^+	5	4	141–150
Ca^{++}	5	3	2
Mg^{++}	2	1	27
Cl^-	104	116	1
HCO_3^-	27	30	10
HPO_4^{--}	2	2	100

13   What are the three principal ions in intravascular fluid? _____ ,
_____ , and _____ .

What are the three principal ions in interstitial fluid? _____ ,
_____ , and _____ .

What are the three principal ions in intracellular fluid? _____ ,
_____ , and _____ .

sodium or Na, chloride or Cl, and bicarbonate or HCO₃
same as in intravascular fluid
potassium or K, phosphate or HPO₄, and magnesium or Mg

■   ■   ■

Figure 3-1 shows the various cations and anions in extracellular and intracellular fluids. Pay special attention to the principal cations and anions in these fluids. Refer to the figure when necessary.

14   The principal cation in extracellular fluid is _____ .

The principal cation in intracellular fluid is _____ .

sodium or Na; potassium or K

■   ■   ■

Figure 3-1.   Anions and cations in body fluid.

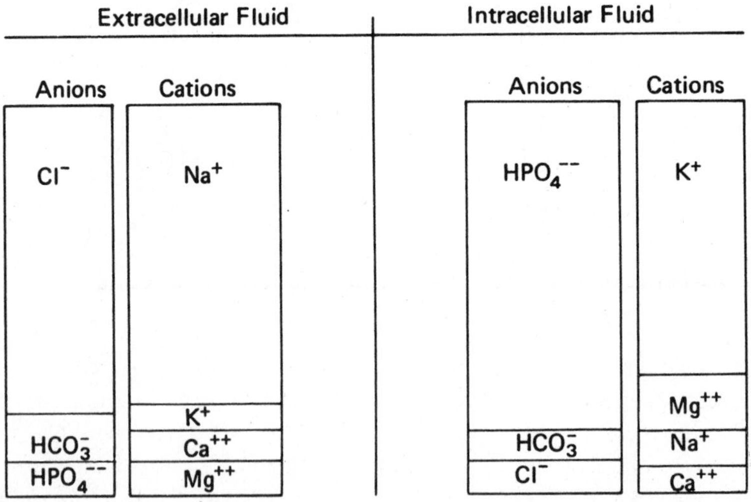

15 The principal anion in extracellular fluid is _____ .

The principal anion in intracellular fluid is _____ .

chloride or Cl; phosphate or HPO$_4$

■   ■   ■

16 a. Choose the three electrolytes having the greatest concentration in extracellular fluid.

___	Na	___	Cl
___	K	___	HCO$_3$
___	Ca	___	HPO$_4$
___	Mg		

b. Choose the three electrolytes having the greatest concentration in intracellular fluid.

___	Na	___	Cl
___	K	___	HCO$_3$
___	Ca	___	HPO$_4$
___	Mg		

a. Na, Cl, HCO$_3$; b. K, Mg, HPO$_4$

■   ■   ■

POTASSIUM

INTRODUCTION

Potassium is the most abundant cation in the body cells. Ninety-seven percent of the body's potassium is found in the intracellular fluid, and 2–3% is found in the extracellular fluid (intravascular and interstitial fluids).

17 Although potassium is present in all body fluids, it is found predominantly in _____ fluid.

What kind of ion is potassium? _____ .

intracellular; cation

■   ■   ■

Figure 3-2 tells the effect of too much potassium or not enough in our body cells. Memorize the normal range of serum potassium. You may wonder why the range of serum potassium and not cell potassium is used to measure the potassium level, since the cells have the highest concentration of potassium. It is easier to aspirate serum from the intravascular fluid than to aspirate potassium from body cells. When you are ready, go ahead to the frames following the figure and refer to the figure when necessary.

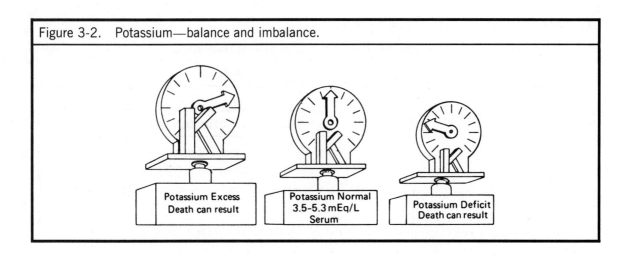

Figure 3-2.   Potassium—balance and imbalance.

18   The normal serum potassium range is _____ mEq/L. The intracellular potassium level is 150 mEq/L, but the concentration is not easily determined.

The kidneys excrete 80–90% of the potassium lost from the body. If the kidneys fail to function, what might result?   *_____ .

3.5–5.3
Excess potassium build up, leading to death.
■   ■   ■

19   Either too much or too little potassium can cause a cardiac arrest. The heart needs potassium for conducting nerve impulses and contracting the heart muscle.

Why do you think too much potassium can cause a cardiac arrest?   *_____

_____ .

Why do you think too little potassium can cause a cardiac arrest?   *_____

_____ .

Too much potassium causes irritability of the heart muscle, increasing and then decreasing the rate.
Too little potassium changes the conduction rate of nerve impulses and weakens the heart muscle, causing the heart to beat irregularly.
■   ■   ■

FUNCTIONS

Table 3-4 gives the various functions of potassium according to body systems. Study the table and refer to it as needed.

Table 3-4. POTASSIUM AND ITS FUNCTIONS	
Body System	**Function**
Neuromuscular	Transmission and conduction of nerve impulses
	Contraction of skeletal and smooth muscles
Cardiac	Nerve conduction and contraction of the myocardium
Cellular	Enzyme action for cellular energy production
	Deposits glycogen in liver cells
	Regulates osmolality of intracellular (cellular) fluids

20 Potassium is needed for transmission and conduction of *_____ . Also potassium is needed for the contraction of *_____ muscles.

nerve impulses; skeletal, smooth, and also the myocardium
■   ■   ■

21 Name two cellular activities of potassium. *_____ , and *_____ .

enzyme action and deposits glycogen in liver, also regulates intracellular osmolality
■   ■   ■

22 The average daily oral intake of potassium is 50–100 mEq per day. Within the first hour, potassium from oral absorption shifts into the cells. Renal excretion is slower in response to increased potassium level. It takes 4–6 hours for the kidneys to excrete potassium.

Identify two ways the body avoids excessive serum potassium levels after large oral potassium consumptions. *_____

_____ and *_____

_____ .

Within an hour of oral potassium intake, potassium shifts into the cells. Also renal excretion of potassium decreases the serum potassium level; however, renal excretion is a slower process.
■   ■   ■

23 Because potassium is not well stored in body cells, a daily potassium intake of 40–60 mEq is needed. Dietary potassium restriction does not necessarily cause a low serum potassium level unless the decreased potassium intake is prolonged or severely deficient.

The average daily oral potassium intake is _____ mEq. The daily potassium intake needed for body function is _____ mEq.

50–100; 40–60

      ■   ■   ■

24 Foods rich in potassium include fruits (fresh, dry, and juices), vegetables, meats, and nuts. Particularly rich sources include bananas, dry fruits, and orange juice. If a person's serum potassium level is slightly decreased (3.4 mEq/L), what would you suggest? *_____

_____.

Consume bananas and other fruits as well as vegetables.

      ■   ■   ■

25 Potassium is continually moving between the intracellular fluid and the extracellular fluid which is controlled by the sodium-potassium pump. Hormones increase the sodium-potassium pump activity. Insulin promotes cellular potassium uptake by shifting glucose and potassium into the cells. Aldosterone promotes potassium excretion and cellular potassium uptake.

The two hormones that can decrease the serum potassium level and increase the cellular potassium level are _____ and _____ .

insulin and aldosterone

      ■   ■   ■

26 Insulin (increases/decreases) _____ the sodium-potassium pump activity.

increases

      ■   ■   ■

PATHOPHYSIOLOGY

27 A serum potassium level below 3.5 mEq/L is known as (hypokalemia/hyperkalemia)
_____ , and a serum potassium level above 5.3 mEq/L is called

_____ .

   Cardiac arrest may occur if the serum potassium level is less than 2.5 mEq/L or greater than 7.0 mEq/L.

   Match the serum potassium levels on the left with the type of potassium imbalance or balance.

   ___ 1. 3.7 mEq/L   a. Hypokalemia
   ___ 2. 4.8 mEq/L   b. Hyperkalemia
   ___ 3. 5.9 mEq/L   c. Normal
   ___ 4. 2.7 mEq/L
   ___ 5. 3.1 mEq/L
   ___ 6. 6.8 mEq/L

   hypokalemia; hyperkalemia
   1. c; 2. c; 3. b; 4. a; 5. a; 6. b
   ▪   ▪   ▪

28 If the client's serum potassium level is less than 2.5 mEq/L, what might occur?
   * _____ .

   cardiac arrest
   ▪   ▪   ▪

29 The assimilative processes involved in the formation of new tissue (the synthesis of complex molecules from simple molecules) are referred to as *anabolism*, and the reactions concerned with tissue breakdown (the breakdown of complex molecules to simple molecules with a release of chemical energy) are referred to as *catabolism*.

   When cellular activity is *anabolic* (state of building up), potassium enters the cells. When cellular activity is *catabolic* (state of breaking down), potassium leaves the cells.

   Potassium enters the cells in _____ states and leaves the cells in
   _____ states.

   anabolic; catabolic
   ▪   ▪   ▪

30   Potassium may leave the cells under various conditions. When tissues are destroyed as a result of trauma, starvation, or wasting diseases, large amounts of potassium
*_____ .

Potassium leaves the cells in _____ states.

leave the cells; catabolic

■   ■   ■

31   During exercise, when muscles contract, the cells lose potassium and absorb a nearly equal quantity of sodium from the extracellular fluid. After exercise, when the muscles are recovering from fatigue, potassium reenters the cells and most of the sodium goes back into the extracellular fluid.

During exercise which ion may be more plentiful in the extracellular fluid—the potassium ion or the sodium ion?   *_____

_____ .

The potassium ion. Of course it depends on how much exercise. The K ion has to go somewhere, so it goes into the extracellular fluid.

■   ■   ■

32   During exercise, potassium leaves the cells, causing muscular fatigue.

After exercise, potassium   *_____ .

Potassium enters the cells in _____ states.

reenters the cells; anabolic

■   ■   ■

33   The muscles, after releasing potassium from the cells, are like "half-filled water bottles" and are soft.

The soft muscles are a result of (hyperkalemia/hypokalemia) _____ .

hypokalemia

■   ■   ■

34   Name as many conditions as you can in which potassium might leave the cells.
_____ ,   _____ ,   _____ , and
*_____ .

trauma, exercise, starvation, wasting disease

■   ■   ■

35 In stress which can be caused by a harmful condition or severe emotional strain, an excessive amount of potassium is lost through the kidneys. The potassium leaves the cells, depleting the cells' supply. From the adrenal gland one of the adrenal cortical hormones, aldosterone, is produced in abundance during stress. This hormone influences the kidneys to excrete potassium and to retain sodium.

Frequently the cations K and Na have an opposing effect on each other in the extracellular fluid. When one is retained, the other is excreted.

Therefore, with an excessive production of aldosterone, what happens to the cations K and Na in the extracellular fluid?   *_____ .

K will be excreted and Na will be retained.

■   ■   ■

36 When kidney function is normal, the excess potassium will be slowly excreted by the kidneys. The range of potassium excreted daily by the kidneys is 20–120 mEq/L.

If potassium intake is decreased or if no potassium is taken orally or given intravenously, potassium is still excreted by the kidneys. More potassium is lost from the cells and the extracellular fluid (ECF) when potassium intake is diminished or absent. What type of potassium imbalance will occur? _____ .

hypokalemia

■   ■   ■

37 With diminished or no potassium intake, the kidneys do which of the following:

( ) a. Continue to excrete potassium
( ) b. Inhibit potassium excretion

Why *_____

_____ .

If the kidneys are injured or diseased and the urine output is markedly decreased, which of the following happen?

( ) a. The potassium piles up in the extracellular fluid
( ) b. The potassium piles up in the intracellular fluid
( ) c. The potassium is excreted through the skin

a. X; b. —. Potassium excretion comes from the cells and ECF even when potassium intake is zero.
a. X; b. —; c. —

■   ■   ■

ETIOLOGY

The causes of hypokalemia and hyperkalemia are divided into two separate tables. Table 3-5 lists the etiology and rationale for hypokalemia and Table 3-6 gives the etiology and rationale for hyperkalemia. Study both tables carefully, noting the causes and reasons for these changes. Then proceed to the frames which follow. Refer to the tables as needed.

Table 3-5. CAUSES OF HYPOKALEMIA (SERUM POTASSIUM DEFICIT)	
Etiology	**Rationale**
Dietary Changes Malnutrition, starvation, alcoholism, unbalanced reducing diets, anorexia nervosa, crash diets	Potassium is poorly conserved in the body. For a potassium deficit to occur, a prolonged, inadequate potassium intake must occur. The body uses all available potassium in the cells and tissues.
Gastrointestinal Losses Vomiting, diarrhea, gastric/intestinal suctioning, intestinal fistula, laxative abuse, bulemia, enemas	Potassium is plentiful in the GI tract. With the loss of GI secretions, large amounts of potassium ions are lost. Diarrhea causes a greater potassium loss than vomiting.
Renal Losses Diuretics, diuretic phase of acute renal failure, hemodialysis and peritoneal dialysis	The kidneys excrete 80–90% of the potassium lost. Diuretics are the major cause of hypokalemia, especially potassium-wasting diuretics (thiazides).
Hormonal Influence Steroids, Cushing's syndrome, licorice abuse, stress	Steroids, especially cortisone and aldosterone, promote potassium excretion and sodium retention. Stress increases the production of steroids in the body. In Cushing's syndrome, there is an excess production of adrenocortical hormones (cortiol and aldosterone). Licorice contains glyceric acid, which has an aldosteronelike effect.
Cellular Damage Trauma, tissue injury, surgery, burns	Cellular and tissue damage cause potassium to be lost. As a result, extra potassium is needed to repair injured tissue.
Redistribution of Potassium Insulin, alkalotic state	Insulin moves glucose and potassium into cells. Metabolic alkalosis promotes the movement of potassium into cells.

38 Name two causes of hypokalemia related to dietary changes. _____ and
_____ .

malnutrition and alcoholism (also reducing diets, anorexia nervosa)
■   ■   ■

39 Why is daily potassium intake necessary? *_____
_____ .

Potassium is poorly conserved in the body. The recommended daily potassium intake is 40–60 mEq.
■   ■   ■

40 The major cause of a potassium deficit is *_____ . Why? *_____
_____ .

potassium-wasting diuretics (especially thiazides)
These diuretics promote loss of water, sodium, and potassium.
■   ■   ■

41 Gastrointestinal (GI) losses account for the second major cause of a potassium deficit. List three GI causes of hypokalemia. _____ , _____ , and
*_____ .

vomiting, diarrhea, and GI suctioning (also laxative abuse, bulemia)
■   ■   ■

42 Trauma and injury to tissues as a result of burns and surgery can cause a potassium
(deficit/excess) _____ . Why? *_____
_____ .

deficit
Potassium is lost from the cells due to tissue injury. Also, great quantities of potassium are needed to repair damaged tissues.
■   ■   ■

43 Excessive ingestion of licorice can cause (hypokalemia/hyperkalemia) _____ .
Why? *_____
_____ .

hypokalemia
Licorice has an aldosteronelike effect, thus promoting potassium excretion and sodium retention.
■   ■   ■

44 How do insulin and alkalotic states affect potassium balance?

*_____

_____ .

Insulin moves potassium into the cells along with glucose, and alkalosis promotes the exchange of potassium ions for hydrogen ions in the cells. Either can cause a low serum potassium level (hypokalemia).

■   ■   ■

45 List six clinical conditions causing a potassium deficit:

a. _____

b. _____

c. _____

d. _____

e. _____

f. _____

a. diarrhea, vomiting, gastric suction

b. starvation, anorexia nervosa, bulemia

c. diuretics—potassium wasting

d. burns

e. trauma or injury

f. surgery

Also: stress; increase of adrenal cortical hormones (steroids); metabolic alkalosis

■   ■   ■

46 The serum potassium level should be monitored for clients taking large doses of a potassium supplement. This is especially true when the daily urine output is diminished.

Why? *_____

_____ .

The kidneys excrete 80–90% of excess potassium. With increased potassium ingestion and poor urine output, hyperkalemia can result.

■   ■   ■

47 Potassium in intravenous (IV) fluids administered at a rate faster than 20 mEq/L per hour for 24–72 hours can result in (hypokalemia/hyperkalemia) _____ .

hyperkalemia

■   ■   ■

Table 3-6.   CAUSES OF HYPERKALEMIA (SERUM POTASSIUM EXCESS)

Etiology	Rationale
Excessive Potassium Intake Oral potassium supplements IV potassium infusions	A potassium consumption rate greater than the potassium excretion rate increases the serum potassium level. Adequate urinary output must be determined when giving a potassium supplement.
Decreased Renal Function Acute renal failure Chronic renal failure Potassium-sparing diuretics	Because potassium is generally excreted in the urine, anuria and oliguria cause a potassium buildup in the plasma. Potassium-sparing diuretics cause an aldosterone deficiency, promoting potassium retention.
Altered Cellular Function Severe traumatic injury Metabolic acidosis	Cellular injury increases potassium loss due to cell breakdown. Potassium excretion may be greater than cellular reabsorption. Potassium can accumulate in the plasma. In acidosis, the hydrogen ion moves into the cells and potassium moves out of the cells, increasing the serum potassium level.
Hormonal Deficiency Addison's disease	Reduced secretion of the adrenocortical hormones causes a retention of potassium and a loss of sodium.
Pseudohyperkalemia Hemolysis Tourniquet application Phlebotomy	With hemolysis, ruptured red blood cells release potassium into the ECF. A tourniquet that has been applied too tightly or rapidly drawing blood with a small needle lumen (<18 gauge) can cause a temporary increase in the serum potassium level.

48 Pseudohyperkalemia may occur due to _____ or *_____

_____ .

hemolysis or a tightly applied tourniquet to obtain blood sample; also, rapidly drawing blood through a small needle lumen

■   ■   ■

49 Which of the following are causes of potassium excess (hyperkalemia)?

( ) a. Potassium-wasting diuretics
( ) b. Potassium-sparing diuretics
( ) c. Adrenal gland insufficiency
( ) d. Vomiting, diarrhea
( ) e. Multiple transfusions of old blood
( ) f. Metabolic acidosis with poor kidney function
( ) g. Renal shutdown

a. —; b. X; c. X; d. —; e. X; f. X; g. X

■   ■   ■

CLINICAL MANIFESTATIONS

50 Although 98% of potassium is found in cells, focus is placed on the extracellular fluid, for it is more readily available for study.

The normal serum potassium level (in extracellular fluid) is _____ mEq/L.

3.5–5.3

■   ■   ■

Table 3-7 lists the signs and symptoms associated with hypokalemia and hyperkalemia. Clinical manifestations can be determined by the serum potassium level, electrocardiography (ECG/EKG) and signs and symptoms related to gastrointestinal, cardiac, renal, and neurological abnormalities. The serum potassium level and the ECG play the most important role in determining the severity of the potassium imbalance.

In Table 3-7, you should become familiar with the signs and symptoms marked with a dagger and those listed with and without an asterisk. Your keen observation and assessment will aid the physician in making a more positive diagnosis. Study the table and refer to it as needed. Clients with hypokalemia and hyperkalemia can be found in many clinical settings. You may save a client's life by recognizing and reporting symptoms of potassium imbalance. If you are not familiar with these words, refer to the glossary.

Table 3-7.   CLINICAL MANIFESTATIONS OF POTASSIUM IMBALANCES

Body Areas	Hypokalemia	Hyperkalemia
Gastrointestinal abnormalities	*Anorexia Nausea *Vomiting Diarrhea †Abdominal distention †Decreased peristalsis or silent ileus	*Nausea *Diarrhea †Abdominal cramps
Cardiac abnormalities	†Dysrhythmias †Vertigo Cardiac arrest when severe	Tachycardia, later †bradycardia, and finally cardiac arrest (severe)
ECG/EKG	†Flat or inverted T wave Depressed ST segment	†Peaked, narrow T wave Shortened QT interval Prolonged PR interval followed by disappearance of P wave Prolonged QRS interval if level continues to rise
Renal abnormalities	Polyuria	†Oliguria or anuria
Neuromuscular abnormalities	†Malaise Drowsiness †Muscular weakness Confusion Mental depression Diminished deep tendon reflexes Respiratory paralysis	Weakness, numbness, or tingling sensation Muscle cramps
Laboratory findings Serum potassium Serum osmolality	<3.5 mEq/L <280 mOsm/L	>5.3 mEq/L >295 mOsm/L

Daggers refer to most commonly seen symptoms of hypo-hyperkalemia. Asterisks refer to commonly seen symptoms of hypo-hyperkalemia.

51   Hypokalemia causes the muscle to become soft, like "half-filled water bottles," and weak. The abdomen becomes bloated due to smooth-muscle weakness and not due to flatus. The blood pressure goes down (hypotension) and dizziness occurs. Malaise or uneasiness occurs.

The heart beat is irregular, known as _____ . Eventually, if the irregularity of the heart beat is not corrected, bradycardia occurs and finally cardiac arrest.

dysrhythmia (arrhythmia)

∎   ∎   ∎

52 A weak grip, an irregular pulse, and dizziness upon standing may be signs of
_____ .

hypokalemia

    ■   ■   ■

53 T wave changes on the ECG/EKG can indicate a potassium imbalance. Match the T wave changes on the left with the type of potassium imbalance.

    ____ 1. Peaked T wave   a. Hypokalemia

    ____ 2. Flat T wave   b. Hyperkalemia

    ____ 3. Inverted T wave

1. b; 2. a; 3. a

    ■   ■   ■

54 Polyuria or excess urine output can be a symptom of hypokalemia. State two *causes* of hypokalemia in which polyuria is involved. (Refer to Table 3-5 if needed.)
*_____ and _____ .

excess aldosterone and diuretics

    ■   ■   ■

55 Name the six most commonly seen symptoms of hypokalemia. *_____ ,
*_____ , _____ , _____ ,
_____ , and *_____ .

abdominal distention, decreased peristalsis or silent ileus, dizziness, dysrhythmia/arrhythmia, malaise, and muscular weakness

    ■   ■   ■

56 With hyperkalemia, the heart beats very fast, which is known as *tachycardia*, and then it slows down (*bradycardia*). The heart goes into a block, with few or no impulses being transmitted, and finally cardiac arrest occurs.

    You recall that the kidneys are responsible for excreting excessive amounts of potassium not needed by the body. If the kidneys excrete a small amount of urine, known as *oliguria*, or no urine, known as *anuria*, what can occur to the potassium level? *_____ .

    What would you think happens to the heart rate? *_____

_____ .

increase or rise in potassium (hyperkalemia); increase (tachycardia) and later decrease (bradycardia)

    ■   ■   ■

57 Name the three most commonly seen symptoms of hyperkalemia. *_____ ,
*_____ , and *_____ .

abdominal cramps, tachycardia and later bradycardia, and oliguria or anuria
        ■   ■   ■

58 Name some other symptoms related to hyperkalemia.

    a. _____
    b. _____
    c. _____
    d. *_____

a. nausea; b. diarrhea; c. weakness; d. numbness or tingling
            ■   ■   ■

59 With prolonged hypokalemia, circulatory failure and eventual heart failure can result. The electrocardiogram frequently shows a flat or inverted T wave. With potassium excess, the electrocardiogram shows a peaked T wave.

    Serum potassium levels below 2.5 mEq/L and above 7.0 mEq/L are extremely dangerous and need immediate attention. Without correction, what type of heart condition can occur?
*_____ .

cardiac arrest
            ■   ■   ■

Figures 3-3 and 3-4 note electrocardiographic changes found with hypo-hyperkalemia. Students who have had a physiology course and/or have a basic knowledge of electrocardiography, also known as ECG or EKG, will find these diagrams most useful when monitoring patients. Students who do not have this basic knowledge should refer to a physiology text and/or a text on electrocardiography. Students who do not need this information to practice nursing may move to Frame 67.

    A brief review of the electrocardiogram. The ECG measures the electrical activity from various areas of the heart and records this as P, QRS, and T waves.

    P wave measures the electrical activity initiating contraction of the atrium or the atrial muscle.

    QRS wave complex measures the electrical activity initiating contraction of the ventricle, which is the thickest part of the heart muscle responsible for forcing blood from the heart into the circulation. A "heart attack," also known as myocardial infarction, frequently affects this part of the heart muscle.

    T wave is the electrical recovery of the ventricles.

    Abnormal potassium levels affect the T wave of the electrocardiogram. Note the normal T wave structure in Figure 3-3 and compare the normal with the abnormal, with patterns 1 and 2. Study this figure and then proceed to the frames.

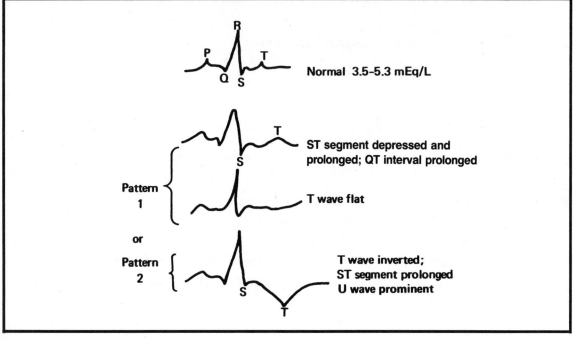

Figure 3-3.   Electrocardiographic changes in serum potassium deficit. (Adapted from H. Statland. (1963). *Fluid and electrolytes in practice,* 3rd ed. Philadelphia, Pa: J. B. Lippincott Co., p. 120.)

60 The two abnormal changes in the T wave that occur with hypokalemia are
*_____ and *_____ .

Abnormal T waves often indicate a potassium (excess/deficit) _____ .

flat T wave and inverted T wave; deficit

■   ■   ■

61 The ST segment is prolonged in both the patterns in Figure 3-3. This change relates to a
*_____ .

potassium deficit

■   ■   ■

62 With a serum potassium *deficit* which of the following electrocardiographic changes may occur?

( ) a. Flat T wave
( ) b. Inverted T wave
( ) c. High-peaked T wave
( ) d. Depressed and prolonged ST segment
( ) e. Absence of the P wave

a. X; b. X; c. —; d. X; e. —

High-peaked T waves are an early electrocardiographic sign of hyperkalemia. Heart block can result from severe hyperkalemia, e.g., 8–10 mEq/L of serum potassium. Study Figure 3-4 carefully, noting especially the T waves, QRS complex, and P wave. If any of the words are unfamiliar, please refer to a physiology text and/or a text on electrocardiography.

Figure 3-4. Electrocardiographic changes in serum potassium concentration. Changes that do occur are most marked in the precordial leads over the right side (V_1–V_4 position) of the heart. (Adapted from H. Statland. (1963). *Fluid and electrolytes in practice.* Philadelphia, Pa: J. B. Lippincott Co., p. 116.)

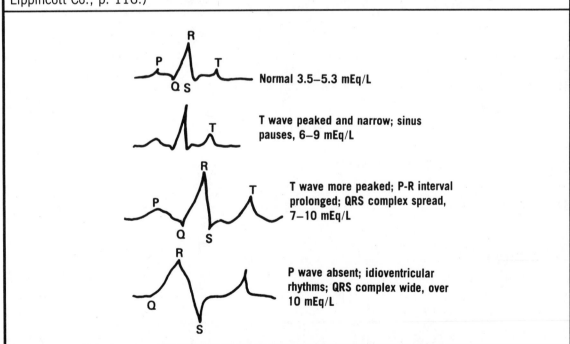

63 Name the abnormal change in the T wave occurring with hyperkalemia. *_____ .

high-peaked T wave

■   ■   ■

64 A flat or inverted T wave on an electrocardiogram frequently indicates a _____ state, whereas a high-peaked T wave can indicate a _____ state.

hypokalemic; hyperkalemia

■   ■   ■

65 Which of the following electrocardiographic changes can occur with a high serum potassium?

( ) a. Flat T wave
( ) b. Inverted T wave
( ) c. High-peaked T wave
( ) d. Depressed and prolonged ST segment
( ) e. QRS complex spread
( ) f. Prolonged P-R interval

a. —; b. —; c. X; d. —; e. X; f. X

■   ■   ■

66. Match the following ECG changes on the left with the electrolyte abnormalities on the right. Refer to Figures 3-3 and 3-4 as needed.

___ 1.

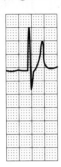

a. Hypokalemia
b. Hyperkalemia

___ 2.

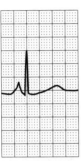

___ 3.

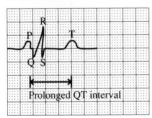

___ 4.

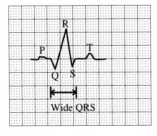

1. b; 2. a; 3. a; 4. b

DRUGS AND THEIR EFFECT ON POTASSIUM BALANCE

67 Diuretics are divided into two categories: potassium wasting and potassium sparing. Potassium-wasting diuretics excrete potassium and other electrolytes such as sodium and chloride in the urine. Potassium-sparing diuretics retain potassium but excrete sodium and chloride in the urine.

Indicate the electrolytes that are lost when potassium-sparing diuretics are taken:

( ) a. Potassium
( ) b. Sodium
( ) c. Chloride

a. —; b. X; c. X

■   ■   ■

Table 3-8 lists the trade and generic names of potassium-wasting and potassium-sparing diuretics and a combination of potassium-wasting and potassium-sparing diuretics. Study the types of diuretic in each category and refer to the table as needed.

Table 3-8. POTASSIUM-WASTING AND POTASSIUM-SPARING DIURETICS	

Potassium-Wasting Diuretics
Thiazides
    Chlorothiazide/Diuril
    Hydrochlorothiazide/Hydrodiuril
 	
Loop diuretics
    Furosemide/Lasix
    Ethacrynic acid/Edecrin
 	
Mercurials
    Mercaptomerin sodium/Thiomerin
 	
Carbonic anhydrase inhibitors
    Acetazolamide/Diamox
 	
Osmotic diuretic
    Mannitol
	Potassium-Sparing Diuretics
	Aldosterone antagonist
	    Spironolactone/Aldactone
	    Triamterene/Dyrenium
	    Amiloride/Midamor
	
	Combination: K-Wasting and K-Sparing Diuretics
	Aldactazide
	Spironazide
	Dyazide
	Moduretic

68 Name the potassium imbalance that is most likely to occur in people taking a potassium-sparing diuretic, who have poor kidney function. *_____ .

potassium excess or hyperkalemia

■   ■   ■

69 Potassium-wasting diuretics can cause (hypokalemia/hyperkalemia) _____ .

hypokalemia

■   ■   ■

70 Enter W for potassium-wasting, S for potassium-sparing, and C for a combination of potassium-wasting and -sparing diuretics for the following drugs. Refer to the table as needed:

( ) a. Chlorothiazide/Diuril
( ) b. Aldactazide
( ) c. Triamterene/Dyrenium
( ) d. Acetazolamide/Diamox
( ) e. Merceptomerin sodium/Thiomerin
( ) f. Mannitol
( ) g. Dyazide
( ) h. Spironolactone/Aldactone
( ) i. Hydrochlorothiazide/Hydrodiuril
( ) j. Furosemide/Lasix
( ) k. Ethacrynic acid/Edecrin
( ) l. Amiloride/Midamor

a. W; b. C; c. S; d. W; e. W; f. W; g. C; h. S; i. W; j. W; k. W; l. S

■   ■   ■

Laxatives, corticosteroids, antibiotics, and potassium-wasting diuretics are the major drug groups that can cause a potassium deficit or hypokalemia. The drug groups attributed to potassium excess or hyperkalemia are oral and intravenous potassium salts, CNS agents, and potassium-sparing diuretics. Table 3-9 lists the drugs that affect potassium balance.

Table 3-9. DRUGS AFFECTING POTASSIUM BALANCE

Potassium Imbalance	Drugs	Rationale
Hypokalemia (serum potassium deficit)	Laxatives Enemas (hyperosmolar)	Laxative abuse can cause potassium depletion.
	Corticosteroids	
	Cortisone	Ion exchange agent.
	Prednisone	Steroids promote potassium loss and sodium retention.
	Kayexalate	Exchange potassium ion for a sodium ion.
	Licorice	Licorice action is similar to aldosterone, promoting K loss and Na retention.
	Levodopa/L-Dopa Lithium	Increases potassium loss via urine.
	Antibiotic I	

	Amphotericin B
	  Polymyxin B
	  Tetracycline (outdated)
	  Gentamicin
	  Neomycin
	  Amikacin
	  Tobramycin
	  Cisplatin
		Toxic effect on renal tubules, thus decreasing potassium reabsorption.

	Antibiotic II	

	Penicillin
	  Ampicillin
	  Carbenicillin
	  Ticarcillin
	  Nafcillin
	  Piperacillin
	  Azlocillin
		Potassium excretion is enhanced by the presence of nonreabsorbable anions.

	Alpha-adrenergic blockers Insulin and glucose	These agents promote movement of potassium into cells, thus lowering the serum potassium level.
	Beta$_2$ Agonists	

	Terbutaline
	  Albuterol
	  Estrogen	

	Potassium-wasting diuretics	See Table 3-8

Table 3-9. (Continued)		
Potassium Imbalance	**Drugs**	**Rationale**
Hyperkalemia (serum potassium excess)	Potassium chloride (oral or IV) Potassium salt (no salt) K penicillin KPO_4 enema	Excess ingestion or infusion of these agents can cause a potassium excess.
	Indomethacin Captopril (Capoten) Heparin	These decrease renal excretion of potassium.

	CNS agents
	  Barbiturates
	  Sedatives
	  Narcotics
	  Heroin
	  Amphetamines
		These CNS agents are usually characterized by muscle necrosis and cellular shift of potassium from cells to serum.

	Nonsteroidal anti-inflammatory drugs (NSAIDS): ibuprofens Alpha agonists Beta blockers	Blocks cellular potassium uptake.
	Succinylcholine Cyclophosphamide	Loss of potassium from cells.
	Potassium-sparing diuretics	See Table 3-8.

71 Enter KD for potassium deficit/hypokalemia and KE for potassium excess/hyperkalemia beside the drugs that can cause a potassium imbalance. Refer to Table 3-9 as needed:

_____ a. Laxatives

_____ b. Corticosteroids

_____ c. Barbiturates

_____ d. Narcotics

_____ e. Indomethacin/Indocin

_____ f. Licorice

_____ g. Antibiotics

_____ h. Levodopa

_____ i. Heparin

_____ j. Potassium chloride

_____ k. Succinylcholine/Anectine

_____ l. Terbutaline/Brethine

a. KD; b. KD; c. KE; d. KE; e. KE; f. KD; g. KD; h. KD; i. KE; j. KE; k. KE; l. KD

72 Digitalis is a drug that strengthens the heart muscle and slows down the heart beat. A serum potassium deficit or hypokalemia enhances the action of digitalis and causes the drug to become more potent. Digitalis toxicity or intoxication (slow and irregular pulse, nausea and vomiting, anorexia) can result from a low serum potassium level.

Thiazides and loop diuretics can cause (hypokalemia/hyperkalemia) _____ .

The nurse needs to be alert for what type of drug toxicity when a client is taking potassium-wasting diuretics and digitalis?   *_____ .

hypokalemia; digitalis toxicity

           ■   ■   ■

73 Common symptoms of digitalis toxicity are bradycardia (slow heart beat) and/or dysrhythmia (arrhythmia.)

Can you name two other symptoms of digitalis toxicity?

a.   *_____

b.   _____

a. nausea and vomiting; b. anorexia

           ■   ■   ■

74 A serum potassium excess (hyperkalemia) inhibits the action of digitalis. If a person has a serum potassium of 5.8 mEq/L, will (more/less) digitalis be needed to obtain the appropriate digitalis dosage?   _____ .

more

           ■   ■   ■

75 Quinidine is an antiarrhythmic drug used to correct irregular heart rates. Hypokalemia blocks the effects of quinidine; therefore more quinidine may be needed to produce therapeutic action. Hyperkalemia enhances the action of quinidine and can produce quinidine toxicity and myocardium depression.

Explain the effect of hypokalemia on digitalis.   *_____ ;
on quinidine   *_____ .

it enhances the action of digitalis; it decreases the action of quinidine

           ■   ■   ■

76 Cortisone causes excretion of potassium and retention of sodium. If a person takes digoxin (digitalis), hydrochlorothiazide/Hydrodiuril, and prednisone/cortisone daily, what type of severe electrolyte imbalance can result? *_____.

Explain the effect this imbalance has on digitalis. *_____

_____.

hypokalemia or potassium deficit
Hypokalemia precipitates digitalis toxicity by enhancing the action of digitalis.
■   ■   ■

77 Calcium gluconate accentuates the effect of a potassium excess on the heart muscle. The effect is transient. When the serum potassium level is high (hyperkalemia), calcium gluconate will decrease the effect on the heart. Calcium gluconate helps the heart rhythm that results from hyperkalemia but it will not correct the potassium level.

How do you think calcium gluconate affects the ECG? *_____

_____.

It improves the ECG and decreases the T wave.
■   ■   ■

CLINICAL MANAGEMENT

Clinical management of hypokalemia consists of oral supplements (tablets, capsules, liquid) and/or intravenous potassium diluted in an IV solution. To correct hyperkalemia, potassium intake is restricted and various drugs can be used to lower the serum potassium level. First, potassium replacement for hypokalemia is discussed and, then, drug modalities are presented for correcting hyperkalemia.

POTASSIUM REPLACEMENT

Oral potassium supplements help to replace potassium losses due to potassium-wasting diuretics, inadequate nutritional intake, and disease entities that increase potassium losses. Table 3-10 contains examples of frequently ordered oral potassium supplements.

78 Name a drug that corrects serum potassium and serum chloride deficits. *_____

_____.

potassium chloride (liquid or tablet)
■   ■   ■

Table 3-10. ORAL POTASSIUM SUPPLEMENTS	
Preparation	**Drug**
Liquid	Potassium chloride 10% = 20 mEq/15 mL; 20% = 40 mEq/15 mL Kay Ciel (potassium chloride) Kaochlor 10% (potassium chloride) Kaon Cl 20 (potassium chloride) Potassium Triplex (potassium acetate, bicarbonate, citrate)
Tablet/capsule	Potassium chloride (enteric-coated tablet) Kaon—plain (potassium gluconate) Kaon Cl (potassium chloride) Slow K (potassium chloride—8 mEq) Kaochlor (potassium chloride) K-Lyte—plain (potassium bicarbonate-effervescent tablet) K-Lyte/Cl (potassium chloride)

79 Oral potassium may be extremely irritating to the gastric mucosa and should be diluted in at least 4–8 ounces of water or juice.

Name two oral potassium supplements that contain bicarbonate. *_____
and *_____ .

potassium triplex and K-Lyte—plain (also Kaon—plain). The gluconate in Kaon is converted to bicarbonate. Kaon comes with or without Cl.
■   ■   ■

80 There have been reports of deaths related to hyperkalemia caused by oral potassium supplements.

Would oral potassium supplements be recommended for a person with poor kidney function?

_____ .

Why? *_____

_____ .

No
Because 80–90% of potassium is excreted from the body by the kidneys; hyperkalemia might result
■   ■   ■

81 Severe serum hyperkalemia may occur from administering an intravenous potassium solution too rapidly, thus not allowing enough time for the potassium to pass into the cells.

The normal dose of intravenous potassium is 20–40 mEq in a liter of solution to run over 8 hours or no more than 10 mEq of KCl per hour. What might result from administering 40 mEq of potassium per hour? _____ .

Why? *_____ .

hyperkalemia; potassium accumulation in the ECF; also ECG changes

■   ■   ■

82 Intravenous (IV) potassium is irritating to blood vessels (can cause phlebitis) and tissues (can cause sloughing and necrosis).

Potassium should NEVER be given as a bolus (injected directly into the vein).

What might happen if a bolus injection of potassium chloride (KCl) is given?

*_____ .

The nurse should assess the infusion site when the client is receiving intravenous KCl for _____ and _____ .

Cardiac arrest. Potassium concentration is extremely irritating to the myocardium (heart muscle).
phlebitis (inflammation of the vein) and infiltration (tissue sloughing or necrosis)

■   ■   ■

83 For severe hypokalemia, 40–60 mEq of KCl can be diluted in 1 liter of IV fluids, and no more than 20 mEq per hour should be given.

For a life-threatening hypokalemic situation, 30–40 mEq of KCl can be diluted in 100–150 mL of D_5W and administered through a central venous line in 1 hour.

What is the recommended KCl dosage to be diluted in 1 liter of IV fluids? *_____ .

20–40 mEq/L

■   ■   ■

84 In hypokalemia, if the serum potassium level is 3.0–3.5 mEq/L, 100–200 mEq of KCl is needed to raise serum level 1 mEq/L. Remember, don't administer the KCl all at once; a high concentration is toxic to the heart muscle and irritating to the blood vessels.

If the serum potassium level is below 3.0 mEq/L, 200–400 mEq of KCl is needed to raise serum level 1 mEq/L.

If an individual has a serum potassium level of 2.7 mEq/L. How much KCl, administered, is needed to raise the serum level to 3.7 mEq/L? *_____ .

200–400 mEq

■   ■   ■

85 The daily potassium requirement is 40–60 mEq. A client with a serum potassium of 3.3 mEq/L must (increase/decrease) _____ daily potassium intake.

increase

■   ■   ■

HYPERKALEMIA CORRECTION

In mild hyperkalemic conditions, correcting the cause of the potassium excess and restricting the potassium intake may correct the hyperkalemic state. Interventions to temporarily correct a moderate hyperkalemic state include: IV sodium bicarbonate infusion, insulin and glucose infusion, and intravenous calcium salt. Correcting the cause of the potassium excess is often successful in lowering the serum potassium level. In severe hyperkalemic conditions, kayexalate and sorbitol are usually prescribed.

Table 3-11 describes various methods used to correct a potassium excess (hyperkalemia). Study the table carefully and refer to it as needed.

86 To correct mild hyperkalemia, restriction of potassium intake is suggested.

Could you correct a hyperkalemia of 7.0 mEq/L by restricting potassium intake? _____ . Why? *_____ .

no
It is severe hyperkalemia, and this method is too slow.

■   ■   ■

Table 3-11. CORRECTION OF POTASSIUM EXCESS (HYPERKALEMIA)

Treatment Methods	Rationale
Potassium restriction	Restriction of potassium intake will slowly lower the serum level. For mild hyperkalemia (slightly elevated K levels), i.e., 5.4–5.6 mEq/L, potassium restriction is normally effective.
IV sodium bicarbonate ($NaHCO_3$)	By elevating the pH level potassium moves back into the cells, thus lowering the serum level. This is a temporary treatment.
10% Calcium gluconate	Calcium decreases the irritability of the myocardium resulting from hyperkalemia. It is a temporary treatment and does not promote K loss. *Caution:* Administering calcium to a patient on digitalis can cause digitalis toxicity.
Insulin and glucose (10–50%)	The combination of insulin and glucose moves potassium back into the cells. It is a temporary treatment, effective for approximately 6 hours, and is not always as effective when repeated.
Kayexalate (sodium polystyrene) and sorbitol 70%	Kayexalate is used as a cation exchange for severe hyperkalemia and can be administered orally or rectally. Approximate dosages are as follows: *Orally:* Kayexalate—10–20 g 3 to 4 times daily Sorbitol 70%—20 mL with each dose *Rectally:* Kayexalate—30–50 g Sorbitol 70%—50 mL; mix with 100–150 mL water (Retention enema—20–30 minutes)

87 For temporary correction of a moderate potassium excess, indicate which methods are most effective:

( ) a. Potassium restriction diet
( ) b. IV sodium bicarbonate
( ) c. 10% Calcium gluconate
( ) d. Insulin and glucose
( ) e. Kayexalate and sorbitol

a. —; b. X; c. X; d. X; e —

88 If a client is taking digitalis and has a serum potassium of 7.4 mEq/L, is 10% calcium gluconate indicated for temporary correction of hyperkalemia? _____ Explain. *_____.

no
Calcium administration enhances the action of digitalis, causing digitalis toxicity.

    ■   ■   ■

89 Drugs such as Kayexalate (sodium polystyrene sulfonate), a cation exchange resin, and sorbitol 70% are given for severe hyperkalemia. They cause a sodium-potassium ion exchange, and the potassium is excreted.

What treatment is suggested for mild hyperkalemia? *_____.

What treatment is suggested for severe hyperkalemia? *_____.

Restrict potassium intake.
Kayexalate and sorbitol—ion exchange

    ■   ■   ■

CLINICAL APPLICATIONS

90 Approximately 2% of healthy adults develop hypokalemia. Twenty to 80% of persons taking potassium-wasting diuretics develop hypokalemia. Hypokalemia is present in about 20% of hospitalized clients, and hyperkalemia occurs in approximately 10% of hospitalized clients.

The most common potassium imbalance in hospitalized clients is (hypokalemia/hyperkalemia) _____ .

hypokalemia

    ■   ■   ■

91 Five percent of hospitalized clients with hypokalemia have a serum potassium level lower than 3.0 mEq/L. One to 2% of hospitalized clients having hyperkalemia have a serum potassium level greater than 6.0 mEq/L.

A client with a serum potassium level below 3.0 mEq/L requires _____ mEq of potassium to raise the serum potassium level 1 mEq/L.

200–400

    ■   ■   ■

92 An example of a severe serum potassium deficit that is life threatening is a serum potassium level of _____ mEq/L. An example of a severe serum potassium excess that is life threatening is _____ mEq/L.

<2.5; >7.0

       ■   ■   ■

93 Eighty to 90% of potassium excretion is lost in the urine, and only a very small percentage is lost in the feces.

Which of the following promotes a greater loss of potassium?

( ) a. An individual taking a laxative
( ) b. An individual taking a diuretic

a. — b. X

       ■   ■   ■

94 Hyperglycemia, an increased blood sugar, is a symptom of diabetes mellitus. Cells cannot utilize glucose; thus, catabolism (cellular breakdown) occurs, and potassium leaves the cells and is excreted by the kidneys. If the kidneys are not functioning adequately (<600 mL per day), potassium can accumulate and serum potassium excess can occur.

When cells do not receive their proper nutrition, what happens to the cells? *_____

_____ .

In hyperglycemia (hypokalemia/hyperkalemia) _____ occurs due to cellular breakdown and polyuria. If there is kidney shutdown, (hypokalemia/hyperkalemia) _____ occurs.

catabolism—cellular breakdown with loss of potassium
hypokalemia; hyperkalemia

       ■   ■   ■

95 Administering glucose and insulin to correct abnormal cellular metabolism in a diabetic client may lead to rapid transfer of potassium from the extracellular fluid to the cell. In this situation, the serum potassium rapidly (increases/decreases) _____ .

decreases

       ■   ■   ■

96 When oliguria develops because of poor renal function, potassium is no longer excreted, which results in a high serum potassium level.

If there is poor renal function, do you think potassium should be administered?
*_____ .

Why?   *_____ .

no, NEVER with poor renal function
Hyperkalemia can be brought to a dangerous level.

■   ■   ■

97 Potassium therapy should not be administered to clients with untreated adrenal insufficiency and   *_____ .

renal failure or poor renal function

■   ■   ■

98 In the cirrhotic client with degenerated liver cells, hypokalemia can precipitate hepatic coma or liver failure.

As a nurse caring for a client with cirrhosis you would alert the physician of any low serum K levels, and you should watch for symptoms of   *_____ .

hypokalemia and hepatic coma

■   ■   ■

99 Potassium is most plentiful in the gastrointestinal tract. Vomiting and diarrhea can cause a potassium (deficit/excess)   *_____ .

deficit

■   ■   ■

100 The serum levels of magnesium, chloride, and protein should be checked when correcting hypokalemia. Low serum levels of Mg, Cl, and protein inhibit potassium utilization by the body.

If hypokalemia and hypomagnesemia (Mg deficit) are present, should a potassium deficit be corrected by giving potassium chloride? _____   Why?   *_____

_____ .

no
Magnesium deficit needs to be corrected first, which may automatically correct potassium deficit by making potassium usable by the body.

■   ■   ■

CASE STUDY REVIEW

Mr. Johnson, 68 years old, has been vomiting and has had diarrhea for 2 days. He takes digoxin, 0.25 mg, and HydroDIURIL, 50 mg, daily. His serum potassium level is 3.2 mEq/L. He complains of being dizzy. The nurse assesses his physiologic status and notes that his muscles are weak and flabby, his abdomen is distended, and peristalsis is diminished.

1. What was his potassium imbalance? *_____ .
2. "Normal" range of potassium balance is *_____ .
3. Should the nurse have checked his pulse rate, since he was receiving digoxin? _____ . Explain. *_____ .
4. Vomiting will cause a potassium (deficit/excess). _____ .
5. Name the signs and symptoms of Mr. Johnson's potassium deficit. _____ , *_____ , *_____ , and *_____ .

Mr. Johnson's heart activity was monitored with an ECG. He received 1 liter of 5% dextrose in water with 40 mEq/L of KCl.

6. A flat T wave would be indicative of _____ .
7. The daily potassium requirement is *_____ .
8. A concentration of KCl in IV fluids higher than 40 mEq/L can cause *_____
_____ .
9. List at least three common symptoms found with hyperkalemia. *_____ , *_____ , and _____ .

A week after his acute illness, his serum potassium was 3.7 mEq/L and his serum chloride was in the "normal" range. The physician ordered Mr. Johnson to take an oral potassium supplement with his daily Digoxin and HydroDIURIL (hydrochlorothiazide). For Mr. Johnson's arthritis, prednisone 4 times a week was ordered.

10. Name an oral potassium supplement that the physician can prescribe. _____
_____ .
11. Explain the effect of cortisone on potassium in the body. *_____ .
12. If a potassium supplement was not prescribed, name a potassium-sparing diuretic that can be taken in conjunction with hydrochlorothiazide _____ .

1. *hypokalemia*
2. *3.5–5.3 mEq/L*
3. *yes; hypokalemia will enhance the action of digoxin, causing digitalis toxicity*
4. *deficit*
5. *dizziness, muscles weak and flabby, distended abdomen, and diminished peristalsis*
6. *hypokalemia*
7. *40–60 mEq/L*
8. *hyperkalemia, which is toxic to heart muscle and can cause phlebitis (irritated blood vessel)*
9. *abdominal cramps, tachycardia and later bradycardia, and oliguria*
10. *Potassium chloride. Also potassium triplex, Kaon, or K-Lyte since the chloride level is normal.*
11. *excretes potassium*
12. *Aldactone or Dyrenium*

HYPOKALEMIA

NURSING ASSESSMENT FACTORS

- Obtain a nursing history observing for a clinical health problem which may cause hypokalemia, i.e., vomiting, diarrhea, fad-reducing diet, potassium-wasting diuretics.
- Assess for signs and symptoms of hypokalemia, i.e., dizziness, dysrhythmia, soft muscles, abdominal distention, and decreased peristalsis or paralytic ileus.
- Check the serum potassium level that can be used as a baseline for comparison of future serum potassium levels. A serum potassium level below 3.5 mEq/L indicates hypokalemia. A serum potassium level below 2.5 mEq/L may cause cardiac arrest.
- Check the ECG/EKG strips for changes in the T wave (flat or inverted) that may indicate hypokalemia.
- Assess the urine output for 24 hours. Excess urine excretion increases the amount of potassium being excreted.
- Assess for signs and symptoms of digitalis toxicity (i.e., nausea, vomiting, anorexia, bradycardia, dysrhythmias) when a client is receiving a potassium-wasting diuretic and/or steroids with a digitalis preparation. Hypokalemia enhances the action of digitalis product.

NURSING DIAGNOSIS 1

High risk for injury: vessels, tissues, or gastric muscosa related to phlebitis from concentrated potassium solution, infiltration of potassium solution into subcutaneous tissues, or ingestion of concentrated oral potassium irritating and damaging to the gastric mucosa.

NURSING INTERVENTIONS AND RATIONALE

1. Dilute oral potassium supplements in at least 4 ounces of water or juice. Concentrated potassium is irritating to the gastric mucosa.
2. Check infusion site for phlebitis or infiltration when KCl is given intravenously. Potassium is irritating to blood vessels and subcutaneous tissue. NEVER administer potassium intravenously as a bolus or IV push.
3. Monitor serum potassium levels. A serum potassium level less than 3.5 mEq/L can cause neuromuscular dysfunction and injury to tissues.
4. Monitor the ECG for changes that indicate hypokalemia such as a flat or inverted T wave. Report changes immediately.

NURSING DIAGNOSIS 2

Nutrition: altered, less than body requirements, related to insufficient intake of foods rich in potassium or potassium losses (gastric suctioning).

NURSING INTERVENTIONS AND RATIONALE

1. Instruct clients to eat foods rich in potassium when hypokalemia is present or when they are taking potassium-wasting diuretics and steroids. Examples of such foods are fresh fruits, fruit juices, dry fruits, vegetables, meats, nuts, cocoa, and cola.

2. Monitor the serum potassium level of clients receiving potassium-wasting diuretics and steroids (cortisone preparations).
3. Irrigate gastrointestinal tube with normal saline solution to prevent electrolyte loss. Gastrointestinal fluid loss from GI suctioning, vomiting, and diarrhea should be measured.
4. Recognize other drugs and substances (i.e., glucose, insulin, laxatives, lithium carbonate, salicylates, tetracycline, and licorice) that decrease serum potassium levels.
5. Monitor serum magnesium, chloride, and protein when hypokalemia is present. Attempts to correct the potassium deficit may not be effective when hypomagnesemia, hypochloremia, and hypoproteinemia are also present.

HYPERKALEMIA

NURSING ASSESSMENT FACTORS

- Obtain a nursing history of clinical health problems or procedures that may cause hyperkalemia (i.e., renal insufficiency or failure, administration of large doses of intravenous potassium or rapid administration of potassium, and Addison's disease).
- Assess for signs and symptoms of hyperkalemia [i.e., cardiac dysrhythmia (tachycardia and later bradycardia), decreased urine output, abdominal cramps].
- Check the ECG/EKG strips for changes in the T wave (peaked) which may indicate hyperkalemia.
- Check the serum potassium level that can be used as a baseline for comparison of future serum potassium levels. A serum potassium level greater than 5.3 mEq/L is indicative of hyperkalemia. A serum potassium level greater than 7.0 mEq/L can be a factor in causing cardiac arrest.
- Assess urine output for 24 hours. A decrease in urine output of less than 600 mL per day can indicate an inadequate fluid intake, decreased cardiac output, or renal insufficiency.
- Check the age of whole blood before administering it to a client with hyperkalemia. Blood, for transfusion, which is 10 or more days old has an elevated serum potassium level due to the hemolysis of aging blood cells.

NURSING DIAGNOSIS 1

High risk for cardiac output: decreased, related to dysrhythmia secondary to hyperkalemia.

NURSING INTERVENTIONS AND RATIONALE
1. Monitor vital signs. Report presence of tachycardia or bradycardia.
2. Monitor ECG strips. Report presence of peaked T wave, wide QRS complex, and prolonged P-R interval.
3. Monitor serum potassium levels. Report precipitous decrease or increase in serum potassium level.

NURSING DIAGNOSIS 2

Urinary elimination: altered, related to renal dysfunction, cardiac insufficiency.

NURSING INTERVENTIONS AND RATIONALE

1. Monitor daily urine output. Urine output that is less than 250 mL per 8 hours should be reported.
2. Monitor urine output for clients receiving potassium supplements (orally or intravenously). If urine output is poor while the client is receiving potassium supplements, the serum potassium level will be increased.
3. Regulate the flow rate of intravenous fluid with potassium so that no more than 10 mEq/L of KCl is administered per hour. Rapidly administered KCl can cause hyperkalemia.
4. Monitor medical treatments for hyperkalemia. Know which corrective treatments are used for mild, moderate, and severe hyperkalemia.
5. Note if the client is on digitalis when calcium gluconate is ordered for temporary correction of hyperkalemia. Hypercalcemia enhances the action of digitalis, causing digitalis toxicity.
6. Administer Kayexalate and sorbitol orally or rectally, according to the amount prescribed by the physician. The serum potassium should be checked frequently during treatment to prevent hypokalemia resulting from overcorrection of hyperkalemia.
7. Administer fresh blood (blood transfusion) to clients with hyperkalemia. The serum potassium level of fresh blood is 3.5–5.5 mEq/L. With blood that is 3 weeks old, the serum potassium level can be as high as 25 mEq/L.

SODIUM

INTRODUCTION

101 Sodium is the main cation found in _____ fluid.

extracellular or intravascular

       ■   ■   ■

102 Sodium loss from the skin is negligible under normal conditions, but with increased environmental temperature, fever, and/or muscular exercise, the loss of sodium increases.

If an individual runs a race and the atmospheric temperature is 100, what do you think happens to the sodium in his or her body? *_____ .

sodium loss

       ■   ■   ■

103 The normal concentration of sodium in the extracellular fluid is 135–146 mEq/L.

The normal concentration of sodium in perspiration is 50–100 mEq, which is less than the concentration found in the *_____ .

extracellular fluid

       ■   ■   ■

104 Perspiration is regarded as a by-product of temperature regulation. Therefore, when the body's sodium level is elevated, perspiration is not a means of regulating sodium excretion.

The concentration of sodium in the extracellular fluid is _____ mEq/L.

135–146

■   ■   ■

105 Bones contain as much as 800–1000 mEq of sodium, but only a portion of the sodium is available for exchange with sodium in other parts of the body.

The concentration of sodium in the extracellular fluid is _____ mEq/L.

135–146

■   ■   ■

106 Bones contain (more/less) _____ sodium than extracellular fluid.

more

■   ■   ■

107 Thirst often leads to the replacement of water, but not of sodium.

One (can/cannot) _____ replace sodium by drinking lots of water.

cannot

■   ■   ■

108 Ocean water is about three times as salty as our body fluid—far too salty for our body organs, i.e., stomach and intestines.

Ocean water is a (hypo-osmolar/hyperosmolar) _____ fluid. Therefore, in cases of ocean water ingestion, the water is drawn from the body fluid into the stomach and intestines by the process of (osmosis/diffusion) _____ .

hyperosmolar; osmosis

■   ■   ■

109 As the stomach and intestines accumulate huge volumes of water, vomiting occurs. Explain why fluids accumulate in the stomach and how this may cause vomiting.

a. *_____ .

b. *_____ .

a. Body fluids accumulate in the stomach due to osmosis (lesser to the greater concentration).
b. Fluids overextend the stomach.

■   ■   ■

110 An elevated serum sodium is known as sodium excess or *hypernatremia* and a decreased serum sodium is known as sodium deficit or *hyponatremia*.

Hypernatremia is also known as *_____ . Hyponatremia is also known as

*_____ .

sodium excess; sodium deficit
∎   ∎   ∎

111 One of the main functions of sodium is to influence the distribution of water in the body. Water accompanies sodium.

A name for a sodium excess is _____ .

A name for a sodium deficit is _____ .

A function of sodium is to influence the distribution of *_____ .

hypernatremia; hyponatremia; body water (water accompanies sodium)
∎   ∎   ∎

FUNCTIONS

Sodium action is influenced by the kidneys, the posterior pituitary gland, and the adrenal glands. The kidneys have an important role in maintaining homeostasis of body sodium. The hypothalamus produces ADH (antidiuretic hormone) and the posterior hypophysis (posterior pituitary gland) stores and secretes ADH. This hormone facilitates the absorption of large quantities of water from the kidneys. The adrenal glands are composed of two sections, the cortex and the medulla, each secreting its own hormones. The hormones from the adrenal cortex are frequently referred to as steroids. Table 3-12 explains how one organ and two glands influence serum sodium. Study this table carefully. Refer to a physiology text for any further clarification.

Table 3-12. INFLUENCES AFFECTING SERUM SODIUM	
Organ Kidneys	The regulators. Kidneys maintain homeostasis through excretion or absorption of water and sodium from renal tubules according to excess or deficit of serum sodium.
Glands 1. Posterior hypophysis or posterior pituitary gland	Pituitary antidiuretic hormone (ADH) favors water absorption from the distal tubules of the kidneys, and thus sodium excretion is restricted.
2. Adrenal cortex of the adrenal glands	Adrenal cortical hormones, e.g., cortisone and aldosterone, favor sodium absorption from the renal tubules. These steroids influence the kidneys to absorb sodium and excrete potassium.

112 The chief regulation of sodium occurs within the _____ .

kidneys

■   ■   ■

113 The amount of water absorbed from the kidneys depends upon the amount of ADH being secreted. If less water is absorbed from the renal tubules, what happens to the sodium?
*_____ .

Less sodium is absorbed.

■   ■   ■

114 Explain the effect of cortisone and aldosterone on the regulation of sodium and potassium.
*_____ .

They influence the kidneys to absorb sodium and excrete potassium.

■   ■   ■

Table 3-13 explains the functions of sodium. The two most important functions of sodium are for water balance and neuromuscular activity. Study Table 3-13 carefully and refer to the table as needed.

Table 3-13. SODIUM AND ITS FUNCTIONS

Body System	Functions
Neuromuscular	Transmission and conduction of nerve impulses (sodium pump—see Cellular).
Body fluids	Largely responsible for the osmolality of vascular fluids. Doubling Na gives the approximate serum osmolality.
	Regulation of body fluid (sodium causes water retention).
Cellular	Sodium pump action. Sodium shifts into cells as potassium shifts out of the cells, repeatedly, to maintain water balance and neuromuscular activity. When Na shifts into the cell, depolarization occurs (cell activity); and when Na shifts out of the cell, K shifts back into the cell, and repolarization occurs.
	Enzyme activity.
Acid-base	Assists with the regulation of acid-base balance. Sodium combines readily with chloride (Cl) or bicarbonate (HCO_3) to promote acid-base balance.

115 An important function of sodium is to aid neuromuscular activity. Name another electrolyte responsible for neuromuscular activity. _____ .

potassium, magnesium, or calcium

■   ■   ■

116 The concentration or tonicity (osmolality) of vascular fluids is determined by which electrolyte?
_____ .

To get a rough estimate of the serum osmolality, what can you do? Refer to Chapter 1 if necessary. *_____ .

sodium; double the serum sodium
∎   ∎   ∎

117 Explain the action of the sodium pump. *_____
_____ .

Name two purposes for the sodium pump. *_____
and *_____ .

Sodium shifts in as potassium shifts out of the cells, and depolarization and cell activity occur. Then K shifts in and Na shifts out for repolarization (cell rest).
water balance and neuromuscular activity
∎   ∎   ∎

118 What are the two anions that combine with sodium to help regulate acid-base balance?
_____ and _____ .

chloride and bicarbonate
∎   ∎   ∎

119 Large amounts of sodium are contained within the following body secretions: saliva, gastric secretions, bile, pancreative juice, and intestinal secretions.

Indicate which of the following body secretions contain large quantities of sodium:

( ) a. Saliva
( ) b. Thyroid secretions
( ) c. Gastric secretions
( ) d. Bile
( ) e. Parathyroid secretions
( ) f. Pancreative juice
( ) g. Intestinal secretions

a. X; b —; c. X; d. X; e. —; f. X; g. X
∎   ∎   ∎

PATHOPHYSIOLOGY

120 The pathophysiologic effects of hyponatremia are evidenced in the membranes of the central nervous system (CNS), the neuromuscular tissues, and the smooth muscles of the gastrointestinal (GI) tract.

The cells of the CNS are more sensitive to a decreased serum sodium level than other cells. The cardiac muscle is usually not affected by changes in the serum sodium level.

Hyponatremia has an effect on the membranes of:

a. * _____

b. * _____

c. * _____

a. central nervous system; b. neuromuscular tissues; c. smooth muscles of the GI tract

■   ■   ■

121 Hyponatremia can occur when the kidneys are unable to excrete enough urine. Reduced urine excretion increases the amount of body water, which in turn dilutes the serum sodium concentration.

The type of electrolyte imbalance that can result when the body fluid volume is increased is known as (hyponatremia/hypernatremia) _____ .

hyponatremia

■   ■   ■

122 When the serum sodium level is increased, sodium passes more freely across the cell membranes, accelerating the rate of depolarization. This can cause (decreased/increased) _____ cellular activity (irritability). As the hypernatremic state intensifies, less sodium passes across the cell membrane, ultimately resulting in (more/less) _____ cellular activity.

increased; less

■   ■   ■

123 An increased serum sodium level (hypernatremia), (increases/decreases) _____ the serum osmolality.

Increases. The serum osmolality is the concentration of solutes in the plasma. An increased serum sodium level increases the serum osmolality.

■   ■   ■

ETIOLOGY

The general causes of hyponatremia are GI losses, altered cellular function, renal losses, electrolyte-free fluids, and hormonal influences. Table 3-14 lists the various causes and gives the rationale concerning the sodium loss. Study this table carefully and refer to it as needed.

124 The hemodilution of body fluids that can cause hyponatremia includes which of the following symptoms:

( ) a. Drinking excessive amounts of plain water
( ) b. Increased adrenocortical hormone
( ) c. SIADH
( ) d. Gastric suction
( ) e. Hypervolemic state due to CHF
( ) f. Increased environmental temperature

a. X; b. —; c. X; d. —; e. X; f. —
                                ■   ■   ■

125 Vomiting and diarrhea can (increase/decrease) _____ the serum sodium
level. Explain *_____

_____ .

decrease
The high concentration of sodium normally present in the GI tract is lost when vomiting/diarrhea occur.
                    ■   ■   ■

126 Name four conditions that cause a large sodium loss through the skin.
_____ , *_____ , _____ , and
*_____ .

sweating, increased environmental temperature, fever, and muscular exercise
                    ■   ■   ■

127 Wound drainage, bleeding, and vomiting postoperatively can cause a sodium (deficit/retention)
_____ .

SIADH may occur following surgery. Explain how it causes a sodium deficit. *_____

_____ .

deficit
Excess or continuous ADH secretion causes water to be reabsorbed from the kidney, thus diluting ECF.
                    ■   ■   ■

Table 3-14.   CAUSES OF HYPONATREMIA (SERUM SODIUM DEFICIT)

Etiology	Rationale
Dietary Changes Low-sodium diet Excessive plain water intake "Fad" diets/fasting Anorexia nervosa	A low-sodium intake over several months can lead to hyponatremia. Drinking large quantities of plain water dilutes the ECF. Administration of continuous intravenous D_5W dilutes the ECF and can cause water intoxication.
Gastrointestinal Losses Vomiting, diarrhea GI suctioning Tap-water enemas GI surgery Bulemia	Sodium concentration is high in the gastric and intestinal mucosas. Sodium losses occur with vomiting, diarrhea, GI suctioning, and GI surgery.
Renal Losses Salt-wasting kidney disease Diuretics	In advanced renal disorders, the tubules do not respond to ADH; therefore, there is a loss of sodium and water. The extensive use of diuretics or excessively potent diuretics can decrease the serum sodium levels.
Hormonal Influences Antidiuretic hormone (ADH), syndrome of inappropriate ADH (SIADH)	ADH promotes water reabsorption from the distal renal tubules. Surgical pain, increased use of narcotics, and head trauma, inappropriately stimulate ADH production (SIADH). This causes more water to be reabsorbed, thus diluting the ECF.
Decreased adrenocortical hormone: Addison's disease	Decreased adrenocortical hormone production related to decreased adrenal gland activity (Addison's disease) causes sodium loss and potassium retention.
Altered Cellular Function Hypervolemic state: CHF, cirrhosis	In hypervolemic states due to CHF, cirrhosis, and nephrosis, the ECF is increased, thus diluting the serum sodium level.
Burns	Great quantities of sodium are lost from burn wounds and from oozing burn surface areas.
Sodium losses from the skin	Large amounts of sodium are lost from the skin due to increased environmental temperature, fever, and large skin wounds.

128 The use of gastric suction for the purpose of drainage can cause (hypernatremia/hyponatremia) _____ . Why? *_____

_____ .

hyponatremia
Gastric and intestinal secretions pass out through the gastric tube.

■   ■   ■

129 Addison's disease occurs when there is an adrenocortical hormone (insufficiency/overproduction) _____ .

   In Addison's disease, there is a sodium (loss/gain) _____ .

insufficiency; loss

■   ■   ■

130 Clients recovering from burn injuries experience numerous fluid shifts as the body attempts to compensate for the trauma to its tissues. Burns promote increased *_____

_____ . Why? *_____ .

   water and sodium loss; due to oozing at the burn surface (or because sodium replaces potassium in the damaged cells)

■   ■   ■

131 Repeated tap-water enemas can result in a *_____ . Why? *_____

_____ .

sodium loss
They wash away intestinal secretions high in sodium.

■   ■   ■

Table 3-15 lists the various causes and gives the rationale concerning sodium excess.

132 Severe vomiting and diarrhea can cause (hyponatremia/hypernatremia) _____ . Why? _____

_____ .

hypernatremia
Water loss is greater than sodium loss (hypovolemic with hypernatremic effect).

■   ■   ■

Table 3-15.   CAUSES OF HYPERNATREMIA (SERUM SODIUM EXCESS)

Etiology	Rationale
Dietary Changes Increased sodium intake Decreased water intake Administration of saline solutions	Inadequate fluid intake and increased use of table salt and canned vegetables and soups increases the serum sodium level. Administration of concentrated saline solutions can cause hypernatremia.
GI Disorders Vomiting Diarrhea	With severe vomiting, water loss can be greater than sodium loss, causing a dangerously high serum sodium level. This is particularly true in babies who have diarrhea. Their loss of water can be greater than their loss of sodium.
Decreased renal function	Reduced glomerular filtration causes an excess of sodium in the body.
Environmental Changes Increased temperature Water loss	Increased environmental and body temperatures may cause profuse perspiration. Water loss can be greater than sodium loss.
Hormonal Influence Increased adrenocortical hormone production: oral or IV cortisone	Excess adrenocortical hormone can cause a sodium excess in the body whether it is due to cortisone ingestion or hyperfunction of the adrenal gland (Cushing's syndrome).
Altered Cellular Function CHF, renal diseases	Usually with CHF and renal disease, the body's sodium is greatly increased. If water retention is greatly enhanced, pseudohyponatremia may result.

133 Which of the following situations can cause an increased serum sodium level:

( ) a. Excessive use of table salt
( ) b. Continuous use of canned vegetables and soups
( ) c. Increased water intake
( ) d. Continuous use of intravenous saline solutions
( ) e. Use of diuretics
( ) f. Large doses or prolonged uses of oral cortisone drug

a. X; b. X; c. —; d. X; e. —; f. X

134 Congestive heart failure (CHF) or obstruction of the arterial blood supply to the kidney can cause sodium (excretion/retention) _____ . Why? *_____
_____ .

retention
Reduced glomerular filtration. Sodium retention usually causes an increase in body fluid and may give a false indication that the serum sodium level is normal or low.

■   ■   ■

135 Cushing's syndrome occurs when there is an adrenocortical hormone (insufficiency/overproduction) _____ .

In Cushing's syndrome, there is a sodium _____ .

overproduction; retention

■   ■   ■

CLINICAL MANIFESTATIONS

The severity of the clinical manifestations of hypo-hypernatremia varies with the onset and extent of sodium deficit or excess. Mild hypernatremia is normally asymptomatic, and early nonspecific symptoms such as nausea and vomiting may be overlooked. Table 3-16 gives the signs and

Table 3-16. CLINICAL MANIFESTATIONS OF SODIUM IMBALANCES		
Body Areas	**Hyponatremia**	**Hypernatremia**
Gastrointestinal abnormalities	*Nausea, vomiting, diarrhea, abdominal cramps	*Nausea, vomiting, anorexia *Rough, dry tongue
Cardiac abnormalities	Tachycardia, hypotension	*Tachycardia, possible hypertension
Central nervous system (CNS)	*Headaches, apprehension, lethargy, confusion, depression, convulsion	*Restlessness, agitation, stupor, *elevated body temperature
Neuromuscular abnormalities	*Muscular weakness	Muscular twitching, tremor, hyperreflexia
Integumentary changes	Dry skin, pale, dry mucous membrane	*Flushed, dry skin, dry, sticky membrane
Laboratory Findings Serum sodium	<135 mEq/L	>146 mEq/L
Urine sodium		<40 mEq/L
Specific gravity	<1.008	>1.025
Serum osmolality	<280 mOsm/kg	>295 mOsm/kg

Note: *Indicates most common clinical manifestations of hyponatremia and hypernatremia.

symptoms associated with hypo-hypernatremia. Memorize the common symptoms which are marked with an asterisk. Study this table carefully. Refer to the glossary for any unknown words. Refer back to this table as needed to complete the frames on hypo-hypernatremia.

136 In hyponatremia, the serum sodium level is below _____ mEq/L. What is the serum value in hypernatremia? *_____ mEq/L.

135; above 146

■   ■   ■

137 Nausea and vomiting may indicate the early stages of which of the following:

( ) a. Hyponatremia
( ) b. Hypernatremia

a. X; b. X

■   ■   ■

138 Headaches, lethargy, depression, and muscular weakness are clinical manifestations of (hyponatremia/hypernatremia) _____ .

hyponatremia

■   ■   ■

139 Which of the following signs and symptoms indicate hypernatremia?

( ) a. Rough, dry tongue
( ) b. Tachycardia
( ) c. Apprehension, confusion
( ) d. Flushed, dry skin
( ) e. Restlessness, agitation
( ) f. Elevated body temperature

a. X; b. X; c. —; d. X; e. X; f. X

■   ■   ■

140 A serum osmolality below 280 mOsm/L may indicate (hyponatremia/hypernatremia) _____ . While a serum osmolality above 295 mOsm/L may indicate _____ .

hyponatremia (also indicates ECF dilution caused by a sodium deficit or excess water retention); hypernatremia

■   ■   ■

DRUGS AND THEIR EFFECT ON SODIUM BALANCE

Diuretics, certain antipsychotics, antineoplastics, and barbiturates can cause a sodium deficit. Corticosteroids and ingestion and infusion of sodium are the major causes of a sodium excess. Table 3-17 lists the drugs that affect sodium balance.

141 Enter SD for sodium deficit/hyponatremia and SE for sodium excess/hypernatremia beside drugs that affect sodium balance. Refer to Table 3-17 as needed.

_____ a. Lithium
_____ b. Cortisone
_____ c. Diuretics
_____ d. Sodium penicillin
_____ e. Antipsychotic agents
_____ f. Ibuprofen/Motrin
_____ g. Amphoterin B
_____ h. Lactulose
_____ i. Barbiturates
_____ j. Cyclophosphamide/Cytoxan
_____ k. Tolbutamide/Orinase

a. SD; b. SE; c. SD; d. SE; e. SD; f. SD; g. SE; h. SE; i. SD; j. SD; k. SD

142 Clients who are receiving steroids, such as cortisone and prednisone, should be cautioned in the use of excess salt. Explain *_____ .

Steroids promote sodium retention (sodium-retaining effect).

143 Hyponatremia enhances the action of quinidine and hypernatremia reduces or decreases the action of quinidine.

With a serum sodium of 156 mEq/L would the action of quinidine be (increased/decreased)? _____ .

decreased

144 Cough medicines, most antibiotics, and sulfonamides can (increase/decrease) _____ the serum sodium level.

increase

Table 3-17. DRUGS AFFECTING SODIUM BALANCE

Sodium Imbalance	Drugs	Rationale
Hyponatremia (serum sodium deficit)	Diuretics	Diuretics, either K wasting or K sparing, cause sodium excretion.
	Lithium	Lithium promotes urinary sodium loss.

	Antineoplastics/Anticancer
	  Vincristine
	  Cyclophosphamide
	  Cisplatin
	Antipsychotics
	  Amitryptyline (Elavil)
	  Thioridazine (Mellaril)
	  Thiothixene (Navane)
	  Tranylcypromine (Parnate)
	Antidiabetics
	  Chlorpropamide
	  Tolbutamide (Orinase)
	CNS depressants
	  Morphine
	  Barbiturates
	  Ibuprofens (Motrin)
	  Nicotine
	  Clonidine (Catapres)
		Anticancer drugs, antipsychotics, and antidiabetics stimulate ADH release and cause hemodilution and decrease sodium level.

Hypernatremia (serum sodium excess)	Corticosteroids
	  Cortisone
	  Prednisone
		Steroids promote sodium retention and potassium excretion.

	Hypertonic saline
	  Sodium salicylate
	  Sodium phosphate
	  Sodium bicarbonate
	  Cough medicines
		Administration of sodium salts in excess.

	Antibiotics
	  Azlocillin Na
	  Penicillin Na
	  Mezlocillin Na
	  Carbenicillin
	  Ticarcillin disodium
	  Cholestyramine
	  Amphotericin B
	  Propoxyphene (Darvon)
	  Demeclocycline
	  Lactulose
		Many of the antibiotics contain the sodium salt which increases drug absorption.
		Ion exchange.
		
		These miscellaneous drugs promote urinary water loss without sodium.
		
		Water loss in excess of sodium via GI.

CLINICAL MANAGEMENT

SODIUM CORRECTION

145 The majority of Americans consume 8–15 g of sodium per day, which is four to five times the amount of sodium required by the body. Daily sodium requirements are 2–4 g. A teaspoon of salt has 2.3 g of sodium.

   When sodium intake increases, what happens to the water intake and to the body fluids? *_____.

Sodium holds water. Extracellular fluid (ECF) is increased.

   ■   ■   ■

146 To restore the sodium balance due to a sodium deficit, either normal saline solution (0.9% NaCl) or a 3% or 5% salt solution is recommended. Several physicians suggest that the serum sodium fall below 130 mEq/L before giving saline and below 120 mEq/L before giving a concentrated salt solution, i.e., 3% saline.

   Remember, a rapid infusion of concentrated salt solutions can result in pulmonary edema. Explain why. *_____

_____.

Sodium retains fluid. A high concentration of sodium pulls intracellular fluid from cells, thus overexpanding the vascular compartment. Fluid collects in the lungs.

   ■   ■   ■

147 Excessive intravenous administration of dextrose and water can cause sodium dilution. Dextrose is metabolized, leaving free water.

   Explain how sodium can be diluted. *_____

_____.

Following the utilization of dextrose, the remaining water dilutes the sodium and other electrolytes.

   ■   ■   ■

CLINICAL APPLICATIONS

148 The majority of laboratory analyses of serum electrolyte content are carried out on the plasma, which represents less than one twelfth of the total body fluid; therefore, results may occasionally be misleading.

   The reason for the use of plasma instead of other body fluid and cells is that *_____

_____ .

it is easier to obtain

   ■   ■   ■

149 You have a cardiac client who has edema and yet his serum sodium concentration is reduced. Why do you think this occurs?   *_____

_____ .

He may be on a low-sodium diet and taking a diuretic. Hyponatremia can result from hemodilution.

∎   ∎   ∎

150 A 24-hour urine sodium test is helpful for determining sodium retention or loss within the body. A normal range for 24-hour urine sodium is 40–220 mEq/L.

If a client's 24-hour urine sodium is 32 mEq/L, the serum sodium level is 133 mEq/L, and the client has symptoms of heart failure, do you think the client is retaining sodium? _____ . Explain.   *_____

_____ .

Yes, very good.
A low urine sodium indicates sodium retention in the body, especially with symptoms of overhydration. A low serum sodium level can be misleading. Hyponatremia can occur with a fluid volume excess (hypervolemia), which causes the sodium to be diluted.

∎   ∎   ∎

151 If your client is vomiting following a surgical intervention and is receiving dextrose and water intravenously, one may expect a sodium (excess/deficit) _____ if the vomiting persists.

A client experiencing severe vomiting without water replacement is at high risk for a sodium (excess/deficit) _____ . Why?   *_____

_____ .

deficit; excess
The loss of water would be greater than the loss of sodium.

∎   ∎   ∎

152 In congestive heart failure, there is sodium (retention/excretion) _____ . Why?   *_____ .

retention
Poor circulation reduces glomerular filtration; therefore, sodium is retained.

∎   ∎   ∎

153 If hyponatremia is due to SIADH (syndrome of inappropriate antidiuretic hormone) secretion or congestive heart failure, which do you think is the treatment of choice?

( ) a. Three percent saline intravenously

( ) b. Water intake restriction

a. —; b. X. Concentrated saline should be administered cautiously because pulmonary edema (lung congestion) can occur.

■   ■   ■

154 If a feeble or debilitated client receives numerous tap-water enemas for the purpose of cleaning the bowel, the enemas can cause a sodium _____ .

loss (deficit)

■   ■   ■

155 Diarrhea can cause either a sodium deficit or a sodium excess. Babies having diarrhea can lose more _____ than the ion, sodium; therefore, a sodium _____ can result.

water; excess

■   ■   ■

CASE STUDY REVIEW

Mrs. Unger has a high temperature and diaphoresis. She has been nauseated and has taken only ginger ale for the last several days. Her serum sodium is 129 mEq/L.

1. What type of sodium imbalance does Mrs. Unger have? *_____

_____   _____ .

2. Give the "normal" serum sodium range. *_____ .
3. Give some of the reasons for Mrs. Unger's imbalance.
   a. *_____
   b. *_____
4. Name some of the clinical signs and symptoms the nurse might observe.
   a. *_____
   b. *_____
   c. *_____
   d. *_____
5. When testing Mrs. Unger's urine, which of the following would the specific gravity be?
   ( ) a. 1.010 or below
   ( ) b. 1.015
   ( ) c. 1.020 or above

Mrs. Unger was given 3% sodium chloride solution. Her serum sodium level rose to 152 mEq/L. She was given quinidine for her irregular pulse rate.

6. Do you think her serum potassium should have been evaluated? _____ . Why?
   * _____ .

7. Name some of the clinical signs and symptoms the nurse observes with hypernatremia.
   a. * _____
   b. * _____
   c. * _____

8. Explain the effect of hypernatremia on quinidine. _____
   _____ .

9. If Mrs. Unger were to receive cortisone and antibiotics, what would this do to her hypernatremic state? * _____
   _____ .

10. Sodium is most plentiful in the extracellular compartment. Explain why sodium might enter the cells. * _____
    _____ .

1. *sodium deficit or hyponatremia*
2. *135–146 mEq/L*
3. *fever; diaphoresis; ginger ale intake for several days (lack of food)*
4. *abdominal cramps; muscular weakness; headaches; nausea and vomiting*
5. *a. 1.010 or below*
6. *Yes. She could have a loss of potassium from lack of food and due to illness. Arrhythmia may be a sign of hypokalemia*
7. *flushed skin; elevated body temperature; rough, dry tongue; and tachycardia*
8. *It reduces or decreases quinidine's action.*
9. *They increase the hypernatremic state. Cortisone causes sodium retention, and antibiotics increase sodium levels.*
10. *During cell catabolism, potassium leaves the cells and sodium enters the cells.*

HYPONATREMIA

NURSING ASSESSMENT FACTORS

- Obtain a history of high-risk factors for a decreased serum sodium level, i.e., GI loss from vomiting, diarrhea, or GI suctioning; eating disorders such as anorexia nervosa and bulimia; SIADH as a result of surgery; hypervolemic state resulting in hemodilution; use of potent diuretics with a low-sodium diet; or continuous use of D_5W.
- Assess for signs and symptoms of hyponatremia, i.e., headaches, nausea, vomiting, lethargy, confusion, tachycardia, and/or muscular weakness.
- Obtain a serum sodium level that may be used as a baseline value for comparison. A serum sodium level less than 135 mEq/L would indicate hyponatremia. A sodium level less than 125 mEq/L should be reported immediately to the physician.
- Check other electrolytes, such as potassium and chloride, when serum sodium levels are not within normal range.
- Check the serum osmolality level and urine specific gravity. A serum osmolality level of less than 280 mOsm/kg can indicate hyponatremia. A specific gravity below 1.010 can indicate hyponatremia.

NURSING DIAGNOSIS 1

Health maintenance: altered, related to vomiting, diarrhea, gastric suction, SIADH resulting from surgery, potent diuretics.

NURSING INTERVENTIONS AND RATIONALE

1. Monitor the serum sodium level. Sodium replacement may be needed if the serum sodium deficit is due to GI losses. Hypervolemic conditions such as CHF could indicate a pseudohyponatremia.
2. Keep an accurate intake and output record. Excess water intake can cause hyponatremia due to hemodilution.
3. Observe changes in vital signs, especially the pulse rate. If hyponatremia is due to hypovolemia (loss of fluid and sodium), shocklike symptoms, such as tachycardia, can occur. Frequently, hyponatremia is due to hemodilution from an excess fluid volume.
4. Check for signs and symptoms of water intoxication, i.e., headaches and behavioral changes, when hyponatremia is due to SIADH.
5. Restrict water when hyponatremia is due to hypervolemia (excess fluid volume).

HYPERNATREMIA

NURSING ASSESSMENT FACTORS

- Obtain a history of high-risk factors for an increased serum sodium level, i.e., increased sodium intake, decreased water intake, administration of concentrated saline solutions, renal diseases, increased adrenocortical hormone production.
- Assess for signs and symptoms of hypernatremia, i.e., nausea, vomiting, tachycardia, elevated blood pressure, flushed-dry skin, dry-sticky membrane, restlessness, elevated body temperature.
- Obtain a serum sodium value. Serum sodium levels greater than 146 mEq/L indicate hypernatremia.
- Check the serum osmolality level and urine specific gravity. A serum osmolality level greater than 295 mOsm/kg can indicate hypernatremia. A specific gravity above 1.025 can indicate hypernatremia.

NURSING DIAGNOSIS 1

Nutrition: altered, more than body requirements, related to excess intake of foods rich in sodium.

NURSING INTERVENTIONS AND RATIONALE

1. Instruct the client with hypernatremia to avoid foods rich in salt, i.e., canned foods, lunch meats, ham, pork, pickles, potato chips, pretzels.
2. Identify drugs that have a sodium-retaining effect on the body, i.e., cortisone preparations, cough medicines, and certain laxatives containing sodium.
3. Monitor the serum sodium level. Check for chest rales and for edema in the lower extremities.
4. Monitor the serum sodium levels daily or as ordered. A serum sodium level above 146 mEq/L can indicate hypernatremia. A serum sodium level above 160 mEq/L should be reported immediately to the physician.

5. Check the serum osmolality level and the urine specific gravity. A serum osmolality level exceeding 295 mOsm/kg can indicate hypernatremia. Sodium is primarily responsible for the serum osmolality value.
6. Check the urine sodium level. A decreased urine sodium (<40 mEq/L) frequently indicates sodium retention in the body, even though the serum sodium level may be within normal range (caused by hemodilution). Also check for rales in the lung and for pitting edema from sodium and fluid retention.
7. Check for signs and symptoms of pulmonary edema when the client is receiving several liters of normal saline (0.9% NaCl) or 3% saline. Sodium holds water in the blood vessels, and when administering a concentrated saline solution, overhydration can occur. Symptoms include dyspnea, cough, chest rales, and neck and hand vein engorgement.
8. Keep an accurate intake and output record. A decrease in urine output could indicate hypervolemia due to sodium excess.

NURSING DIAGNOSIS 2

Skin integrity: impaired, related to peripheral edema secondary to sodium and water excess.

NURSING INTERVENTIONS AND RATIONALE

1. Provide skin care to the body, especially the edematous areas.
2. Change the client's positions frequently to maintain skin integrity.
3. Promote increased mobility.
4. Use lotions as needed to keep skin moist.

CALCIUM

INTRODUCTION

156 Calcium (Ca) is a(n) (anion/cation) _____ found in the
(extracellular/intracellular/both) _____ body fluids.

Which body fluid has the greater calcium concentration? *_____

_____ . (Refer to Table 3-3 as needed).

cation; both; extracellular fluid

■   ■   ■

157 Calcium is a durable chemical substance of the body that is the last element to find its place in the adult body composition and the last element to leave after death.

The element that preserves the bony remains of dead creatures and is responsible for the x-ray photograph of bones is _____ .

calcium

■   ■   ■

158 The serum (plasma) calcium concentration level in the blood is 4.5–5.5 mEq/L or 9–11 mg/dL. Approximately 99% of the body's calcium is in teeth and bones; the remaining 1% is in the extracellular and intracellular fluids.

    Most of the body's calcium is in the _____ and _____ .

teeth and bones

        ■   ■   ■

159 About one-half of the body's serum calcium is bound to plasma proteins and the other half is free, ionized calcium that serves as a catalyst to stimulate a physiologic cellular response. Do you think the calcium that is bound to protein can cause a cellular response? _____ .

    The serum calcium level is _____ mEq/L _____ mg/dL.

No. For calcium to cause a physiologic response, it must be free, ionized calcium.
4.5–5.5; 9–11

        ■   ■   ■

160 When calcium becomes unbound from the plasma protein, the calcium is free, active calcium. This free calcium (can/cannot) _____ cause a physiologic cellular response.

can

        ■   ■   ■

161 Today's blood analyzers allow the ionized calcium (iCa) level to be measured. The normal serum ionized calcium level is 2.2–2.5 mEq/L or 4.5–5.0 mg/dL.

    Certain changes in the blood composition can either increase or decrease the serum iCa level. During acidosis, decreased pH, calcium is released from the plasma proteins, which (increases/decreases) _____ the serum iCa level.

    With alkalosis, there is an increased pH level which (increases/decreases) _____ calcium bound to protein. This results in a(n) (increase/decrease) _____ in the amount of free serum calcium, and thus, the serum iCa level is (increased/decreased) _____ .

increases; increases; decrease; decreased

        ■   ■   ■

162 The normal serum calcium (Ca) level is _____ mEq/L or
_____ mg/dl.

The normal ionized calcium (iCa) level is _____ mEq/L or
_____ mg/dL.

4.5–5.5; 9–11
2.2–2.5; 4.5–5.0

■   ■   ■

FUNCTIONS

163 Vitamin D is an element that is needed for calcium absorption from the gastrointestinal tract. The anion phosphorus (P) inhibits calcium absorption. Thus the actions of these two ions on the body have an opposite physiologic effect. When the serum calcium level is increased, the serum phosphorus level is (increased/decreased) _____ . However, both calcium and phosphorus are stored in the bone and excreted by the kidneys.

decreased

■   ■   ■

164 The parathyroid glands, which are four small oval-shaped glands located on the posterior thyroid gland, regulate the serum level of calcium. These glands secrete the parathyroid hormone, which is responsible for the homeostatic regulation of the calcium ion in the body fluids.

When the serum calcium level is low, the parathyroid glands secretes more parathyroid hormone. Explain what happens when the serum calcium level is high. *_____

_____ .

It inhibits or limits the secretion of the parathyroid hormone.

■   ■   ■

165 Calcitonin from the thyroid gland increases calcium return to the bone, thus decreasing the serum calcium level.

The parathyroid hormone (PTH) can (increase/decrease) _____ the serum calcium level by promoting calcium release from the bone as needed.

Indicate which of the hormones listed on the left increase or decrease the serum calcium levels.

_____ 1. Calcitonin   a. Increase
_____ 2. PTH   b. Decrease

increase; 1. b; 2. a

■   ■   ■

166 The regulation of serum calcium is maintained by the negative-feedback system. A low serum calcium stimulates the parathyroid gland to   *_____ . What do you think happens when there is a high serum calcium?   *_____

_____ .

secret parathyroid hormone
It inhibits the secretion of parathyroid hormone from the parathyroid gland.
            ▪   ▪   ▪

167 A low serum calcium level tells the parathyroid gland to secrete more parathyroid hormone. The parathyroid hormone increases serum calcium by mobilizing calcium from the bone, increasing renal absorption of calcium and promoting calcium absorption from the intestine in the presence of vitamin D.

   Parathyroid hormone increases serum calcium by which of the following mechanisms:

( ) a. Mobilizing calcium from the bone
( ) b. Decreasing renal absorption of calcium
( ) c. Increasing renal absorption of calcium
( ) d. Promoting calcium absorption from the intestine with vitamin D

a. X; b. —; c. X; d. X
            ▪   ▪   ▪

Table 3-18 explains the functions of calcium. Calcium is needed for neuromuscular activity, contraction of the myocardium, normal cellular permeability, coagulation of blood, and bone and teeth formation. Study the table carefully, and refer to it as needed.

Table 3-18. CALCIUM AND ITS FUNCTIONS	
Body System	**Functions**
Neuromuscular	Normal nerve and muscle activity. Calcium causes transmission of nerve impulses and contraction of skeletal muscles.
Cardiac	Contraction of heart muscle (myocardium).
Cellular and blood	Maintenance of normal cellular permeability. ↑ calcium decreases cellular permeability and ↓ calcium increases cellular permeability. Coagulation of blood. Calcium promotes blood clotting by converting prothrombin into thrombin.
Bones and teeth	Formation of bone and teeth. Calcium and phosphorus make bones and teeth strong and durable.

168 Name five functions of calcium in the body. Refer to Table 3-18 as needed.

a. * _____

b. * _____

c. * _____

d. * _____

e. * _____

a. normal nerve and muscle activity, b. contraction of myocardium, c. maintenance of normal cellular permeability, d. coagulation of blood, and formation of bone and teeth

■   ■   ■

169 A high serum concentration of calcium (increases/decreases) _____ the permeability of membranes, whereas a low serum concentration of calcium (increases/decreases) _____ the permeability of membranes.

decreases; increases

■   ■   ■

170 A calcium deficit causes neuromuscular excitability (tetany symptoms). How does calcium promote blood clotting? * _____ .

Explain how tetany occurs. * _____ .

calcium converts prothrombin into thrombin; calcium deficit causes neuromuscular excitability

■   ■   ■

PATHOPHYSIOLOGY

171 A decrease in the serum calcium level is known as *hypocalcemia*. What do you think an increase in the serum calcium level would be called? _____ .

The normal serum calcium level is * _____ .

hypercalcemia; 4.5–5.5 mEq/L or 9–11 mg/dL

■   ■   ■

172 A serum calcium level less than 4.5 mEq/L is (hypocalcemia/hypercalcemia/normal)
_____ .

A serum calcium level greater than 5.5 mEq/L is known as
(hypocalcemia/hypercalcemia/normal) _____ .

hypocalcemia; hypercalcemia

■   ■   ■

173 Match the serum calcium levels on the left with the type of calcium imbalance or balance.

___ 1. 5.0 mEq/L   a. Hypocalcemia
___ 2. 6.5 mEq/L   b. Hypercalcemia
___ 3. 5.8 mEq/L   c. Normal
___ 4. 4.2 mEq/L
___ 5. 8.2 mg/dL
___ 6. 9.6 mg/dL
___ 7. 11.8 mg/dL

1. c; 2. b; 3. b; 4. a; 5. a; 6. c; 7. b

■   ■   ■

174 When the parathyroid hormone (PTH) level is low, calcium release from the bones is
(increased/inhibited) _____ .

What type of calcium imbalance can occur? _____ .

inhibited; hypocalcemia

■   ■   ■

175 Tissues most affected by hypocalcemia include: peripheral nerves, skeletal and smooth
muscles, and the cardiac muscle.

A prolonged serum calcium deficit leads to osteoporosis, and a marked serum calcium deficit
impairs the clotting time (clot formation).

Neuromuscular excitability of the skeletal, smooth, and cardiac muscles can result from
(hypocalcemia/hypercalcemia) _____ .

A decrease in blood coagulation resulting in bleeding may be due to a serum calcium
(deficit/excess) _____ .

hypocalcemia; deficit

■   ■   ■

176 Hypercalcemia is frequently the result of calcium loss from the bones. Hypophosphatemia (serum phosphorus deficit) promotes calcium retention.

As a result of hypercalcemia, cellular permeability is _____ . (Refer to Table 3-18 as needed.)

decreased

■   ■   ■

177 Increased calcium enhances hydrochloric acid, gastrin, and pancreatic enzyme release. Hypercalcemia decreases GI peristalsis; thus gastrointestinal motility would be (increased/decreased) _____ .

decreased

■   ■   ■

178 Hypercalcemia can decrease the activity of the smooth muscles in the GI system as well as the cardiac muscle activity. Dysrhythmias, heart block, and ECG/EKG changes are likely to occur from hypercalcemia.

Indicate the effects of a calcium deficit (CD) or calcium excess (CE) for the following physiologic changes:

_____ a. Impaired clotting time
_____ b. Decreased GI perstalsis
_____ c. Increased capillary permeability
_____ d. Neuromuscular excitability of skeletal, smooth, and cardiac muscles
_____ e. Decreased cardiac muscle activity
_____ f. Decreased capillary permeability

a. CD; b. CE; c. CD; d. CD; e. CE; f. CE

■   ■   ■

ETIOLOGY

The causes of hypocalcemia and hypercalemia are presented in two separate tables. Table 3-19 lists the etiology and rationale for hypocalcemia and Table 3-20 gives the etiology and rationale for hypercalcemia. Proceed to the frames and refer to the tables as needed.

179 Name three causes of hypocalcemia related to dietary changes.

a. * _____

b. * _____ .

c. * _____ .

lack of calcium intake, inadequate vitamin D intake, and lack of protein in the diet

■   ■   ■

Table 3-19. CAUSES OF HYPOCALCEMIA (SERUM CALCIUM DEFICIT)	
Etiology	**Rationale**
Dietary Changes Lack of calcium intake, inadequate vitamin D, and/or lack of protein in diet	A calcium (Ca) deficit resulting from lack of Ca intake is rare. Vitamin D must be present for calcium absorption from GI tract. Inadequate protein intake inhibits the body's utilization of calcium.
Chronic diarrhea	Chronic diarrhea interferes with adequate calcium absorption.
Renal Dysfunction Renal failure	Renal failure causes phosphorus and calcium retention. Lack of PTH decreases renal calcium absorption.
Hormonal and Electrolyte Influence Decreased PTH Increased serum phosphorus Increased serum magnesium Severe decreased magnesium Increased calcitonin	With hypoparathyroidism, there is less parathyroid hormone (PTH) secreted. Secondary hypoparathyroidism may be caused by sepsis, burns, surgery, or pancreatitis. Overuse of phosphate laxatives can decrease calcium retention. Magnesium imbalances inhibit PTH secretion.
Calcium Binders or Chelators Citrated blood transfusions Alkalosis Increased serum albumin level	Rapid administration of citrated blood binds with calcium, inhibiting ionized (free) Ca. Alkalosis increases calcium protein binding. With an increase in serum albumin, more calcium is bound and less calcium is free and active.

180 What effect does vitamin D insufficiency have on calcium? * _____

_____ .

Vitamin D needs to be present for calcium absorption.

∎   ∎   ∎

181 What effect does an inadequate protein diet have on calcium? * _____

_____ .

It inhibits the body's utilization of calcium.

∎   ∎   ∎

182 Hypoparathyroidism can cause a calcium (deficit/excess) _____ . How?
*_____ .

deficit
Less parathyroid hormone (PTH) is secreted.
       ■   ■   ■

183 Which of the following are effects of insufficient PTH level?

____ a. Calcium release from the bone is inhibited.
____ b. Less calcium is absorbed from the kidney tubules.
____ c. Calcium release from the bone is promoted.
____ d. Calcium absorption from the kidneys is promoted.

a. —; b. X; c. X; d. —
       ■   ■   ■

184 Calcium and phosphorus are regulated by the parathyroid gland, found in many foods, and absorbed together. The serum values of calcium and phosphate (ionized phosphorus) are opposites. With hyperphosphatemia, (hypocalcemia/hypercalcemia) _____ is more likely to occur.

hypocalcemia
       ■   ■   ■

185 What effect does prolonged immobilization have on calcium? *_____
_____ .

It increases serum calcium level by releasing Ca from the bones.
       ■   ■   ■

186 Hypercalcemia occurs because of increased amounts of calcium being released from the bone due to which of the following conditions:

____ a. Fractures
____ b. Immobilization
____ c. Decreased parathyroid hormone (PTH) secretion
____ d. Bone cancer
____ e. Malignancies promoting PTH production

a. X; b. X; c. —; d. X; e. X
       ■   ■   ■

Table 3-20. CAUSES OF HYPERCALCEMIA (SERUM CALCIUM EXCESS)	
Etiology	**Rationale**
Dietary changes: increased calcium salts (supplements)	Excessive use of calcium supplements, calcium salts and antacids can increase the serum calcium level.
Renal impairment, diuretics: thiazides	Kidney dysfunction and use of thiazide diuretics decrease the excretion of calcium.

Cellular destruction
  Bone
  Immobility
	A malignant bone tumor, a fracture, and/or a prolonged immobilization can cause loss of calcium from the bone. Some malignancies cause an ectopic PTH production. Increased immobility promotes calcium loss from the bone.

Hormonal and drug influence
  Increased PTH
  Decreased serum phosphorus
  Steroid therapy
  Thiazide diuretics
	Hyperparathyroidism increases the production of PTH and increased PTH, then promotes the release of calcium from the bone.
	A decreased phosphorus level can increase the serum calcium level to the extent that the kidneys are unable to excrete excess calcium.
	Thiazides increase the action of PTH on kidneys, promoting calcium reabsorption.
	Steroids such as cortisone mobilize calcium absorption from the bone.

187 Multiple fractures cause the release of calcium into the intravascular fluid, thus (increasing/decreasing) _____ the serum calcium level.

increasing

■   ■   ■

188 Loop or high ceiling diuretics (furosemide) decrease the serum calcium level. Thiazide diuretics such as HydroDiuril, (increase/decrease) _____ the serum calcium level.

Hypercalcemia (increases/decreases) _____ cellular permeability.

increase; decreases

■   ■   ■

189 Hypercalcemia occurs in 25–50% of malignancies occurring in the lung, breast, ovaries, prostate, and bladder. These cancers can cause bone destruction due to metastasis or (increased/decreased) _____ ectopic PTH secretion. Why? *_____

_____ .

increased
PTH promotes calcium release from the bones.

■   ■   ■

190 Prolonged steroid therapy can cause increased serum calcium levels. Explain. *_____

_____ .

Prolonged use of steroids mobilizes calcium release from the bone.

■   ■   ■

CLINICAL MANIFESTATIONS

191 Clinical manifestations of hypocalcemia and hypercalcemia are determined by the signs and symptoms of calcium imbalance, ECG/EKG changes, and the serum calcium level.

The normal serum calcium level is _____ mEq/L or _____ mg/dL. Levels less than _____ mEq/L indicate hypocalcemia and those greater than _____ mEq/L indicate hypercalcemia.

4.5–5.5; 9–11; 4.5; 5.5

■   ■   ■

192 A commonly seen clinical manifestation of hypocalcemia is tetany. A calcium deficit causes neuromuscular excitability. With hypocalcemia, the amount of circulating free, ionized calcium is (increased/decreased) _____ .

decreased

■   ■   ■

Table 3-21 lists the clinical manifestations of hypocalcemia and hypercalcemia according to the body areas that are affected. The serum calcium level and the specific ECG changes determine the severity of the calcium imbalance. Study the table and refer to it as needed.

Table 3-21. CLINICAL MANIFESTATIONS OF CALCIUM IMBALANCES

Body Areas	Hypocalcemia	Hypercalcemia

CNS and muscular abnormalities	Anxiety, irritability
	Tetany
	    Twitching around mouth
	    Tingling and numbness of fingers
	    Carpopedal spasm
	    Spasmodic contractions
	    Laryngeal spasm
	    Convulsions
	Abdominal cramps
	Muscle cramps
		Depression/apathy
		Muscles are flabby

Chvostek's sign	Positive	
Trousseau's sign	Positive	
Cardiac abnormalities	Weak cardiac contractions	Signs of heart block Cardiac arrest in systole
ECG/EKG	Lengthened ST segment Prolonged QT interval	Decreased or diminished ST segment Shortened QT interval
Blood abnormalities	Blood does not clot normally, reduction of prothrombin.	
Skeletal abnormalities	Fractures occur if deficit persists.	Pathologic fractures Deep pain over bony areas Thinning of bones apparent
Renal abnormalities		Flank pain Calcium stones formed in the kidney
Milliequivalents per liter	Below 4.5 mEq/L	Above 5.5 mEq/L
Milligrams per deciliter	Below 9.0 mg/dL	Above 11.0 mg/dL

193 Tetany symptoms are due to a decrease in free, (ionized/nonionized) _____
circulating calcium. Symptoms of tetany include which of the following:

____ a. Twitching around the mouth
____ b. Tingling and numbness of the extremities
____ c. Carpopedal spasms
____ d. Laryngeal spasm
____ e. Spasmodic contractions
____ f. Muscular hypertrophy

ionized; a. X; b. X; c. X; d. X; e. X; f. —

■   ■   ■

194 Tetany symptoms are (present/absent) _____ when the client with
hypocalcemia is in an acidotic state (metabolic acidosis). Explain your response. *_____

_____ .

absent
*With metabolic acidosis, more calcium is freed from protein-binding sites. When the acidotic
state is corrected, calcium will bind again with albumin/protein and the tetany symptoms can
occur.*

■   ■   ■

195 Two tests that can confirm severe hypocalcemia with tetany are *_____ and
*_____ .

the Chvostek test and the Trousseau test

■   ■   ■

196 Two tests may be used to test for severe hypocalcemia and presence of tetany. Descriptions of
these are:

Chvostek's sign: The face is tapped over the facial nerve (2 cm anterior to the earlobe). A
positive test results when the facial muscle twitches.
Trousseau's sign: Inflate a blood pressure cuff (20–30 mm Hg) on the upper arm to constrict
circulation. A positive Trousseau is evidenced as the occurrence of a carpopedal spasm of
the fingers and hands within 1–5 minutes.

A positive test for Chvostek and/or Trousseau indicates a calcium (deficit/excess)

_____ .

deficit

■   ■   ■

197 Match the symptoms of hypocalcemia on the left with the appropriate test for tetany.

    ___ 1. Carpopedal spasm   a. Chvostek's sign
    ___ 2. Facial muscle twitching   b. Trousseau's sign

1. b; 2. a

           ■   ■   ■

198 With hypercalcemia, kidney stones (calcium) may occur. This may result when calcium leaves the bones due to immobilization, bone tumors, or increased PTH associated with a secondary malignancy. Increased PTH promotes *_____.

calcium release from the bone

           ■   ■   ■

199 For the following clinical manifestations, indicate which is the result of a calcium deficit (CD) or a calcium excess (CE).

    ___ a. Muscles are flabby
    ___ b. Tetany symptoms
    ___ c. Muscle cramps
    ___ d. Positive Chvostek's sign
    ___ e. Deep pain over bony areas
    ___ f. Kidney stones
    ___ g. Blood does NOT clot normally

a. CE; b. CD; c. CD; d. CD; e. CE; f. CE; g. CD

           ■   ■   ■

The diagrams below note the electrocardiographic changes found with hypocalcemia and hypercalcemia. The normal ECG/EKG tracing is found on pages 102 and 103.
   Note the following ECG changes that may occur with hypocalcemia.

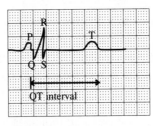

Lengthened ST segment
Prolonged QT interval

Note the following ECG change that may occur with hypercalcemia.

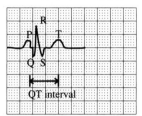

Decreased ST segment
Shortened QT interval

200 The hypocalcemia effect on the ECG causes the ST segment to be _____
and the QT interval to be _____ .

lengthened; prolonged
■   · ■   ■

201 The hypercalcemia effect on the ECG causes the ST segment to be _____
and the QT interval to be _____ .

decreased; shortened
■   ■   ■

DRUGS AND THEIR EFFECT ON CALCIUM BALANCE

Phosphate preparations, corticosteroids, loop diuretics, aspirin, anticonvulsants, magnesium sulfate, and mithramycin are some of the groups of drugs that can lower the serum calcium level. Excess calcium salt ingestion and infusion, and thiazide and chlorthalidone diuretics are drugs that can increase the serum calcium level. Table 3-22 lists drugs that affect calcium balance.

202 Enter CD for calcium deficit/hypocalcemia and CE for calcium excess/hypercalcemia opposite the following drugs. Refer to the table as needed.

(   ) a. Magnesium sulfate
(   ) b. Aspirin
(   ) c. Anticonvulsants
(   ) d. Calcium sulfates
(   ) e. Thiazide diuretics
(   ) f. Corticosteroids
(   ) g. Loop diuretics
(   ) h. Vitamin D
(   ) i. Aminoglycosides

a. CD; b. CD; c. CD; d. CE; e. CE; f. CD; g. CD; h. CE; i. CD
■   ■   ■

Table 3-22.   DRUGS AFFECTING CALCIUM BALANCE

Calcium Imbalance	Drugs	Rationale
Hypocalcemia (serum calcium deficit)	Magnesium sulfate Propylthiouracil/Propacil Colchicine Plicamythin/Mithramycin Neomycin Excessive sodium citrate	These agents inhibit parathyroid hormone/PTH secretion and decrease the serum calcium level.

	Acetazolamide
	Aspirin
	Anticonvulsants
	Glutethimide/Doriden
	Estrogens
	Aminoglycosides
	   Gentamicin
	   Amikacin
	   Tobramycin
		These agents can alter the vitamin D metabolism that is needed for calcium absorption.

	Phosphate preparations:
	oral, enema, and intravenous
	   Sodium phosphate
	   Potassium phosphate
		Phosphates can increase the serum phosphorus level and decrease the serum calcium level.

	Corticosteroids
	   Cortisone
	   Prednisone
		Steroids decrease calcium mobilization and inhibit the absorption of calcium.

	Loop diuretics Furosemide/Lasix	Loop diuretics reduce calcium absorption from the renal tubules.
Hypercalcemia (serum calcium excess)	Calcium salts Vitamin D	Excess ingestion of calcium and vitamin D and infusion of calcium can increase the serum Ca level.
	IV lipids	Lipids can increase the calcium level.

	Kayexalate androgens
	Diuretics
	   Thiazides
	   Chlorthalidone/Hygroten
		These agents can induce hypercalcemia.

203 Mithramycin, an antineoplastic antibiotic, is used to treat hypercalcemia. This agent lowers the serum calcium level.

   Steroids and mithramycin (increase/decrease) _____ the serum calcium level.

decrease

■   ■   ■

204 Hypercalcemia can cause cardiac dysrhythmias. An elevated serum calcium enhances the effect of digitalis and can cause digitalis toxicity.

   Give three signs and symptoms of digitalis toxicity. *_____ , _____ , and _____ .

bradycardia with or without dysrhythmias (slow heart rate), nausea and vomiting, and anorexia

■   ■   ■

205 During a hypercalcemic state should the dose of digitalis preparations, e.g., digoxin, be (increased/decreased)? _____ .

decreased

■   ■   ■

206 Steroids such as cortisone tend to decrease calcium mobilization and inhibit the absorption of calcium.

   Steroids (increase/decrease) _____ the serum calcium level.

decrease

■   ■   ■

207 A loop (high ceiling) diuretic affects the renal tubules by reducing the absorption of calcium and increasing calcium excretion. Identify the name of a loop diuretic.

_____ .

   Name two other electrolytes that are excreted by loop diuretics. _____ and _____ .

Furosemide/Lasix; potassium and sodium

■   ■   ■

CLINICAL MANAGEMENT

Clinical management of hypocalcemia consists of oral supplements and intravenous calcium diluted in 5% dextrose in water (D_5W). Calcium should not be diluted in normal saline solution (0.9% NaCl) since the sodium encourages calcium loss.

The goal of management for hypercalcemia is to correct the underlying cause of the serum calcium excess. Drugs such as calcitonin or IV saline solution administered rapidly and followed by a loop diuretic can be used to promote urinary excretion of calcium. First, calcium replacement for hypocalcemia is discussed and then drug modalities are presented for correcting hypercalcemia.

CALCIUM REPLACEMENT

208 Identify food products high in calcium that can be used to prevent or correct the body's calcium deficit. *_____ .

milk and milk products with vitamin D

■   ■   ■

209 Normally, calcium is not required for IV therapy since there is a tremendous reservoir in the bone. However, the body needs vitamin D for the utilization of dietary calcium.

What other essential composition of the diet is needed for calcium utilization?

_____ .

protein

■   ■   ■

Table 3-23 lists the oral and intravenous preparations of calcium salts and their dosages and drug form. The drugs are listed in alphabetic order. The drug dosage is given in milligrams per gram and indicates the elemental calcium amount within that gram. Study the table carefully and refer to it as needed.

Table 3-23. CALCIUM PREPARATIONS		
Calcium Name	**Drug Form**	**Drug Dose**
Orals		
Calcium carbonate	650–1500 mg tablets	400 mg/g*
Calcium citrate	950 mg tablet	211 mg/g*
Calcium lactate	325–650 mg tablets	130 mg/g*
Calcium gluconate	500–1000 mg tablets	90 mg/g*
Intravenous		
Calcium chloride	10 mL size	272 mg/g*; 13.5 mEq
Calcium gluceptate	5 mL size	90 mg/g*; 4.5 mEq
Calcium gluconate	10 mL size	90 mg/g*; 4.5 mEq

* Elemental calcium is 1 gram (1 g).

210 Asymptomatic hypocalcemia is normally corrected with oral calcium gluconate, calcium lactate, and calcium carbonate. For better calcium absorption, the calcium supplement should be given 30 minutes before meals with a glass of milk. Why milk? *_____

_____ .

Milk contains vitamin D and vitamin D is needed for calcium absorption from the intestine.

∎   ∎   ∎

211 Acute hypocalcemia with tetany symptoms needs immediate correction. Intravenous 10% calcium chloride and 10% calcium gluconate is given slowly, 1–3 mL per minute, to avoid hypotension, bradycardia, and other dysrhythmias.

Calcium chloride provides more ionized calcium than calcium gluconate; however, it is more irritating to the subcutaneous tissue, and if calcium chloride infiltrates, sloughing of the tissue results.

For intravenous administration calcium salts should be diluted in which of the following solution(s):

( ) a. Normal saline (0.9% NaCl)
( ) b. Five percent dextrose in water

a. —; b. X

∎   ∎   ∎

212 When tetany symptoms are present, the physician may order calcium to be administered by a slow intravenous push. Infiltration of intravenous calcium chloride can cause
*_____ .

sloughing of the subcutaneous tissue

∎   ∎   ∎

213 The suggested rate of IV flow for a calcium solution is *_____ . If the rate of IV flow is too rapid, what might occur? *_____ .

1–3 mL per minute; cardiac dysrhythmias (bradycardia), hypotension

∎   ∎   ∎

214 Care should be taken when administering calcium to a client who is taking digoxin daily (digitalis preparation). An elevated serum calcium level enhances the action of digoxin; thus digitalis toxicity can result.

A decreased calcium level (can/cannot) _____ cause digitalis toxicity.

cannot (elevated calcium level enhances the action of digoxin)

∎   ∎   ∎

215 Intravenous calcium salts may be used to counteract the effect of a potassium excess on the heart muscle (myocardium). Would IV calcium (increase/decrease) _____ the effect of hyperkalemia?

What type of ECG improvement should the nurse observe when using calcium supplements to correct hyperkalemia?   *_____ .

decrease; a decrease in the T wave

■   ■   ■

216 Match the calcium preparations on the left with the route of administration. In some cases the calcium salt may be given by more than one route.

____ 1. Calcium citrate   a. Oral
____ 2. Calcium chloride   b. Intravenous
____ 3. Calcium carbonate
____ 4. Calcium lactate
____ 5. Calcium gluconate

1. a; 2. b; 3. a; 4. a; 5. b

■   ■   ■

HYPERCALCEMIA CORRECTION

217 Immediate correction of a moderate and severe serum calcium excess is essential. An intravenous normal saline solution is given rapidly with furosemide (Lasix) to prevent a fluid overload. Explain how this increases the calcium loss.   *_____ .

It promotes urinary calcium excretion.

■   ■   ■

218 Which diuretic promotes urinary calcium excretion?

____ a. Hydrochlorothiazide (HydroDiuril)
____ b. Furosemide (Lasix)

a. —; b. X

■   ■   ■

219 Other drugs that can decrease the serum calcium level are:

a. Calcitonin, a thyroid hormone that inhibits the effects of PTH on the bone and increases urinary calcium excretion

b. Glucocorticoids (Cortisone), which compete with vitamin D, thus decreasing the intestinal absorption of calcium

c. Intravenous phosphates, which promote calcium excretion

The four drugs that may be used to treat hypercalcemia are _____ , _____ , _____ , and *_____ .

furosemide, calcitonin, cortisone, and IV phosphate

■   ■   ■

220 Malignancies are a common cause of hypercalcemia. A metastatic bone lesion can destroy the bone, which releases calcium into the circulation, thus (increasing/decreasing) _____ serum calcium level.

Some cancers promote the secretion of the parathyroid hormone (PTH) and may be referred to as tumor-secreting (ectopic) PTH production. The most common types of cancer that can cause hypercalcemia are lung, breast, ovary, prostate, leukemia, and gastrointestinal cancers.

Parathyroid hormone (increases/decreases) _____ the release of calcium from the _____ .

increasing; increases; bone

■   ■   ■

221 The antitumor antibiotic plicamycin (mithramycin) inhibits the action of PTH on osteoclasts in bone. The result of this drug action is a(n) (increase/decrease) _____ in serum calcium level.

decrease

■   ■   ■

CLINICAL APPLICATIONS

222 For body utilization, calcium must be in the ionized form. In body fluids, calcium is found in both ionized and nonionized (bound to plasma proteins) forms.

In an alkalotic state (body fluids are more alkaline), large amounts of the calcium become protein bound and cannot be utilized. If the body fluids were more acid (acidotic state), calcium is more likely to be (ionized/nonionized)? _____ .

ionized (hence calcium could be utilized)

■   ■   ■

223 Calcium acts like a sedative on the central nervous system (CNS).

Let us say you are caring for a debilitated client who becomes severely agitated. You notice the client's hands trembling and mouth twitching. These symptoms may indicate a calcium (excess/deficit) _____ .

Identify three important nursing actions.

a. * _____

b. * _____

c. * _____ .

deficit;
a. check the lab report on serum calcium
b. notify physician of symptoms and lab report
c. check client's dietary intake of Ca

■   ■   ■

224 Lack of calcium causes neuromuscular irritability. Explain. * _____

_____ .

What does hypocalcemia do to blood clotting? * _____ .

It leads to hyperactivity of the nervous system and painful muscular contractions (symptoms of tetany).
It decreases clotting and causes bleeding.

■   ■   ■

225 Prolonged vomiting leads to alkalosis due to the loss of hydrogen and chloride ions from the stomach.

When the body fluids are alkaline, what happens to calcium? * _____

_____ .

Calcium is ionized poorly and hypocalcemia can occur, especially with a decrease in calcium intake

■   ■   ■

226 Acidosis (increases/decreases) _____ the ionization of calcium.

increases

■   ■   ■

227 Describe a positive Trousseau's sign.

*_____

_____ .

Describe a positive Chvostek's sign.

*_____

_____ .

positive Trousseau's sign—_carpopedal spasm after blood pressure cuff is inflated for 3 minutes or a similar response_
positive Chvostek's sign—_spasms of the cheek and corner of the lip after tapping the facial nerve or a similar response_
■ ■ ■

228 The kidneys excrete approximately 50–250 mg/dL of calcium in the urine daily. If the kidneys excrete less than 50 mg/dL, what type of calcium imbalance is likely to occur?

_____ .

hypercalcemia
■ ■ ■

229 The nursing action for a client with hypercalcemia is to prevent renal calculi. There are three ways this can be accomplished:

a. Drink at least 12 glasses of fluid a day.
b. Keep urine acid.
c. Prevent urinary tract infections.

How do you think the urine can be kept acid? *_____

_____ .

Eat foods that are high in acid content (meat, fish, poultry, eggs, cheese, peanuts, cereals) and/or drink at least 1 pint (2 glasses) or cranberry juice daily. Orange juice does not make the urine acid.
■ ■ ■

CASE STUDY REVIEW

Mr. Morgan, age 58, has had a gastric upset for the past 6 weeks. He has been taking antacids and drinking several glasses of milk each day. His stomach discomfort was not relieved and he was admitted to the hospital for further diagnostic study. A possible malignant neoplasm was to be determined. His serum calcium was 5.9 mEq/L.

1. His serum calcium level indicates what type of calcium imbalance? _____ .
2. The "normal" range for calcium balance is *_____ .

3. Explain what happens to body calcium when there is a decrease in gastric acidity and an increase in body alkaline fluids. *_____

_____ .

4. Give four functions of calcium in the body.
   a. *_____
   b. *_____
   c. *_____
   d. *_____

5. If Mr. Morgan was bedridden, would you expect his serum calcium to be (elevated/decreased)? _____ . Explain. *_____

_____ .

6. Identify a symptom that can occur from immobilization. *_____ .

7. Identify three nursing interventions to prevent renal calculi resulting from hypercalcemia.
   a. *_____
   b. *_____
   c. *_____

8. Previously, Mr. Morgan has a "heart condition" and he was started on digoxin. What effect does hypercalcemia have on digoxin?
   *_____ .

   Should his Digoxin dosage be (increased/decreased) _____ until his hypercalcemic state is corrected?

9. If Mr. Morgan's serum calcium became 3.9 mEq/L, what type of calcium imbalance would be present? _____ .

10. Identify five common signs and symptoms of hypocalcemia. _____ ,
   *_____ , *_____ , *_____ , and
   *_____ .

1. hypercalcemia
2. 4.5–5.5 mEq/L or 9–11 mg/dL
3. Decrease in ionized calcium for utilization. In alkaline fluids, calcium is nonionized and protein bound. An elevated serum calcium can result from large amounts of milk intake and from a malignant neoplasm. A variety of neoplasms (tumors) can cause hypercalcemia.
4. a. maintenance of normal cell permeability
   b. formation of bone and teeth
   c. normal clotting mechanism
   d. normal muscle and nerve activity
5. Elevated. Prolonged immobilization would increase the serum calcium by releasing calcium from the bones
6. kidney stones
7. a. drink at least 12 glasses of fluid a day
   b. eat foods high in acid content to keep urine acid
   c. prevent urinary tract infections
8. Hypercalcemia enhances the action of digoxin, making it more powerful; decreased.
9. hypocalcemia
10. Carpopedal spasm, twitching of the mouth, tingling of the fingers, spasm of the larynx, and abdominal cramps, also muscle cramps

HYPOCALCEMIA

NURSING ASSESSMENT FACTORS

- Obtain a nursing history to identify potential causes of hypocalcemia: insufficient diet in protein and calcium, lack of vitamin D intake, chronic diarrhea, hormonal influence [decreased parathyroid hormone (PTH)], drug influence, hypoparathyroidism, metabolic alkalotic state, and rapid administration of a blood transfusion that contains citrate.
- Assess for signs and symptoms of hypocalcemia, i.e., tetany symptoms (twitching around mouth, carpopedal spasms, laryngospasms), abdominal cramps, and muscle cramps.
- Obtain a serum calcium level that can be used as a baseline for comparison of future serum calcium levels. A serum calcium level below 4.5 mEq/L or 9 mg/dL indicates hypocalcemia.
- Check the ECG/EKG strips for changes in the QT interval. A prolonged QT interval may indicate a serum calcium deficit.
- Identify drugs the client is taking that may cause a serum calcium deficit, such as, furosemide (Lasix), cortisone preparations, phosphate preparations, and massive use of antacids that can interfere with calcium absorption.
- Determine the acid-base status when hypocalcemia is present. In an acidotic state, calcium is ionized and can be utilized by the body even though there is a calcium deficit. This is not true when alkalosis occurs. Calcium is not ionized in an alkalotic state; and if a calcium deficit is present, tetany symptoms occur.
- Assess for positive Trousseau's and Chvostek's signs of hypocalcemia. For Trousseau's sign, inflate the blood pressure cuff for 3 minutes and observe for a carpopedal spasm. For Chvostek's sign, tap the facial nerve in front of the ear for spasms of the cheek and mouth.

NURSING DIAGNOSIS 1

Nutrition: altered, less than body requirements, related to insufficient calcium intake, poor calcium absorption due to insufficient vitamin D and protein intake, or drugs (antacids, cortisone preparation) that interfere with calcium ionization.

NURSING INTERVENTIONS AND RATIONALE

1. Monitor serum calcium levels. A serum calcium level under 4.5 mEq/L can cause neuromuscular excitability. Tetany symptoms may occur.
2. Monitor ECG and note changes related to hypocalcemia, i.e., prolonged QT interval and lengthened ST segment.
3. Monitor IV solutions containing calcium frequently to prevent infiltration. Calcium is irritating to the subcutaneous tissues and can cause tissue sloughing.
4. Administer oral calcium supplements an hour before meals to enhance intestinal absorption.
5. Regulate IV 10% calcium gluconate or chloride in a liter of 5% dextrose in water (D_5W) to run 1–3 mL per minute, or according to the physician's order. Do not administer calcium salts in a normal saline solution (0.9% NaCl). The sodium encourages calcium loss.
6. Teach clients to eat foods rich in calcium, vitamin D, and protein, especially the older adult. Explain the importance of calcium in the diet to prevent osteoporosis and to aid normal clot formation. Tell the client that protein is needed to aid in calcium absorption. Nonfat dry milk can be used to meet calcium requirements.

7. Teach "bowel-conscious" persons that chronic use of laxatives can increase intestinal motility, which prevents calcium absorption from the intestine. Suggest fruits for bowel elimination, instead of laxatives.
8. Explain to persons using antacids that constant use of antacids can decrease calcium in the body. Antacids decrease acidity, which decreases calcium ionization.
9. Monitor the pulse regularly for bradycardia when the client is receiving digitalis and calcium, either orally or intravenously. Increased serum calcium enhances the action of digitalis, and digitalis toxicity can result.

NURSING DIAGNOSIS 2

High risk for injury: bleeding, related to the interference with blood coagulation secondary to calcium loss.

NURSING INTERVENTIONS AND RATIONALE

1. Check for prolonged bleeding or reduced clot formation. A low serum calcium level inhibits the production of prothrombin, which is needed in clot formation.
2. Observe for symptoms of hypocalcemia in clients receiving massive transfusions of citrated blood. The serum calcium level may not be affected, but the citrates prevent calcium ionization.

HYPERCALCEMIA

NURSING ASSESSMENT FACTORS

- Obtain a nursing history to identify probable causes of hypercalcemia, such as excessive use of calcium supplements, bone destruction due to cancer, cancer of the breast, lung, or prostate (ectopic PTH production), prolonged immobilization, multiple fractures, hormone influence (increased PTH, steroid therapy), hyperparathyroidism, and thiazide diuretics. Approximately 20–25% of hypercalcemia is due to continuous use of large doses of thiazide diuretics.
- Assess for signs and symptoms of hypercalcemia, i.e., flabby muscles, pain over bony areas, renal calculi, and pathologic fractures.
- Check ECG/EKG strips for changes in the QT interval. A shortened QT interval may indicate a serum calcium excess.
- Obtain a serum calcium level that can be used as a baseline for comparison of future serum calcium levels. A serum calcium level above 5.5 mEq/L or 11 mg/dL indicates hypercalcemia.
- Assess for fluid volume depletion and changes in the state of the client's sensorium. These changes may be indicators of hypercalcemia.

NURSING DIAGNOSIS 1

High risk for injury, related to pathologic fractures due to bone destruction from bone cancer, prolonged immobilization.

NURSING INTERVENTIONS AND RATIONALE

1. Monitor serum calcium levels. Report increased serum calcium levels. Levels exceeding 13.0 mg/dL can be life threatening.

2. Monitor ECG and note changes related to hypercalcemia, i.e., shortened QT interval and decreased ST segment.
3. Monitor client's state of sensorium. Extreme lethargy, confusion, and a comatose state may be the result of hypercalcemia. Safety precautions may be needed.
4. Promote active and passive exercise for bedridden clients. Immobilization promotes calcium loss from the bone.
5. Handle clients gently who have long-standing hypercalcemia and bone demineralization to prevent fractures.
6. Identify symptoms of digitalis toxicity . When the client has an elevated serum calcium level and is receiving a digitalis preparation such as digoxin, digitalis toxicity may occur. Elevated serum calcium enhances the action of digitalis. Symptoms of digitalis toxicity include: bradycardia, nausea, and/or vomiting.

NURSING DIAGNOSIS 2

Nutrition: altered, more than the body requirements, related to excess calcium intake.

NURSING INTERVENTIONS AND RATIONALE

1. Instruct clients with hypercalcemia to avoid foods rich in calcium and to avoid taking massive amounts of vitamin D supplements.
2. Teach clients with hypercalcemia to keep hydrated, in order to increase calcium dilution in the serum and urine and to prevent renal calculi formation.
3. Explain to clients with hypercalcemia that the purpose for maintaining an acid urine is to increase solubility of calcium. An acid-ash diet may be ordered that includes meats, fish, poultry, eggs, cheese, cereals, nuts, cranberry juice, and prune juice. Orange juice will not change the urine pH.

NURSING DIAGNOSIS 3

Urinary elimination, altered patterns of urinary excretion, related to causes of hypercalcemia.

NURSING INTERVENTIONS AND RATIONALE

1. Monitor urinary output and urine pH. Calcium precipitates in alkaline urine and renal calculi may result. Acid-ash foods and juices such as cranberry and prune juices should be encouraged to increase the acidity of the urine.
2. Instruct clients to increase fluid intake to dilute the serum and urine levels of calcium to prevent formation of renal calculi.
3. Administer prescribed loop diuretics to enhance calcium excretion. Thiazide diuretics inhibit calcium excretion and are not indicated in hypercalcemia.

MAGNESIUM

INTRODUCTION

230 Magnesium (Mg), the second most plentiful intracellular cation, has similar functions, causes of imbalances, and clinical manifestations as potassium. Approximately one half (50%) of the body's magnesium is contained in the bone, 49% in the body cells (intracellular fluid), and 1% in the extracellular fluid. The normal serum magnesium level is 1.5–2.5 mEq/L or 1.8–3.0 mg/dL.

Magnesium is a(n) (anion/cation) _____ . Its highest concentration is found in what type of body fluid? _____ .

cation; intracellular

  ■   ■   ■

231 What other cation has its highest concentration in the intracellular fluid? _____ .

potassium

  ■   ■   ■

232 Magnesium is widely distributed throughout the body. Half of the body magnesium is in the bone. What other ion is found plentifully in the bone? _____ .

calcium

  ■   ■   ■

233 Magnesium has a higher concentration in the cerebrospinal fluid, also known as spinal fluid, than in the blood plasma. The serum concentration of magnesium is *_____.

1.5–2.5 mEq/L or 1.8–3.0 mg/dL

  ■   ■   ■

234 One third of magnesium is protein bound and approximately two thirds is ionized, free magnesium that can be utilized by the body. Magnesium is absorbed from the small intestine. Sixty percent of magnesium is excreted in the feces (magnesium that was not absorbed) and 40% is excreted through the kidneys.

Magnesium is excreted via _____ and _____ .

feces and kidneys

  ■   ■   ■

235 The minimum daily magnesium requirement is 200–300 mg for an adult and 150 mg for an infant. Many of the same foods that are rich in potassium are also rich in magnesium. These foods include: green vegetables, whole grains, fish and seafood, and nuts.

If your client has a magnesium deficit, name three foods rich in magnesium that the client should include in his or her diet.

a. *_____ .

b. *_____ .

c. *_____ .

a. green vegetables; b. whole grains; c. and fish and seafood

      ■   ■   ■

236 A serum magnesium level of less than 1.5 mEq/L is known as (hypomagnesemia/hypermagnesemia) _____ . A serum magnesium level of greater than 2.5 mEq/L is called _____ .

hypomagnesemia; hypermagnesemia

      ■   ■   ■

FUNCTIONS

Table 3-24 describes the various functions of magnesium. Study the table and refer to it as needed.

Table 3-24. MAGNESIUM AND ITS FUNCTIONS	
Body System	**Functions**
Neuromuscular	Transmits neuromuscular activity. Important mediator of neural transmission in CNS.
Cardiac	Contracts the heart muscle (myocardium).
Cellular	Activates many enzymes for proper carbohydrate and protein metabolism. Responsible for the transportation of sodium and potassium across cell membranes. Influences utilization of potassium, calcium, and protein. When there is a magnesium deficit, there is frequently a potassium and/or calcium deficit.

237 Magnesium plays an important role in enzyme activity. An *enzyme* is a catalyst capable of inducing chemical changes in other substances. Magnesium acts as a coenzyme in the metabolism of carbohydrates and protein.

Magnesium is also involved in maintaining neuromuscular stability. What other ion has this similar function? _____ .

calcium

      ■   ■   ■

238 Indicate which of the following are functions of magnesium:

( ) a. Neuromuscular activity
( ) b. Contraction of the myocardium
( ) c. Exchange of CO_2 and O_2
( ) d. Enzyme activity
( ) e. Responsibility (partial) for Na and K crossing cell membranes

a. X; b. X; c. —; d. X; e. X

■   ■   ■

239 When there is a magnesium deficit, what two other cations may also be decreased?
_____ and _____ .

potassium and calcium

■   ■   ■

PATHOPHYSIOLOGY

240 Magnesium maintains neuromuscular function. A serum magnesium deficit increases the release of acetylcholine from the presynaptic membrane of the nerve fiber. This increases neuromuscular excitability.

A serum magnesium excess has a sedative effect on the neuromuscular system which may result in a loss of deep tendon reflexes.

Indicate which neuromuscular function may occur from the magnesium imbalances listed on the left.

___ 1. Hypomagnesemia   a. Hyperexcitability
___ 2. Hypermagnesemia   b. Inhibition

1. a (due to increased release of acetylcholine); 2. b (causing a sedative effect)

■   ■   ■

241 Cardiac dysrhythmias can result from a serum magnesium deficit. Tachycardia, hypertension, and ventricular fibrillation may result from hypomagnesemia. Hypotension and heart block may result from hypermagnesemia.

What is the most serious cardiac dysfunction that might occur from hypomagnesemia?
*_____ .

From hypermagnesemia? *_____ .

ventricular fibrillation; heart block

■   ■   ■

242 In the gastrointestinal tract, an increase in calcium absorption causes a decrease in magnesium absorption and an increase in magnesium excretion.

What is likely to occur with decreased calcium absorption? *_____

magnesium absorption is increased

■   ■   ■

243 Magnesium inhibits the release of the parathyroid hormone (PTH). A decrease in the release of PTH (increases/decreases) _____ the amount of calcium released from the bone. This can cause a calcium (excess/deficit) _____ .

decreases; deficit

■   ■   ■

244 Match the serum magnesium levels on the left with the type of magnesium imbalance or balance.

___ 1. 1.2 mEq/L   a. Normal serum magnesium level
___ 2. 2.0 mEq/L   b. Hypomagnesemia
___ 3. 2.3 mEq/L   c. Hypermagnesemia
___ 4. 2.9 mEq/L
___ 5. 1.0 mEq/L
___ 6. 3.6 mEq/L

1. b; 2. a; 3. a; 4. c; 5. b; 6. c

■   ■   ■

ETIOLOGY

Hypomagnesemia is probably the most undiagnosed electrolyte deficiency. This is most likely due to the fact that hypomagnesemia is asymptomatic until the serum magnesium level approaches 1.0 mEq/L. The total serum magnesium concentration is not representative of the cellular magnesium levels. This is why many clients with hypomagnesemia are asymptomatic. Clients with hypokalemia or hypocalcemia who do not respond to potassium and/or calcium replacement may also have hypomagnesemia. Correction of the magnesium deficit is necessary when correcting serum potassium and serum calcium imbalances.

The causes of hypomagnesemia and hypermagnesemia are presented in two tables. Table 3-25 lists the etiology and rationale for hypomagnesemia and Table 3-26 lists the etiology and rationale for hypermagnesemia. After studying the tables, proceed to the frames. Refer to the tables as needed.

245 Magnesium is found in various foods, but prolonged inadequate nutrient intake can cause (hypomagnesemia/hypermagnesemia) _____ .

hypomagnesemia

■   ■   ■

Table 3-25.   CAUSES OF HYPOMAGNESEMIA (SERUM MAGNESIUM DEFICIT)

Etiology	Rationale
Dietary Changes Inadequate intake, poor absorption. GI losses Malnutrition, Starvation	Magnesium is found in various foods, e.g., green, leafy vegetables and whole grains. Inadequate nutrition can result in a magnesium deficit.
Total parenteral nutrition (TPN, hyperalimentation)	Continuous use of TPN without magnesium supplement can cause a magnesium deficit.
Chronic alcoholism Increased calcium intake	Alcoholism promotes inadequate food intake and GI loss of magnesium. Calcium absorption promotes magnesium loss in feces.
Chronic diarrhea, intestinal fistulas, chronic use of laxatives	Chronic diarrhea impairs magnesium absorption. Prolonged use of laxatives can cause a magnesium deficit.
Renal Dysfunction Diuresis: diabetic ketoacidosis	Diuresis due to diabetic ketoacidosis causes magnesium loss via the kidneys.
Acute renal failure (ARF)	ARF in the diuretic phase promotes magnesium loss.
Cardiac Dysfunction Acute myocardial infarction (AMI)	Hypomagnesemia may occur during the first to the fifth day post-acute MI.
Congestive heart failure (CHF)	Prolonged diuretic therapy for CHF can cause a magnesium deficit.
Electrolyte Influence Hypokalemia Hypocalcemia	The cations potassium and calcium are interrelated with magnesium action. Hypomagnesemia can occur with hypokalemia and hypocalcemia.
Drug Influence Aminoglycosides, potassium-wasting diuretics, cortisone, amphotericin B, digitalis	These drugs promote the loss of magnesium. Hypomagnesemia enhances the action of digitalis; digitalis toxicity may result.

246 Chronic alcoholism is a leading cause and problem of hypomagnesemia. This results from GI losses due to diarrhea and poor absorption and is due to *_____ .

Chronic diarrhea is attributed to hypomagnesemia. Why? *_____

_____ .

inadequate nutritional intake; because of impaired magnesium absorption

    ■   ■   ■

247 The diuretics that promote magnesium loss are the (potassium-wasting diuretics/potassium sparing diuretics) _____ .

When does acute renal failure cause hypomagnesemia? *_____ .

potassium-wasting diuretics; during the diuretic phase of acute renal failure (ARF)

    ■   ■   ■

248 Two cardiac causes of hypomagnesemia are acute myocardial infarction (AMI) and
*_____ .

During what period of time during the AMI does a serum magnesium deficit occur?
*_____ .

congestive heart failure (CHF); 1–5 days post-AMI

    ■   ■   ■

249 Hypokalemia and hypocalcemia may be present along with hypomagnesemia. Can hypokalemia and hypocalcemia be corrected without correcting hypomagnesemia? _____ .
Explain. *_____

_____ .

No. Large doses of potassium and calcium supplements do not fully correct hypokalemia and hypocalcemia unless the magnesium deficit is also being corrected with a magnesium supplement.

    ■   ■   ■

250 Indicate which of the following are causes of hypomagnesemia.

_____ 1. Chronic alcoholism

_____ 2. Chronic use of laxatives

_____ 3. Potassium-sparing diuretics

_____ 4. Hyperkalemia

_____ 5. Increased calcium intake

_____ 6. Malnutrition

_____ 7. Diuresis due to diabetic ketoacidosis

_____ 8. Magnesium-containing antacids

_____ 9. Continuous TPN or salt-free IV fluids

1. X; 2. X; 3. —; 4. —; 5. X; 6. X; 7. X; 8. —; 9. X

Table 3-26. CAUSES OF HYPERMAGNESEMIA (SERUM MAGNESIUM EXCESS)	
Etiology	**Rationale**
Dietary Changes Excessive administration of magnesium products IV Magnesium sulfate Antacids with magnesium Laxatives with magnesium	Hypermagnesemia rarely occurs unless there is a prolonged excess use of magnesium-containing antacids (Maalox), laxatives (milk of magnesia), and IV magnesium sulfate.
Renal Dysfunction Renal insufficiency Renal failure	Renal insufficiency or failure inhibits the excretion of magnesium.
Severe Dehydration Diabetic ketoacidosis	Loss of body fluids due to diuresis from diabetic ketoacidosis causes a hemoconcentration of magnesium. This can result in an increased magnesium level.

251 When magnesium-containing antacids and laxatives are taken continuously for a prolonged period of time, what type of magnesium imbalance is likely to occur? _____ .

   Name an antacid that can cause magnesium excess when used for a prolonged period of time or in conjunction with renal impairment? _____ .

   Name a laxative that if used constantly can cause magnesium excess, especially if there is renal impairment? *_____

_____ .

hypermagnesemia or magnesium excess; Maalox (also Mylanta); milk of magnesia (MOM), also magnesium sulfate (Epsom salt)

■   ■   ■

252 Approximately one half of magnesium is excreted via the kidneys. With renal insufficiency, the serum magnesium level is (increased/decreased) _____ .

   What other electrolyte is primarily excreted in the urine? _____ .

increased; potassium

■   ■   ■

253 Place a D for magnesium deficit and an E for magnesium excess in the following:

( ) a. Renal insufficiency
( ) b. Prolonged diuresis
( ) c. Constant use of Epsom salt or milk of magnesia
( ) d. Chronic alcoholism
( ) e. Malnutrition
( ) f. Prolonged inadequate nutrient intake
( ) g. Severe diarrhea
( ) h. Constant use of antacids with magnesium hydroxide

a. E; b. D; c. E; d. D; e. D; f. D; g. D; h. E

■   ■   ■

CLINICAL MANIFESTATIONS

254 The normal serum magnesium level is *_____ .

   A serum magnesium level less than _____ mEq/L is known as hypomagnesemia.

   For hypermagnesemia to occur, the serum magnesium level should be greater than _____ mEq/L.

1.5–2.5 mEq/L or 1.8–3.0 mg/dL; 1.5; 2.5

■   ■   ■

255 Severe magnesium imbalance occurs when the serum magnesium level is below 1.0 mEq/L and above 10.0 mEq/L. A cardiac arrest may result with a severe magnesium imbalance.

Severe serum magnesium deficit and excess are life threatening and need immediate action. Would a serum magnesium deficit of 1.3 mEq/L be life threatening? _____ .

For severe hypermagnesemia to be life threatening, the serum magnesium level is

* _____ .

no; greater than 10 mEq/L

■   ■   ■

Table 3-27 lists the clinical manifestations of hypomagnesemia and hypercalcemia according to the body area affected. The serum magnesium level and the ECG determine the severity of the magnesium imbalance. Study the table carefully and refer to it as needed.

Table 3-27. CLINICAL MANIFESTATIONS OF MAGNESIUM IMBALANCE		
Body Areas	**Hypomagnesemia**	**Hypermagnesemia**

Neuromuscular abnormalities	Hyperirritability
	Tetanylike symptoms
	    Tremors
	    Twitching of face
	    Spasticity
	    Increased tendon reflexes
		CNS depression
		    lethargy, drowsiness, weakness,
		    paralysis
		    Loss of deep tendon reflexes

Cardiac abnormalities	Hypertension
	Cardiac dysrhythmias
	    Premature ventricular contractions
	    Ventricular tachycardia
	    Ventricular fibrillation
		Hypotension (if severe, profound hypotension)
		Complete heart block

ECG/EKG	Flat or inverted T wave Depressed ST segment	Widening QRS complex Prolonged QT interval
Others		Flushing Respiratory depression

256 Magnesium influences the nervous system; too much or not enough magnesium affects the neuromuscular function.

Hyperirritability, tremors, and twitching of the face are signs and symptoms of

_____ .

Lethargy, drowsiness, and loss of deep tendon reflexes are signs and symptoms of

_____ .

hypomagnesemia; hypermagnesemia

■   ■   ■

257 Central nervous system depression, inhibited neuromuscular transmission, decreased respiration, and lethargy are signs and symptoms of _____ .

hypermagnesemia

■   ■   ■

258 Match the cardiac signs and symptoms on the left to a magnesium deficit or excess:

_____ 1. Hypotension   a. Hypomagnesemia
_____ 2. Ventricular tachycardia   b. Hypermagnesemia
_____ 3. PVC (Premature ventricular contraction)
_____ 4. Heart block

1. b; 2. a; 3. a; 4. b

■   ■   ■

259 Place a D for hypomagnesemia and an E for hypermagnesemia beside the following signs and symptoms:

( ) a. Hyperirritability
( ) b. CNS depression
( ) c. Lethargy
( ) d. Tremors
( ) e. Twitching of the face
( ) f. Convulsion
( ) g. Decreased respiration
( ) h. Loss of deep tendon reflexes
( ) i. Ventricular fibrillation

a. D; b. E; c. E; d. D; e. D; f. D; g. E; h. E; i. D

■   ■   ■

DRUGS AND THEIR EFFECT ON MAGNESIUM BALANCE

260 Long-term administration of saline infusions may result in magnesium and calcium loss.

Can you explain why long-term or excessive use of saline infusions can cause magnesium and calcium deficits? *_____

It expands the extracellular fluid (ECF), causes dilution, and inhibits tubular absorption of Mg and Ca.

■   ■   ■

Diuretics, antibiotics, laxatives, and digitalis are groups of drugs that promote magnesium loss (hypomagnesemia). Excess intake of magnesium salts is the major cause of serum magnesium excess (hypermagnesemia). Table 3-28 lists drugs that affect magnesium balance.

Table 3-28.   DRUGS AFFECTING MAGNESIUM BALANCE

Magnesium Imbalance	Drugs	Rationale

Hypomagnesemia (serum magnesium deficit)	Diuretics
	  Furosemide/Lasix
	  Ethacrynic acid/Edecrin
	  Mannitol
		Diuretics promote urinary loss of magnesium.

	Antibiotics
	  Gentamicin
	  Tobramycin
	  Carbenicillin
	  Capreomycin
	  Neomycin
	  Polymyxin B
	  Amphotericin B
	Digitalis
	Calcium gluconate
	Insulin
		These agents can cause magnesium loss via kidney.

	Laxatives Cisplatin	Laxative abuse causes magnesium loss via GI.

	Corticosteroids
	  Cortisone
	  Prednisone
		Steroids can decrease serum magnesium level.

Hypermagnesemia (serum magnesium excess)	Magnesium salts:
	Oral and enema
	  Magnesium hydroxide/MOM
	  Magnesium sulfate/Epsom salt
	  Magnesium citrate
	  Magnesium sulfate (maternity)
		Excess use of magnesium salts could increase serum magnesium level.

		Use of excess $MgSO_4$ in treatment of toxemia could cause hypermagnesemia.
	Lithium	Hypermagnesemia associated with lithium.

261 Place MD for magnesium deficit/hypomagnesemia and ME for magnesium excess/hypermagnesemia beside the following drugs:

___ a. Furosemide/Lasix
___ b. Tobramycin
___ c. Magnesium hydroxide/MOM
___ d. Digitalis
___ e. Magnesium sulfate for toxemia
___ f. Laxatives
___ g. Cortisone
___ h. Lithium

a. MD; b. MD; c. ME; d. MD; e. ME; f. MD; g. MD; h. ME
∎   ∎   ∎

262 Excessive use of steroids (corticosteroids) can cause hypomagnesemia.

A decrease in the adrenal cortical hormone can cause (hypomagnesemia/hypermagnesemia).

_____ .

hypermagnesemia. GOOD.
∎   ∎   ∎

263 Hypomagnesemia enhances the action of digitalis and causes digitalis toxicity. Magnesium sulfate will correct hypomagnesemia and symptoms of digitalis toxicity.

Give at least three symptoms of digitalis toxicity.   *_____ ,
_____ , and _____ .

What other electrolyte (cation) deficit can cause digitalis toxicity? _____ .

nausea and vomiting, anorexia, and bradycardia; potassium
∎   ∎   ∎

CLINICAL MANAGEMENT

Clinical management of hypomagnesemia may be corrected by a diet consisting of green vegetables, legumes, nuts (peanut butter), and fruits. Oral or intravenous magnesium salts may be prescribed when there is a marked to severe magnesium deficit.

For hypermagnesemia, correcting the underlying cause and using intravenous saline or calcium salts decreases the magnesium level. First, magnesium replacement for hypomagnesemia is discussed and then drug modalities are presented for correcting hypermagnesemia.

MAGNESIUM REPLACEMENT

264 Oral magnesium comes as sulfate, gluconate, chloride, citrate, and hydroxide in liquid, tablet, and powder form.

For magnesium supplement for maintenance or replacement, magnesium gluconate/Magonate and magnesium-protein complex/Mg-PLUS may be ordered by the physician.

For severe hypomagnesemia do you think the physician would order magnesium replacement to be administered (orally/intramuscularly/intravenously)? _____ . Why?

_____ .

intravenously
It is a direct and quick method for replacing serum magnesium deficit.

      ■   ■   ■

265 Magnesium sulfate is the parenteral replacement for hypomagnesemia and can be administered intramuscularly or intravenously. The drug is available in strengths of 10, 12.5, and 50%. Many physicians order 10 mL of a 50% solution for adults.

For intramuscular injections the dosage is divided and for intravenous infusion the dosage is diluted into 1 liter of solution. The two injectable routes in which magnesium sulfate can be delivered to the body are _____ and _____ .

intramuscular and intravenous

      ■   ■   ■

HYPERMAGNESEMIA CORRECTION

266 For temporary correction of a serum magnesium excess, the intravenous electrolytes _____ or *_____ may be prescribed.

If hypermagnesemia is due to renal failure, dialysis may be necessary. Ventilatory assistance may be needed if respiratory distress is present.

saline (sodium chloride); calcium salt

      ■   ■   ■

267 Intravenous calcium is an (agonist/antagonist) _____ to magnesium; therefore, calcium can (increase/decrease) _____ the symptoms of hypermagnesemia.

antagonist; decrease

      ■   ■   ■

268 If renal failure is the cause of the severe hypermagnesemia, what is the best course to correct this imbalance? _____ .

dialysis

■   ■   ■

CLINICAL APPLICATIONS

Hypomagnesemia is frequently an undiagnosed problem which surfaces when the client is hospitalized, critically ill, or not responding to correction of hypokalemia or hypocalcemia. Approximately 65% of clients with normal renal function in intensive care units (ICUs) have a low serum magnesium level. Over 40% of the clients with hypomagnesemia also have hypokalemia. Twenty percent of the elderly have a decreased serum magnesium level.

269 When a client is being treated for hypokalemia and is not responding to therapy, the serum magnesium should be checked. If a magnesium deficit is present, hypokalemia (will/will not) _____ be completely corrected.

will not

■   ■   ■

270 The kidneys regulate the concentration of magnesium in the body. When there is a slight increase in the magnesium concentration, the kidneys will excrete the excess. If there is a decreased serum magnesium level, what do you think the kidneys will do? *_____
_____ .

If a client has renal insufficiency and is receiving magnesium sulfate, what type of magnesium imbalance can occur? _____ .
Why? *_____ .

Kidneys conserve Mg or Mg is reabsorbed from the kidney tubules—not excreted;
hypermagnesemia;
Kidneys regulate Mg balance—cannot excrete it.

■   ■   ■

271 For clients on prolonged hyperalimentation (TPN), the serum magnesium level should be checked.

What type of magnesium imbalance can occur when magnesium is not included in the solutions for TPN? _____ .

hypomagnesemia

■   ■   ■

272 Magnesium is needed by the heart for myocardial contractions. It is said that magnesium slows the rate of the atrium and corrects atrial flutter.

Electrocardiographic changes due to magnesium imbalances are similar to potassium imbalances. With hypomagnesemia, the T wave can be *_____ and the ST segment _____ .

flat or inverted; depressed

■   ■   ■

273 In diabetic acidosis, magnesium leaves the cells. When insulin and dextrose are given intravenously, magnesium returns to the cells.

If the diabetic condition is corrected too fast, then (hypomagnesemia/hypermagnesemia) _____ occurs. Why? *_____
_____ .

hypomagnesemia
Magnesium leaves the ECF rapidly and returns to the cells.

■   ■   ■

CASE STUDY REVIEW

Mrs. Landis has had diuresis for several days. In the hospital her diagnoses were prolonged diuresis, severe dehydration, and malnutrition. She received 3 liters of 5% dextrose in ½ of normal saline (0.45% NaCl). Her serum magnesium was 1.3 mEq/L.

1. What is the "normal" serum magnesium range? *_____ .
2. Name the type of magnesium imbalance present. _____ .
3. Mrs. Landis received fluids intravenously. Explain the relationship of IV fluids to magnesium deficit. *_____
_____ .
4. Name two clinical causes of hypermagnesemia. *_____ , and
   *_____ .

Mrs. Landis's pulse was irregular. She developed tremors and twitching of the face. The physician ordered 10 mL of magnesium sulfate IV to be diluted in 1 liter of solution. Other drugs that she was receiving included digoxin and Lasix.

5. Name Mrs. Landis's clinical signs and symptoms of hypomagnesemia.
   a. *_____
   b. _____
   c. *_____
6. What cation, in a *hypo* state, causes CNS abnormalities similar to hypomagnesemia?

   _____ .
7. Name at least two symptoms of hypermagnesemia. *_____ , and
   *_____ .

8. The physician ordered IV magnesium sulfate diluted in 1 liter of IV fluids. The nursing implication is first to check Mrs. Landis's urinary output. Explain the rationale. *_____

_____ .

9. The nurse should be assessing digitalis toxicity while Mrs. Landis's serum magnesium is low. Explain. *_____

_____ .

10. Lasix can cause (hypomagnesemia/hypermagnesemia) _____ .

1. 1.5–2.5 mEq/L
2. hypomagnesemia
3. It causes dilution of magnesium in the ECF.
4. renal insufficiency and use of Epsom salt (MgSO₄) as a laxative (also magnesium containing antacids)
5. a. irregular pulse (dysrhythmia); b. tremors; c. twitching of the face
6. calcium
7. CNS depression (lethargic, drowsiness) and decrease in respiration
8. Kidneys excrete excess magnesium and kidney impairment can cause hypermagnesemia.
9. Hypomagnesemia enhances the action of digitalis.
10. hypomagnesemia

HYPOMAGNESEMIA

NURSING ASSESSMENT FACTORS

- Obtain a nursing history and identify which findings are associated with hypomagnesemia, such as malnutrition, chronic alcoholism, chronic diarrhea, laxative abuse, TPN with magnesium, and electrolyte imbalance (hypokalemia, hypocalcemia).
- Assess for signs and symptoms of hypomagnesemia (neuromuscular and cardiac abnormalities), i.e., tetanylike symptoms due to hyperexcitability (tremors, twitching of the face), cardiac dysrhythmias (ventricular tachycardia leading to ventricular fibrillation), and hypertension.
- Assess dietary intake and use of intravenous therapy without magnesium. Prolonged intravenous therapy including total parenteral nutrition (TPN, hyperalimentation) may be a cause of hypomagnesemia.
- Check the ECG/EKG strips for changes in the T wave (flat or inverted) and ST segment (depressed) that may indicate hypomagnesemia.
- Check serum magnesium level. Frequently the serum magnesium level is not ordered and is usually not part of the routine chemistry test. If a potassium deficit does not respond to potassium replacement, hypomagnesemia should be suspected.

NURSING DIAGNOSIS 1

Nutrition: altered, less than body requirements, related to poor nutritional intake, chronic alcoholism, chronic laxative abuse, and chronic diarrhea.

NURSING INTERVENTIONS AND RATIONALE

1. Instruct the client to eat foods rich in magnesium (green vegetables, fruits, fish and seafood, grains, and nuts (peanut butter).
2. Report to physicians when clients receive continuous magnesium-free intravenous fluids. Solutions for hyperalimentation should contain some magnesium.
3. Administer intravenous magnesium sulfate diluted in solution slowly unless the client has a severe deficit. Rapid infusion can cause a hot or flushed feeling.
4. Have IV calcium gluconate available for emergency to reverse hypermagnesemia from overcorrection of a magnesium deficit.

NURSING DIAGNOSIS 2

Cardiac output: decreased, related to a serum magnesium deficit.

NURSING INTERVENTIONS AND RATIONALE

1. Monitor vital signs and ECG strips. Report abnormal findings to the physician.
2. Monitor serum electrolyte results. Report a low serum potassium and/or calcium level. Low serum magnesium level may be attributed to hypokalemia or hypocalcemia. When correcting a potassium deficit, potassium is not replaced in the cells until magnesium is replaced. A serum magnesium level of 1.0 mEq/L or less can cause cardiac arrest.
3. Check clients with hypomagnesemia who are taking digoxin for digitalis toxicity, e.g., nausea and vomiting, bradycardia. Magnesium deficit enhances the action of digoxin (digitalis preparations).
4. Report urine output of less than 25 mL per hour or 600 mL per day when the client is receiving magnesium supplements. Magnesium excess is excreted by the kidneys. With a poor urine output, hypermagnesemia can occur.
5. Check for positive Trousseau's and Chvostek's signs of severe hypomagnesemia. Tetany symptoms occur in both magnesium and calcium deficits.

HYPERMAGNESEMIA

NURSING ASSESSMENT FACTORS

- Assess, via nursing history, for possible causes of hypermagnesemia, i.e., renal insufficiency or failure and chronic use of antacids and laxatives containing magnesium salts.
- Assess for signs and symptoms of hypermagnesemia, such as decreased neuromuscular activity, lethargy, decreased respiration, and hypotension.
- Obtain a serum magnesium level that can be used as a baseline for comparison of future serum magnesium levels. A serum calcium level above 2.5 mEq/L or 3.0 mg/dL is indicative of hypermagnesemia.

NURSING DIAGNOSIS 1

Nutrition: altered, more than body requirements, related to oral and intravenous magnesium supplements and chronic use of drugs containing magnesium.

NURSING INTERVENTIONS AND RATIONALE

1. Monitor urinary output for clients taking magnesium-containing drugs. Urine output, 600–1200 mL per day, allows for the excretion of magnesium. A poor urine output can result in hypermagnesemia.
2. Observe for signs and symptoms of hypermagnesemia, such as decreased neuromuscular activity, decreased reflexes, lethargy and drowsiness, decreased respirations, and hypotension.
3. Monitor serum magnesium levels. A serum magnesium level exceeding 10 mEq/L can precipitate cardiac arrest.
4. Monitor for ECG changes. A wide QRS complex and a prolonged QT interval can suggest hypermagnesemia.
5. Instruct the client to avoid prolonged use of antacids and laxatives containing magnesium. Suggest that the client check drug labels for magnesium.
6. Suggest that the client increase fluid intake unless contraindicated. Fluids will dilute the serum magnesium level and should increase urine output.

PHOSPHORUS

INTRODUCTION

274 Phosphorus is a major anion. It is found in high concentration in the (extracellular/intracellular) _____ fluid (Refer to Table 3-3).

The ions phosphorus (P) and phosphate (PO_4) are used interchangeably. Phosphorus is measured in the serum; in the cells it appears as a form of phosphate.

intracellular (highest concentration)

■   ■   ■

275 Approximately 85% of phosphorus is located in the bones and the remaining 15% is located in the intracellular fluid. The normal serum phosphorus level is 1.7–2.6 mEq/L or 2.5–4.5 mg/dL.

A serum phosphorus level below 1.7 mEq/L or 2.5 mg/dL is identified as hypophosphatemia. A serum level above 2.6 mEq/L or 4.5 mg/dL is labeled _____

_____ .

hyperphosphatemia

■   ■   ■

276 The normal serum phosphorus range in adults is _____ mEq/L or _____ mg/dL.

The serum phosphorus level is usually higher in children: 4.0–7.0 mg/dL.

1.7–2.6; 2.5–4.5

■   ■   ■

277 Like potassium, 90% of the phosphorus compound is excreted by the kidneys and 10% is excreted by the gastrointestinal tract.

Potassium is a(n) (anion/cation) _____ , and phosphorus is a(n) (anion/cation) _____ . Both potassium and phosphorus are most plentiful in the (extracellular/intracellular) _____ fluid.

cation; anion; intracellular

■   ■   ■

278 Phosphorus balance is influenced by the parathyroid hormone (PTH). PTH stimulates calcitriol, a vitamin D derivative, which increases phosphorus absorption from the gastrointestinal tract. The PTH also stimulates the proximal renal tubules to increase phosphate excretion.

The two hormones that influence phosphorus/phosphate balance are _____ and *_____ .

calcitriol and parathyroid hormone or PTH

■   ■   ■

FUNCTIONS

Phosphorus has many functions. It is a vital element needed in bone formation, a component of the cell (nucleic acids and cell membrane), and is incorporated into the enzymes needed for metabolism, e.g., adenosine triphosphate (ATP), and acts as an acid-base buffer. Table 3-29 explains the functions of phosphorus according to the body system and structure it affects. Study the table carefully and refer to the table as needed.

Table 3-29. PHOSPHORUS AND ITS FUNCTIONS	
Body System and Structure	**Function**
Neuromuscular	Normal nerve and muscle activity.
Bones and teeth	Bone and teeth formation, strength, and durability.
Cellular	Formation of high-energy compounds (ATP, ADP). Phosphorus is the backbone of nucleic acids and stores metabolic energy.
	Formation of the red-blood-cell enzyme 2,3-diphosphoglycerate (2,3-DPG) is responsible for oxygen delivery to tissues.
	Utilization of B vitamins.
	Transmission of hereditary traits.
	Metabolism of carbohydrates, proteins, and fats.
	Maintenance of acid-base balance in body fluids.

279 An important function of phosphorus is neuromuscular activity. Name at least two cations that play an important role in neuromuscular activity. _____ and

_____ .

potassium and sodium (answers could also include calcium and magnesium)
 ■   ■   ■

280 Phosphorus, like calcium, is needed for strong, durable teeth and _____ .

bones
 ■   ■   ■

281 Intracellular ATP is needed for cellular energy.

The red-blood-cell enzyme 2,3-DPG is responsible for *_____ .

oxygen delivery to tissues
 ■   ■   ■

282 Other functions of phosphorus include which of the following:

( ) a. Utilization of vitamin A
( ) b. Utilization of B vitamins
( ) c. Metabolism of carbohydrates, proteins, and fats
( ) d. Maintenance of acid-base balance in body fluids
( ) e. Transmission of hereditary traits

a. —; b. X; c. X; d. X; e. X.
 ■   ■   ■

PATHOPHYSIOLOGY

283 Hypophosphatemia occurs approximately 3–4 days after inadequate nutrient intake. The kidneys compensate by decreasing urinary phosphate excretion; however, a continuous inadequate intake of phosphorus results in an extracellular fluid shift to the cells in order to replace the phosphorus loss.

What happens to the serum phosphorus level with this shift? *_____

_____ .

The serum phosphorus level decreases, resulting in hypophosphatemia.
 ■   ■   ■

284 Indicate the type of phosphorus imbalance based upon the serum phosphorus level listed on the left:

    ___ 1. 3.0 mg/dL   a. Hypophosphatemia
    ___ 2. 6.8 mg/dL   b. Hyperphosphatemia
    ___ 3. 1.5 mg/dL   c. Normal
    ___ 4. 1.2 mEq/L
    ___ 5. 3.2 mEq/L
    ___ 6. 2.0 mEq/L

1. c; 2. b; 3. a; 4. a; 5. b; 6. c

■   ■   ■

ETIOLOGY

Table 3-30 lists the causes of hypophosphatemia and Table 3-31 lists the causes of hyperphosphatemia. Study the tables and then proceed to the frames that follow. Refer to the tables as needed.

285 A decreased serum phosphorus level is known as a phosphorus deficit or

_____ .

Name two dietary changes that can cause a decreased serum phosphorus level.
_____ and _____ .

hypophosphatemia; malnutrition and chronic alcoholism (also the use of phosphorus-poor or -free IV solutions including those for TPN)

■   ■   ■

286 Alcoholism can cause severe hypophosphatemia. The phosphorus loss is the result of a
*_____ and _____ .

poor diet (malnutrition) and diuresis

■   ■   ■

287 Name the vitamin that is necessary for phosphorus absorption in the small intestines.

_____ .

vitamin D

■   ■   ■

Table 3-30. CAUSES OF HYPOPHOSPHATEMIA (SERUM PHOSPHORUS DEFICIT)

Etiology	Rationale
Dietary Changes	
Malnutrition	Poor nutrition results in a reduction of phosphorus intake.
Chronic alcoholism	Alcoholism contributes to dietary insufficiencies and increased diuresis.
Total parenteral nutrition (TPN, hyperalimentation)	TPN is usually a phosphorus-poor or -free solution. IV concentrated glucose and protein given rapidly shift the phosphorus into the cells, thus causing a serum phosphorus deficit.
Gastrointestinal Abnormalities	
Vomiting, anorexia	Loss of phosphorus through the GI tract decreases
Chronic diarrhea	cellular ATP (energy) stores.
Intestinal malabsorption	A vitamin D deficiency inhibits phosphorus absorption. Phosphorus is absorbed in the jejunum in the presence of vitamin D.
Hormonal Influence	
Hyperparathyroidism (increased PTH)	Parathyroid hormone (PTH) production enhances renal phosphate excretion and calcium reabsorption.
Drug Influence	
Aluminum-containing antacids	Phosphate binds with aluminum to decrease the serum phosphorus level.
Diuretics	Most diuretics promote a decrease in the serum phosphorus level.
Cellular Changes	
Diabetic ketoacidosis	Glycosuria and polyuria increase phosphate excretion. A dextrose infusion with insulin causes a phosphorus shift into the cells; decreasing the serum phosphorus level.
Burns	Phosphorus is lost due to its increased utilization in tissue building.
Acid-base disorders	Respiratory alkalosis from prolonged hyperventilation decreases the serum phosphorus level by causing an intracellular shift of phosphorus. Metabolic alkalosis can also cause this shift.

288 Gastrointestinal abnormalities that may cause hypophosphatemia include:

a. _____

b. _____

c. *_____

d. *_____

a. vomiting; b. anorexia; c. chronic diarrhea; d. intestinal malabsorption

■ ■ ■

289 In parathyroid disorders the parathyroid hormone (PTH) influences phosphorus balance. Increased PTH secretion causes a phosphorus (loss/excess) _____ .

loss

■ ■ ■

290 An increased calcium level is usually accompanied by a decreased serum phosphorus level. Aluminum-containing antacids decrease the serum phosphorus level. Explain how.

*_____ .

Phosphate binds with aluminum.

■ ■ ■

291 A client in diabetic ketoacidosis may have severe hypophosphatemia. Give two reasons why the phosphorus deficit occurs.

a. *_____

b. *_____

a. Glycosuria and polyuria increase phosphorus excretion.
b. Dextrose infusions with insulin cause a phosphorus shift from the serum into cells.

■ ■ ■

292 Explain how hypophosphatemia occurs as a result of prolonged hyperventilation.

*_____ .

What type of acid-base imbalance can result from prolonged hyperventilation

*_____ .

phosphorus shifts into cells (intracellular fluid); respiratory alkalosis (Good.)

■ ■ ■

Table 3-31. CAUSES OF HYPERPHOSPHATEMIA (SERUM PHOSPHORUS EXCESS)	
Etiology	**Rationale**
Dietary Changes Oral phosphate supplements Intravenous phosphate	Excessive administration of phosphate-containing substances increases the serum phosphorus level.
Hormonal Influence Hypoparathyroidism (lack of PTH)	Lack of PTH causes a calcium loss and a phosphorus excess.
Renal Abnormalities Renal insufficiency	Renal insufficiency or shutdown decreases phosphorus excretion.
Drug Influence Laxatives containing phosphate	Frequent use of phosphate laxatives increases the serum phosphorus level.

293 An elevated serum phosphorus level is known as phosphorus excess or _____ .

   With a decrease in the serum calcium level, the serum phosphorus level (increases/decreases) _____ .

   hyperphosphatemia; increases
   ▪   ▪   ▪

294 Hypoparathyroidism causes a(n) (increase/decrease) _____ in the secretion of the parathyroid hormone (PTH).

   A decrease in PTH secretion causes a calcium (loss/excess) _____ and a phosphorus (loss/excess) _____ .

   decrease; loss; excess
   ▪   ▪   ▪

295 Certain groups of drugs affect phosphorus balance. Enter PD for phosphorus deficit and PE for phosphorus excess against the drug groups that can cause phosphorus imbalance.

   ____ a. Aluminum antacids
   ____ b. Phosphate-containing laxatives
   ____ c. Thiazide diuretics
   ____ d. Oral phosphate ingestion
   ____ e. Intravenous phosphate administration

   a. PD; b. PE; c. PD; d. PE; e. PE
   ▪   ▪   ▪

CLINICAL MANIFESTATIONS

296 Clinical manifestations of hypophosphatemia and hyperphosphatemia are determined by signs and symptoms of phosphorus imbalances, particularly neuromuscular irregularities, hematologic abnormalities, and an abnormal serum phosphorus level.

A normal serum phosphorus level is   *_____ .

A serum phosphorus level of less than _____ mg/dL indicates hypophosphatemia, and one greater than _____ mg/dL indicates hyperphosphatemia.

1.7–2.6 mEq/L or 2.5–4.5 mg/dL; 2.5; 4.5

∎   ∎   ∎

Table 3-32 lists the clinical manifestations of hypophosphatemia and hyperphosphatemia according to the body areas that are affected. Study the table carefully and refer to it as needed.

Table 3-32. CLINICAL MANIFESTATIONS OF PHOSPHORUS IMBALANCES		
Body Areas	**Hypophosphatemia**	**Hyperphosphatemia**
Neuromuscular abnormalities	Muscle weakness Tremors Paresthesia Bone pain Hyporeflexia Seizures	Tetany (with decreased calcium) Hyperreflexia Flaccid paralysis Muscular weakness
Hematologic abnormalities	Tissue hypoxia (decreased oxygen-containing hemoglobin and hemolysis) Possible bleeding (platelet dysfunction) Possible infection (leukocyte dysfunction)	
Cardiopulmonary abnormalities	Weak pulse (myocardial dysfunction) Hyperventilation	Tachycardia
GI abnormalities	Anorexia Dysphagia	Nausea, diarrhea Abdominal cramps
Milliequivalents per liter	Below 1.7 mEq/L	Above 2.6 mEq/L
Milligrams per deciliter	Below 2.5 mg/dL	Above 4.5 mg/dL

297 Indicate which of the following signs and symptoms relate to hypophosphatemia:

( ) a. Muscle weakness
( ) b. Paresthesia
( ) c. Bone pain
( ) d. Flaccid paralysis
( ) e. Tissue hypoxia
( ) f. Tachycardia
( ) g. Hyporeflexia

a. X (also could occur with hyperphosphatemia); b. X; c. X; d. —; e. X; f. —; g. X
∎   ∎   ∎

298 Indicate which of the following signs and symptoms relate to hyperphosphatemia:

( ) a. Muscle weakness
( ) b. Paresthesia
( ) c. Hyperreflexia
( ) d. Flaccid paralysis
( ) e. Tachycardia
( ) f. Abdominal cramps
( ) g. Bone pain

a. X (more common with hypophosphatemia; b. —; c. X; d. X; e. X; f. X; g. —.
∎   ∎   ∎

299 Symptoms of phosphorus imbalance are very often vague; therefore serum values are needed.

Hypophosphatemia is present when the serum phosphorus level is less than
_____ mEq/L or _____ mg/dL. Hyperphosphatemia is
present when the serum phosphorus level is greater than _____ mEq/L or
_____ mg/dL.

1.7; 2.5; 2.6; 4.5
∎   ∎   ∎

DRUGS AND THEIR EFFECT ON PHOSPHORUS BALANCE

The major drug group that causes hypophosphatemia is aluminum antacids; the drug groups responsible for hyperphosphatemia are phosphate laxatives, phosphate enemas, and oral and intravenous phosphates. Table 3-33 lists the names and rationales for drugs that affect phosphorus balance.

Table 3-33. DRUGS THAT AFFECT PHOSPHORUS BALANCE

Phosphorus Imbalance	Drugs	Rationale

Hypophosphatemia (serum phosphorus deficit)	Sucralfate
	Aluminum antacids
	    Amphojel
	    Basaljel
	Aluminum/magnesium antacid
	    Di-Gel
	    Gelusil
	    Maalox
	    Maalox Plus
	    Mylanta
	    Mylanta II
	
	Calcium antacids
	    Calcium carbonate
		Aluminum-containing antacids bind with phosphorus; therefore the serum phosphorus level is decreased. Calcium promotes phosphate loss.

	Diuretics
	    Thiazide
	    Loop (high ceiling)
	    Acetazolamide
		Phosphorus can be lost in diuresis when diuretics are used.

	Androgens
	Corticosteroids
	    Cortisone
	    Prednisone
	Glucagon
	Gastrin
	Epinephrine
	Mannitol
	
	Salicylate overdose
	Insulin and glucose
		These agents have a mild to moderate effect on phosphorus loss.

Hyperphosphatemia (serum phosphorus excess)	Oral phosphates
	    Sodium phosphate/
	    Phospho-Soda
	    Potassium phosphate/
	    Neutra-Phos K
	
	Intravenous phosphates
	    Sodium phosphate
	    Potassium phosphate
		Excess oral ingestion and IV infusion can increase the serum phosphorus level.

Table 3-33. (Continued)

Phosphorus Imbalance	Drugs	Rationale

	Phosphate laxatives
	  Sodium phosphate
	  Sodium biphosphate/
	  Phospho-Soda
	  Phosphate enema
	  Fleet sodium phosphate
		Continuous use of phosphate laxatives and enemas can increase the serum phosphorus level.

	Excessive vitamin D
	Antibiotics
	  Tetracyclines
	  Methicillin	

300 Prolonged intake of aluminum antacids, with or without magnesium, decreases the serum phosphorus level. Why?   *_____

_____ . The phosphorus imbalance that results is _____ .

Aluminum-containing antacids bind with phosphorus; hypophosphatemia.
　　　　　　　　　■　　　　　　　　　■　　　　　　　　　■

301 Aluminum antacids may be ordered for hyperphosphatemia. Do you know why?

*_____ .

Aluminum binds with phosphorus to decrease the serum phosphorus level.
　　　　　　　　　■　　　　　　　　　■　　　　　　　　　■

302 Enter PD for phosphorus deficit and PE for phosphorus excess beside the drugs that can cause a phosphorus imbalance:

____ a. Amphojel
____ b. Cortisone
____ c. Phospho-Soda
____ d. Fleet's sodium phosphate
____ e. Epinephrine/adrenalin
____ f. Diuretics
____ g. IV potassium phosphate

a. PD; b. PD; c. PE; d. PE; e. PD; f. PD; g. PE
　　　　　　　　　■　　　　　　　　　■　　　　　　　　　■

CLINICAL MANAGEMENT

When the serum phosphorus level falls below 1.5 mEq/L or 2 mg/dL, oral and/or intravenous phosphate-containing solutions are usually ordered.

If the serum phosphorus level falls below 0.5 mEq/L or 1 mg/dL, severe hypophosphatemia occurs. Intravenous phosphate-containing solutions are indicated.

PHOSPHORUS REPLACEMENT

303 Name two drugs, oral or intravenous, that are administered to replace the phosphorus deficit (refer to Table 3-33).   *_____ and *_____ .

sodium phosphate/Phospho-Soda and potassium phosphate/Neutra-Phos K
   ∎   ∎   ∎

304 Concentrated IV phosphates are hyperosmolar and must be diluted. If IV potassium phosphate (K PO$_4$) is given in intravenous solution, the IV rate should be no more than 10 mEq per hour to avoid phlebitis.

If an intravenous potassium phosphate solution infiltrates, what happens to the tissue?

*_____ .

Necrosis or sloughing of tissue. Potassium is extremely irritating to subcutaneous tissue.
   ∎   ∎   ∎

305 Foods rich in phosphorus include milk (especially skin milk), milk products, meat (beef and pork), whole grain cereals, and dried beans.

Phosphorus-rich foods are indicated if the serum phosphorus level is which of the following:

( ) a. 0.3 mEq/L or 1 mg/dL
( ) b. 0.9 mEq/L or 1.5 mg/dL
( ) c. 1.6 mEq/L or 2.4 mg/dL

a. —; b. —; c. X
   ∎   ∎   ∎

CLINICAL APPLICATIONS

306 Severe hypophosphatemia results from hyperalimentation/TPN. Two reasons for a serum phosphorus deficit related to hyperalimentation are

a. *_____

b. *_____

a. phosphate-poor or -free solution; b. concentrated glucose and/or protein, given too rapidly, causes phosphorus to shift from serum into cells.
   ∎   ∎   ∎

307 If a severely malnourished patient is receiving a 25% dextrose solution (TPN), the infusion rate should be (fast/slow) _____ when first administered? What type of serum phosphorus imbalance can occur if the infusion rate was faster than 80 mL per hour? _____ . Why? *_____

_____ .

slow; hypophosphatemia
Concentrated glucose tends to shift phosphorus into cells; the result is a serum phosphorus deficit.

■　　　　　　　■　　　　　　　■

308 Any carbohydrate-loading diet can cause a phosphorus shift from the serum into the cells.

During tissue repair following trauma, phosphorus shifts into the cells. The serum phosphorus imbalance that occurs is called _____ .

hypophosphatemia

■　　　　　　　■　　　　　　　■

CASE STUDY REVIEW

Mrs. Peterson had a history of alcohol abuse. She was admitted for GI bleeding. In her own words she had not eaten a balanced diet for 2 months and had been taking Amphojel to relieve an "upset stomach." Mrs. Peterson complained of hand paresthesias and "overall" muscle weakness.

1. What type of phosphorus imbalance could Mrs. Peterson have? _____ .
2. Give the "normal" serum phosphorus range. _____ mEq/L; _____ mg/dL.
3. Give two reasons for Mrs. Peterson's imbalance: *_____ and *_____ .
4. What among Mrs. Peterson's signs and symptoms indicated a phosphorus deficit?
   a. *_____ .
   b. *_____ .
5. Name other clinical signs and symptoms of hypophosphatemia: *_____ , *_____ , *_____ , and _____ .
6. Explain how aluminum hydroxide lowers the serum phosphorus level. *_____ .

Mrs. Peterson was given a 10% dextrose solution intravenously. Her serum phosphorus level was 1.5 mg/dL and her potassium level, 3.0 mEq/L. Several hours later potassium phosphate was added to her intravenous solution.

7. What effect does concentrated dextrose (glucose) solution have on the serum phosphorus level? *_____ .
8. What is the responsibility of the nurse who is attending Mrs. Peterson while she is receiving IV potassium phosphate diluted in this solution?
   *_____ .
9. Name two oral phosphate drugs: *_____ and _____ .

1. *hypophosphatemia*
2. *1.7–2.6; 2.5–4.5*
3. *poor diet (possible malnutrition) and ingestion of aluminum hydroxide antacid, Amphojel*
4. *a. hand paresthesias; b. muscle weakness*
5. *bone pain, tissue hypoxia, weak pulse, and hyperventilation*
6. *Phosphorus binds with aluminum, thus lowering the serum phosphorus level.*
7. *Concentrated glucose causes a shift of phosphorus from the serum into the cells.*
8. *monitor IV rate so Mrs. Peterson receives approximately 10 mEq per hour of KPO$_4$; check infusion cite frequently for signs of infiltration*
9. *sodium phosphate/Phospho-Soda and potassium phosphate/NeutraPhos K*

HYPOPHOSPHATEMIA

NURSING ASSESSMENT FACTORS

- Obtain a nursing history of clinical problems. Note if the health problem is related to hypophosphatemia, i.e., malnutrition, chronic alcoholism, chronic diarrhea, vitamin D deficit, continuous use of IV solutions without a phosphate additive (including TPN), hyperparathyroidism, continuous use of aluminum-containing antacids, and alkalotic state due to hyperventilation (respiratory alkalosis).
- Assess for signs and symptoms of hypophosphatemia, i.e., muscle weakness, paresthesia, hyporeflexia, weak pulse, and overbreathing (tachypnea).
- Check serum phosphorus level. The serum phosphorus level can act as a baseline level for assessing future serum phosphorus levels.
- Check serum calcium level and, if elevated, report findings to the physician. An elevated calcium level causes a decreased phosphorus level.

NURSING DIAGNOSIS

Nutrition: altered, less than body requirements, related to inadequate nutritional intake, chronic alcoholism, vomiting, chronic diarrhea, lack of vitamin D intake, intravenous fluids, including TPN with lack of phosphate additive.

NURSING INTERVENTIONS AND RATIONALE

1. Monitor neuromuscular and cardiopulmonary abnormalities related to a decreased phosphorus level, such as muscle weakness, tremors, paresthesia, hyporeflexia, bone pain, weak pulse, and tachypnea.
2. Monitor serum phosphorus and calcium levels. Report abnormal findings to the physician. An increase in the serum calcium level results in a decrease in the serum phosphorus level and vice versa.
3. Monitor oral and IV phosphorus replacements. Some of the oral phosphate salts (Neutrophos) come in capsules, which are indicated if nausea is present. Administer IV phosphate [potassium phosphate (KPO$_4$)] slowly to prevent hyperphosphatemia and irritation of the blood vessel. The suggested amount of KPO$_4$ to be administered per hour is 10 mEq. Rapidly administered KPO$_4$ and/or high concentrations of phosphate can cause phlebitis.
4. Check for signs of infiltration at the IV site; KPO$_4$ is extremely irritating to subcutaneous tissue and can cause sloughing of tissue and necrosis.

5. Inform the physician if your client is receiving a phosphorus-poor or -free solution for TPN.
6. Instruct the client to eat foods rich in phosphorus, i.e., meats (beef, pork, turkey), milk, whole grain cereals, and nuts. Most carbonated drinks are high in phosphates.
7. Instruct the client not to take antacids that contain aluminum hydroxide (Amphojel). Phosphorus binds with aluminum products; a low serum phosphorus level results.

HYPERPHOSPHATEMIA

NURSING ASSESSMENT FACTORS

- Obtain a nursing history of clinical problems; associate the health problems to hyperphosphatemia, i.e., continuous use of phosphate-containing laxatives, hypoparathyroidism, and renal insufficiency.
- Assess for signs and symptoms of hyperphosphatemia, i.e., hyperreflexia, tachycardia, abdominal cramps, and tetany symptoms which can also indicate a low serum calcium level.
- Check serum phosphorus level. A serum phosphorus level greater than 4.5 mg/dL or greater than 2.6 mEq/L indicates hyperphosphatemia. A serum phosphorus level exceeding 10 mg/dL can result in cardiac distress.
- Check urinary output. A decrease in urine output, <25 mL (cc) per hour or <600 mL per day, increases the serum phosphorus level. This is especially true if the client is receiving a phosphate-containing product.

NURSING DIAGNOSIS

Nutrition: altered, more than body requirements, related to excess intake of phosphate-containing compounds such as some laxatives, intravenous potassium phosphate, and others.

NURSING INTERVENTIONS AND RATIONALE

1. Monitor neuromuscular, cardiac, and GI abnormalities related to an increased phosphorus level.
2. Monitor serum phosphorus and calcium levels. A decreased calcium level can result in an increase in the phosphorus level. Report abnormal findings to the physician.
3. Observe the client for signs and symptoms of hypocalcemia (e.g., tetany) when phosphate supplements are being administered. An increase in the serum phosphorus level decreases the calcium level.
4. Instruct the client to eat foods that are low in phosphorus, such as vegetables. Instruct the client to avoid drinking carbonated beverages that contain phosphates.
5. Instruct client with hyperphosphatemia or poor renal output to read labels on over-the-counter medications and canned foods that may contain phosphate ingredients.
6. Monitor urine output. Report inadequate urine output to the physician. Phosphorus is excreted by the kidneys and poor renal function can cause hyperphosphatemia.

CHLORIDE

INTRODUCTION

309 Chloride is a(n) (anion/cation) _____ .

The chloride ion frequently appears in combination with the sodium ion. Which fluid has the greatest concentration of chloride—intracellular or extracellular?   *_____ .

anion; extracellular fluid

■ ■ ■

310 The normal serum chloride (Cl) range is 95–108 mEq/L. The chloride concentration in the intracellular fluid is 1 mEq/L.

A serum chloride level less than 95 mEq/L is called (hypochloremia/hyperchloremia) _____ .

A serum chloride level greater than 108 mEq/L is called _____ .

hypochloremia; hyperchloremia

■ ■ ■

FUNCTIONS

Table 3-34 lists the four functions of the chloride ion. Study the table and refer to it as needed.

Table 3-34. CHLORIDE AND ITS FUNCTIONS	
Body Involvement	**Functions**
Osmolality (tonicity) of ECF	Chloride, like sodium, changes the serum osmolality. When serum osmolality is increased (>295 mOsm/L), there are more sodium and chloride ions in proportion to the water. With a decreased serum osmolality (<280 mOsm/L), there are less sodium and chloride ions.
Body water balance	When sodium is retained, chloride is frequently retained, causing an increase in water retention.
Acid-base balance	The kidneys excrete the anion chloride or bicarbonate, and sodium reabsorbs either chloride or bicarbonate to maintain acid-base balance.
Acidity of gastric juice	Chloride combines with the hydrogen ion in the stomach to form hydrochloric acid (HCl).

311 Chloride, like sodium, influences the serum osmolality.

What two ions are usually increased when the serum osmolality is elevated?

_____ and _____ .

sodium and chloride

■   ■   ■

312 When there is a body water deficit, what occurs to the:

    a. Serum sodium and serum chloride levels? _____ .

    b. Serum osmolality? _____ .

    c. Body water? _____ .

a. increases; b. increases; c. is reabsorbed

■   ■   ■

313 For every sodium ion absorbed from the renal tubules, a chloride or bicarbonate ion is also absorbed; thus the proportion of sodium and chloride lost can differ.

The organs responsible for electrolyte homeostasis by the excretion and absorption of ions are the _____ .

kidneys

■   ■   ■

314 If metabolic alkalosis is present, the kidneys excrete the bicarbonate ion and sodium is reabsorbed with the (bicarbonate/chloride) _____ ions.

If metabolic acidosis is present, the kidneys excrete (bicarbonate/chloride) _____ ion, and the sodium is reabsorbed with which ion?

_____ .

chloride; chloride; bicarbonate

■   ■   ■

315 Chloride plays a part in the oxygen and carbon dioxide exchange in the red blood cells. When the red blood cells are oxygenated, chloride travels from the red blood cells to the plasma, and bicarbonate leaves the plasma to the red blood cells. This is called the *chloride shift*.

This chloride shift is necessary in maintaining _____ .

homeostasis or equilibrium

■   ■   ■

316 The four functions of chloride are for the maintenance of

a. *_____

b. *_____

c. *_____

d. *_____

a. osmolality of extracellular fluid (serum osmolality)
b. body water balance
c. acid-base balance
d. acidity of the gastric juice (HCl)

■   ■   ■

317 The name for a chloride deficit is hypochloremia; therefore, the name for a chloride excess is

_____ .

hyperchloremia

■   ■   ■

PATHOPHYSIOLOGY

318 A chloride deficiency can lead to a potassium deficiency and vice versa. Usually chloride losses follow sodium losses. Most chloride ingestion is in combination with sodium.

The chloride ion is mostly found in combination with a _____ ion.

What is the common name for sodium chloride? _____ .

sodium; salt

■   ■   ■

319 Indicate the type of chloride imbalance according to the serum chloride levels listed on the left:

___ 1. 112 mEq/L   a. Hypochloremia
___ 2. 93 mEq/L   b. Hyperchloremia
___ 3. 98 mEq/L   c. Normal
___ 4. 89 mEq/L
___ 5. 109 mEq/L

1. b; 2. a; 3. c; 4. a; 5. b

■   ■   ■

ETIOLOGY

Table 3-35 lists the causes of hypochloremia with rationale, and Table 3-36 lists the causes of hyperchloremia with rationale. Study the tables carefully noting the rationale for each cause of chloride imbalance. Refer to the tables as needed.

Table 3-35.   CAUSES OF HYPOCHLOREMIA (SERUM CHLORIDE DEFICIT)

Etiology	Rationale
Dietary Changes Low-sodium diet	A decrease in the serum sodium level can cause a decrease in the serum chloride level.
Prolonged use of IV dextrose in water (D_5W)	Dextrose in water dilutes the serum levels of chloride, sodium, and potassium.
Gastrointestinal Abnormalities Continuous vomiting; gastric suction	Gastric juice is composed of the acid hydrogen chloride (HCl). Loss of gastric juice via vomiting or through gastric suction can cause a chloride deficit.
Diarrhea	Loss of gastrointestinal salty secretions can cause a chloride deficit.
Loss of potassium	Loss of potassium is accompanied by loss of chloride.
Renal Abnormality Prolonged use of diuretics	Most diuretics interfere with the absorption of chloride ions from the renal tubules.
Skin Excessive sweating	Chloride combines with sodium and is lost via the skin. This can result from increased body temperature, fever, or muscular exercise.
Acid-Base Imbalance Metabolic alkalosis	An increase in the concentration of bicarbonate ions is associated with a decrease in the concentration of chloride ions.

320 Name the two ions that influence the acidity of the gastric juice. _____
and _____ .

What gastrointestinal conditions can cause a chloride deficit?

a. * _____
b. * _____
c. _____

hydrogen and chloride
a. continuous vomiting; b. gastric suction; c. diarrhea

■   ■   ■

321 The loss of chloride is frequently accompanied by the loss of what other ion?
_____ .

potassium (yes, sodium could be an answer too)

■   ■   ■

322 Chloride is frequently combined with the _____ ion.

Name at least two causes for sodium and chloride loss or salt loss through the skin.
_____ and _____ .

sodium (yes, hydrogen is also correct)
fever and muscular exercise (also increased environmental temperature)

■   ■   ■

323 What type of chloride imbalance occurs with excessive use of diuretics?
_____ . Why? * _____ .

Name the chloride imbalance occurring with continuous use of IV dextrose in water?
_____ . Why? * _____ .

hypochloremia (chloride deficit); diuretics interfere with chloride absorption
hypochloremia; dextrose in water dilutes the serum chloride level

■   ■   ■

324 Increased bicarbonate ion concentration (HCO_3) is associated with a(n) (increased/decreased)
_____ chloride ion concentration.

What type of acid-base imbalance results? * _____ .

decreased; metabolic alkalosis

■   ■   ■

Table 3-36.   CAUSES OF HYPERCHLOREMIA (SERUM CHLORIDE EXCESS)

Etiology	Rationale
Body fluid loss: dehydration	Serum solutes, including chloride, become concentrated when there is a body water (ECF) deficit.
Hormonal influence: excessive adrenocortical hormone production	Excessive adrenal cortical hormone causes an excess of sodium in the body. Sodium combines with chloride, increasing the concentration of the chloride ion in blood.
Trauma: head injury	Chloride ions are frequently retained with sodium.
Acid-base imbalance: metabolic acidosis	Increased chloride (Cl) ion concentration is associated with a decreased bicarbonate ion concentration.

325 Excessive adrenal cortical hormones can cause a sodium excess and a chloride

_____ ? Why? *_____

_____ .

excess
Cortisone has a sodium-retaining effect. Sodium combines with chloride, increasing the
chloride ion concentration in the blood.
     ■   ■   ■

326 With severe dehydration, what happens to the chloride level? _____ .

Explain. *_____ .

increases; ECF deficit increases chloride concentration, or hemoconcentration causes chloride
excess, or a similar response
     ■   ■   ■

327 An increased chloride level is associated with a(n) (increased/decreased) _____

bicarbonate (HCO_3) level. What type of acid-base imbalance occurs?

*_____ .

decreased; metabolic acidosis
     ■   ■   ■

328 Place D for chloride deficit and E for chloride excess in the following:

( ) a. Vomiting
( ) b. Diarrhea
( ) c. Gastric suction
( ) d. Excessive adrenal cortical hormone production
( ) e. Sweating
( ) f. Diuretics
( ) g. Potassium loss
( ) h. Severe dehydration
( ) i. Head injury

a. D; b. D; c. D; d. E; e. D; f. D; g. D; h. E; i. E

CLINICAL MANIFESTATIONS

329 The normal serum chloride level is *_____ .

A serum chloride level less than _____ mEq/L is known as hypochloremia.

For hyperchloremia to occur, the serum chloride level should be greater than
_____ mEq/L.

95–108 mEq/L; 95; 108

Table 3-37 lists the clinical manifestations of hypochloremia and hyperchloremia according to the body areas affected. Hypochloremic symptoms are similar to metabolic alkalosis, and hyperchloremic symptoms are similar to metabolic acidosis. Study the table carefully and refer to it as needed.

Table 3-37. CLINICAL MANIFESTATIONS OF CHLORIDE IMBALANCES

Body Areas	Hypochloremia	Hyperchloremia
Neuromuscular abnormalities	Hyperexcitability of the nerves and muscles (tremors, twitching)	Weakness Lethargic Unconsciousness (later)
Respiratory abnormalities	Slow and shallow breathing	Deep, rapid, vigorous breathing
Cardiac abnormalities	↓ Blood pressure with severe Cl and ECF losses	
Milliequivalent per liter	↓ 95 mEq/L	↑ 108 mEq/L

330 Hypochloremic neuromuscular abnormalities are similar to tetany symptoms. Tetany symptoms are evidenced as (hypo/hyper) _____ excitability of the nerves and muscles. Examples of these symptoms are _____ and _____ .

hyper; tremors and twitching
■   ■   ■

331 With hyperchloremic neuromuscular abnormalities, there is a decrease in nerve and muscle activity. Two examples of these symptoms are _____ and _____ .

weakness and lethargy
■   ■   ■

332 In hypochloremia, the respiratory symptom is similar to metabolic alkalosis.

Indicate which type of breathing occurs with a chloride deficit.

( ) a. Slow, shallow breathing
( ) b. Deep, rapid, vigorous breathing
Explain why. *_____

_____ .

a. X; b. —
The lungs conserve carbon dioxide (CO_2 + H_2O = H_2CO_3) or carbonic acid to increase acid and restore pH. Very good.
■   ■   ■

333 In hyperchloremia, the respiratory symptom is similar to metabolic acidosis.

Indicate which type of breathing occurs with a chloride excess.

( ) a. Slow, shallow breathing
( ) b. Deep, rapid, vigorous breathing

Do you know why? *_____

_____ .

a. —; b. X
The lungs blow off carbon dioxide to prevent the formation of H_2CO_3—carbonic acid. Very good.
■   ■   ■

CLINICAL APPLICATIONS

334 Hypochloremia usually indicates alkalosis (hypochloremic alkalosis) due to increased levels of bicarbonate.

Persistent vomiting and gastric suction cause a loss of hydrogen and chloride ions. A loss in hydrogen and chloride results in *_____ .

hypochloremic alkalosis

■   ■   ■

335 With vomiting, a hypokalemic state can also occur.

Name four clinical symptoms of hypokalemia. _____ ,
_____ , *_____ , and *_____ .

dizziness; dysrhythmia; muscular weakness; and abdominal distention

■   ■   ■

336 A potassium deficit cannot be fully corrected until a chloride deficit is corrected.

With vomiting, what type of potassium supplement (Kaon/K-Lyte/potassium chloride) _____ is needed to replace ion deficits.

Explain. *_____ .

potassium chloride
Both chloride and potassium are lost due to vomiting.

■   ■   ■

337 Hypochloremia can result from excessive IV administration of 5% dextrose in water. How can hypochloremia be prevented?

*_____ .

by administering 5% dextrose in normal saline or in ½ normal saline

■   ■   ■

338 One liter of normal saline contains 154 mEq/L of chloride, which exceeds the daily amount needed; however, with severe hypochloremic alkalosis, normal saline is the solution of choice.

What is the "normal" serum chloride range? *_____ .

95–108 mEq/L

■   ■   ■

339 A normal urine chloride level in 24 hours is 150–250 mEq/L. The amount of chloride excreted depends on the amount of salt intake, body fluid imbalance, and acid-base imbalance.

With a body fluid deficit, the serum chloride and sodium levels are increased due to hemoconcentration. What would you expect the urine chloride level to be (increased/decreased)? _____ .

decreased

■   ■   ■

340 Nursing responsibilities for hypochloremia include:

a. *_____

b. *_____

a. *assessing the serum chloride level*
b. *suggesting that normal saline or ½ NSS (half normal saline solution) be included with the IV orders*

■   ■   ■

CASE STUDY REVIEW

Mr. Reynolds, 68 years old, has been vomiting for several days. In the hospital, a nasogastric tube was inserted. His serum electrolytes were as follows: serum chloride, 94 mEq/L; serum sodium, 132 mEq/L; and serum potassium, 3.2 mEq/L. Dextrose, 5% in 0.45% normal saline, with 40 mEq/L of KCl was started.

1. What are the four main functions of the chloride ion?
   a. *_____ .
   b. *_____ .
   c. *_____ .
   d. *_____ .
2. According to Mr. Reynolds' serum electrolytes, what three imbalances were present?
   _____ , _____ , and _____ .
3. The acidity of Mr. Reynolds' gastric juice was decreased because of vomiting and nasogastric suctioning. Name the clinical condition that occurs due to the loss of hydrogen and chloride ions. *_____ .
4. What is the "normal" range of serum chloride? *_____ .
5. Most of the chloride ingested is in combination with the ion _____ .
6. With hypokalemia and hypochloremia, explain what can occur if only potassium is replaced.
   *_____
   _____ .

7. Mr. Reynolds received 5% dextrose in 0.45% NaCl or ½ normal saline and KCl as the IV fluid. How many mEq/L does 1 liter of ½ normal saline contain? *_____ .

8. Nursing implications in caring for Mr. Reynolds include:

   a. * _____ .

   b. * _____ .

   c. * _____ .

1. a. serum osmolality, b. acid-base balance, c. body water balance, and d. acidity of the gastric juice
2. hypochloremia; hyponatremia, and hypokalemia
3. hypochloremic alkalosis
4. 95–108 mEq/L
5. sodium
6. A potassium deficit cannot be fully corrected without a correction of chloride deficit.
7. 77 mEq/L
8. a. assessing Mr. Reynolds's serum electrolyte values
   b. assessing for signs and symptoms of hypokalemia and hyponatremia
   c. checking the pH for acid-base imbalance
      Others: measure GI loss (vomiting and gastric drainage for suction)

HYPOCHLOREMIA

NURSING ASSESSMENT FACTORS

- Obtain a nursing history and identify findings that are associated with hypochloremia, i.e., continuous vomiting, gastric suctioning, diarrhea, prolonged use of diuretics, excessive sweating, prolonged use of IV fluids without saline content, metabolic alkalosis.
- Assess for signs and symptoms of hypochloremia (neuromuscular and respiratory abnormalities), i.e., tetanylike symptoms due to hyperexcitability (tremors, twitching), and slow, shallow breathing. As the chloride deficit decreases, the blood pressure decreases.
- Check serum chloride level to be used as a baseline for comparison with future serum chloride levels. A serum chloride level below 95 mEq/L is indicative of hypochloremia.

NURSING DIAGNOSIS

Health maintenance: altered, related to dietary changes, gastrointestinal abnormalities, and acid-base imbalance.

NURSING INTERVENTIONS AND RATIONALE

1. Monitor the serum chloride levels. Report abnormal findings, serum chloride level less than 95 mEq/L.
2. Report serum potassium loss as well as serum chloride loss. A potassium deficit cannot be fully corrected until the chloride deficit is corrected.
3. Monitor serum CO_2 or arterial HCO_3. An increased serum CO_2, >32 mEq/L, and/or increased arterial HCO_3, >28 mEq/L, can indicate metabolic alkalosis and hypochloremia (hypochloremic alkalosis).
4. Observe for respiratory difficulties, i.e., slow, shallow breathing due to hypochloremic alkalosis.
5. Interpret the types of intravenous fluids ordered; and if continuous IV dextrose in water is administered, notify the physician.

6. Record the amount of gastric secretions from gastric suction, and report continuous and excessive losses.
7. Check the client's medications. If the client is taking potassium bicarbonate (Kaon without Cl) and has a chloride deficit, the nurse should notify the physician. Giving bicarbonate increases the chloride deficit.

HYPERCHLOREMIA

NURSING ASSESSMENT FACTORS

- Obtain a nursing history and identify findings that are associated with hyperchloremia, i.e., severe dehydration, head injury, excessive use of steroids (cortisone preparation), and metabolic acidosis.
- Assess for signs and symptoms of hyperchloremia (neuromuscular and respiratory abnormalities), i.e., weakness and lethargy and deep, rapid, vigorous breathing.
- Check serum chloride level to be used for comparison with future serum chloride levels. A serum chloride level greater than 108 mEq/L is indicative of hyperchloremia.

NURSING DIAGNOSIS

Health maintenance: altered, related to severe dehydration, head injury, excessive use of steroids, and acid-base imbalance.

NURSING INTERVENTIONS AND RATIONALE

1. Monitor the serum chloride levels. Report abnormal findings, e.g., serum chloride level greater than 108 mEq/L.
2. Monitor serum CO_2 or arterial HCO_3. A decreased serum CO_2 level, <22 mEq/L, and/or decreased arterial HCO_3, <24 mEq/L, can indicate metabolic acidosis and hyperchloremia.
3. Observe for respiratory difficulties, i.e., deep, rapid, vigorous breathing due to hyperchloremia and an acidotic state (metabolic acidosis).
4. Instruct the client with hyperchloremia to avoid foods rich in sodium (salt), e.g., ham, bacon, pickles, potato chips, and pretzels. Most of the chloride ion in food is combined with sodium.
5. Check the 24-hour urine chloride value and compare to the 24-hour urine sodium value. In acidosis, the kidneys excrete the chloride ion and conserve the bicarbonate ion. Sodium is reabsorbed and combined with bicarbonate to correct the acidosis.

FOODS RICH IN ELECTROLYTES

Table 3-38 lists by name the foods that are rich in electrolyte content, according to class. If no foods are listed, all in that class are low in that electrolyte. You will, no doubt, have to refer to this table. It is important, however, to memorize the foods rich in potassium. Because potassium deficits frequently occur, you must remember foods rich in this electrolyte. Again, study this table carefully before proceeding to the next frames.

Classes	Potassium	Sodium	Calcium	Magnesium	Chloride	Phosphorus
Table 3-38.	**FOODS RICH IN POTASSIUM, SODIUM, CALCIUM, MAGNESIUM, CHLORIDE AND PHOSPHORUS**					
Daily requirements	3–4 g	2–4 g	800 mg	300 mg	3–9 g	800 mg
Beverages	Cocoa, Coca Cola, coffee, wines	Pepsi-Cola, tea, decaffeinated coffee		Cocoa		
Fruit and fruit juices	Citrus fruits: oranges, grapefruit Juices: grapefruit (canned), orange (canned), prune (canned), tomato (canned)					
	Fruits: apricots (dry), bananas, cantaloupe, dates, raisins (dry), watermelon, prunes			Average	High only in dates and bananas	
Bread products and cereal	Average to low amount	White bread, soda crackers, and wheat flakes		Cereals with oats		Whole grain cereal
Dairy products	Average to low—milk, buttermilk	Butter, cheese, and margarine	Milk, cheese	Milk (average)	Cheese, milk	Cheese, milk
Nuts	Almonds, Brazil nuts, cashews, and peanuts	Low, except if salted	Brazil nuts (moderate)	Almonds, Brazil nuts, peanuts, and walnuts		Peanuts
Vegetables	Baked beans, carrots (raw), celery (raw), dandelion greens, lima beans (canned), mustard greens, tomatoes, spinach NOTE: Nearly all vegetables are rich in potassium when raw, but K will be lost if water used in cooking is discarded.	Average to low Celery (high average)	Baked beans, kale, mustard and turnip greens, broccoli	Green, leafy	Spinach, celery	Dry beans
Meat, fish, and poultry	Average—meats High average— sardines, codfish, scallops	Corned beef, bacon, ham, crab, tuna fish, sausage (pork) Low in poultry	Salmon, meats	Fish, shrimp Low in poultry Low in meats Egg, average	Eggs, crabs, fish (average), turkey	Beef, pork, fish, chicken, turkey
Miscellaneous	Catsup (average), spices, potato chips, and peanut butter	Catsup, mayonnaise, potato chips, pretzels, pickles, dill, olives, mustard, Worcestershire sauce, celery salt, salad dressing—French and Italian	Molasses	Chocolate and chocolate bars, chocolate syrup Molasses Table salt		

341 What classes of food are rich in potassium?

    a. _____

    b. _____

    c. _____

    d. _____

    e. * _____

a. fish; b. nuts; c. vegetables; d. fruits; e. fruit juice (see Table 3-38)
      ■   ■   ■

342 Foods with the highest concentration of potassium are nuts and dried fruits. Juices, such as orange juice, are a quick source of potassium. Bananas, dates, prunes, and apricots have a greater concentration of potassium than have oranges and orange juice.

    A quick source of potassium is *_____ .

    Name four fruits containing a high concentration of potassium. _____ ,

_____ , _____ , and _____ .

orange juice; bananas, dates, prunes, and apricots
      ■   ■   ■

343 Many Americans consume 5–10 g of sodium chloride per day, which is more than needed.

    The daily requirement for sodium per day is *_____ .

    The daily requirement for potassium per day is *_____ .

2–4 g; 3–4 g
      ■   ■   ■

344 Name the classes of food that are rich in sodium.

    a. * _____

    b. * _____

    c. _____

    d. _____

a. bread products; b. dairy products; c. meat; d. fish
      ■   ■   ■

345 The classes of food that are rich in calcium are:

a. * _____
b. * _____
c. _____
d. _____

a. baked beans; b. dairy products; c. fish (salmon); d. meat

■   ■   ■

346 The classes of food that are rich in magnesium are oats from bread products, shrimp, fish, and

_____ .

nuts

■   ■   ■

347 Give examples of foods that are rich in chloride.

a. Fruits: * _____
b. Meats: _____
c. Fish: _____
d. Dairy products: _____ and _____
e. Vegetables: _____ and _____

a. dates or bananas
b. turkey
c. crab
d. cheese and milk
e. spinach and celery

■   ■   ■

348 Name five foods that are rich in phosphorus. _____ ,
_____ , _____ , _____ , and
* _____ .

milk, beef, pork, fish, and whole grain cereal (also chicken, turkey, peanuts, and dried beans)

■   ■   ■

349 Check the classes of food that are rich in K (potassium), Na (sodium), Ca (calcium), Mg (magnesium), Cl (chloride), and P (phosphorus).

	K	Na	Ca	Mg	Cl	P	
a.	( )	( )	( )	( )	( )	( )	Fruits
b.	( )	( )	( )	( )	( )	( )	Fruit juices
c.	( )	( )	( )	( )	( )	( )	Bread products
d.	( )	( )	( )	( )	( )	( )	Dairy products
e.	( )	( )	( )	( )	( )	( )	Nuts
f.	( )	( )	( )	( )	( )	( )	Vegetables
g.	( )	( )	( )	( )	( )	( )	Meat
h.	( )	( )	( )	( )	( )	( )	Fish

a. *K, Cl (dates)*
b. *K*
c. *Na, Mg, P*
d. *Na, Ca, Cl, P*

e. *K, Mg, P*
f. *K, Ca, Mg, Cl*
g. *Na, Cl, Ca, P*
h. *K, Na, Ca, Mg, Cl, P*

CHAPTER 4

ACID-BASE BALANCE AND IMBALANCE

Behavioral Objectives

Upon completion of this chapter, you will be prepared to:

- Explain the influence of the hydrogen ion (H^+) on body fluids.
- Identify the pH ranges for acidosis and alkalosis.
- Discuss the four regulatory mechanisms for pH control and how the regulatory mechanisms can maintain acid-base balance.
- Explain how various clinical conditions can cause metabolic acidosis and alkalosis and respiratory acidosis and alkalosis.
- Identify clinical symptoms of metabolic acidosis and alkalosis and respiratory acidosis and alkalosis. (You may need some assistance in recognizing all these symptoms.)
- Discuss the body's defense action and the clinical management for acid-base balance and be able to apply this information to various clinical situations.

Introduction

Our body fluid must maintain a balance between acidity and alkalinity in order for life to be maintained. *Acid* comes from the Latin word meaning "sharp," and acid is frequently referred to as being sour. On the other hand, alkaline is referred to as being sweet. According to the Bronsted-Lowry concept of acids and bases, an "*acid* is any molecule or ion that can *donate a proton* to any other substance, whereas a *base* is any molecule or ion that can *accept a proton.*" The more readily an acid gives up its protons, the stronger it is as an acid. Acids and bases are not synonymous with anions and cations.

Other theories state that the concentration of hydrogen ions (plus or minus) determine either the acidity or the alkalinity of a solution. The amount of ionized hydrogen in extracellular fluid is extremely small; around 0.0000001 g/liter. Instead of using this cumbersome figure, the symbol pH is used, which stands for the negative logarithm (exponent) of the hydrogen ion concentration. Mathematically, it is expressed as 10^{-7}, the base being 10 and the power -7, the logarithm of the number. In this example the minus sign is dropped and the symbol used to designate the hydrogen ion concentration is pH 7. As the hydrogen ion concentration rises (in solution), the pH value falls, indicating a decreased negative logarithm of the hydrogen ion concentration, thus indicating increased acidity. As the hydrogen concentration falls, the pH rises, thus indicating increased alkalinity.

The hydroxyl ions (OH^-) are base ions and, when in excess, increase the alkalinity of the solution. A solution of pH 7 is neutral since at this concentration the number of hydrogen ions (H^+) is exactly balanced by the number of hydroxyl ions (OH^-).

The above information will help you in the basic understanding of acidity and alkalinity. This will aid in understanding the material presented in this chapter: the regulatory mechanism for pH control; the clinical conditions causing metabolic acidosis and alkalosis and respiratory acidosis and alkalosis (etiology); clinical manifestations and clinical management of acidosis and alkalosis; and clinical applications.

There are two case reviews and two sets of nursing diagnoses with nursing interventions.

Refer to the Introduction as needed to answer the first six frames. An asterisk (*) on an answer line indicates a multiple-word answer. The meanings for the following symbols are: ↑ increased, ↓ decreased, > greater than, < less than.

1   According to the Bronsted-Lowry concept of acids and bases, an acid is a proton (donor/acceptor) _____ and a base is a proton (donor/acceptor)

_____ .

donor; acceptor

      ■   ■   ■

2   For our purposes, consider that the acidity or alkalinity of a solution depends on the concentration of the   *_____ .

    An increase in concentration of the hydrogen ions makes a solution more _____ and a decrease in the concentration of hydrogen ions makes it more

_____ .

hydrogen ions; acid; alkaline

      ■   ■   ■

3   Explain the meaning of the pH symbol. *_____ .
    What effect does this have on a solution? *_____ .

negative logarithm of the hydrogen ion
It determines the acidity or alkalinity of a solution.

      ■   ■   ■

4   As the hydrogen ion concentration increases, the pH value _____

_____ . What does this indicate? _____ .

As the hydrogen ion concentration falls, the pH value _____

_____ . What does this indicate? _____ .

falls or decreases; acidity
rises or increases; alkalinity

■   ■   ■

5   A pH of 7 represents 10 times the number of hydrogen ions, as does a pH of 8. Which of the two pH's would be considered alkaline? _____ .

pH 8

■   ■   ■

6   A solution at pH 7 is neutral. Why? *_____

_____ .

The symbol for the hydrogen ion is _____ and the symbol for the hydroxyl ion is _____ .

A hydroxyl ion and CO_2 yields _____ , which is known as a

_____ .

The number of hydrogen ions is balanced by the number of hydroxyl ions.
H^+; OH^-; HCO_3; bicarbonate

■   ■   ■

7   The pH of extracellular fluid in health is maintained at a level between 7.35 and 7.45. Thus the body fluid is slightly (acid/alkaline) _____ .

alkaline

■   ■   ■

8   With a pH higher than this range (7.35–7.45), the body is considered to be in a state of alkalosis.

What would you call a state in which the pH is below 7.35? _____ .

acidosis

■   ■   ■

9   The pH norm of blood serum is 7.4; a variation of 0.4 of a pH unit in either direction can be fatal.

In a healthy individual, the pH range of blood serum is _____ .

7.35–7.45

        ■   ■   ■

10   Within our bodies, the pH of the different body fluids varies. The normal pH for urine is 6.0; for gastric juice, 1.0–2.0; for bile, 5.0–6.0; and for intracellular fluid, 6.9–7.2. These body fluids are (acidic/alkaline) _____ .

Why? * _____ .

The normal pH for intestinal juice is 6.5–7.6. The fluids from the intestinal tract can be which of the following:

( ) a. Acidic
( ) b. Alkaline
( ) c. Neutral

acidic; the pH is below 7.35
a. X; b. X; c. X

        ■   ■   ■

11   Whether a substance is acid, neutral, or alkaline depends on the number of
_____ ions present in a given weight or volume.

hydrogen

        ■   ■   ■

12   When the number of hydrogen ions increases in the body fluid, the body fluid becomes
_____ .

When the number of hydrogen ions decreases, the body fluid becomes
_____ .

acid; alkaline

        ■   ■   ■

13   In health, there are $1\frac{1}{3}$ mEq/L of acid to each 27 mEq of alkali for each liter of extracellular fluid, which represents a ratio of 1 part of acid to 20 parts of alkali.

Why do you think the measurement of acid and alkali is based on the extracellular fluid?

*_____ .

If the ratio of $1:20$ is maintained, the client is said to be in acid-base (balance/imbalance)

_____ .

more easily accessed for analysis; balance

∎   ∎   ∎

Figure 4-1 demonstrates by the arrow that the body is in acid-base balance when there is 1 part acid to 20 parts alkali. A pH of 7.4 represents this balance. If the arrow tilts left due to an alkali deficit or acid excess, then acidosis occurs, and if the arrow tilts right due to an alkali excess or acid deficit, then alkalosis occurs. Carbonic acid is H_2CO_3.

Study this diagram carefully. Know what happens when the arrow tilts either left or right. Refer to the figure when needed.

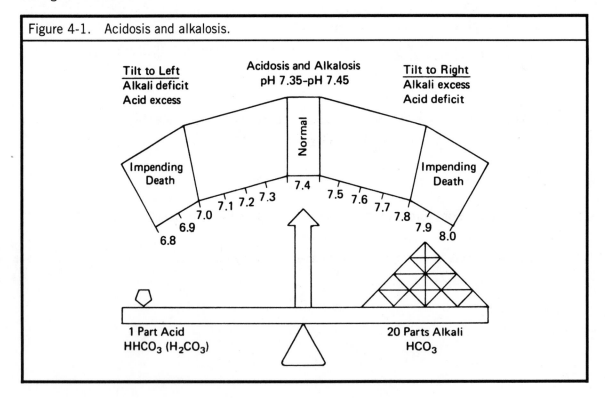

Figure 4-1.   Acidosis and alkalosis.

14 Your client's serum pH is 7.1. Tell everything you can about the client's condition on the basis of Figure 4-1. *_____

_____ .

An acidotic condition has occurred. It is due to either too much acid or too little alkali in the extracellular fluid.

■   ■   ■

15 Another client's serum pH is 7.8. Tell everything you can about the client's condition on the basis of the diagram. *_____

_____ .

Disturbance causing alkalosis. It is due to too much alkali or to too little acid. Borderline on impending death.

■   ■   ■

16 If the ratio 1 : 20 of the extracellular fluid is no longer present and the acid is increased or the alkali is decreased, then we say the client suffers from _____ .

If the alkaline reserve is increased or the acid decreases, then he suffers from

_____ .

acidosis; alkalosis

■   ■   ■

17 When there is acidosis, the balance is tilted _____ .

Which of the following occur:

( ) a. Alkali deficit
( ) b. Alkali excess
( ) c. Acid deficit
( ) d. Acid excess

The pH is below _____ .

left
a. X; b. —; c. —; d. X
7.35

■   ■   ■

18 When there is alkalosis, the balance is tilted _____ .

Which of the following occur:

( ) a. Alkali deficit
( ) b. Alkali excess
( ) c. Acid deficit
( ) d. Acid excess

The pH is below _____ .

right
a. —; b. X; c. X; d. —
7.45

■   ■   ■

19 The body is provided with several mechanisms for controlling its pH even though considerable amounts of acid or alkali enter the body.

The pH of blood serum in a healthy individual is between *_____ .

The pH norm of blood serum is _____ .

7.35 and 7.45; 7.4

■   ■   ■

REGULATORY MECHANISMS FOR pH CONTROL

20 The main regulatory mechanisms for pH control are:

1. The buffer system
2. The ion exchange
3. The respiratory regulation
4. The renal regulation

Name the four regulatory mechanisms for pH control. *_____ ,
*_____ , *_____ , and *_____ .

buffer system, ion exchange, respiratory regulation, and renal regulation

■   ■   ■

Table 4-1 is divided into three parts. Part A explains the buffer system. Buffers maintain the acid-base balance of body fluids by protecting the fluids against changes in pH. They act like chemical sponges, by either soaking up surplus hydrogen ions or releasing them.

There are four main examples of the buffer system, including bicarbonate–carbonic acid; phosphate; hemoglobin-oxyhemoglobin; and protein. They are shown in Table 4-1A along with their interventions—their action as a buffer—and the rationale—the reason for their action. The bicarbonate–carbonic acid buffer system is more readily available and acts within a fraction of a second to prevent excessive changes in H^+ concentration, and therefore it is the principal buffer

Table 4-1A. REGULATORY MECHANISM FOR pH CONTROL: BUFFER SYSTEMS

Regulatory Mechanism	Intervention	Rationale
a. Bicarbonate—carbonic acid buffer system (principal buffer system of body)	Acids combine with bicarbonates in blood to form neutral salts (bicarbonate salt) and carbonic acid (weak acid). Carbonic acid (H_2CO_3) is weak and unstable acid, changing to water and carbon dioxide in fluid ($H_2CO_3 \rightleftharpoons H_2O + CO_2$). A strong base combines with weak acid, e.g., H_2CO_3	When a strong acid such as HCl enters body, H^+ ions combine with HCO_3^- ions of $NaHCO_3$, yielding carbonic acid and neutral salt. (HCl + $NaHCO_3 \rightarrow H_2CO_3 + NaCl$). Weak acid, e.g., H_2CO_3, does not release H^+ as readily as does a strong acid, e.g., HCl, and thus ionizes less effectively. When a strong base such as NaOH is added to the system, it is neutralized by carbonic acid, yielding water and HCO_3^- from a salt (NaOH + $H_2CO \rightarrow H_2O + NaHCO_3$)
b. Phosphate buffer system	The phosphate buffer system increases the amount of sodium bicarbonate ($NaHCO_3$) in extracellular fluids, making extracellular fluids more alkaline. The H^+ is excreted as NaH_2PO_4 and Na and bicarbonate ions combine.	Excess H^+ combines in renal tubules with Na_2HPO_4 (disodium phosphate), forming NaH_2PO_4 ($H^+ + Na_2HPO_4 \rightarrow Na^+ + NaH_2PO_4$); Na^+ is reabsorbed ($Na^+ + HCO_3^- \rightarrow NaHCO_3$) and H^+ is passed into urine.
c. Hemoglobin-oxyhemoglobin buffer system	Maintains same pH level in venous blood as in arterial blood.	Venous blood has higher CO_2 content and bicarbonate ion concentration than arterial blood. The pH is the same since oxyhemoglobin (acid) in erythrocyte has taken over some anion function which was provided by excess bicarbonate in venous plasma.
d. Protein buffer system	Proteins can exist in form of acids (H protein) or alkaline salts (B protein) and in this way are able to bind or release excess hydrogen as required.	Proteins are amphoteric, carrying both acidic and basic charge.

system of the body. Strong acids, when added, combine with the bicarbonate ion to form carbonic acid, which is a weak acid. This prevents the fluids from becoming strongly acid.

Remember that bicarbonate and phosphates are anions. Refer to the glossary for unknown words. Study the table carefully and refer to it as needed.

21 (Refer to the Introduction of Table 4-1A if necessary.)

Explain the purpose of the buffer systems. *_____ .

How do the buffer systems accomplish their purpose? *_____

_____ .

They protect fluids against changes in pH.
They soak up surplus H^+ and release them as needed.

■   ■   ■

22 What is the principal buffer system of the body? *_____ .

the bicarbonate—carbonic acid buffer system

■   ■   ■

23 When acid enters the body, the H^+ is picked up by the bicarbonate, changing it to
*_____ .

A base added to the body is neutralized by carbonic acid to form _____
and _____ .

carbonic acid (H_2CO_3); water; bicarbonate

■   ■   ■

24 The bicarbonate—carbonic acid buffer system is the most important buffer system in the body. It maintains acid-base balance 55% of the time. Give an example with a formula of how a strong acid combines with a bicarbonate to yield a weak acid. *_____ .

Write an example with a formula of how a strong base is neutralized by a weak acid to yield water and bicarbonate from a weak salt. *_____ .

$HCl + NaHCO_3 \rightarrow H_2CO_3 + NaCl$
$NaOH + H_2CO_3 \rightarrow H_2O + NaHCO_3$

■   ■   ■

25 The phosphate buffer system maintains the acid-base balance by combining the excess H^+ with sodium salts, forming *_____ .

   The H^+ is excreted in _____ .

   This system (excretes/retains) _____ excess acid in the body.

   NaH_2PO_4; urine; excretes

   ■   ■   ■

26 What is the function of the hemoglobin-oxyhemoglobin buffer system? *_____
_____ .

   It maintains the same pH level in the venous blood and the arterial blood.

   ■   ■   ■

27 What is unique about the protein buffer system? *_____
_____ .

   This system carries a(n) _____ and a(n) _____ charge.

   It is amphoteric—it has the ability to bind or release excess H^+.
   acidic; basic

   ■   ■   ■

28 The four buffer systems in the body are: *_____ , _____ ,
   *_____ , and _____ .

   bicarbonate—carbonic acid, phosphate, hemoglobin-oxyhemoglobin, and protein

   ■   ■   ■

   Table 4-1B gives an explanation of the ion exchange in the respiratory regulation of ions as regulatory mechanisms for pH control. The ion exchange is frequently referred to as the *chloride shift*. Refer to Chapter 3 for clarification of the chloride shift if needed. The respiratory regulation depends on the lungs to exhale CO_2 or retain CO_2 for the control of pH. Again, the interventions refer to the action, and the rationale refers to the reason.
   Study this table carefully and refer to it as needed.

29 When carbon dioxide enters the red blood cell, what happens to the bicarbonate and chloride anions? *_____ .

   This ion exchange is frequently called the *_____ .

   Bicarbonate diffuses out of the cell and the chloride ion enters the cell.
   chloride shift

   ■   ■   ■

Table 4-1B. REGULATORY MECHANISM FOR pH CONTROL: ION EXCHANGE AND RESPIRATORY REGULATION

Regulatory Mechanism	Intervention	Rationale
Ion exchange	Ion exchange of HCO_3 and Cl occurs in red blood cell as result of O_2 and CO_2 exchange. There is redistribution of anions in response to increase in CO_2. Chloride ion enters red blood cell (RBC) as bicarbonate ion and diffuses into plasma in order to restore ionic balance.	Increase in serum carbon dioxide causes CO_2 to diffuse into red blood cells combining with H_2O to form H_2CO_3. This weak acid dissociates, forming acid and base ions, $H_2CO_3 \rightarrow H^+ + HCO_3^-$. Hydrogen ion is buffered by hemoglobin, and HCO_3^- ion moves into plasma as chloride ion (Cl^-) shifts into cell to replace it.

Regulatory Mechanism	Intervention	Rationale
Respiratory regulation (acts quickly in case of emergency)	For regulation of acid balance, the lungs blow off more CO_2 and for regulation of alkaline balance, the respiratory center depresses respirations in order to retain CO_2. It takes 1–3 min for the respiratory system to readjust H^+ concentration.	Respiratory center in medulla controls the rate and depth of respiration and is sensitive to changes in blood pH or CO_2 concentration. When pH is decreased, carbonic acid is exhaled in the form of carbon dioxide and moist air ($H_2CO_3 \rightarrow H_2O + CO_2$); thus acid is eliminated.

Note: Illustration from "Blood-Gases and Blood-Gas Transport," by J. L. Keyes, 1974, *Heart and Lung,* pp. 945–954. Copyright 1982. Adapted by permission.

30 When the red blood cells are oxygenated, what anion is commonly present? _____ .

When carbon dioxide enters the red blood cells, what anion also enters? _____ .

What anion leaves as carbon dioxide enters? _____ .

bicarbonate (HCO_3); chloride (CI); bicarbonate (HCO_3)
■   ■   ■

31 How does the respiratory regulatory mechanism control the serum pH?   * _____

_____ .

When the serum pH is decreased, the lungs blow off CO_2. With an increased pH, the lungs retain CO_2.
■   ■   ■

32 Where is the respiratory center located? _____ . What does the respiratory center control? * _____ .

medulla; rate and depth of respirations
■   ■   ■

33 How do the two mechanisms in Table 4-1B deal with an increased CO_2?

a. * _____

b. * _____

a. As the CO_2 enters the red cells, HCO_3 leaves the red cell and Cl enters.
b. The lungs blow off more CO_2.
■   ■   ■

Table 4-1C describes how the kidneys regulate pH in the body. The kidneys compensate for an excess production of acid by excreting the acid and returning the bicarbonate to the extracellular fluid. The acid occurs as the result of normal metabolism.

Study the table carefully, noting how, in each instance, the excess H^+ ions are neutralized. When you think you understand the renal regulatory mechanism described in the table, answer the frames that follow. Refer to the table when needed.

34 Name the three renal regulatory mechanisms for pH control. * _____ ,
* _____ , and * _____ .

acidification of phosphate buffer salts, reabsorption of bicarbonate, and secretion of ammonia
■   ■   ■

| Table 4-1C.   REGULATORY MECHANISM FOR pH CONTROL: RENAL REGULATION |

Regulatory Mechanism	Intervention	Rationale
a. Acidification of phosphate buffer salts	Exchange mechanism occurs between H^+ of renal tubular cells and disodium salt (Na_2HPO_4) in tubular urine.	Sodium salt (Na_2HPO_4) dissociates into Na^+ and $NaHPO_4^-$; Na^+ moves into tubular cell and hydrogen unites with $NaHPO_4$, forming dihydrogen phosphate salt, NaH_2PO_4, which is excreted.

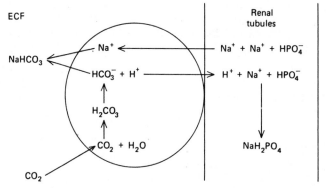

| b. Reabsorption of bicarbonate | Carbon dioxide is absorbed by tubular cells from blood and combines with water present in cells to form carbonic acid, which in turn ionizes, forming H^+ and HCO_3^-. Na^+ of tubular urine exchanges with H^+ of tubular cells and combines with HCO_3^- to form sodium bicarbonate and is reabsorbed into blood. | The enzyme carbonic anhydrase is responsible for formation of carbonic acid H_2CO_3.

Ionization of $H_2CO_3 \rightarrow H^+ + HCO_3^-$. Free H^+ exchanges with Na^+.

Exchange of H^+ and Na^+ permits reabsorption of bicarbonate with sodium.

($NaHCO_3$) and excretion of an acid or H^+. |

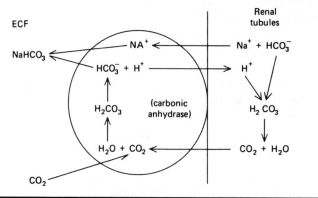

Table 4-1C.   (Continued)

Regulatory Mechanism	Intervention	Rationale
c. Secretion of ammonia	Ammonia (NH_3) unites with HCl in renal tubules and H^+ is excreted as NH_4Cl (ammonium chloride).	Almost half of H^+ excretion is from this method—HCl + $NH_3 \rightarrow NH_4Cl$.
		Ammonia is formed in renal tubular cells by oxidative breakdown of amino acid glutamine in presence of enzyme glutanimase.
		Ammonia can also be converted into urea by the liver and excreted as urea by the kidneys.

Note: Illustrations from *Textbook of Medical Physiology*, ed 8, by A. C. Guyton, 1991, Philadelphia: W. B. Saunders Co. Copyright 1991 by W. B. Saunders Co. Adapted by permission.

35 Hydrogen ions exist largely in the renal tubules in the buffered state. They are excreted indirectly by replacing a cation in excretion.

Explain how the hydrogen ion is excreted after it combines with the sodium salt Na_2HPO_4.

*_____ .

The H^+ replaces a Na^+, forming a dihydrogen phosphate salt, NaH_2PO_4. This salt is excreted.

■   ■   ■

36 The kidneys regulate the H$^+$ levels in the body by varying the excretion and reabsorption of H$^+$ and HCO$_3^-$.

Explain how the H$^+$ is derived from carbonic acid. *_____.

Explain how the bicarbonate ion is reabsorbed. *_____

_____.

by the ionization of $H_2CO_3 \rightarrow H^+ + HCO_3^-$
The Na$^+$ exchanges with the H$^+$ in renal tubules and the Na$^+$ combines with HCO$_3^-$ and is reabsorbed into the blood.

■   ■   ■

37 Explain the formation of ammonia in the renal tubular cells. *_____

_____.

How does ammonia aid in the excretion of the hydrogen ion? *_____

_____.

It is formed from the breakdown of amino acid glutamine.
NH$_3$ unites with HCl and is excreted as NH$_4$Cl (ammonium chloride).

■   ■   ■

38 Which one of the three methods in Table 4-1C is responsible for nearly half of the hydrogen ion excretion? *_____ .

secretion of ammonia

■   ■   ■

SUMMARY

The three major mechanisms that regulate pH or the hydrogen ion concentration in the body fluids are chemical buffers, pulmonary (respiration) exchange, and renal (kidney) regulation. The action time that it takes to maintain acid-base balance (homeostasis) varies.

Regulatory Mechanisms	Action time
Chemical buffers	Immediate
Pulmonary exchange	Minutes
Renal regulation	Hours to days

39 The chemical buffers combine with acids or bases to maintain acid-base balance. Their action time is _____ .

immediate

■   ■   ■

40 The lungs control the carbon dioxide (CO_2) concentration by increasing or decreasing the rate of respirations. The action time occurs in _____ .

minutes

  ▪   ▪   ▪

41 The kidneys control bicarbonate ion (HCO_3^-) concentration by reabsorption of HCO_3 or excretion of hydrogen ion (H^+) and the production of ammonia.

   The action time for the kidneys to maintain this acid-base balance is

_____ .
*

hours to days

  ▪   ▪   ▪

42 Match the regulatory mechanisms on the left according to their action times for maintaining acid-base balance.

   ___ 1. Chemical buffers   a. Minutes
   ___ 2. Respiratory action   b. Hours to days
   ___ 3. Kidney action   c. Immediate

   1. c; 2. a; 3. b

  ▪   ▪   ▪

PRINCIPLES OF ACID-BASE IMBALANCES

43 Hydrogen ions circulate throughout the body fluids in two forms, namely, *volatile acid* and *nonvolatile acid*.

   A volatile acid (carbonic acid—H_2CO_3) circulates as CO_2 and H_2O and is excreted as a gas. The gas excreted is (HCO_3/CO_2) _____ , which helps maintaining acid-base balance.

   A nonvolatile acid (fixed acid, e.g., lactic, pyruvic, sulfuric, phosphoric acids) is produced as the result of various organic acids within the body. It must be excreted from the body in water, e.g., urine. What regulatory mechanism is responsible for excreting nonvolatile acids?

_____ .

CO_2; kidney or renal

  ▪   ▪   ▪

44 The lungs excrete (volatile/nonvolatile) _____ acids and the kidneys excrete (volatile/nonvolatile) _____ acids.

Renal Regulation   *Respiratory Regulation*

$H^+ + HCO_3^- \leftrightharpoons$ $|H_2CO_3| \leftrightharpoons H_2O + CO_2$
(excreted as nonvolatile acid)   (excreted as volatile acid)

volatile; nonvolatile

■   ■   ■

45 The kidneys and lungs aid in acid-base balance. Label the chemical formula according to the organ that is responsible for acid-base regulation.

_____ $H^+ + HCO_3^- \leftrightharpoons |H_2CO_3| \leftrightharpoons H_2O + CO_2$ _____
(organ)   (organ)

kidneys; lungs

■   ■   ■

Figure 4-2 demonstrates the normal acid-base balance and the three blood tests (pH, arterial CO_2 concentration [$Paco_2$], HCO_3 or serum CO_2) that can indicate acid-base imbalance. The top scale shows acid-base balance with 1 part acid and 20 parts base. The middle two scales indicate acidosis, either respiratory (excess carbonic acid [H_2CO_3]) or metabolic (bicarbonate deficit). The lower two scales indicate alkalosis, either respiratory (deficit of carbonic acid) or metabolic (excess bicarbonate).

46 When the acid-base scale tips to the left, it is an indication that an (acidotic/alkalotic) _____ state is present.

When the scale tips to the right, the type of acid-base imbalance is (acidosis/alkalosis) _____ .

acidotic; alkalosis

■   ■   ■

To determine the type of acid-base imbalance, the following blood tests are essential:

1. Normal pH level: adult, 7.35–7.45; newborn, 7.27–7.47; child, 7.33–7.43.
2. $Paco_2$ level (respiratory component): adult and child, 35–45 mm Hg; newborn, 27–40 mm Hg; infant, 27–41 mm Hg.
   Increased $Paco_2$: hypoventilation (respiratory acidosis).
   Decreased $Paco_2$: hyperventilation (respiratory alkalosis).

Figure 4-2. Acid-base balance and imbalance.

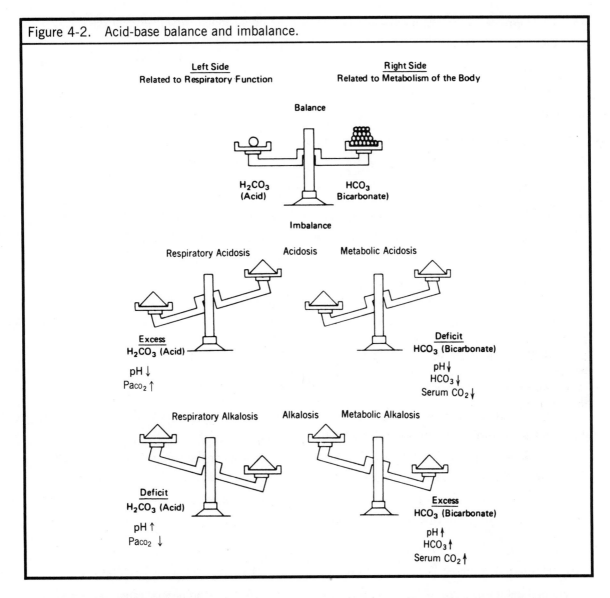

3. HCO₃ and base excess levels (metabolic or renal component): HCO₃—adult and child, 24–28 mEq/L; newborn, 22–30 mEq/L. Base excess (BE): adult and child, +2 to −2. Also serum CO₂ is 22–32 mEq/L.* Increased HCO₃, BE, and/or serum CO₂ is metabolic alkalosis. Decreased HCO₃, BE, and/or serum CO₂ is metabolic acidosis.

*Serum CO₂ is a serum bicarbonate determinant and is frequently called *CO₂ combining power*. It refers to the amount of cations, e.g., H⁺, Na⁺, K⁺, and so on, available to combine with HCO₃. The level of HCO₃ in the blood is determined by the amount of CO₂ dissolved in the blood.

47 To determine if acidosis or alkalosis is present, the nurse should *first* check for the ($pH/Paco_2/HCO_3$) _____ of the arterial blood gas results.

pH

■   ■   ■

48 If the pH is less than 7.35, the acid-base imbalance is _____ .

 If the pH is greater than 7.45, the acid-base imbalance is _____ .

acidosis; alkalosis

■   ■   ■

49 To determine if the acid-base imbalance is respiratory acidosis or alkalosis, the $Paco_2$ should be checked. If $Paco_2$ is within normal range, the imbalance is not respiratory.

 If the $Paco_2$ is greater than 45 mm Hg and the pH is less than 7.35, the type of acid-base imbalance is *_____ .

 If the $Paco_2$ is less than 35 mm Hg and the pH is greater than 7.45, the type of acid-base imbalance is *_____ .

respiratory acidosis; respiratory alkalosis

■   ■   ■

50 The third step to determine the type of acid-base imbalance is to check the bicarbonate (HCO_3) and base excess (BE) levels of the arterial blood gas and the serum CO_2 level (either one of the levels or all of them if available).

 If the HCO_3 is less than 24 mEq/L, the BE is −2 or less, or the serum CO_2 is less than 22 mEq/L, the type of acid-base imbalance is *_____ .

 If the HCO_3 is greater than 28 mEq/L, the BE is +2 or more, or the serum CO_2 is greater than 32 mEq/L, the type of acid-base imbalance is *_____ .

metabolic acidosis; metabolic alkalosis

■   ■   ■

51 The normal range for pH in blood is _____ . The normal range for $Paco_2$ in arterial blood is *_____ . The normal range of HCO_3 in arterial blood is *_____ . The normal range of serum CO_2 in venous blood is *_____ .

7.35–7.45; 35–45 mm Hg; 24–28 mEq/L; 22–32 mEq/L

■   ■   ■

52 To determine acidotic and alkalotic states, the nurse must first assess the _____ level; second the _____ of arterial blood; and third the _____ of arterial blood or _____ of venous blood.

pH; $Paco_2$; HCO_3; serum CO_2
　　　　　　　■　　　　　　　　　　■　　　　　　　　　■

53 Respiratory acidosis and alkalosis are determined by which of the following:

( ) a. pH
( ) b. $Paco_2$
( ) c. HCO_3
( ) d. BE

a. X; b. X; c. —; d. —
　　　　　　　■　　　　　　　　　　■　　　　　　　　　■

54 Metabolic acidosis and alkalosis are determined by which of the following:

( ) a. pH
( ) b. $Paco_2$
( ) c. HCO_3
( ) d. BE
( ) e. serum CO_2

a. X; b. —; c. X; d. X; e. X
　　　　　　　■　　　　　　　　　　■　　　　　　　　　■

55 Place R. Ac for respiratory acidosis, R. Al for Respiratory alkalosis, M. Ac for metabolic acidosis, and M. Al for metabolic alkalosis beside the following laboratory determinants.

_____ ,	_____	a. pH ↑
_____ ,	_____	b. pH ↓
	_____	c. $Paco_2$ ↑
	_____	d. HCO_3 ↑
	_____	e. $Paco_2$ ↓
	_____	f. HCO_3 ↓
	_____	g. serum CO_2 ↓
	_____	h. serum CO_2 ↑

a. R. Al, M. Al
b. R. Ac, M. Ac
c. R. Ac
d. M. Al
e. R. Al
f. M. Ac
g. M. Ac
h. M. Al

■   ■   ■

COMPENSATION FOR pH BALANCE

56 There are specific compensatory reactions in response to metabolic acidosis and alkalosis and respiratory acidosis and alkalosis. The pH returns to normal or close to normal by changing the component, e.g., $Paco_2$ or HCO_3 and/or BE, that originally was not affected.

The respiratory system can compensate for metabolic acidosis and alkalosis. With metabolic acidosis, the lungs (stimulated by the respiratory center) hyperventilate to decrease CO_2 level.

A pH of 7.34, $Paco_2$ of 24, and HCO_3 of 15 indicate metabolic acidosis, since the pH is slightly acid and the HCO_3 is definitely low (acidosis). The $Paco_2$ should be normal (35–45); however, it is low since the respiratory center compensates for the acidotic state by "blowing off" CO_2 (hyperventilating); respiratory compensation occurs. Without compensation, the pH would be extremely low, e.g., pH 7.2.

For metabolic alkalosis, the lungs (hypoventilate/hyperventilate) _____ to conserve _____ .

With a pH of 7.48, $Paco_2$ of 46, and HCO_3 of 39, the pH and HCO_3 indicate
* _____ .

The $Paco_2$ indicates respiratory compensation. Explain. * _____

_____ .

hypoventilate; CO_2; metabolic alkalosis
The lungs compensate for the alkalotic state by conserving CO_2 (respiratory compensation).
■　　　　　■　　　　　■

57 With respiratory acidosis, the kidneys excrete more acid, H^+, and conserve HCO_3^-.

With a pH of 7.35, $Paco_2$ of 68, and HCO_3 of 35, the pH is low normal, borderline acidosis, and the $Paco_2$ is highly elevated, indicating CO_2 retention—respiratory acidosis. The HCO_3 indicates * _____

_____ .

kidney or metabolic compensation. Without this compensation the pH is lower.
■　　　　　■　　　　　■

58 With respiratory alkalosis, the kidneys excrete _____ ions and conserve _____ ions.

A pH of 7.46, $Paco_2$ of 20, and HCO_3 of 22, the pH and $Paco_2$ indicate
* _____ . The HCO_3 indicates renal or metabolic compensation.

Explain how. * _____

_____ .

bicarbonate (HCO_3^-); acid (H^+); respiratory alkalosis
The kidneys compensate for the alkalotic state by excreting HCO_3 (metabolic compensation).
■　　　　　■　　　　　■

59 When the body is in a state of metabolic acidosis, an excess of nonvolatile acid is retained in body fluids.

What do you suppose occurs in metabolic alkalosis * _____

_____ .

How is a nonvolatile acid excreted from the body? _____ .

a decrease in nonvolatile acid in body fluids; in the urine
■　　　　　■　　　　　■

60 With respiratory acidosis, there is an excess of volatile acid. In what form do you think a volatile acid is excreted from the body? _____ .

   With respiratory alkalosis, there is a(n) (increase/decrease) _____ in volatile acid.

gas (lungs); decrease

■   ■   ■

61 Identify the type of acid-base imbalance and if there is compensation, indicate which kind, metabolic or respiratory. Memorize the norms for pH, Pa_{CO_2}, and HCO_3.

	pH	Pa_{CO_2}	HCO_3	Type	Compensation Metabolic	Compensation Respiratory
a.	7.33	62	32	_____	_____ _____	_____
b.	7.50	29	25	_____	_____ _____	_____
c.	7.26	59	27	_____	_____ _____	_____
d.	7.21	40	19	_____	_____ _____	_____
e.	7.53	39	36	_____	_____ _____	_____
f.	7.40	40	26	_____	_____ _____	_____
g.	7.32	79	41	_____	_____ _____	_____
h.	7.1	16	6	_____	_____ _____	_____
i.	7.57	48	40	_____	_____ _____	_____
j.	7.23	23	10	_____	_____ _____	_____

a. respiratory acidosis with metabolic compensation
b. respiratory alkalosis with NO compensation
c. respiratory acidosis with NO compensation
d. metabolic acidosis with NO compensation
e. metabolic alkalosis with NO compensation
f. normal arterial blood gases
g. respiratory acidosis with metabolic compensation
h. metabolic acidosis with respiratory compensation
i. metabolic alkalosis with respiratory compensation
j. metabolic acidosis with respiratory compensation

■   ■   ■

METABOLIC ACIDOSIS AND ALKALOSIS

PATHOPHYSIOLOGY

62   Metabolic acidosis is characterized by a(n) (increased/decreased) _____
bicarbonate concentration or acid (deficit/excess) _____ in the extracellular
fluid.

The pH is (less/more) _____ than 7.35.

decreased; excess; less (<)
■   ■   ■

63   With metabolic acidosis, the HCO$_3$ level is _____ mEq/L, the base excess
(BE) is (>+2/<−2) _____ , and the serum CO$_2$ is _____
mEq/L.

<24; <−2; <22
■   ■   ■

64   Metabolic alkalosis is characterized by a(n) (increased/decreased) _____
bicarbonate concentration or loss of the hydrogen ion (strong acid) in the extracellular fluid.

The pH is _____ .

increased; greater than (>) 7.45
■   ■   ■

65   With metabolic alkalosis, the bicarbonate level is _____ mEq/L; BE is
_____ ; and the serum CO$_2$ is _____ mEq/L.

>28; >+2; >32
■   ■   ■

ETIOLOGY

The causes of metabolic acidosis and metabolic alkalosis are described in Tables 4-2 and 4-3.
The rationale is given with each of the causes. Study the tables and then proceed to the frames.
Refer to the tables as needed.

66   With severe or chronic diarrhea, the anion that is lost from the small intestine is
_____ . The sodium ion is also lost in excess of the chloride ion. The chloride
ion combines with the hydrogen ion to produce the acid *_____ .

bicarbonate; hydrochloric acid
■   ■   ■

Table 4-2. CAUSES OF METABOLIC ACIDOSIS

Etiology	Rationale
Gastrointestinal Abnormalities Starvation Severe malnutrition	Nonvolatile acids, i.e., lactic and pyruvic acids, occur as the result of an accumulation of acid products from cellular breakdown due to starvation and/or severe malnutrition.
Chronic diarrhea	Loss of bicarbonate ions in the small intestines is in excess. Also, the loss of sodium ions exceeds that of chloride ions. Cl^- combines with H^+, producing a strong acid (HCl).
Renal Abnormalities Kidney failure	Kidney mechanisms for conserving sodium and water and for excreting H^+ fail.
Hormonal Influence Diabetic ketoacidosis	Failure to metabolize adequate quantities of glucose causes the liver to increase metabolism of fatty acids. Oxidation of fatty acids produces ketone bodies which cause the ECF to become more acid. Ketones require a base for excretion.
Hyperthyroidism, thyrotoxicosis	An overactive thyroid gland can cause cellular catabolism (breakdown) due to a severe increase in metabolism which increases cellular needs.
Others Trauma, shock	Trauma and shock cause cellular breakdown and the release of nonvolatile acids.
Excess exercise, severe infection, fever	Excessive exercise, fever, and severe infection can cause cellular catabolism and acid accumulation.

67 How does starvation cause metabolic acidosis? *_____.

Nonvolatile acids such as lactic acid result from cellular breakdown.

■   ■   ■

68 With uncontrolled diabetes mellitus, glucose cannot be metabolized; therefore, what occurs?
*_____.

The liver produces fatty acids, which leads to ketone body production.

■   ■   ■

69 Shock, trauma, severe infection, and fever can cause cellular (anabolism/catabolism) _____ . The acid products frequently released from the cells are *_____

_____ .

catabolism; nonvolatile acids such as lactic acid

      ■   ■   ■

70 Indicate which of the following conditions can cause metabolic acidosis:

( ) a. Starvation
( ) b. Gastric suction
( ) c. Excessive exercise
( ) d. Mercurial diuretics
( ) e. Shock
( ) f. Uncontrolled diabetes mellitus (ketoacidosis)

a. X; b. —; c. X; d. —; e. X; f. X

      ■   ■   ■

Table 4-3 lists the causes of metabolic alkalosis with the rationale. Refer to the table as needed.

Table 4-3. CAUSES OF METABOLIC ALKALOSIS	
Etiology	**Rationale**
Gastrointestinal Abnormalities	
Vomiting, gastric suction	With vomiting and gastric suctioning, large amounts of chloride and hydrogen ions that are plentiful in the stomach are lost. Bicarbonate anions increase to compensate for chloride loss.
Peptic ulcers	Excess of alkali in ECF occurs when a client takes excessive amounts of acid neutralizers such as $NaHCO_3$ to ease ulcer pain.
Others	
Mercurial diuretics	Loss of potassium, chloride, and other electrolytes.
Hypokalemia	Loss of potassium from the body is accompanied by loss of chloride (see Chapter 3, on chloride).

71 Name the anion that is lost in great quantities due to vomiting, gastric suction, or mercurial diuretics. _____ .

chloride

      ■   ■   ■

72 Name the conditions that cause metabolic alkalosis.

a. *_____

b. *_____

c. *_____

d. *_____

e. *_____

a. treated peptic ulcer; b. vomiting; c. gastric suction; d. mercurial diuretics; e. loss of potassium

       ▪   ▪   ▪

73 For causes of metabolic acidosis and alkalosis, place M. Ac for metabolic acidosis and M. Al for metabolic alkalosis for the appropriate condition.

____ a. Diabetic ketoacidosis

____ b. Treated peptic ulcer

____ c. Severe diarrhea

____ d. Shock, trauma

____ e. Vomiting, gastric suction

____ f. Mercurial diuretics

____ g. Fever, severe infection

____ h. Excessive exercise

a. M. Ac; b. M. Al; c. M. Ac; d. M. Ac; e. M. Al; f. M. Al; g. M. Ac; h. M. Ac

       ▪   ▪   ▪

CLINICAL APPLICATIONS

Anion gap is a useful indicator for determining the presence or absence of metabolic acidosis. Anion gap can be obtained by completing the following steps:

1. Adding the serum chloride/Cl and serum CO_2 values
2. Subtracting the sum of serums Cl and CO_2 from the serum sodium/Na value

The difference is the anion gap.

74 If the anion gap is >16 mEq/L, metabolic acidosis is suspected. The acid in the body would be stronger than the carbonic acid.

Which of the following acid-base imbalances are indicated by an anion gap that exceeds 16 mEq/L:

( ) a. Metabolic acidosis
( ) b. Metabolic alkalosis
( ) c. Respiratory acidosis

a. X; b. —; c. —

■   ■   ■

75 A client's serum values are Na, 142 mEq/L; Cl, 102 mEq/L; and CO_2, 18 mEq/L.

The anion gap is   *_____ .

Is metabolic acidosis present? _____ Why? *_____

_____ .

142 − 120 = 22 mEq/L; yes
The anion gap is greater than 16 mEq/L.

■   ■   ■

76 Conditions associated with an anion gap that is greater than 16 mEq/L are diabetic ketoacidosis, lactic acidosis, poisoning, and renal failure.

Indicate which of the following conditions might apply to an anion gap of 25 mEq/L:

( ) a. Diabetic ketoacidosis   ( ) d. Renal failure
( ) b. COPD   ( ) e. Poisoning
( ) c. Respiratory failure   ( ) f. Lactic acidosis

a. X; b. —; c. —; d. X; e. X; f. X

■   ■   ■

77 When a client takes excessive amounts of baking soda or commercially prepared acid neutralizers to ease indigestion or stomach ulcer pain, what imbalance will most likely occur?
*_____ . Why? *_____ .

metabolic alkalosis
There is excess alkali in the extracellular fluid.

■   ■   ■

CLINICAL MANIFESTATIONS

When metabolic acidosis occurs, the central nervous system (CNS) is depressed and symptoms can include apathy, disorientation, weakness, and stupor. Deep rapid breathing is a respiratory compensatory mechanism for the purpose of decreasing acid content in the blood.

With metabolic alkalosis, excitability of the CNS occurs. These symptoms may include irritability, mental confusion, tetanylike symptoms, and hyperactive reflexes. Hypoventilation may occur and it acts as a compensatory mechanism for metabolic alkalosis; conserves the hydrogen ions and carbonic acid.

Table 4-4 lists the clinical manifestations related to metabolic acidosis and alkalosis. Study the table and refer to it as needed when answering the frames.

Table 4-4. CLINICAL MANIFESTATIONS OF METABOLIC ACIDOSIS AND METABOLIC ALKALOSIS

Body Areas	Metabolic Acidosis	Metabolic Alkalosis
CNS abnormalities	Restlessness, apathy, weakness, disorientation, stupor, coma	Irritability, confusion, tetanylike symptoms, hyperactive reflexes
Respiratory abnormalities	Kussmaul breathing: deep, rapid, vigorous breathing	Shallow breathing
Skin changes	Flushing and warm skin	
Cardiac abnormalities	Cardiac dysrhythmias, decrease in heart rate and cardiac output	
Gastrointestinal abnormalities	Nausea, vomiting, abdominal pain	Vomiting with loss of chloride and potassium
Laboratory Tests		
pH	<7.35	>7.45
HCO_3, BE	<24 mEq/L; <−2	>28 mEq/L; >+2
Serum CO_2	<22 mEq/L	>32 mEq/L

Note: <=less than; >=greater than.

78 With metabolic acidosis, the CNS is (depressed/excited) _____ .

With metabolic alkalosis, the CNS is (depressed/excited) _____ .

depressed; excited

■ ■ ■

79 Indicate which of the following CNS abnormalities are associated with metabolic acidosis (M. Ac) and metabolic alkalosis (M. Al):

_____ a. Irritability
_____ b. Apathy
_____ c. Disorientation
_____ d. Tetanylike symptoms
_____ e. Hyperactive reflexes
_____ f. Stupor

a. M. Al; b. M. Ac; c. M. Ac; d. M. Al; e. M. Al; f. M. Ac

   ■   ■   ■

80 Metabolic acidosis results from a   *_____ .
In metabolic acidosis, the HCO_3 and BE are (decreased/increased) _____
and the serum CO_2 is (decreased/increased) _____ .

bicarbonate deficit or acid excess; decreased; decreased

   ■   ■   ■

81 With metabolic acidosis, the renal and respiratory mechanisms try to reestablish balance.

 Explain how the renal mechanism works to reestablish balance.
*_____ .

 Explain how the respiratory mechanism works to reestablish balance.
*_____ .

 When these two mechanisms fail, what happens to the plasma pH?
*_____ .

The H^+ exchange with the Na^+ and thus H^+ is excreted.
As the result of the Kussmaul breathing, CO_2 is blown off; decreasing carbonic acid (H_2CO_3).
It decreases.

   ■   ■   ■

82 Metabolic alkalosis results from a   *_____ .
In metabolic alkalosis, the HCO_3 and BE are (decreased/increased) _____
and the serum CO_2 is (decreased/increased) _____ .

bicarbonate excess; increased; increased

   ■   ■   ■

83 With metabolic alkalosis, the buffer, renal, and respiratory mechanisms try to reestablish balance. With the buffer mechanism, the excess bicarbonate reacts with buffer acid salts; thus, there is a decrease in bicarbonate ions in the extracellular fluid and an increase in the concentration of carbonic acid.

Explain how the renal mechanism works to reestablish balance.

* _____ .

Explain how the respiratory mechanism works to reestablish balance.

* _____ .

When these three mechanisms fail, what happens to the plasma pH?

* _____ .

H^+ is conserved and Na^+ and K^+ are excreted with HCO_3.
Pulmonary ventilation is decreased; therefore, CO_2 is retained, increasing H_2CO_3.
It increases.

■   ■   ■

CLINICAL MANAGEMENT

Figure 4-3 outlines the body's normal defense actions and various methods of treatment for restoring balance in metabolic acidosis and alkalosis. Study this figure carefully, with particular attention to the cause of each imbalance, the body's defense action, the pH of the urine as to whether it is acidic or alkaline, and the treatment for these imbalances. Refer to the figure whenever you find it necessary.

Figure 4-3. Body's defense action and treatment for metabolic acidosis and alkalosis.

Metabolic Acidosis (Deficit of bicarbonate or excess acid in the extracellular fluid)

Lungs   Kidney

Lungs "blow off" acid. Respirations are increased.

Urine is acid. Kidneys conserve alkali and excrete acid.

Treatment: Remove the cause. Administer an IV alkali solution, e.g., sodium bicarbonate or sodium lactate. Restore water, electrolytes, and nutrients.

Metabolic Alkalosis (Excess of bicarbonate in the extracellular fluid)

Lungs   Kidney

Breathing is suppressed.

Urine is alkaline. Kidneys excrete alkali ions, and retain hydrogen ions and nonbicarbonate ions.

Treatment: Remove the cause. Administer an IV solution of chloride, e.g., sodium chloride. Replace potassium deficit.

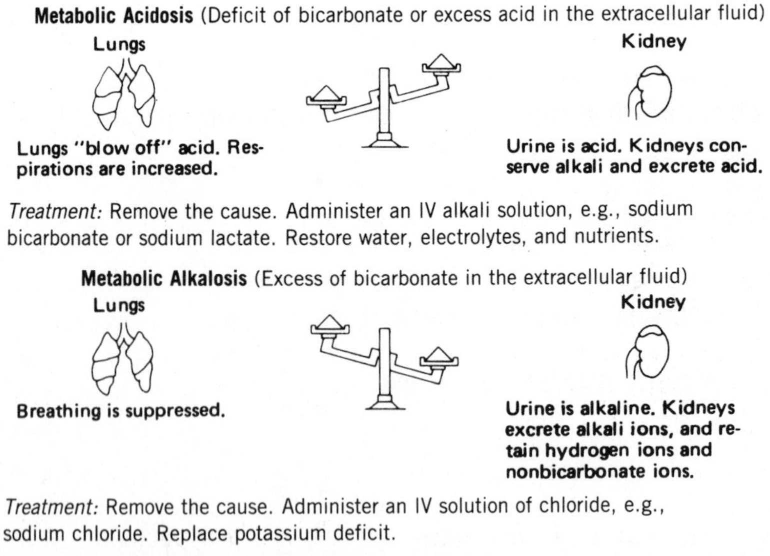

84 What is metabolic acidosis? *_____ .
Is the urine (acid/alkaline)? _____ .
What are the body's defense actions against it?

a. *_____

b. *_____

bicarbonate deficit or acid excess; acid
a. lungs blow off CO_2 or acid
b. kidneys excrete acid or H^+ and conserve alkali
■   ■   ■

85 Identify three treatment modalities for metabolic acidosis.

*_____ , *_____ , and *_____ .

remove cause, administer IV alkali solution (e.g., $NaHCO_3$), and restore H_2O and electrolyte
■   ■   ■

86 What is metabolic alkalosis? *_____ .
Is the urine (acid/alkaline)? _____ .
What are the body's defense actions against it?

a. *_____

b. *_____

bicarbonate excess; alkaline
a. breathing is suppressed
b. kidneys excrete alkali ions (e.g., HCO_3) and retain H^+ and nonbicarbonate ions
■   ■   ■

87 Identify three treatment modalities for metabolic alkalosis.

*_____ , *_____ , and *_____ .

remove cause, administer IV chloride solution (e.g., NaCl), and replace K deficit
■   ■   ■

CASE STUDY REVIEW

Mrs. Brush, age 56, has chronic renal disease. Her respirations are rapid and vigorous. She is restless. Her urine pH is 4.5 and urine output is decreased. Her laboratory results are pH of 7.2, $Paco_2$ of 38, and HCO_3 of 14.

1. The "normal" extracellular level of pH is _____ . The average range of $Paco_2$ is *_____ , and that of HCO_3 is *_____ .

2. According to Mrs. Brush's pH and HCO_3, her acid-base imbalance is
*_____ .

3. Is there effective respiratory compensation? _____ .
4. Identify two symptoms related to her acid-base imbalance. *_____ and
_____ .

5. Identify the source of the imbalance.

( ) a. Bicarbonate excess
( ) b. Bicarbonate deficit
( ) c. Carbonic acid excess
( ) d. Carbonic acid deficit

6. How are Mrs. Brush's lungs and kidneys compensating for the acid-base imbalance?
*_____ and _____ .

7. Her chronic renal disease (failure) can cause an acid-base imbalance due to
*_____ .

Later Mrs. Brush's pH is 7.34, $Paco_2$ is 31, and HCO_3 is 20. Fluid with sodium bicarbonate is given IV. As a nurse, you should reassess her laboratory findings.

8. Her pH and HCO_3 indicate *_____ .
9. Is there effective respiratory compensation? _____ . Explain how. *_____
_____ .

10. Why are IV fluids with sodium bicarbonate administered? *_____ .

1. 7.35–7.45; 36–44 mm Hg; 24–28 mEq/L
2. metabolic acidosis
3. no
4. rapid, vigorous breathing and restlessness
5. b. bicarbonate deficit
6. rapid, vigorous breathing and excretion of acid urine
7. retention or buildup of nonvolatile acids
8. metabolic acidosis
9. Yes. Lungs were blowing off CO_2 ($CO_2 + H_2O \rightarrow H_2CO_3$ [acid]).
10. Sodium bicarbonate restores the bicarbonate level in ECF.

NURSING ASSESSMENT FACTORS

- Obtain a client history of clinical problems that are occurring. Recognize the client's health problems that are associated with metabolic acidosis, i.e., starvation, severe or chronic diarrhea, kidney failure, diabetic ketoacidosis, severe infection, trauma, and shock, and with metabolic alkalosis, i.e., vomiting, gastric suction, peptic ulcer, and electrolyte imbalance (hypokalemia, hypochloremia).
- Check the arterial bicarbonate and serum CO_2 levels for metabolic acid-base imbalance. Decreased HCO_3 (<24 mEq/L) and serum CO_2 (<22 mEq/L) are indicative of metabolic acidosis, and increased HCO_3 (>28 mEq/L) and serum CO_2 (>32 mEq/L) are indicative of metabolic alkalosis.
- Obtain baseline vital signs for comparison with future vital signs. Note if there are any cardiac dysrhythmias and/or bradycardia that may result from a severe acidotic state. Check respirations for Kussmaul breathing. This is a sign of metabolic acidosis; also may be due to diabetic ketoacidosis.
- Check laboratory results, especially blood sugar and electrolytes.

METABOLIC ACIDOSIS

NURSING DIAGNOSIS 1

Nutrition, Altered: less than body requirements, related to starvation, diabetic ketoacidosis, and shock.

NURSING INTERVENTIONS AND RATIONALE

1. Monitor dietary intake and report inadequate nutrient and fluid intake.
2. Check the laboratory results regarding electrolytes, blood sugar, and arterial blood gases (ABGs). Some abnormal findings associated with metabolic acidosis are hyperkalemia, decreased serum CO_2, elevated blood sugar (slightly elevated with trauma and shock and highly elevated with uncontrolled diabetes mellitus), and decreased arterial bicarbonate level and pH (HCO_3 <24 mEq/L and pH <7.35).
3. Monitor vital signs. Report the presence of Kussmaul respirations that relate to diabetic ketoacidosis or severe shock. Compare results of vital signs with baseline findings.
4. Monitor signs and symptoms related to metabolic acidosis, i.e., CNS depression (apathy, restlessness, weakness, disorientation, stupor); deep, rapid, vigorous breathing (Kussmaul respirations): and flushing of the skin (vasodilation resulting from sympathetic nervous system depression).
5. Administer adequate fluid replacement with sodium bicarbonate as prescribed by the physician to correct severe acidotic state.

NURSING DIAGNOSIS 2

Cardiac output decreased, related to severe metabolic acidotic state.

NURSING INTERVENTIONS AND RATIONALE

1. Monitor the heart rate closely and note any cardiac dysrhythmia. During severe acidosis, the heart rate decreases and dysrhythmias can occur, causing a decrease in cardiac output.
2. Provide comfort and alleviate anxiety when possible.

NURSING DIAGNOSIS 3

High risk for injury, related to disorientation, weakness, and stupor.

NURSING INTERVENTIONS AND RATIONALE

1. Monitor client's sensorium and note changes, i.e., increased disorientation and stupor.
2. Provide safety measures such as bedside rails.
3. Assist the client in meeting physical needs.

METABOLIC ALKALOSIS

NURSING DIAGNOSIS 1

Fluid volume deficit, related to vomiting or nasogastric suctioning.

NURSING INTERVENTIONS AND RATIONALE

1. Monitor fluid intake and output. Record the amount of fluid loss via vomiting and gastric suctioning. Hydrogen and chloride are lost with the gastric secretions, which increases the pH level, causing metabolic alkalosis.
2. Administer intravenous fluids as ordered; fluids should contain 0.45–0.9% sodium chloride (normal saline). Encourage oral fluids if able to retain and as prescribed by the physician.
3. Monitor the serum electrolytes. If the serum chloride is decreased and the serum CO_2 is decreased, an alkalotic state is present.
4. Monitor vital signs. Note if the respirations remain shallow and slow.
5. Report if the client is consuming large quantities of acid neutralizers that contain bicarbonate compounds such as Bromo-Seltzer.
6. Monitor signs and symptoms of metabolic alkalosis, i.e., CNS excitability (tetanylike symptoms, irritability, confusion, hyperactive reflexes) and shallow breathing.

NURSING DIAGNOSIS 2

High risk for injury, related to CNS excitability secondary to metabolic alkalosis.

NURSING INTERVENTIONS AND RATIONALE

1. Provide safety measures while the client is confused and irritable, such as bedside rails and assistance with basic needs.
2. Monitor the client's state of CNS excitability. Report tetanylike symptoms.

RESPIRATORY ACIDOSIS AND ALKALOSIS

PATHOPHYSIOLOGY

88 Respiratory acidosis is characterized by a(n) (increase/decrease) _____ of carbon dioxide (CO_2) and carbonic acid ($CO_2 + H_2O \rightarrow H_2CO_3$) concentration in the extracellular fluid.

   The pH is (<7.35/>7.45) _____ .

   increase; <7.35

   ■   ■   ■

89 Respiratory alkalosis is characterized by a decrease in the *_____ concentration in the extracellular fluid. The pH is _____ .

   carbonic acid; >7.45

   ■   ■   ■

90 With respiratory acidosis, the $Paco_2$ is _____ mm Hg.

   With respiratory alkalosis, the $Paco_2$ is _____ mm Hg.

   >45; <35

   ■   ■   ■

ETIOLOGY

The causes of respiratory acidosis and alkalosis are described in Tables 4-5 and 4-6. Study the tables and then proceed to the frames. Refer to the tables as needed.

Table 4-5. CAUSES OF RESPIRATORY ACIDOSIS	
Etiology	**Rationale**
CNS Depressants Drugs: narcotics [morphine, meperidine (Demerol)], anesthetics, barbiturates	These drugs depress the respiratory center in the medulla, causing retention of CO_2 (carbon dioxide), which results in hypercapnia (increased partial pressure of CO_2 in the blood).
Pulmonary Abnormalities Chronic obstructive pulmonary disease (COPD: emphysema, severe asthma)	Inadequate exchange of gases in the lungs due to a decreased surface area for aeration causes retention of CO_2 in the blood.
Pneumonia, pulmonary edema	Airway obstruction inhibits effective gas exchanges, resulting in a retention of CO_2.
Poliomyelitis, Guillain-Barré syndrome, chest injuries	Weakness of the respiratory muscles decreases the excretion of CO_2; thus, increasing carbonic acid concentration.

91 Explain how an inadequate exchange of gases in the lungs can cause respiratory acidosis?

* _____ .

It causes a retention of CO_2 in the blood: $H_2O + CO_2 \rightarrow H_2CO_3$.

■   ■   ■

92 Narcotics, sedatives, chest injuries, respiratory distress syndrome, pneumonia, and pulmonary edema can cause acute respiratory acidosis (ARA). ARA results from the rapidly increasing CO_2 level and retention of CO_2 in the blood.

With chronic obstructive pulmonary disease (COPD), the body compensates for CO_2 accumulation by excreting excess hydrogen ions and conserving the bicarbonate ion. The type of respiratory acidosis that occurs with COPD is (acute/chronic) _____ .

chronic

■   ■   ■

93 Explain how poliomyelitis and Guillain-Barré syndrome can cause CO_2 retention. *_____

_____ .

These conditions weaken the respiratory muscles, thus inhibiting CO_2 excretion.

■   ■   ■

Table 4-6.   CAUSES OF RESPIRATORY ALKALOSIS

Etiology	Rationale

Hyperventilation
  Psychologic effects: anxiety, hysteria,
  overbreathing
Pain
	Excessive blowing off of CO_2 through the lungs results in hypocapnia (decreased partial pressure of CO_2 in the blood).

Fever Brain tumors, meningitis, encephalitis Early salicylate poisoning Hyperthyroidism	Overstimulation of the respiratory center in the medulla results in hyperventilation.

---

94 Respiratory alkalosis occurs as the result of a carbonic acid deficit due to   *_____

_____ .

The kidneys compensate for the alkalotic state by (excreting/retaining) _____ bicarbonate ions in the plasma to maintain the bicarbonate-to-carbonic-acid ratio.

blowing off of CO_2, which results in a lack of H_2CO_3; excreting

■   ■   ■

95 Indicate which of the following conditions can cause respiratory alkalosis:

____ a. Early aspirin toxicity
____ b. Emphysema
____ c. Anxiety
____ d. Encephalitis
____ e. Narcotics
____ f. Pneumonia
____ g. Pain and fever

a. X; b. —; c. X; d. X; e. —; f. —; g. X

■   ■   ■

96 Explain the difference between respiratory alkalosis and respiratory acidosis according to $Paco_2$ and carbonic acid levels.   *_____

_____ .

respiratory alkalosis ↓ $Paco_2$, carbonic acid deficit
respiratory acidosis ↑ $Paco_2$, carbonic acid excess

■   ■   ■

CLINICAL APPLICATIONS

97 For 25 years your client has been a heavy smoker. The client has been diagnosed as having COPD, which stands for
*_____ .

chronic obstructive pulmonary disease.

■   ■   ■

98 COPD frequently causes (acute/chronic) _____ respiratory acidosis.

chronic

■   ■   ■

99 The client's blood gases are pH, 7.21; $Paco_2$, 98 mm Hg; HCO_3, 40 mEq/L. The type of acid-base imbalance is *_____ . Is there metabolic (renal) compensation?
*_____ .

respiratory acidosis
Yes, there is metabolic compensation (bicarbonate is conserved).

■   ■   ■

100 Frequently, with respiratory alkalosis, you notice that sufferers are very apprehensive and anxious. They hyperventilate to overcome their anxiety. Many times this occurs for a psychological reason, e.g., giving a speech for the first time or fear of failing an exam. How do you think you might help with respiratory compensation for this imbalance?   *_____

_____ .

Encourage the client to breathe slowly and deeply. There is a lack of CO_2, so giving CO_2 (e.g., rebreathing CO_2 from a paper bag) stimulates the lungs to breathe more deeply and then more slowly.

■   ■   ■

CLINICAL MANIFESTATIONS

With respiratory acidosis, an increase in hypercapnia causes dyspnea (difficulty in breathing), an increased pulse rate, and an elevated blood pressure. The skin may be warm and flushed due to vasodilation from the increased CO_2 concentration.

When respiratory alkalosis occurs, there is CNS hyperexcitability and a decrease in cerebral blood flow. Tetanylike symptoms and dizziness frequently result.

Table 4-7 lists the clinical manifestations related to respiratory acidosis and alkalosis. Study the table carefully. Refer to the table as needed when answering the frames.

Table 4-7.   CLINICAL MANIFESTATIONS OF RESPIRATORY ACIDOSIS AND RESPIRATORY ALKALOSIS

Body Areas	Respiratory Acidosis	Respiratory Alkalosis
Cardiopulmonary abnormalities	Dyspnea Tachycardia Blood pressure	Rapid shallow breathing Palpitations
CNS abnormalities	Disorientation Depression, paranoia Weakness Stupor (later)	Tetany symptoms: numbness and tingling of fingers and toes, positive Chvostek and Trousseau signs Hyperactive reflexes Vertigo (dizziness) Unconsciousness (later)
Skin	Flushed and warm	Sweating may occur
Laboratory Tests		
pH	<7.35 (when compensatory mechanisms fail)	>7.45 (when compensatory mechanisms fail)
Pa_{CO_2}	>45 mm Hg	<35 mm Hg

Note: <=less than; >=greater than.

101 Respiratory patterns of breathing are clues to the type of respiratory acid-base imbalance.

The characteristic breathing pattern associated with respiratory acidosis is _____ , and for respiratory alkalosis, the breathing pattern is   *_____

_____ .

dyspnea (labored or difficulty in breathing); rapid shallow breathing (hyperventilating or overbreathing)

■   ■   ■

102 Indicate which CNS abnormalities are associated with respiratory acidosis (R. Ac) and respiratory alkalosis (R. Al).

___ a. Tetanylike symptoms
___ b. Disorientation
___ c. Dizziness or lightheadedness
___ d. Depression, paranoia
___ e. Hyperactive reflexes
___ f. Positive Chvostek's sign

a. R. Al; b. R. Ac; c. R. Al; d. R. Ac; e. R. Al; f. R. Al

■   ■   ■

103 Respiratory acidosis results from a(n) (deficit/excess) _____ of carbonic acid.

The Pa_{CO_2} is *_____.

excess; greater than (>) 45 mm Hg

■   ■   ■

104 With respiratory acidosis, the buffer, renal, and respiratory mechanisms try to reestablish balance. As a result of the chloride shift, bicarbonate ions are released to neutralize carbonic acid excess.

With an increased CO_2, explain how the respiratory mechanism works to compensate for this imbalance. *_____

_____.

Explain how the renal mechanism works to compensate for this imbalance.

a. *_____.
b. *_____.

When these mechanisms fail, what happens to the blood pH? *_____.

CO_2 stimulates the respiratory center to increase the rate and depth of respiration. CO_2 is blown off with water. $H_2O + CO_2 \rightarrow H_2CO_3$.
a. the H^+ exchanges with Na^+, and the Na^+ is reabsorbed with the HCO_3
b. an increased secretion of ammonium chloride
It is decreased.

■   ■   ■

105 Respiratory alkalosis results from a(n) (deficit/excess) _____ of carbonic acid.

The Pa_{CO_2} is *_____ .

deficit; <35 mm Hg

■   ■   ■

106 The buffer mechanism produces more organic acids, in respiratory alkalosis, which react with the excess bicarbonate ions.

How do you think the renal mechanism works to compensate for this imbalance?
* _____ .

When these mechanisms fail, what happens to the blood pH?
* _____ .

an increased HCO_3 excretion and a H^+ retention
It increases.

■   ■   ■

CLINICAL MANAGEMENT

Figure 4-4 outlines the body's normal defense actions and various methods of treatment for restoring balance in respiratory acidosis and alkalosis. Study the figure carefully, with particular attention to the factors causing the acid-base imbalances, the pH of the urine as to whether it is acid or alkaline, and the treatment for these imbalances. Refer to the figure as needed.

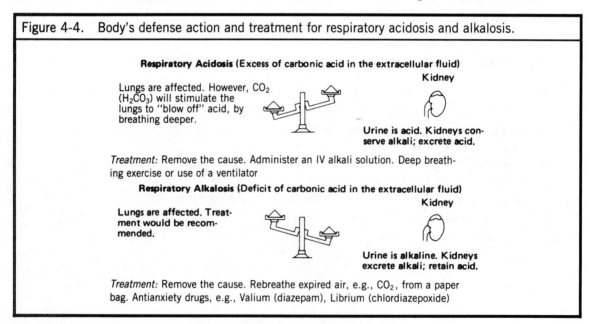

Figure 4-4. Body's defense action and treatment for respiratory acidosis and alkalosis.

Respiratory Acidosis (Excess of carbonic acid in the extracellular fluid)

Lungs are affected. However, CO_2 (H_2CO_3) will stimulate the lungs to "blow off" acid, by breathing deeper.

Kidney

Urine is acid. Kidneys conserve alkali; excrete acid.

Treatment: Remove the cause. Administer an IV alkali solution. Deep breathing exercise or use of a ventilator

Respiratory Alkalosis (Deficit of carbonic acid in the extracellular fluid)

Lungs are affected. Treatment would be recommended.

Kidney

Urine is alkaline. Kidneys excrete alkali; retain acid.

Treatment: Remove the cause. Rebreathe expired air, e.g., CO_2, from a paper bag. Antianxiety drugs, e.g., Valium (diazepam), Librium (chlordiazepoxide)

107 What is the basic cause of respiratory acidosis? *_____ .

    Is the urine (acidic/alkaline)? _____ .

    What are the body's defense actions (lung and kidney)?

    a. *_____

    b. *_____

carbonic acid excess; acidic
a. Excess CO_2 accumulation stimulates the lung to blow off CO_2 or acid.
b. Kidneys conserve alkali and excrete H^+ or acid urine.

    ■   ■   ■

108 Identify three treatment modalities for respiratory acidosis.

    *_____ , *_____ and _____ .

removal of cause, deep breathing exercise, and ventilator

    ■   ■   ■

109 What is the basic cause of respiratory alkalosis? *_____ .

    Is the urine (acidic/alkaline)? _____ .

    Identify the body's defense action against it? *_____

    _____ .

carbonic acid deficit; alkaline
Kidneys excrete alkaline HCO_3 and retain acid, H^+.

    ■   ■   ■

110 Identify three treatment modalities for respiratory alkalosis.

    *_____ , *_____ , and *_____ .

removal of cause, rebreathing expired air, and antianxiety drugs, e.g., chlordiazepoxide
(Librium) and diazepam (Valium)

CASE STUDY REVIEW

Mr. Swift, age 46, has a history of respiratory problems. His latest problem was pneumonia. He smokes two to three packs of cigarettes a day. His condition indicates an acid-base imbalance.

1. The acidity or alkalinity of a solution depends on the concentration of the (hydrogen/bicarbonate) _____ ions.
2. With respiratory regulation, for acid-base balance the lungs blow off or conserve CO_2 by _____ or _____ .

3. The kidney maintains the acid-base balance by excreting _____ or _____ and by retaining _____ or _____ .

4. Which acts faster in regulating or correcting acid-base imbalance (kidneys/lungs)? _____ .

5. Respiratory acidosis has a carbonic acid (excess/deficit) _____ , whereas respiratory alkalosis has a carbonic acid (excess/deficit) _____ .
   Mr. Swift's blood gases are a pH of 7.29, $Paco_2$ of 54, and HCO_3 of 25.

6. Mr. Swift's pH and $Paco_2$ indicate *_____ .

7. Is there any renal (metabolic) compensation? _____ .

   Two days later Mr. Swift's blood gases had a pH of 7.34, Pco_2 of 62, and HCO_3 of 30.

8. Mr. Swift has been (hyperventilating/hypoventilating)? _____ .

9. Is there metabolic (renal) compensation? _____ .

10. Complete the following chart on acid-base imbalance as to pH, $Paco_2$, and HCO_3. Use the arrow pointed upward for increase, the arrow pointed downward for decrease, and—for not involved (except with compensation).

Metabolic Acidosis	Metabolic Alkalosis
pH	pH
$Paco_2$	$Paco_2$
HCO_3 or serum CO_2	HCO_3 or serum CO_2

Respiratory Acidosis	Respiratory Alkalosis
pH	pH
$Paco_2$	$Paco_2$
HCO_3 or serum CO_2	HCO_3 or serum CO_2

1. *hydrogen*
2. *hyperventilating or hypoventilating*
3. *hydrogen or bicarbonate; bicarbonate or hydrogen*
4. *lungs*
5. *excess; deficit*
6. *respiratory acidosis*
7. *no*
8. *hypoventilating. It causes CO_2 retention—respiratory acidosis.*
9. *Yes, if compensation was not present, the pH would be greatly decreased, causing more H^+ concentration.*
10.

Metabolic Acidosis	Metabolic Alkalosis
pH ↓	*pH ↑*
$Paco_2$—	*$Paco_2$—*
HCO_3 or serum CO_2 ↓	*HCO_3 or serum CO_2 ↑*

Respiratory Acidosis	Respiratory Alkalosis
pH ↓	*pH ↑*
$Paco_2$ ↑	*$Paco_2$ ↓*
HCO_3 or serum CO_2—	*HCO_3 or serum CO_2—*

NURSING ASSESSMENT FACTORS

- Obtain a client history of clinical problems. Recognize the client's health problems that are associated with respiratory acidosis, i.e., CNS depressant drugs (narcotics, sedatives, anesthetics), pneumonia, pulmonary edema, and chronic obstructive pulmonary (lung) disease (COPD or COLD) such as emphysema, chronic bronchitis, bronchiectasis, and severe asthma, and those associated with respiratory alkalosis, i.e., anxiety, hysteria, fever, severe infection, aspirin toxicity, and deliberate overbreathing.
- Check for signs and symptoms of respiratory acidosis, i.e., dyspnea, tachycardia, disorientation, weakness, stupor, and flushed and warm skin, and signs and symptoms related to respiratory alkalosis, i.e., apprehension, rapid shallow breathing, palpitations, tetanylike symptoms such as numbness and tingling of the toes and fingers, hyperactive reflexes, and dizziness.
- Obtain vital signs for a baseline record to compare with future vital signs.
- Check arterial blood gas report, particularly the $Paco_2$ result. An increased $Paco_2$ that exceeds 45 mm Hg is indicative of respiratory acidosis and a decreased $Paco_2$ of less than 35 mm Hg is indicative of respiratory alkalosis. Report abnormal findings.

RESPIRATORY ACIDOSIS

NURSING DIAGNOSIS 1

Gas exchange impaired, related to inadequate ventilation (hypoventilation) secondary to COPD.

NURSING INTERVENTIONS AND RATIONALE

1. Monitor client's respiratory status for changes in respiratory rate, distress, and breathing pattern.
2. Monitor arterial blood gases (ABGs), especially the pH, $Paco_2$, and HCO_3. A pH of less than 7.35 indicates acidosis and a $Paco_2$ of greater than 45 mm Hg indicates respiratory acidosis. If the bicarbonate level (HCO_3) is greater than 28 mEq/L, then there is metabolic (renal) compensation. With compensation, the respiratory acidotic state is most likely to be chronic rather than acute.
3. Auscultate breath sounds periodically to determine wheezing, rhonchi, or crackles (rales) that indicate poor gas exchange.
4. Monitor vital signs for tachycardia or cardiac dysrhythmias associated with hypercapnia and hypoxemia (oxygen deficit in the blood).
5. Monitor mechanical ventilator use for a client having respiratory distress due to impaired gas exchange.

NURSING DIAGNOSIS 2

Airway clearance ineffective, related to thick bronchial secretions and/or bronchial spasms.

NURSING INTERVENTIONS AND RATIONALE

1. Assist client with self-care.
2. Encourage client to deep breathe and cough. This helps to eliminate bronchial secretions and improve gas exchange.
3. Assist the client with use of an inhaler containing a bronchodilator drug. Explain the use and frequency of medications.

4. Administer chest clapping on COPD clients to break up mucous plugs and secretions in the alveoli.
5. Teach breathing exercises and postural drainage to clients with chronic obstructive pulmonary disease (COPD). Mucous secretions are trapped in overextended alveoli (air sacs), and breathing exercises and postural drainage help to remove secretions and restore gas exchange (ventilation).
6. Monitor oxygen administration. Too high a concentration of oxygen intake such as greater than 3 liters may depress respirations and increase the severity of the respiratory acidosis. Hypercapnia (increased partial pressure of carbon dioxide) stimulates the respiratory center in the brain; however, after the $Paco_2$ level becomes highly elevated, it is no longer a stimulus. The hypoxemia continues to stimulate the respiratory center. Too much oxygen inhibits the respiratory stimulus effect.
7. Encourage the client to increase fluid intake in order to decrease tenacity of the secretions.

NURSING DIAGNOSIS 3

High risk for injury, related to hypoxemia and hypercapnia.

NURSING INTERVENTIONS AND RATIONALE

1. Monitor the client's state of sensorium for signs of disorientation due to a lack of oxygen to the brain.
2. Provide safety measures, such as bedside rails when the client is disoriented or in a stuporous state.

NURSING DIAGNOSIS 4

Activity intolerance, related to dyspnea secondary to poor gas exchange.

NURSING INTERVENTIONS AND RATIONALE

1. Assist the client with activities of daily living.
2. Plan daily activities that follow his or her breathing exercises as indicated by the physician.
3. Encourage the client to participate in a pulmonary rehabilitation program.

OTHER POTENTIAL NURSING DIAGNOSIS

Breathing pattern ineffective, related to inadequate ventilation.

RESPIRATORY ALKALOSIS

NURSING DIAGNOSIS 1

Anxiety related to hyperventilation secondary to behavioral problems and stressful situations.

NURSING INTERVENTIONS AND RATIONALE

1. Encourage the client who is overanxious and hyperventilating to take deep breaths and breathe slowly. Proper breathing prevents respiratory alkalosis.
2. Listen to client who is emotionally distressed. Encourage the client to seek professional help for psychological problems.

NURSING DIAGNOSIS 2

Breathing pattern ineffective, related to hyperventilation and anxiety.

NURSING INTERVENTIONS AND RATIONALE

1. Demonstrate a slow, relaxed breathing pattern to decrease overbreathing, which causes respiratory alkalosis.
2. Administer a sedative as prescribed to relax client and restore a normal breathing pattern.

NURSING DIAGNOSIS 3

High risk for injury, related to dizziness, lightheadedness, and syncope or unconsciousness.

NURSING INTERVENTIONS AND RATIONALE

1. Instruct the client to be seated when feeling dizzy or lightheaded.
2. Remove objects that may harm the client if dizziness leads to syncope (fainting).
3. Provide side rails if unconsciousness occurs due to severe respiratory alkalosis.

Behavioral Objectives

Upon completion of this chapter, you will be prepared to:

- Explain five basic purposes of intravenous (IV) therapy.
- List five basic classifications of IV fluids.
- Discuss the indications for selections from each classification of IV fluids.
- List four important considerations associated with the transfusion of blood and blood components.
- Calculate the flow rate for IV fluids using macro- and minidrop administration sets.
- Discuss the three most common infusion devices used for short-term IV therapy.
- Describe central venous catheters and four common reasons for their use.
- Describe complications that can occur with central venous line placement and long-term maintenance.
- Discuss the purpose of total parenteral nutrition (TPN).
- List four nursing considerations and five potential complications of (TPN).
- Describe nursing assessment factors for IV transfusion therapy.
- Describe complications associated with different modes of IV therapy.
- List selected nursing diagnoses and corresponding interventions for clients receiving IV therapy.
- List selected nursing diagnoses and corresponding interventions for the clients receiving TPN.

Introduction

This chapter discusses general purposes for intravenous (IV) therapy, selected IV therapy solutions, the classification of IV fluids including transfusion of blood and blood products, calculation of prescribed flow rates for IV infusions, types of intravenous infusion devices, and total parenteral nutrition (TPN). The assessment of clients receiving IV therapy, nursing diagnoses associated with IV therapy, and nursing interventions with rationale are summarized at the end of the chapter. Clinical applications throughout the chapter allow students to apply the nursing process with specific clients receiving IV therapies.

Refer to the text as needed.

An asterisk (*) indicates a multiple word answer. The meaning of the following symbols are:

↑ increased, ↓ decreased, > greater than, < less than.

BASIC PURPOSES OF IV THERAPY

The five purposes of IV therapy are to:

1. Provide maintenance requirements for fluids and electrolytes
2. Replace previous losses
3. Meet concurrent losses
4. Provide nutrition
5. Provide a mechanism for the administration of medications and/or the transfusion of blood and blood components

   Healthy persons can normally preserve their fluid and electrolyte balance; however, certain illnesses and conditions compromise the body's ability to adapt to fluid changes. When a client cannot maintain this balance, IV therapy may be indicated.

1   List the five basic purposes of administering fluids and electrolytes by IV therapy.

*_____

*_____

*_____

*_____

*_____

to provide maintenance requirements for fluids and electrolytes, replace previous fluid losses, meet concurrent fluid losses, provide nutrition, provide a mechanism for the administration of medications and/or blood and blood products

■   ■   ■

2   People requiring intravenous therapy may depend on this route to meet daily maintenance needs for water, electrolytes, calories, vitamins, and other nutritional substances.

   The first purpose in administering IV therapy is to *_____ .

provide daily maintenance requirements

■   ■   ■

3   It is necessary for a client to have adequate kidney function while receiving IV fluids and electrolytes. Renal dysfunction may result in electrolyte (retention/excretion) _____ .

retention

■   ■   ■

4 Multiple electrolyte solutions are also helpful in accomplishing the second purpose for IV therapy. The second purpose for IV therapy is *_____ .

to replace previous (past) fluid losses

■   ■   ■

5 Fluid and electrolyte losses that occur from diarrhea, vomiting, and/or gastric suction are an indication for the third purpose of administering fluids and electrolytes intravenously. The third purpose of IV therapy is *_____ .

to meet concurrent fluid losses

■   ■   ■

6 In situations when a client is unable to meet his or her nutritional needs through oral intake, total parenteral nutrition (TPN) may be used to meet the client's _____ needs.

nutritional

■   ■   ■

7 There are many clinical situations in which the IV route is preferable for medication administration. This fifth purpose of intravenous therapy is *_____

_____ .

    To meet client needs for blood losses or conditions such as anemia, IV therapy meets another purpose. The last purpose of IV therapy is *_____

_____ .

to provide a mechanism for the administration of medications; to transfuse blood or blood products

■   ■   ■

SOLUTIONS FOR IV THERAPY

Many of the solutions supplied for IV therapy are produced commercially to meet specific types of needs. Table 5-1 lists commonly used IV solutions and the rationale for their use.

The osmolality (tonicity) of IV solutions may be hypo-osmolar (hypotonic), iso-osmolar (isotonic), or hyperosmolar (hypertonic). The concentration of solutions is determined by the number of osmols (particles) suspended in the solution.

Study Table 5-1 carefully. It will be referred to throughout the chapter. Then proceed to the frames that follow, referring to the table as necessary.

Table 5-1. SELECTED SOLUTIONS COMMONLY USED IN IV THERAPY

Solution Classifications	Osmolality (Tonicity)	Caloric Value	Na$^+$	K$^+$	Cl$^+$	Miscellaneous	Rationale for Use of Selected IV Fluids
Protein Solutions Aminosyn RF 5.2%	Hyper	175	0	5.4	0	Amino acids	Provides protein and fluid for the body and promotes wound healing.
Aminosyn II 3.5% with dextrose 5%	Hyper	345	18	0	—	Amino acids	Provides protein, calories, and fluid; especially helpful for clients who are elderly and malnourished and for clients with hypoproteinemia due to other causes. Not to be used in severe liver damage.
Plasma Expander Dextran 40 10% in normal saline (0.9%) or 5% dextrose in water (500-mL bottle)	Iso						Dextran is a colloidal solution used to increase plasma volume. Dextran 40 is a short-lived plasma volume expander (4–6 h). It is useful in early shock by helping to correct hypovolemia, increasing arterial pressure, pulse pressure, and cardiac output. It improves microcirculation by reducing red blood cell (RBC) aggregation in the capillaries (increases small-vessel perfusion). *Caution:* It should not be used for clients who are severely dehydrated, have renal disease, have thrombocytopenia, or are actively hemorrhaging.
Dextran 70 6% in normal saline (0.9%)	Iso						Dextran 70 is a long-lived plasma volume expander (20 h). It is useful for shock or impending shock due to hemorrhage, surgery, or burns. It can interfere with platelet function causing prolonged bleeding. Blood for type and cross-match should be drawn before starting dextran since it coats RBCs.

Solution	Osmolality (Tonicity)	Caloric Value	Na$^+$	K$^+$	Ca^{2+}	Cl	Lactate	Mg^{++}	P	Rationale for Use of Selected IV Fluids
										The blood type is difficult to obtain. Overhydration may occur if oliguria or heart failure is present. Allergic reactions can occur, i.e., nausea, vomiting, dyspnea, wheezing, hypotension.
Hydrating Solution Sodium chloride 0.45%	Hypo	—	77	—		77		—		Useful for daily maintenance of body fluid but is of less value for replacement of NaCl deficits. It is helpful for establishing renal function.

Table 5-1.   (Continued)

Solution	Osmolality (Tonicity)	Caloric Value	Na+	K+	Ca2+	Cl	Lactate	Mg++	P	Rationale for Use of Selected IV Fluids
			mEq/L							
Dextrose 2.5% in 0.45% saline	Iso	85	77		—	77		—		Helpful in establishing renal function/urine output.
Dextrose 5% in 0.2% saline	Iso	170	38		—	38		—		Useful for daily maintenance of body fluids when less Na and Cl are required.
Dextrose 5% in 0.33% saline	Hyper	170	51		—	51		—		
Dextrose 5% in 0.45% saline	Hyper	170	77		—	77		—		Useful for daily maintenance of body fluids and nutrition and for treating fluid volume deficits.
Dextrose 5% in water (50 g) (dextrose 10% is occasionally used)	Iso	170	—		—	—		—		Helpful in rehydration and elimination. May cause urinary sodium loss. Good vehicle for IV potassium.
Replacement Solutions										
Dextrose 5% in saline 0.9%	Hyper	170	154	—	—	154	—	—	—	Replacement of fluid, sodium, chloride, and calories.
Dextrose 10% in saline 0.9%	Hyper	340	154	—	—	154	—	—	—	Replacement of fluid, sodium, chloride, and calories.
Lactated Ringer's	Iso	0	130	4	3	109	28	—	—	This solution resembles the electrolyte composition of normal blood serum and plasma. The amount of potassium available is not sufficient for the body's daily potassium requirement.
Dextrose 5% in lactated Ringer's	Hyper	180	130	4	3	109	28	—	—	Same contents as lactated Ringer's plus calories.
Ringer's solution	Iso	—	147	4	5	156	—	—	—	Does not contain lactate, which can be harmful to people who cannot metabolize lactic acid.
Dextrose 5% Ringer's solution	Hyper	170	147	4	4	156	—	—	—	Same contents as Ringer's solution plus calories.

			mEq/L							
Solution	Osmolality (Tonicity)	Caloric Value	Na+	K+	Ca2+	Cl	Lactate	Mg++	P	Rationale for Use of Selected IV Fluids
M/6 sodium lactate	Iso	56	167	—	—	—	167	—	—	Supplies sodium without chloride. Lactate has some caloric value and is metabolized to CO_2 for excretion or increases bicarbonate in alkalosis.
Normal saline (0.9%)	Iso	—	154	—	—	154	—	—	—	Restores extracellular fluid volume and replaces sodium chloride deficit.
Hyperosmolar saline 3% and 5% NaCl	Hyper	—	856	—	—	856	—	—	—	Helpful in hyponatremia by raising Na osmolality of the blood. Helpful in eliminating intracellular fluid excess.
Ionosol B with dextrose 5%	Hyper	178	57	25	—	49	25	5	7	Useful in treating clients requiring polyionic parenteral replacement, e.g., alkalosis due to vomiting, diabetic acidosis, fluid losses due to burns, and postoperative fluid volume deficit.
Ionosol D-CM with dextrose 5%	Hyper	186	138	12	5	108	50	3	—	Useful for electrolyte replacement of duodenal fluid losses because of intestinal suction or biliary or pancreatic drainage and to correct mild acidosis.

Source: Solution chart reviewed by Abbott Laboratories Clinical Research Associate and Baxter Laboratories Clinical Information Manager. Selected portions from Abbott Laboratories: *Wall Chart, Intravenous and Other Solutions,* North Chicago, October 1968, H. Statland: *Fluid and Electrolytes in Practice,* Philadelphia, J.B. Lippincott Co., 1963; McGaw Laboratories: *Guide to Parenteral Fluid Therapy,* CA Glendale, 1963; Travenol Laboratories, Inc.: *Guide to Fluid Therapy,* Deerfield, IN, 1970; N. Methaney, W. Shively: *Nurses' Handbook of Fluid Balance,* Philadelphia, W. B. Saunders, Co, 1983.

BASIC CLASSIFICATIONS OF IV SOLUTIONS

The five basic classifications of IV solutions are (1) sources of free water and calories, (2) crystalloids, (3) colloids, (4) blood and blood components, and (5) hypertonic-hyperosmolar solutions.

8   The five basic classifications of intravenous solutions are: *_____ ,

_____ , _____ , *_____ , and

*_____ .

source of free water and calories, crystalloids, colloids, blood and blood components, and hypertonic-hyperosmolar solutions

■   ■   ■

9   The most commonly used free water and caloric solution is the iso-osmolar (isotonic) solution of dextrose 5% and water (D_5W). When the glucose in D_5W is metabolized, free water is available to the body. Solutions used to provide free water and calories are often referred to as hydrating solutions.

Dextrose 5% in water is an example of an (iso-osmolar/hypo-osmolar/hyperosmolar) _____ solution. It provides the client with *_____.

iso-osmolar; free water and calories

■   ■   ■

Commonly used crystalloid solutions include sodium chloride and lactated Ringer's (or Ringer's lactate). Crystalloid solutions can be iso-osmolar (approximately equal to the sodium chloride concentration of blood, which is 0.9%), hypo-osmolar (less than the sodium chloride concentration of blood), and hyperosmolar (greater than the sodium chloride concentration of blood). Sodium chloride 0.9% or normal physiologic saline (NS) is an example of an iso-osmolar saline solution. Hypo-osmolar solutions include 0.2% or ¼ NS, 0.33% or ⅓ NS, and 0.45% or ½ NS. Hyperosmolar saline solutions include 3 and 5% sodium chloride. Saline solutions may or may not include dextrose.

10   Crystalloid solutions can be (iso-osmolar/hypo-osmolar/hyperosmolar) *_____ in nature.

Two common examples of iso-osmolar crystalloid solutions are: *_____ , and *_____ .

Identify three examples of hypo-osmolar crystalloid solutions: *_____ , *_____ , and *_____ .

Identify two examples of hyperosmolar crystalloid solutions: *_____ _____ .

Saline solutions (may/may not) *_____ include dextrose.

iso-osmolar, hypo-osmolar, or hyperosmolar
0.9% NS and lactated Ringer's
0.2% or ¼ NS, 0.33% or ⅓ NS, and 0.45% or ½ NS
3% and 5% NS, 10% dextrose in water ($D_{10}W$), also D_5/0.9% NS
may or may not

■   ■   ■

Colloids are frequently called volume expanders or plasma expanders; they physiologically function like plasma proteins in blood by maintaining oncotic pressure. Commonly used colloids include albumin, dextran, Plasmanate, and hetastarch (artificial blood substitute). Hypotension and allergic reactions can occur with the use of colloid solutions.

11   Colloids function like _____ and are often called volume or plasma
       _____ .

       Identify four examples of commonly used colloid solutions: _____ ,
       _____ , _____ , and _____ .

       Identify two possible adverse reactions to colloid solutions: _____ and
       *_____ .

       plasma; expanders
       albumin, dextran, Plasmanate, and hetastarch
       hypotension and allergic reactions
                              ■   ■   ■

Total parenteral nutrition (TPN) utilizes hyperosmolar (hypertonic) IV solutions. TPN is designed to
meet the complete nutritional needs of selected clients who cannot maintain their nutrition via the
enteral route. TPN is a mixture of a 25% glucose solution containing proteins, selected electrolytes,
vitamins, and trace elements. TPN therapy is covered more extensively later in this chapter.

12   Hyperosmolar solutions are used in _____ therapy.

       Four major components of TPN solutions are: _____ ,
       _____ , _____ , and _____ .

       TPN (total parenteral nutrition)
       glucose, proteins (amino acids), electrolytes, and vitamins. Trace elements are a small part of
       these solutions.
                              ■   ■   ■

13   Blood and blood components are another type of intravenous therapy. Whole blood, packed red
      cells (whole blood minus the plasma), plasma, and platelets can be administered
      intravenously. Intravenous therapy in relation to blood and blood components is covered more
      extensively later in this chapter.

       Four examples of commonly used blood products are: *_____ ,
       *_____ , _____ , and _____ .

       whole blood, packed cells (whole blood minus the plasma), plasma, and platelets
                              ■   ■   ■

14   Successful fluid and electrolyte therapy often depends upon satisfying all five purposes of IV
      therapy, which are: *_____ , *_____ ,
       *_____ , *_____ , *_____ .

       to provide maintenance requirements, replace previous losses, meet concurrent losses, provide
       a mechanism for administering medications and/or blood or blood products, and provide
       nutrition
                              ■   ■   ■

15   The five main classifications of parenteral solutions designed to address these purposes are:
*_____ , _____ , _____ ,
*_____ , and *_____ .

sources of free water and calories, crystalloids, colloids, blood and blood products, and hyperosmolar (hypertonic) solutions
        ■   ■   ■

16   Dextran is a colloidal solution that is used to expand the *_____ . Dextran 40 remains in the circulatory system _____ hours and dextran 70 remains in the circulation for _____ hours.

plasma volume; 4–6; 20
        ■   ■   ■

17   Identify two ways that dextran 40 is useful in correcting hypovolemia in early shock:
*_____ , and *_____ .

How does dextran 40 improve the microcirculation? *_____
_____ .

increases arterial blood pressure and increases cardiac output (also increases pulse pressure) reduces red blood cell (erythrocyte) aggregation in the capillaries
        ■   ■   ■

18   Identify three clinical conditions in which dextran 40 is contraindicated. Provide a rationale related to each condition:
*_____
_____

*_____
_____

*_____
_____

Severe dehydration: Dextran 40 increases dehydration by pulling more fluid from the cells and tissue space and into the vascular space. If urine output is good, the vascular fluid is excreted. Both cellular and extracellular dehydration can occur.
Renal disease: If oliguria is due to hypovolemia, dextran 40 may improve urine output; but if renal damage is present, dextran 40 may cause renal failure.
Thrombocytopenia: Dextran 40 tends to clot platelets and prolong bleeding time.
Active hemorrhaging: Dextran 40 improves microcirculation, which can cause additional blood loss from the capillaries if hemorrhage is prolonged.
        ■   ■   ■

19 Discuss why blood is typed and cross-matched before administering dextran 70. *_____

_____ .

The nurse should stay with the client receiving dextran 70 for 30 minutes to observe for allergic reactions. Name two allergic reactions. _____ and

_____ .

Dextran 70 tends to coat red blood cells, which makes it difficult to accurately type and cross-match the blood specimen
urticaria (hives) and wheezing (also dyspnea, hypotension, nausea, and vomiting). Very good.
■   ■   ■

20 Identify an IV solution resembling the electrolyte composition of plasma. *_____

_____ .

lactated Ringer's or Ringer's solution
■   ■   ■

21 Hydrating solutions are helpful for daily maintenance of body fluid, rehydration, and establishing effective renal output.

Indicate which of the following are hydrating solutions:

(   ) a. Dextrose 2½% in 0.45% saline
(   ) b. Ringer's solution
(   ) c. Dextrose 5% in water
(   ) d. Sodium chloride 5%
(   ) e. Dextrose 5% in 0.45% saline
(   ) f. Sodium chloride 0.45%
(   ) g. Dextrose 5% in 0.2% saline

a. X; b. —; c. X; d. —; e. X; f. X; g. X
■   ■   ■

22 Dextrose solutions for IV therapy are prepared in two strengths: 5 and 10%. Five percent dextrose means that there are 5 g of dextrose in 100 mL of solution. If the IV container contains 1000 mL of 5% dextrose, how many grams are in this solution? _____ .

Ratio: 5 : 100 :: X : 1000

   100X = 5000
   X = 50 g

Fraction:

$$\frac{5}{100} = \frac{X}{1000}$$

   100X = 5000
   X = 50 g   ■   ■   ■

23 Potassium is often administered intravenously by diluting the potassium chloride in an IV solution. A good vehicle for IV potassium is the hydrating solution, *_____ .

5% dextrose in water   ■   ■   ■

24 Replacement solutions are used to replace fluid, calories, and electrolyte deficits resulting from injury or illness.

   Indicate which of the following solutions are considered to be replacement solutions:

( ) a. Sodium chloride 0.45%
( ) b. Dextrose 5% in normal saline
( ) c. Lactated Ringer's
( ) d. Ringer's
( ) e. Dextrose 5% in water
( ) f. M/6 sodium lactate
( ) g. Hypertonic (3 or 5%) saline
( ) h. Dextrose 5% in 0.45% saline
( ) i. Multiple electrolyte or polyionic solutions (Ionosol B or D-CM solutions and Isolyte E).

a. —; b. X; c. X; d. X; e. —; f. X; g. X; h. —; i. X   ■   ■   ■

25 Identify an IV solution that contains sodium but not chloride. *_____ .

M/6 sodium lactate   ■   ■   ■

26 Hyperosmolar (hypertonic) saline (3 or 5%) is used in the treatment of (hypernatremia/hyponatremia) _____ . It is not usually administered until the serum Na is below 115 mEq/L.

This solution raises the _____ of sodium in the blood.

hyponatremia; osmolality

■   ■   ■

27 The multiple electrolyte replacement solution most helpful in treating severe vomiting, diabetic acidosis, postoperative dehydration, and fluid loss due to burns is *_____

_____ .

Ionosol B with 5% dextrose or Isolyte E with 5% dextrose (Ionosol B and Isolyte E comes without dextrose)

■   ■   ■

28 The multiple electrolyte replacement solution most helpful in correcting electrolyte imbalance due to losses from the gastrointestinal tract is *_____ . Explain why?
*_____ .

Ionosol D-CM
The electrolyte content of this solution is similar to the gastrointestinal fluid.

■   ■   ■

29 Should lactated Ringer's solution be administered to replace a potassium deficit? Why or why not? *_____

_____ .

No! The amount of potassium in lactated Ringer's is not sufficient to replace potassium deficits.

■   ■   ■

30 Name three purposes of hydrating solutions. *_____ , _____ , and *_____ .

daily maintenance, rehydration, and maintenance of renal output

■   ■   ■

31 Three types of intravenous fluids that are used in restoring body fluids are:

Crystalloids (lactated Ringer's, saline, and dextrose)

Blood (whole blood and red blood cells)

Colloids (albumin, plasma, Plasmanate, and dextran)

Dextrose, saline, and lactated Ringer's are considered (crystalloids/colloids)

_____ .

crystalloids

■   ■   ■

32 The first step in the treatment of fluid and electrolyte disturbances is the reconstitution of the extracellular fluid and blood volume. This can best be accomplished by iso-osmolar saline (normal saline), lactated Ringer's, or M/6 sodium lactate.

The iso-osmolar solutions used in the reconstitution of the extracellular fluid and blood volume are: * _____ , * _____ , and * _____ .

normal saline, lactated Ringer's, and M/6 lactated sodium

■   ■   ■

33 Does the volume of urine increase or decrease following the administration of these iso-osmolar solutions? _____ . Why? * _____ .

increase
There is more fluid in the body to be excreted.

■   ■   ■

WHOLE BLOOD AND BLOOD PRODUCTS

34 The hematocrit is the volume of red blood cells (RBCs) in proportion to the extracellular fluid. It is one indication of a gain or loss of fluid. An increased hematocrit reading can indicate an extracellular fluid loss. Why? * _____

_____ .

Extracellular fluid loss increases the number of RBCs in proportion to the fluid volume.

■   ■   ■

35 The concentration of red blood cells is known as *hemoconcentration.*

A high hematocrit reading can be an indication of an extracellular fluid volume (deficit/excess) _____ .

deficit

■   ■   ■

36 Giving whole blood or plasma decreases the hemoconcentration, lowers the hematocrit, raises the blood pressure, and establishes renal flow.

Does whole blood dilute the hemoconcentration? _____ . Why? *_____

_____ .

Yes. There is a slight increase in the extracellular fluid, since 55% of whole blood is plasma; however, plasma or crystalloids may be a better choice depending on the reason for the hemoconcentration.

■   ■   ■

37 For best results, whole blood should be given following initial dilution by an iso-osmolar solution.

Explain why you think an iso-osmolar solution should be given for hemoconcentration before blood is administered. *_____

_____ .

It aids in extracellular dilution and helps to prevent clotting of the blood.

■   ■   ■

38 Various components of whole blood can be fractionated and administered separately. These components include RBCs, plasma, platelets, white blood cells (WBCs) (leukocytes), albumin, and blood factors II, VII, VIII, IX, and X.

Name three blood components that can be fractionated from whole blood.

_____ , _____ , and _____ .

RBCs, plasma, and platelets (also WBCs, albumin, and blood factors)

■   ■   ■

39 Red blood cells are known as *packed cells*. A unit (200–250 mL) of RBCs (packed cells) is composed of whole blood minus the plasma.

Should a unit of RBCs be administered to dilute hemoconcentration? _____ . When are packed RBCs instead of whole blood indicated? *_____

_____ .

no; to restore RBCs and not the fluid volume

■   ■   ■

40 The shelf life of refrigerated whole blood is 35 days. Red blood cells and plasma can be frozen to extend their shelf life to at least 3 years. Platelets must be administered within 3 days after they have been extracted from whole blood.

As whole blood ages, potassium leaves the RBCs (increasing the K level in the serum). The platelets and RBCs are destroyed. After 3 weeks of shelf life, serum potassium (in whole blood) can be increased to 20–25 mEq/L.

The shelf life of refrigerated whole blood is _____ days; the shelf life of frozen RBCs and plasma is _____ years; the shelf life of platelets is _____ days.

35; 3; 3

   ■   ■   ■

41 Identify four important considerations when administering blood products.
_____ , _____ , * _____ , and
_____ .

match/type, purpose, age/shelf life, osmolality, and electrolytes (Na, K)

   ■   ■   ■

42 The serum potassium level in 3-week-old whole blood (increases/decreases) _____ .

What can happen if a critically ill client with poor renal function is given 3 or more units (pints) of "aging" whole blood? * _____ .

If a client has a serum potassium of 6.0 mEq/L, should the client receive a transfusion of 3-week-old whole blood? _____ . Why? * _____
_____ .

increases; cardiac arrest or extreme hyperkalemia
No. The serum potassium level of old blood is increased and a further increase in the client's serum potassium level can cause cardiac dysrhythmias or a cardiac arrest.

   ■   ■   ■

43 As blood volume is being restored, attention is directed to the osmolal changes and correcting the osmolality. A solution of 5% dextrose in water is effective in correcting a water deficit.

Should 5% dextrose be administered to a client with hyponatremia? _____ .
Why or why not? * _____ .

No. Body sodium is further diluted.

   ■   ■   ■

COLLOIDS

44 Name four colloids used to restore body fluids. (Refer to Frame 11.) _____ ,
_____ , _____ , and _____ .

albumin, plasma, Plasmanate, and dextran
     ■   ■   ■

45 Albumin concentrate is helpful in restoring body protein. It is considered to be a plasma volume expander. Too much albumin, or albumin administered too rapidly, can cause fluid to be retained in the pulmonary vasculature.

 Albumin is used to restore *_____ and is considered a
*_____ .

 What should the nurse assess when the client is receiving albumin? *_____ .

body protein; plasma volume expander; lung sounds for fluid congestion (rales)
     ■   ■   ■

46 Dextran, in saline or dextrose, is another plasma volume expander. Dextran comes in two concentrations, dextran 40 and 70. The stronger concentration is a colloid hyperosmolar solution. If large quantities are administered too rapidly, fluid leaves the cells and intestine, thus causing an intracellular fluid volume deficit.

 Dextran can affect clotting by coating the platelets, which reduces their ability to clot. Dextran also interferes with blood typing and cross-matching.

 If your client is to receive dextran and his blood is to be typed and cross-matched, what is the corresponding nursing action? *_____
_____ .

Draw blood for type and cross-match before administering dextran.
     ■   ■   ■

47 Plasmanate is a commercially prepared protein product that is used instead of plasma and albumin to replace body protein.

 Name the commercially prepared solution that resembles plasma and albumin.
_____ .

Plasmanate
     ■   ■   ■

A laboratory test used by physicians to determine the need for IV therapy is the BUN (blood urea nitrogen) and creatinine. The BUN is a serum test to determine the amount of urea, a by-product of protein metabolism, remaining in the blood that is normally excreted by the kidneys. The normal range for the BUN level is 10–25 mg/dL.

An elevated BUN frequently indicates poor renal function; however, a slightly elevated BUN may also indicate a decrease in the extracellular fluid (ECF) volume (dehydration).

The normal range for the creatinine-BUN ratio is $1:10-1:20$. A ratio of $1:20$ or greater is indicative of dehydration or a fluid volume deficit. For example, if a client's creatinine-BUN ratio is $0.9:9$, the client's creatinine-BUN ratio is within the normal $1:10$ ratio. However, if a client's ratio is $1.4:60$, this is well beyond the $1:10-1:20$ ratio and is considered to be a fluid volume deficit. When the creatinine-BUN ratio increases to the point of extreme imbalance, the client can go into renal failure. For example, a $2.4:40$ ratio is indicative of an extreme imbalance as seen in renal failure. The creatinine level is elevated.

48   After the client has been rehydrated, the elevated BUN should return to a normal range; if the BUN does not return to normal, it can be an indication of (poor renal function/decrease in body fluids)?   *_____ .

poor renal function

■   ■   ■

49   Mary Jones has a creatinine of 0.8 and a BUN of 30. This creatinine-BUN ratio is indicative of
*_____ .

Paul Thomas has a ratio of $2.8:50$. His creatinine-BUN ratio is indicative of
*_____ .

a fluid volume deficit or dehydration; renal failure

■   ■   ■

50   A third method of determining the need for IV therapy is through checking the serum electrolytes.

Three methods to determine the necessity of IV therapy are: *_____ ,
*_____ , and   *_____ .

hematocrit level, BUN-creatinine ratio, and serum electrolyte levels

■   ■   ■

51   Fluids and electrolytes for maintenance therapy should be administered continuously for at least 24 hours and then ordered on a daily basis.

Normally, the administration of IV fluids results in prompt excretion of excess water and electrolytes. This response defends the body against   *_____ in water and electrolyte balance.

How should fluids and electrolytes for maintenance therapy be scheduled?
*_____ . Why?   *_____.

excess or significant alterations; CONTINUOUSLY on a daily basis
This defends the body against significant alterations in fluid and electrolyte balance.

        ■   ■   ■

52   If a client receives his full 24-hour maintenance parenteral therapy in 8 hours, two thirds of the water and electrolytes are in (excess/deficit) _____ of the client's current needs. Normally, a large quantity of the excess maintenance fluid are (excreted/retained) _____ .

excess; excreted

        ■   ■   ■

53   Tolerance for sudden changes in water and electrolytes is limited for very ill clients, clients following major surgery, elderly clients, small children, and infants.

Rapid administration of fluids which exceeds one's physiologic tolerance can cause hyponatremia, pulmonary edema (accumulation of fluid in the lungs), and other complications.

Maintenance parenteral therapy should be administered over a period of
*_____ .

Two possible complications of rapid administration of maintenance fluids are
_____ , and   *_____ .

24 hours; hyponatremia and pulmonary edema

        ■   ■   ■

IV FLOW RATE

54   Hyperosmolar IV solutions (those having an osmolality greater than the osmolality of body fluids) should be infused no faster than 2 to 4 mL per minute or as ordered by the physician.

List at least five hyperosmolar solutions to which this might apply. Refer back to Table 5-1 if needed.

* _____

* _____

* _____

* _____

* _____

dextrose 5% in normal saline, dextrose 10% in water, dextrose 10% in normal saline, dextrose 5% in lactated Ringer's solution, hyperosmolar saline, and multiple electrolyte replacement solutions

■   ■   ■

Table 5-2 outlines three types of IV therapy. The table includes the desired amount of solution and the recommended rate of flow. The symbol mL (milliliter) has the same equivalence as cc (cubic centimeter). The symbol for drops is gtt.

Today many institutions use IV controllers or pumps to deliver most IV fluids, but the nurse still needs to know how to calculate the flow rate and regulate various types of infusion devices.

Take several minutes to study this table carefully. Know the three purposes of therapy and the recommended drip rates. Refer to this table as needed.

Table 5-2. RATES OF IV ADMINISTRATION		
Type of Therapy	**Amount of Solution Desired (mL)**	**Rate of Flow**
Maintenance therapy	1500–2000	62–83 mL/h or 1–1.5 mL/min if given over 24 h
Replacement with maintenance therapy	2000–3000	83–125 mL/h or 1.5–2 mL/min (depends on individual)
Hydration therapy	1000–3000	60–120 cc/h or 1–2 mL/min

Note: These guidelines may be adapted to individual circumstances. The physician orders the 24-h requirements and the registered nurse computes 1-h requirements from this. The amount of solution to be administered and the rate of flow can vary greatly with the very sick, the elderly, the small child, the infant, and the postsurgical client.

55   The five purposes of IV therapy are: *_____ ,   *_____ ,
*_____ ,   *_____ , and   *_____ .

maintenance therapy, replacement therapy, hydration therapy, nutritional therapy, and a mechanism for the administration of medications and/or blood and blood products

■   ■   ■

56 The type of solution most frequently suggested in hydration therapy is (hyper/hypo/iso) _____ -osmolar.

Once urinary output is reestablished, then (maintenance/replacement hydration) _____ therapy is started.

iso-osmolar; maintenance

■   ■   ■

57 Identify four types of clients for which the amount of solution to be administered and the rate of flow can vary greatly. *_____ , *_____ , *_____ , and *_____ .

a very sick client, an elderly client, a small child, an infant, and a postsurgical client

■   ■   ■

58 The physician's order determines the 24-hour fluid requirements, and the registered nurse computes the *_____ and calculates the *_____ .

hourly volume; flow rate

■   ■   ■

CALCULATION OF IV INFUSION FLOW RATES

The physician's order for IV therapy includes the type of fluid for infusion and the amount to be administered in a specified period of time. The nurse must compute the number of cubic centimeters per hour and then calculate the drops per minute for the infusion. Volume and pressure infusion pumps are frequently used to administer IV fluids and are considered essential if the client is receiving continuous heparin, aminophylline, medications that affect blood pressure and pulse, and infusions where continuous blood levels are required, as with insulin.

The first step in calculating the drip rate (drops per minute) is to check the manufacturer's specifications for how many drops (gtt) per cubic centimeter (cc) or milliliter (mL) that the infusion set delivers. The number of drops per cubic centimeter varies with each manufacturer and ranges from 8 to 20 gtt/cc for macrodrip chambers and from 50 to 60 gtt/cc for microdrip chambers.

Example. Physician's order: 3000 cc D$_5$W to run over 24 hours. The nurse must compute the number of milliliters (mL) per hour for the infusion and then calculate the drops per minute. A commonly used formula for this conversion is

Two-Step Method:

(a)
$$\frac{\text{Total volume}}{\text{Time in hours}} = \text{volume per hour}$$

In the above order the formula becomes:

$$\frac{3000 \text{ mL}}{24 \text{ h}} = 125 \text{ mL/h}$$

To convert the milliliters/hours (mL/h) to drops/minute (gtt/minute), the second part of the formula is:

(b) $$\frac{\text{Volume to be infused (mL/h)} \times \text{gtt/mL (IV set)}}{\text{Time in minutes [e.g., 60 min (1 h)]}} = \text{gtt/min}$$

In the above order, if the drip factor is 15 gtt/mL (IV set instruction), the second part of the formula is:

$$\frac{125 \text{ mL/h} \times 15 \text{ gtt/mL (IV set)}}{60 \text{ min (1 h)}} = \frac{1875}{60} = 31 \text{ gtt/min}$$

The nurse may compute calculations in one step using only the second part of the formula if the mL/h is known.

Instead of the two-step formula, a one-step formula may be used:

One-Step Method:

$$\frac{\text{Volume to be infused (mL)} \times \text{gtt/mL (IV set)}}{\text{Hours to administer (h)} \times \text{min/h (60)}} =$$

$$\frac{3000 \text{ mL/24 h} \times 15 \text{ gtt/mL}}{24 \text{ h} \times 60 \text{ min}} = \frac{45,000}{1,440} \frac{\text{gtt}}{\text{min}} = 31 \text{ gtt/min}$$

If the nurse were to use an IV infusion pump or controller, it would only be necessary to calculate the volume per hour (in this case 125 mL) and enter that number on the pump.

Practice the necessary calculations on the following orders for IV therapy.

59 Mr. Dean is ordered 1000 mL of $D_5/0.9\%$ NS to infuse over 10 hours. The drip factor is 10 gtt/mL. Using the two-step method, how many drops per minute would you regulate the IV?

a. $\dfrac{\text{Volume in mL}}{\text{Time in h}} = \text{mL/h}$ a. $\underline{\hspace{3cm}} = \text{mL/h}$

b. $\dfrac{\text{Volume in mL} \times \text{gtt/mL}}{\text{Time in minutes}} = \text{gtt/min}$ b. $\dfrac{\times}{\underline{\hspace{2cm}}} = \underline{\hspace{1cm}} \text{gtt/min}$

a. $\dfrac{1000 \text{ mL}}{10 \text{ h}} = 100 \text{ mL/h}$ b. $\dfrac{100 \text{ mL/h} \times 10 \text{ gtt/mL}}{60 \text{ min/h}} = \dfrac{1000}{60} = 16.6 \text{ or } 17 \text{ gtt/min}$

60 Mr. Dean is to have a secondary infusion of 50 mL of dextran to run for 1 hour. The drip factor is 20 gtt/mL (IV set instruction). How many drops per minute would you regulate the IV? Remember mL/h is known, so calculating part one of the two-step method is not necessary.

$$\frac{\text{Volume in mL} \times \text{gtt/mL}}{\text{Time in min}} = \frac{\times}{} = \underline{\quad} \text{ gtt/min}$$

$$\frac{50 \text{ mL} \times \overset{1}{\cancel{20}} \text{ gtt/mL}}{\underset{3}{\cancel{60} \text{ min}}} = \frac{50}{3} = 16.6 \text{ or } 17 \text{ gtt/min}$$

■   ■   ■

61 When the dextran infusion is completed on Mr. Dean, he is to receive erythromycin, 1000 gm in 250 mL of D_5W to infuse over 1 hour. The drip factor is 15 gtt/mL. How many drops per minute would you give?

$$\frac{\text{Volume in mL} \times \text{gtt/mL}}{\text{Time in minutes}} = \frac{\times}{} = \underline{\quad} \text{ gtt/min}$$

$$\frac{250 \text{ mL} \times \overset{1}{\cancel{15}} \text{ gtt/mL}}{\underset{4}{\cancel{60} \text{ min (1 h)}}} = \frac{250}{4} = 62.5 \text{ or } 63 \text{ gtt/min}$$

■   ■   ■

62 The reason Mrs. Beare had a KVO (keep vein open) infusion was for the intermittent administration of medications and electrolytes. The physician's order reads potassium chloride 40 mEq in 150 mL D_5W to infuse over 3 hours. Drip factor is 15 gtt/mL. How many drops per minute would you give?

$$\frac{\text{Volume in mL} \times \text{gtt/mL}}{\text{Time in minutes}} = \underline{\quad}.$$

$$\frac{150 \text{ mL} \times 15 \text{ gtt/mL}}{180 \text{ min (3 h)}} = \frac{2250}{180} = 12.5 \text{ gtt/min}$$

■   ■   ■

63 Instead of using the macrodrip chamber of 15 gtt/mL for Mrs. Beare's potassium chloride, you decide to use a microdrip chamber of 60 gtt/mL. How many drops per minute would you give?

$$\frac{\text{Volume in mL} \times \text{gtt/mL}}{\text{Time in minutes}} = \underline{\quad}.$$

$$\frac{150 \text{ mL} \times \overset{\overset{1}{\cancel{60}}}{\cancel{1}} \text{ gtt/mL}}{\underset{\underset{3}{\cancel{180}}}{\cancel{3} \text{ min (3h} \times 60 \text{ min)}}} = \frac{150}{3} = 50 \text{ gtt/min}$$

■   ■   ■

64 Mr. Shirtzer is to receive 1500 mL of D$_5$/0.2% NS to infuse over 24 hours. The drip factor is 15 gtt/mL. How many drops per minute would you give?

$$\frac{\text{Volume in mL} \times \text{gtt/mL}}{\text{Time in minutes}} = \underline{\hspace{2cm}} .$$

$$\frac{1500 \text{ mL} \times 15 \text{ gtt/mL}}{1440 \text{ min (24 h)}} = \frac{22,500}{1440} = 15.6 \text{ or } 16 \text{ gtt/min}$$

■ ■ ■

TYPES OF IV INFUSION DEVICES FOR SHORT-TERM IV THERAPY

There are three common types of infusion devices for routine short-term IV therapy: the butterfly, the over-needle-catheter, and the in-needle-catheter.

The first type is a winged-tip or butterfly set which consists of a wing-tip needle with a metal cannula, plastic or rubber wings, and a plastic catheter or hub. The needle is $\frac{1}{2}$–$1\frac{1}{2}$ inches long with needle gauges of 16–26. The infusion needle and clear tubing are bonded into a single unit.

A second type of commonly used IV device is the over-needle-catheter (ONC). The bevel of the needle extends beyond the catheter, which is $1\frac{1}{4}$–8 inches in length. The needle is available in gauges of 8–22.

A third type of commonly used IV device is the in-needle-catheter (INC), which is constructed exactly opposite the ONC. Needle length is $1\frac{1}{2}$–3 inches with a catheter length of 8–36 inches. The catheter is available in gauges of 8–22. The INC set comes with a catheter sleeve guard which must be secured over the needle bevel to prevent severing the catheter.

Catheters used in INCs and ONCs are constructed of silicone, Teflon, polyvinyl chloride, or polyethylene.

65 Three common types of IV infusion devices for short-term intravenous therapy are:

* _____ , * _____ , and * _____ .

Identify three to four types of materials used to make ONC and INC devices.

_____ , _____ , * _____ , and

_____ .

butterfly (wing-tipped), over-needle-catheter (ONC), and in-needle catheter (INC)
silicone, Teflon, polyvinyl chloride, and polyethylene

■ ■ ■

Some advantages of the butterfly infusion set are that it is a one-piece apparatus, has a short beveled needle, and is easy to tape securely. The butterfly reduces the risk of secondary puncture and infiltration on puncture. A disadvantage of this IV apparatus is that the butterfly wings prevent manipulation and rotation of the needle in the vein. The butterfly infusion set is commonly used in children and the elderly, whose veins are likely to be small or fragile.

The ONC with its short large cannula is preferable for rapid IV infusion and is more comfortable for the client.

In INC with its longer narrower catheter is preferred when vein catheterization is necessary for prolonged infusions.

66 Three advantages of the butterfly (winged-tip) infusion device are: *_____ ,
*_____ , *_____ .

A disadvantage of the butterfly device is *_____ .

The butterfly is most commonly used for _____ and
_____ whose veins are (large/small) _____ or
(fragile/durable) _____ .

one-piece apparatus, short bevel needle, easy to secure, and decreased risk of puncture
limited manipulation/rotation of needle
children and the elderly; small; fragile

       ■   ■   ■

67 Two advantages of the ONC device are: *_____ , and *_____ .

The cannula in the ONC device is (short and large/long and narrow) *_____ .

good for rapid intravenous infusion of fluids and more comfortable for client
short and large

       ■   ■   ■

68 INC devices are preferred for (short/prolonged) _____ infusions.

The cannula in the INC device is (short and large/long and narrow) *_____ .

prolonged; long and narrow

       ■   ■   ■

Factors to consider in the needle selection for IV therapy include (1) the nurse's preference, (2) the client's condition, and (3) the type or amount of IV solution to be administered.

69 Identify three factors for the nurse to consider when selecting a needle for an IV infusion.
*_____ , *_____ , and _____ .

nurse's preference, client's condition, and type/amount of solution to be infused

       ■   ■   ■

CENTRAL VENOUS CATHETERS AND LONG-TERM IV THERAPY

Central venous catheters are another type of IV device. These catheters are radiopaque and may have a single, double, or triple lumen. Since the insertion of a central venous catheter presents critical risks, their insertion is followed by an x-ray to confirm the position of the catheter.

70 Central venous catheters are _____ so they may be visualized in x-rays to determine their _____ . Identify the three types of lumen that may be present in a central venous catheter: _____ , _____ , and

_____ .

radiopaque; position; single, double, and triple

■   ■   ■

71 Four common reasons for using a central venous catheter are (1) measuring the central venous pressure, (2) infusion of TPN, (3) infusion of multiple IV fluids and/or medications, and (4) infusion of chemotherapeutic or irritating medications. Most IV fluids can be infused through a central venous line.

Identify four reasons central venous lines are used.

*_____ .

*_____ .

*_____ .

*_____ .

to measure the central venous pressure, to infuse TPN, to infuse multiple IV fluids and/or medications, and to infuse chemotherapeutic or irritating medications

■   ■   ■

72 Heckman and Groshong are examples of central venous catheters that must be inserted in the operating room. The implantable vascular access device (IVAD) is another example of a central venous line that must be surgically inserted in the operating room.

Name three types of central venous lines that must be inserted in the operating room.

_____ , _____ , and *_____ .

Heckman, Goshong, and implantable venous access devices (IVAD)

■   ■   ■

73 Polyethylene, silicone, and polyvinyl chloride central venous lines can be inserted at the bedside under sterile conditions.

Name three types of central venous catheters that can be inserted under sterile conditions at the bedside. _____ , _____ , and *_____ .

polyethylene, silicone, and polyvinyl chloride

■   ■   ■

74 Veins commonly used to insert central venous lines are the subclavian vein, internal jugular vein, femoral vein, and the antecubital vein. A procedure called venous cutdown may be used to insert central venous lines.

Name four veins commonly used for access when inserting a central venous catheter.
_____ , *_____ , _____ , and

_____ .

subclavian, internal jugular, femoral, and antecubital

■   ■   ■

75 Complications that can occur with insertion of a central venous line into the subclavian and internal jugular veins are pneumothorax, hemorrhage, air embolism, thrombus dislodgement, and cardiac dysrhythmias. Long-term complications that occur with central venous lines include hemorrhage, phlebitis, air embolism, thrombus formation, infection, dislodgement, cardiac dysrythmias, and circulatory impairment.

Refer to Table 5-5 for the causes, nursing assessment, and interventions related to central venous lines.

Identify five complications associated with inserting a central venous catheter.
_____ , _____ , *_____ ,

*_____ , and *_____ .

Identify four to five complications associated with the long-term use of central venous catheters. _____ , _____ , _____ ,

_____ , and *_____ .

pneumothorax, hemorrhage, air embolism, thrombus dislodgement, and cardiac dysrhythmias
hemorrhage, phlebitis, infection, dislodgement, cardiac dysrhythmias, and circulatory impairment

■   ■   ■

TOTAL PARENTERAL NUTRITION

Total parenteral nutrition (TPN), sometimes referred to as hyperalimentation, is the infusion of amino acids, hypertonic glucose, and additives such as vitamins, electrolytes, minerals, and trace elements. TPN can meet a client's total nutritional needs and is commonly used for clients whose caloric intake is insufficient, clients with severe burns who are in negative nitrogen balance, clients who cannot take enteral feedings, and clients with gastrointestinal disorders such as ulcerative colitis, gastrointestinal fistulas and other conditions where the GI tract needs complete rest. Table 5-3 identifies additional indications for TPN.

76 Nutritional solutions for TPN contain glucose, amino acids, trace elements, vitamins, minerals, lipids, and electrolytes.

Are hyperalimentation solutions (hypo-osmolar/hyperosmolar)? _____ .
Explain the effects that this concentration can have on body cells. *_____

_____ .

hyperosmolar
It can pull fluid from the intracellular compartment (cells) into the extracellular compartment, thus causing a cellular fluid volume deficit.

■   ■   ■

77 A solution of 2500 mL of 10% dextrose in water provides 1000 calories. Concentrations of sugar higher than 10% dextrose can cause severe peripheral vein damage. Continuous use of 10% dextrose in water or dextrose solutions >10% increases the risk for developing phlebitis and should be administered via a central venous line.

Is 1000 calories daily sufficient for a client following major surgery? _____
Explain why/why not. *_____

_____ .

No. Following surgical treatment 2500–3500 calories are needed daily. One thousand (1000) calories does not meet daily maintenance requirements for the client following major surgery.

■   ■   ■

78 Glucose concentrations higher than 10% can cause venous damage when infused peripherally. Identify the type of vein damage which occurs with irritating concentrations of glucose.
*_____ .

phlebitis or thrombophlebitis (clots)

■   ■   ■

Subclavian veins, internal jugular veins, femoral veins, and venous cutdowns are used when administering hyperosmolar solutions.

79 Indicate which veins can be used for hyperalimentation.

( ) a. Peripheral arm veins
( ) b. Internal jugular veins
( ) c. Leg veins
( ) d. Subclavian veins
( ) e. Femoral veins
( ) f. Venous cutdowns

a. —; b. X; c. —; d. X; e. X; f. X

■   ■   ■

When clients do not receive enough protein-sparing calories in the form of amino acids, fat, and carbohydrates (CHO), the body's protein and fat are converted into carbohydrates. To prevent this conversion, the body needs 600–800 calories daily during the resting state, approximately 1600 calories daily for the sitting state, and 2500–3500 calories daily following major surgical procedures.

If a client receives 2500 mL ($2\frac{1}{2}$ liters) of 5% dextrose in water, the caloric intake is 500 calories (CHO: 1 g = 4 calories; 50 g = 5% dextrose per 1000 mL).

$$1000 \text{ mL } 5\% \text{ dextrose} = 50 \text{ g} \times 4 = 200 \text{ calories}$$
$$200 \times 2\tfrac{1}{2} \text{ liters} = 500 \text{ calories}$$

80 Is this a sufficient number of calories for the resting state? _____
Why? *_____ .

No. In the resting state 600–800 calories are needed.

  ∎   ∎   ∎

81 The average percentage of dextrose used in TPN is between 25 and 30%. This high glucose concentration is mixed with commercially prepared protein sources. Vitamins and electrolytes are added prior to administration. Electrolytes are frequently added immediately before the infusion according to the client's serum electrolyte levels.

Since high glucose concentrations are irritating to peripheral veins, such concentrations are administered through *_____ . Identify two large veins commonly used in the administration of TPN. _____ and *_____ .

central venous lines; subclavian and internal jugular

  ∎   ∎   ∎

82 Why is it recommended that electrolytes be added to the solution immediately before administration? *_____

_____ .

The amount of electrolytes needed are determined by the client's daily serum electrolyte levels. Frequently, electrolytes are added with the other nutrients, 12–24 hours before infusion, according to the client's serum electrolyte levels.

  ∎   ∎   ∎

Table 5-3 gives the indications for TPN. Study the table carefully before proceeding. Refer to the table as needed.

Table 5-3. INDICATIONS FOR TPN/HYPERALIMENTATION	
Indications	**Rationale**
Oral or nasogastric feedings are contraindicated or not tolerated	Long-term use of IV glucose solutions can cause protein wasting. TPN maintains a positive nitrogen balance.
Severe malnutrition	Malnutrition can cause severe protein loss and wasting syndrome. Negative nitrogen (protein) balance occurs. TPN restores positive nitrogen balance.
Malabsorption syndrome	The inability to absorb nutrients in the small intestine requires nutrients to be offered intravenously.
Dysphagia	Difficulty in masticating and swallowing due to pharyngeal radiation treatment prevents clients from breaking down food sufficiently for digestion.
Gastrointestinal fistula	Fistulas promote protein losses. TPN allows the intestine to rest and decreases gall bladder, pancreas, and small intestine secretions.
Major bowel resection and ulcerative colitis	These disorders reduce the absorptive area of the small intestine. TPN increases the intestine's ability to absorb nutrients more quickly than oral feedings and it permits the bowel to rest.
Extensive surgical trauma and stress	Extensive surgery requires 3500–5000 calories a day to maintain protein balance. TPN lowers the chance for infection and provides a positive nitrogen balance to aid in wound healing.
	TPN before surgery improves the nutritional status so that the client can withstand surgery and its stresses.
Extensive burns	Extensive burns require 7500–10,000 calories daily. TPN improves wound healing and formation of granulation tissue and promotes successful skin grafting.
Metastatic cancer with anorexia and weight loss	Clients with waꞁting syndrome and debilitating diseases, such as cancer ᴏr AIDS, frequently are in negative nitrogen balance. TPN restores protein balance and tissue synthesis.

83 Indications for hyperalimentation, or TPN, include which of the following:

( ) a. Major bowel resection
( ) b. Minor surgical procedures
( ) c. Gastrointestinal fistula
( ) d. Severe malnutrition
( ) e. Contraindicated or intolerable oral and gastric feedings
( ) f. Severe congestive heart failure
( ) g. Extensive burns
( ) h. Metastatic cancer with weight loss
( ) i. Malabsorption syndrome
( ) j. Aquired immunodeficiency syndrome (AIDS) with wasting syndrome

a. X; b. —; c. X; d. X; e. X; f. —; g. X; h. X; i. X; j. X
■   ■   ■

84 In clients who are unable to tolerate oral or gastric feeding and suffer from severe malnutrition, TPN helps in restoring *_____ .

a positive nitrogen balance
                      ■   ■   ■

85 What happens to the intestinal area in relationship to nutrient absorption following major bowel resection? *_____ .

reduced absorptive area of the intestine
                      ■   ■   ■

86 What benefit does TPN provide for clients who have a gastrointestinal fistula and/or a major bowel resection? *_____ .

It allows the intestine (bowel) to rest.
                      ■   ■   ■

87 The trauma and stress related to an extensive surgical procedure (increases/decreases) _____ the body's daily caloric needs. Is 3000 mL (3 liters) of 10% dextrose in saline adequate to meet the client's daily caloric requirement following an extensive surgical procedure? _____ Explain why. *_____

_____ .

increases
No. One liter of 10% dextrose is 400 calories; 3 liters is 1200 calories, thus less than the caloric need of clients undergoing stress.
                      ■   ■   ■

88   What purpose does TPN provide prior to surgery   *_____

_____ .

It improves the client's nutritional status so that he or she can withstand the surgical procedure and its stresses.

        ■   ■   ■

89   What is the caloric need of clients with extensive burns?   *_____ .

    Give two ways that TPN aids in healing extensive burns.

*_____

*_____ .

7500–10,000 calories daily
It promotes wound healing and formation of granulation tissue and enhances successful skin grafting.

        ■   ■   ■

90   Clients suffering from metastatic cancer with anorexia and weight loss frequently experience a negative nitrogen balance. Explain how TPN helps to remedy this clinical problem.   *_____

_____ .

Protein replacement restores the positive nitrogen (protein) balance and promotes tissue synthesis.

        ■   ■   ■

COMPLICATIONS OF TPN

Major complications that can result from TPN therapy are air embolism, phlebitis, thrombus, infection, hyper/hypoglycemia, and fluid overload.

TPN is an excellent medium for organisms, bacteria, and yeast to grow. Strict asepsis is necessary when medications are added to the solution, when IV tubing is changed, and when dressings are changed. Most hospitals have a procedure for changing dressings in which strict aseptic technique (i.e., gloves, masks, and antibiotic ointment) is mandated.

When IV tubing is changed at the central venous catheter site, the client must lie flat and perform the Valsalva maneuver (take a breath, hold it, and bear down) to prevent air from being sucked into the circulation. The Valsalva maneuver increases intrathoracic pressure.

Increased blood glucose (hyperglycemia) occurs as a result of hyperosmolar dextrose solutions used when TPN is infused rapidly. An elevated blood glucose level may occur during early TPN until the pancreas adjusts to the hyperglycemic load. Regular insulin, either in the IV solution or by subcutaneous injection, may be required to prevent or control hyperglycemia. Other complications that can occur include hypoglycemia from abruptly discontinuing hyperosmolar dextrose solutions, fluid volume excess from the infusion of an excessive amount of fluid, or a fluid shift from intracellular to extracellular compartments.

Table 5-4.   COMPLICATIONS OF TPN

Problems	Causes	Symptoms	Actions
Air embolism	IV tubing disconnected Catheter not clamped Injection port fell off Improper changing of IV tubing (no Valsalva procedure)	Coughing Shortness of breath Chest pain Cyanosis	Clamp catheter Client must lie on left side with head down Check VSs Notify physician
Infection	Poor aseptic technique when catheter inserted Contamination when changing tubing Contamination when solution mixed Contamination when dressing changed	Temperature above 100° (37.7°C) Pulse increased Chills Sweating Redness, swelling, drainage at insertion site Pain in neck, arm, or shoulder Lethargy Urine: glycosuria Bacteria Yeast growth	Notify physician Change dressing every 24–48 h according to agency policy Change solution every 24 h Change tubing every 24 h according to agency policy Check VSs q 4 h
Hyperglycemia	Fluid infused rapidly Insufficient insulin coverage Infection	Nausea Weakness Thirst Headache Blood glucose elevated	Monitor blood glucose Notify physician Decrease infusion rate Regular insulin as required Monitor blood glucose every 4 h and prn
Hypoglycemia	Fluids stopped abruptly Too much insulin infused	Nausea Pallor Cold, clammy Increased pulse rate Shaky feeling Headache Blurred vision	Notify physician Increase infusion rate with NO insulin, as per physician order or hospital policy *or* Orange juice with 2 teaspoons of sugar if client can tolerate fluids *or* Glucose IV, as per physician order or hospital policy *or*

Table 5-4. (Continued)			
Problems	**Causes**	**Symptoms**	**Actions**
			Glucagon, as per physician order or hospital policy
Fluid overload (hypervolemia)	Increased rate of IV infusions Fluid shift from cellular to vascular due to hyperosmolar solutions	Cough Dyspnea Neck vein engorgement Chest rales Weight gain	Check VSs q 4 h Weigh daily Monitor intake and output Check neck veins for engorgement Check chest sounds Monitor electrolytes Monitor BUN and creatinine

Note: From "Helping Your Client Settle in with TPN" by L. Wilhelm, 1985, *Nursing 85, 15*(4), p. 63. Copyright 1985 by Springhouse Corporation. Reprinted by permission.

Table 5-4 lists the five major complications associated with TPN hyperalimentation and the related causes, symptoms, and corresponding nursing actions.

91 To prevent an air embolism when changing IV tubing with clients receiving TPN therapy, the Valsalva maneuver is performed. Explain how it is done (see introduction to TPN). *_____

_____ .

Take a deep breath, hold it, and bear down.
■   ■   ■

92 Identify two immediate nursing interventions when an air embolism is suspected?
*_____ and *_____ .

clamp catheter and position client on left side with head down
■   ■   ■

93 Hyperosmolar dextrose in a protein hydrolysate solution promotes yeast and bacteria growth. It has been reported that these organisms do not grow as rapidly in a crystalline amino acid solution as they do in protein hydrolysate solution.

Name three symptoms indicative of infection:

a. *_____
b. *_____
c. *_____ .

a. elevated temperature; b. chills; redness, swelling, and drainage at insertion site;
c. sweating and pain in arm or shoulder

      ■   ■   ■

94   Usually 1 liter of solution is ordered for the first 24 hours when initiating TPN therapy. This allows the pancreas to accommodate the increased glucose concentration of the solution. Additional daily increases of 500–1000 mL per day are ordered until the desired daily volume is reached.

    A usual maintenance volume of $2\frac{1}{2}$–3 liters of the hyperosmolar dextrose solution for TPN is administered over 24 hours. A continuous infusion rate is important to prevent fluctuations in blood glucose levels.

    What test is suggested to assess for, prevent, and control hyperglycemia?

* _____ .

    How often should the test be performed? *_____ .

finger stick for blood sugar level (Chemistrip bG); every 4–6 hours

      ■   ■   ■

95   It is suggested that an iso-osmolar dextrose solution be administered for 12–24 hours after TPN therapy is discontinued. A gradual decrease in the hourly infusion rate of TPN may also be used to discontinue TPN therapy.

    If the hyperosmolar dextrose solution is discontinued abruptly what complication may develop? _____ .

    What signs and symptoms should the nurse be aware of? _____ ,

* _____ , * _____ , and _____ .

hypoglycemia; pallor, cold and clammy skin, increased pulse, and shakiness (also nausea and blurred vision)

      ■   ■   ■

96   Medications should not be infused with TPN. A multilumen catheter or supplemental peripheral site must be used if the client requires IV fluids, TPN, blood products, and medications.

    What must the nurse do when medications are given parenterally with TPN? *_____

_____ .

start a supplemental peripheral site and use a multilumen central venous catheter

      ■   ■   ■

97 Fat emulsion supplement therapy provides an increased number of calories and is a carrier of fat-soluble vitamins.

The two solutions that can provide nutrients, calories, and vitamins for TPN are
*_____ and *_____ .

TPN solution or hyperosmolar dextrose/protein solution and fat emulsion solution

■   ■   ■

NURSING ASSESSMENT IN IV THERAPY

Table 5-5 presents nursing responsibilities in the assessment of IV therapy. Once the physician orders the IV fluids, the nurse must know and understand the various solutions, needles, catheters, tubings, IV sites, and potential complications in order to accurately assess, initiate, and monitor IV infusions. Table 5-5 provides the assessment, nursing interventions, and rationale related to IV therapy. Study the table carefully and refer to it as needed.

Table 5-5. NURSING ASSESSMENT OF IV THERAPY		
Assessment	**Nursing Interventions**	**Rationale**
Types of IV solutions	Note the types of IV fluid ordered, hypo-osmolar, iso-osmolar, or hyperosmolar solution.	An excessive use of hypo-osmolar solutions can cause a fluid volume excess and excess use of hyperosmolar solutions may cause a fluid volume deficit. An iso-osmolar solution has 240–340 mOsm/L; less than 240 is hypo-osmolar, and greater than 340 is hyperosmolar (see Chapter 1).
	Report extended use of continuous IVs of dextrose in water.	Dextrose 5% in water administered continuously becomes a hypo-osmolar solution. Dextrose is metabolized rapidly and the water remaining decreases the serum osmolality. Alternate use of D/W with D/NSS (saline) can prevent such complications.

Table 5-5.   (Continued)

Assessment	Nursing Interventions	Rationale
	Observe for signs and symptoms of fluid volume deficit, i.e., dry mucous membranes, poor skin turgor, and increased pulse and respiration rates, when using hyperosmolar solutions. Creatinine/BUN ratio, 1 : 10/20; hemoconcentration, 1 : 20 or greater.	Continuous use of hyperosmolar solutions pulls fluid from intracellular compartments to the extracellular compartments. The fluid is excreted by the kidneys. Poor kidney function causes fluid retention, increasing the risk for a fluid volume excess.
Intravenous tubing and bag	Inspect IV bags for leaks by gently squeezing.	Microorganisms can enter IV bags through small leak sites, contaminating the fluid.
	Check drop size on the equipment box. Use IV tubing with macrodrip chamber (10–20 gtt/mL) for administering IV fluids at a rate of 50 cc/h or greater.	Use of a microdrip chamber (IV tubing) for fluids that are ordered to run at a rate greater than 50 mL/h is too slow and inaccurate.
	Use microdrip chamber (60 gtt/mL) for administering IV fluids at a rate under 50 mL/h.	Infusion pumps increase the accuracy and decrease the risks associated with IV fluids that are to run for 12–24 h and meet specific client fluid needs.
	Change IV tubing every 24–48 h at time of new hanging.	Studies have shown that IV tubing left hanging for 48 h is free of bacteria when proper aseptic technique is used.
	New IV containers are hung according to agency policy.	An IV bag should not be used for longer than 24 h. If the order is for KVO (keep vein open) a 250–500 mL container with a microdrip chamber set is suggested.

Table 5-5. (Continued)		
Assessment	**Nursing Interventions**	**Rationale**

Needles and IV catheters (cannulas)	Recognize the types of IV needles and catheters used for IV fluids:
	    Straight needles
	    Scalp vein needles (butterfly needles)
	    Heparin lock
	    Over-needle-catheter (ONC)
	    Through-the-needle catheter
		Needles (straight and scalp vein) are used for short-term IV therapy and for clients with autoimmune problems. Catheters made of silicone and Teflon are less irritating than polyvinylchloride and polyethylene catheters.

	Change IV site every 2–3 days according to agency policy.	Needles and catheters in longer than 72 h increase the risk of phlebitis.
	Check the ONC for placement and function.	There are many types of ONCs, i.e., Angiocath, A-Cath, Vicra Quik-Cath, etc. Catheter length can be 2.5–36 inches. Care should be taken to avoid severing the catheter with the needle tip.
	Check for fluid leaks at the insertion site after the insertion of an in-needle-catheter (INC).	An INC is used for central venous pressure monitoring, TPN (hyperalimentation), etc. It is frequently inserted in large veins, i.e., subclavian vein, internal jugular or femoral vein. Leaks result from needle punctures that are larger than the catheter.
Injection site	Insert needle or catheter in the hand or the distal veins of the arm. Use the antecubital fossa (elbow) site last.	The upper extremity is preferred for the infusion site, since the occurrence of phlebitis and thrombosis in the upper extremities is not as prevalent as it is in the lower extremities.
	Avoid using the leg veins if possible.	Circulation in the leg veins is reduced and thrombus formation can occur.
	Avoid using limbs affected by a stroke or mastectomy for IV sites.	Circulation is usually decreased in affected extremities.

Table 5-5.　(Continued)

Assessment	Nursing Interventions	Rationale
	Apply arm board and/or soft restraints to the extremity with the IV when the client is restless or confused.	Prevention of extremity movement with an IV decreases the chance of dislodging the needle and phlebitis.
Flow rate and irrigation	Check types of solutions clients are receiving.	Knowledge of tonicity (osmolality) of fluids aids in determining rate of flow. Rate of hyperosmolar solutions should be slower than iso-osmolar solutions.
	Observe drip chamber and regulate accordingly.	Regulation of IV fluids is important to prevent overhydration, i.e., cough, dyspnea, neck vein engorgement, and chest rales. Do not play "catch-up" with IV fluids.
	Regulate KVO (keep vein open) rate to run 10–25 mL/h or according to agency policy or use an infusion pump.	KVO IVs should run approximately 10–25 mL/h.
	Label IV bag for milliliters (mL) to be received per hour. Check rate of flow every 30 min to 1 h with hyperosmolar and toxic solutions and every hour with iso-osmolar solutions.	Hyperosmolar solutions administered rapidly can cause cellular dehydration and, if the kidneys are properly functioning, vascular dehydration. Hyperosmolar fluids act as an osmotic diuretic and can cause diuresis; when administered rapidly, speed shock can occur; and if infiltration occurs, necrotic tissue can result.

Table 5-5.   (Continued)

Assessment	Nursing Interventions	Rationale
	Restore IV flow if stopped by opening flow clamp, milking the tubing, raising the height of IV bag, or repositioning the extremity.	If IV flow has stopped and does not start by opening clamp, milking tubing, raising the bag, or repositioning extremity, then the IV catheter should be removed. Irrigating IV catheters is prohibited in some institutions. Forceful irrigation can dislodge clot(s) and cause the movement of an embolus to the lungs.
Position of IV line	Position and tape IV tubing to prevent kinking.	Kinking of the tubing may cause the IV to be discontinued and to be restarted at a different site.
	Hang IV bag 2½–3 feet above client's infusion site.	The higher the IV bag, the faster the flow rate. If the IV bag is too low, IV fluids may stop or the client may receive an insufficient amount of fluids.
Infusion problems and complications		
1. Infiltration	Observe insertion site for infiltration, i.e., swelling, coolness, and soreness.	Infiltration is accumulation of fluid in the subcutaneous tissue. When infiltration occurs, the IV should be discontinued and restarted at a different site.
2. Phlebitis	Observe insertion site for phlebitis, i.e., red, swollen, hard, pain, and warm to touch. Apply warm, moist heat to area as ordered.	Phlebitis is an inflammation of the vein that can be caused by irritating substances. Drugs and hyperosmolar solutions may cause phlebitis. Application of moist heat decreases inflammation.
3. Systemic infection	Observe for pyrogenic reactions (septicemia), i.e., chills, fever, headache, fast pulse rate. Check vital signs q4h for shocklike symptoms. Utilize aseptic technique when inserting IV catheters and changing IV tubing and IV bag.	Aseptic technique should be used at all times with IV therapy. Prevention of systemic infections is of primary importance.

Table 5-5. (Continued)

Assessment	Nursing Interventions	Rationale
4. Speed shock	Observe for signs and symptoms of speed shock, i.e., tachycardia, syncope, decreased blood pressure.	Speed shock occurs when solutions with drugs are given rapidly. High drug concentration accumulates rapidly in the body and can cause shocklike symptoms.
5. Air embolism	Remove air from tubing to prevent air embolism.	Air can be removed from tubing by (1) inserting a needle with syringe into side arm of tubing set and withdrawing the air and (2) placing pen or pencil on tubing, distal to the air, and rolling tubing until air is displaced into the drip chamber.
	Observe for signs and symptoms of air embolism. These include pallor, dyspnea, cough, syncope, tachycardia, decreased blood pressure.	Air embolism occurs when air inadvertently enters the vascular system. Injection of more than 50 mL of air can be fatal. It occurs more frequently in the central veins, and symptoms usually appear within 5 min.
	Immediately place client on left side in Trendelenburg position.	Air is trapped in the right atrium, which prevents it from going to the lungs.
6. Pulmonary embolism	Report signs and symptoms of pulmonary embolism, i.e., restlessness, chest pain, cough, dyspnea, tachycardia.	Thrombus originating in the peripheral vein becomes an embolus and can lodge in a pulmonary vessel.
	Administer oxygen, analgesics, anticoagulants, and IV fluids as ordered.	Preventive measures should be taken, such as *never* forcefully irrigating an IV catheter to reestablish flow and avoiding the use of veins in the lower extremities.
7. Pulmonary edema	Check breath sounds for rales. Check neck veins for engorgement. Decrease IV flow rate.	IV fluids administered too rapidly or in large amounts can cause overhydration. Fluids "back up" into lung tissue.

Table 5-5. (Continued)		
Assessment	**Nursing Interventions**	**Rationale**
8. "Runaway" IV fluids	Monitor IV fluid every hour even if on an IV controller.	Flow value on IV tubing is opened.
	Check IV controllers: flow rate and alarm set.	Alarm was not set properly on IV controller.
9. Hematoma	Observe for hematoma with unsuccessful attempts to start IV therapy.	Hematoma (blood tumor) is a raised ecchymosed area.
	Apply warm compresses after 1 h.	Warm compresses cause vasodilation and improves blood flow and healing.
Additives to IV fluids	Recognize the untoward reactions of drugs in IV fluids: potassium, Levophed, low-pH drugs, vitamins, antibiotics, antineoplastic drugs.	Potassium, antineoplastic drugs, and Levophed irritate the blood vessels and body tissue. Phlebitis is common with these drugs; and if infiltration occurs, sloughing of tissues may result. Vitamins and antibiotics should not be mixed together. They are incompatible. Always check compatibility charts before adding medications to IV fluids.
	Stay with the client 10–15 min when the client is receiving drugs intravenously.	Allergic reactions often occur within the first 15 min when drugs are administered by IV.
	Inject drugs into IV container and invert several times before administering.	Equal drugs distribution throughout the solution insures proper dilution. *Do not* inject drugs, i.e., potassium, into the IV bag while it is being administered unless the IV is temporarily stopped and the bag is inverted several times to promote equal distribution.
Intake and output	Check urine output every 4–8 h. If a critically ill client is receiving potassium, urine output should be checked every hour.	If urine output is poor, overhydration can occur when excessive or continuous IV fluids are given. Potassium is excreted by the kidneys; thus, a decreased urine output can result in hyperkalemia.

98 When a client receives IV therapy, the nursing responsibility begins with assessment of the solutions ordered.

Intravenous solutions with less than 240 mOsm are considered (hypo-osmolar/hyperosmolar) _____ solutions. Continuous use of this type of solution can cause
* _____ . Give an example of a solution that can become hypo-osmolar if its contents are metabolized. * _____ .

hypo-osmolar; water intoxication; 5% dextrose in water
■   ■   ■

99 Continuous use of hyperosmolar solutions can cause which of the following:

( ) a. Overhydration/fluid volume excess
( ) b. Dehydration/fluid volume deficit
( ) c. Water intoxication

It is usually recommended that IV solutions with different osmolality be alternated. Give an example of an appropriate alternating solution. * _____ .

a. —; b. X; c. —
5% D/W, 5% D/NSS, or 5% D/½ NSS (0.45% NaCl)
■   ■   ■

100 IV containers should be inspected for _____ . If IV fluids are to run for less than 50 mL per hour for 12 hours, IV tubing with a (macrodrip/microdrip) _____ chamber should be used.

The macrodrip chamber delivers * _____ gtt (drops) per milliliter. The microdrip chamber delivers _____ gtt/mL.

leaks or flaws; microdrip; 10 or 20; 60
■   ■   ■

101 IV tubing should be changed at least every _____ hours. KVO means
* _____ . An IV container should not hang longer than _____ hours.

24–48; keep vein open; 24
■   ■   ■

102 Needles or IV catheters should be changed every _____ days. Which of the following needles/catheters are irritating to the veins and can cause phlebitis?

( ) a. Scalp vein needles
( ) b. Straight needles
( ) c. Polyvinyl chloride catheters
( ) d. Polyethylene catheters
( ) e. Teflon catheters
( ) f. Silicone catheters

3
a. —; b. —; c. X; d. X; e. —; f. —
■   ■   ■

103 A problem with ONCs is *_____.
What can happen at the skin site with INCs?

*_____.

severing the catheter with the needle tip
A leak can occur at the infusion insertion site.
■   ■   ■

104 Which of the following body areas are preferred for the insertion of IV devices?

( ) a. Hand veins
( ) b. Distal arm veins
( ) c. Leg veins

What body sites should be avoided? *_____ and *_____ .
Identify at least two client conditions when an upper extremity should not be used.
*_____ and *_____ .

a. X; b. X; c. —
leg veins and affected limbs resulting from a stroke or mastectomy
poor circulation, burns, scleroderma, and rashes
■   ■   ■

105 IV fluids running too fast can cause (dehydration/overhydration) _____ . Give two symptoms of a fluid volume excess. _____ , and _____ .

overhydration; cough and dyspnea, also neck vein engorgement, and chest rales
■   ■   ■

106 KVO should run approximately _____ mL per hour. Name two types of solutions whose flow rate should be checked every 30 minutes to 1 hour:
* _____ and * _____ .

10–25; hyperosmolar solutions and solutions with potassium or medications that affect the pulse and blood pressure (e.g., Levophed, epinephrine)

■   ■   ■

107 Identify two methods of restoring IV fluids that have stopped running. *_____ and * _____ .

   Explain the danger of forcefully irrigating the catheter when the IV fluid has stopped dripping. *_____

_____ .

opening flow clamp, milking the tubing, raising bag, and repositioning extremity
Irrigation can dislodge clot(s) and cause an embolus (emboli) to travel to the lungs, brain, or heart.

■   ■   ■

108 Indicate how high an IV bag should hang above the infusion site:

( ) a. $2\frac{1}{2}$–3 inches
( ) b. $2\frac{1}{2}$–3 feet
( ) c. 5–6 feet

a. —; b. X; c. —

■   ■   ■

109 Indicate which of the following problems/complications can result from intravenous therapy:

( ) a. Infiltration
( ) b. Phlebitis
( ) c. Infections (septicemia)
( ) d. Bradycardia
( ) e. Speed shock
( ) f. Air embolus
( ) g. Pulmonary embolus
( ) h. Hematoma
( ) i. Pulmonary edema

a. X; b. X; c. X; d. —; e. X; f. X; g. X; h. X; i. X

■   ■   ■

110 When an IV infiltrates, the nurse should do which of the following:

( ) a. Decrease the flow rate
( ) b. Discontinue and restart the IV fluids

Phlebitis (inflammation of the vein) can result from an IV needle or catheter that has been in the vein too long, solutions with irritating drugs (potassium, Levophed), or hyperosmolar solutions (25% dextrose) for TPN. Give three symptoms of phlebitis. _____ , _____ , and * _____ .

a. —; b. X
redness, edema (swelling), skin warm to touch, and pain
■   ■   ■

111 How can pyrogenic reactions (septicemia) be prevented? * _____ .

Give two symptoms of systemic infections: _____ , and

_____ .

good aseptic technique; chills, fever, also headache, and tachycardia
■   ■   ■

112 What is speed shock? * _____ .
What is a hematoma? * _____ .

Drugs given rapidly in solution. This increases the drug concentration in the body and produces shocklike symptoms.
blood tumor or raised ecchymosed area
■   ■   ■

113 An air embolus can be fatal if more than _____ mL of air is injected into the vein.

If an air embolus is expected, what should be done? * _____

_____ .

50
Immediately place the client on left side in Trendelenburg position.
■   ■   ■

114 A pulmonary embolus results when a thrombus in the peripheral veins becomes an embolus and travels to the _____ .

Identify two ways in which a pulmonary embolus can occur.

* _____ and * _____ .

lungs; forcefully irrigating a clotted IV needle or catheter and IV fluids given in the lower extremities

       ■   ■   ■

115 Match the symptoms of an air embolus on the right with the pulmonary embolus. Refer to Table 5-5 as needed.

1. Air embolus   (   ) a. Restlessness
2. Pulmonary embolus   (   ) b. Chest pain
3. Both 1 and 2   (   ) c. Pallor
                          (   ) d. Cough
                          (   ) e. Dyspnea
                          (   ) f. Tachycardia

a. 2; b. 2; c. 1; d. 3; e. 3; f. 3

       ■   ■   ■

116 Which of the following drug additives in IV solutions can cause phlebitis or, if infiltrated, can cause sloughing off of the tissue?

(   ) a. Potassium
(   ) b. Decadron (cortisone)
(   ) c. Antineoplastic agents
(   ) d. Low-pH drugs (tetracycline)
(   ) e. Levophed

a. X; b. —; c. X; d. X; e. X

       ■   ■   ■

117 In critically ill clients who are receiving potassium in IV solutions, the urine output is monitored hourly. Why?   *_____.

   Explain why potassium should not be injected into an IV bag while it is being administered.

   *_____

   _____.

To determine kidney function. Eighty to 90% of body potassium is excreted by the kidney. With kidney impairment or shutdown, hyperkalemia can occur.
If the potassium is not properly distributed in the IV container and its highest concentration is in the lower part of the container, it can be toxic to the myocardium (heart) and irritating to the peripheral veins.

■   ■   ■

CASE STUDY REVIEW A

Mrs. Ryan, age 60, was admitted to the hospital for a possible intestinal obstruction. Diagnostic studies were ordered. Food, except for soup and tea, nauseated her. She had not had a bowel movement for a week. An IV infusion of 2000 mL of 5% dextrose/0.33% saline with 20 mEq/L of KCl in 1 liter (1000 mL) was ordered for the first 24 hours.

1. The purpose of Mrs. Ryan's IV therapy was   *_____

   _____.

2. Five percent (5%) dextrose/0.33% saline is what type of solution?   *_____

   _____.

3. What is the rationale for using 5% dextrose/0.33% saline?   *_____

   _____.

4. Was Mrs. Ryan's fluid and nutrient intake completely dependent on IV therapy?

   _____ . Explain   *_____

   _____.

   After 2 days, Mrs. Ryan vomited when she took any oral fluid. Her IV fluid order for the day was 1 liter of 5% dextrose in lactated Ringer's, followed by 1 liter of 5% dextrose in water.

5. Identify the classifications of solutions ordered:
   a. 5% dextrose in water: *_____ .
   b. 5% dextrose in lactated Ringer's: *_____ .
6. Explain the relationship of lactated Ringer's to body fluids.   *_____

   _____.

7. Is the potassium in lactated Ringer's sufficient to meet the daily requirement?

   _____ Explain.   *_____

   _____

   _____.

8. During IV administration of fluid and electrolytes, adequate kidney function is extremely important. Why?   *_____

_____

_____ .

Mrs. Ryan's clinical condition did not improve. Her x-ray showed a complete intestinal obstruction. The following day, a major bowel resection was performed. TPN was started with a hyperosmolar solution containing dextrose 25% per liter, protein hydrolysate, vitamins, and electrolytes.

9. One liter of dextrose 25% has 850 mOsm. The osmolality of this solution is (hypo-osmolar/hyperosmolar) _____ (mOsm and osmolality are explained in Chapter 1).

10. Why is TPN indicated following a major bowel resection?   *_____

_____ .

11. Mrs. Ryan should receive TPN therapy in what blood vessel?   *_____

_____ . Explain your reason.

    *_____

_____

_____ .

12. Name four major complications that can result from TPN therapy.   *_____ ,

_____ , _____ , and _____ .

13. Name at least two nursing interventions that are necessary when caring for Mrs. Ryan as she receives TPN.

    a. *_____
    b. *_____

14. How can an air embolus be prevented?   *_____

_____

_____

1. to provide fluid maintenance requirements
2. hydrating solution/crystalloid
3. daily maintenance of body fluid when minimal sodium and chloride are required
4. No. She was taking soup and tea.
5. a. hydrating solution/free water and calories
   b. replacement solution/crystalloid
6. Lactated Ringer's resembles the electrolyte structure of normal blood serum plasma.
7. No. The potassium is 4 mEq/L. Daily requirement is approximately 40–45 mEq/L.
8. Renal dysfunction can result in electrolyte retention.
9. hyperosmolar
10. TPN increases the intestine's ability to absorb nutrients and allows the intestines to rest.
11. Central vein: subclavian or internal jugular veins. Femoral vein cutdown: high concentration of glucose is not as irritating to large veins and there is a decreased risk of phlebitis.
12. air embolism, infection, hyperglycemia, and hypoglycemia (also fluid overload or fluid volume excess)

13. a. Observe for sepsis due to infection. Nutrient-rich TPN solution provides a good medium for growth of bacteria and yeast.
    b. Monitor blood glucose level with Dextrostix or chemstrip bb. A rapid rate of infusion can cause hyperglycemia.
    Others: Observe for electrolyte imbalance, prevent air embolus, and use strict aseptic technique when dressing and tubing or infusion containers are changed.
14. Valsalva maneuver: taking a breath, holding it, and bearing down

CASE STUDY REVIEW B

Mr. Deale, age 84, was admitted to the hospital because of malnutrition. His hematocrit and BUN were elevated and his serum electrolytes were decreased. His blood gases were pH of 7.3, $Paco_2$ of 40, and HCO_3 of 19. Mr. Deale's urine output was decreased. He was to receive 3 liters of fluid for 24 hours, 2000 mL of 5% dextrose in lactated Ringer's, and 1000 mL of 5% dextrose in 0.2% saline with 30 mEq/L of KCl.

1. The first step in treating Mr. Deale's nutritional, fluid, and electrolyte deficits should be the restoration of *_____ and *_____ .
2. Along with the fluid replacement, name two other nutritional replacements that Mr. Deale needs. *_____ , and _____ .
3. Mr. Deale's elevated hematocrit and BUN may be indicative of *_____.
4. After hydration Mr. Deale's BUN does not return to normal. What does the elevated BUN indicate? *_____

_____ .
5. Mr. Deale's blood gases show a low pH and HCO_3. These findings may indicate
   *_____ .
6. If the IV fluids were administered at a rapid rate, what could happen to Mr. Deale taking into consideration his age and his state of dehydration? *_____

_____ .
7. Mr. Deale's IV fluid orders were 3000 mL (3 liters) in 24 hours or 1000 mL (1 liter) in 8 hours. Using an IV with a drip factor of 10 gtt/mL, calculate the number of drops per minute.

_____ .
8. The physician determines the need for IV therapy by checking on which blood studies?
   a. _____
   b. _____
   c. * _____
9. Mr. Deale was ordered to receive a plasma volume expander. Name three solutions that can be used. _____ , _____ , and _____ .
10. Identify two potential adverse effects that can occur with dextran. *_____
    and *_____ .

1. extracellular fluid volume and blood volume
2. nutrients such as glucose and electrolytes
3. dehydration or a fluid volume deficit
4. renal impairment or failure
5. acidosis (metabolic)
6. pulmonary edema and fluid volume excess

7. a. *1000 ÷ 8 h = 125 mL/h*

b. $\dfrac{125\ mL/h \times 10\ gtt/mL\ (IV\ set)}{60\ min} = \dfrac{1250}{60} = 20\text{–}21\ gtt/min$

8. a. *hematocrit; b. BUN; c. serum electrolytes*
9. *albumin, plasma or Plasmanate, and dextran*
10. *reduces clotting ability and interferes with type and cross-matching*

CASE STUDY REVIEW C

Ms. McCann, age 74, has orders to receive 2 liters of 5% dextrose in normal saline (0.9% NaCl) daily. After several days, Ms. McCann's skin turgor was poor and her mucous membranes were dry. Her pulse rate had increased 26 beats per minute.

1. Identify the type of solution osmolality (tonicity) of 5% dextrose in saline.

   _____ .

2. What type of fluid imbalance did Ms. McCann have according to her symptoms?
   * _____ .

   Give three symptoms that were indicative of the fluid imbalance. * _____ ,
   * _____ and * _____ .

The nurse has many responsibilities with assessment and monitoring of IV therapy. Describe the nursing interventions related to the following:

3. Needle or catheter: * _____

   _____ .

4. IV tubing: * _____

   _____ .

5. Flow rate: * _____

   _____ .

6. Intravenous insertion site: * _____

   _____ .

7. Prevention of infection: * _____

   _____ .

8. Prevention of air and pulmonary emboli:
   a. * _____
   b. * _____
9. Drug additives: * _____

   _____ .

10. Urine output: * _____

    _____ .

1. *hyperosmolar*
2. *dehydration or fluid volume deficit; poor skin turgor, dry mucous membrane, and increased heart rate*

3. *Needles and catheters should be changed every 3 days (with some exceptions). Check for leaks when using INCs and severing the catheter with ONCs.*
4. *Change IV tubing every 2 days or according to agency policy.*
5. *Regulate drip chamber to deliver specified drops per minute with macrodrip or microdrip chambers.*
6. *Use hands or distal veins in the arm. Avoid using leg veins, antecubital fossa (elbow), or limbs affected with paralysis or impaired circulation.*
7. *Use aseptic technique when administering and caring for IV therapy.*
8. *a. Remove air from the IV tubing. b. Do not irrigate an IV that has stopped dripping.*
9. *Check for infiltration and phlebitis.*
10. *Monitor urine output every 4–8 hours, every hour when potassium is in the solution.*

NURSING ASSESSMENT FACTORS FOR CLIENTS RECEIVING TPN

Total parenteral nutrition is a complex form of IV therapy intended to meet the complete nutritional needs of selected clients. Nurses are responsible for the coordination of activities needed to ensure the proper use of solutions, maintain a continuous infusion, and monitor the effectiveness of the TPN therapy. The nurse coordinating the TPN must have keen assessment skills and a thorough understanding of the physiologic factors related to nutrition and the fluid and electrolyte needs of clients receiving hyperosmolar solutions over an extended period of time. Before beginning TPN therapy the placement of the central venous catheter must be confirmed with an x-ray report.

Nursing assessment factors for TPN therapy include the various observations necessary with any IV therapy as well as some specific assessments focused on issues important to TPN therapy. Assess fluid balance: Monitor intake and output closely to assess for signs of fluid (volume excess or fluid volume deficit) retention or fluid overload. Daily weights provide a good measure of the effectiveness of treatment, and any sudden weight gain or loss can alert the nurse to problems related to fluid volume retention or deficits.

- Monitor laboratory studies. Laboratory studies provide essential information about electrolyte and blood glucose levels associated with fluid balance. Important laboratory values include Na, K, HCO_3, Cl, Ca, phosphorus, Mg, serum glucose, serum creatinine, and the total protein level. The nurse can monitor glucose levels with the blood Dextrostix or blood glucose scanner. Blood glucose levels should be measured every 4 hours in the acute stages of illness. Serum albumin and globulin should be monitored every 72 hours or per the physician's orders.
- Monitor vital signs. Temperature, pulse, respirations, and blood pressure readings alert the nurse to potential fluid volume problems and impending infections.
- Monitor TPN solutions and maintain infusion lines. TPN solutions are usually prepared by the pharmacy under a laminar airflow hood. TPN lines are not to be interrupted except for lipids that may be piggybacked into the TPN line. All solutions must be verified before hanging. Solution containers should be checked for leaks and for clarity. Cloudy solutions may be defective and must be approved before hanging (unless lipids are added directly to the TPN solution). Strict aseptic techniques must be maintained when changing solutions and tubing. The physician prescribes the amount of fluid per 24 hours, and the nurse calculates the related flow rate depending upon the type of drip chamber and company specifications for number of drops per milliliter. It is highly recommended that flow rates be maintained by an infusion pump; some literature states this as mandatory. Infusion rates must remain constant. The TPN port is not used for anything except TPN infusions and lipid infusions. If TPN therapy is interrupted for any reason, infuse 10% D/W at the same rate ordered for the TPN therapy.

- Intravenous tubing is changed according to agency policy (usually every 24–48 hours). To prevent an air embolus when changing the IV tubing, either clamp the central venous line using plastic or padded clamps only or have the client perform the Valsalva maneuver while tubing is being changed. Assist the client if necessary by pressing down on the abdomen. If an air embolus is suspected, immediately place the client in a Trendelenburg position on his or her left side. Additional precautions to prevent an air embolism include using leur-lock connections on all-IV tubing, taping catheter and tubing connections securely, and suturing the central venous line in place. The tubing or filter should be anchored to prevent pulling on the central venous line, skin sutures, and catheter.
- Central venous line dressings are changed according to hospital policy, usually every 24–48 hours (regular IVs are changed every 48 hours), using strict sterile technique. Never use an existing TPN line for blood samples. All bags, IV lines, and dressings are to be labeled and dated accordingly with documentation on the client's chart.
- Each agency usually develops its own procedure for monitoring TPN therapy. Prepared solutions not in use are usually refrigerated and should be removed 2 hours before hanging. TPN is usually started at 1000 mL for the first 24 hours and is increased at a rate of 500–1000 mL daily until the desired volume is reached. When discontinuing TPN, decrease the daily rate gradually over 12–72 hours according to the volume prescribed and the physician's orders.
- Observe client and central venous line infusion site for signs of infection. Generalized symptoms of infection can indicate sepsis, requiring the discontinuation of the solutions along with the removal of cannulas. Complaints of pain, numbness, or tingling in the fingers, neck, or arm on the same side as the catheter may indicate thrombus formation and must be reported immediately.
- Monitor nutritional status—daily weights, physical assessment observations of skin, energy level, nitrogen balance (healing/tissue growth), etc.—as needed to determine adequacy of prescribed solutions.

TPN is a complex medical intervention requiring astute observations and reporting skills on the part of the nurse. Many complications of this complex treatment modality are life threatening.

NURSING DIAGNOSES AND INTERVENTIONS FOR TPN

Diagnoses related to nutritional status associated with TPN are collaborative problems since the physician manages the fluid and nutritional replacement therapy.

NURSING DIAGNOSIS 1

High risk for infection, related to TPN therapy, concentrated glucose solutions, and invasive lines requiring dressing and tubing changes.

NURSING INTERVENTIONS AND RATIONALE

1. Assess source and extent of infection. TPN solutions are a prime medium for bacteria growth. Observing bags for leaks and solutions for clarity may provide clues to the source of infection when the solution is the medium. Infusion sites must also be observed for signs of redness and swelling and drainage that may indicate an infection. When an infection is suspected, cannulas are removed and may be cultured according to agency procedure. Environmental and personal contacts must be assessed as other sources of infection.

2. Reduce risks for infection. Use good surgical asepsis when changing solutions and tubing. Use sterile techniques with dressing changes. Invasive therapies increase the client's risk of infection; thus the nurse must maintain a sterile technique when providing invasive treatments.
3. Monitor vital signs. Assess for symptoms of infection. Elevated temperature, pulse, and respiration may indicate an impending infection.
4. Refrigerate TPN solutions not in use. High glucose concentration is an excellent medium for bacteria growth.

NURSING DIAGNOSIS 2

Nutrition: altered, less than body requirements, related to inadequate intake of calories and proteins.

NURSING INTERVENTIONS AND RATIONALE

1. Monitor client's caloric intake in relation to changes in exercise and supplemental nutritional intake in addition to TPN calories and proteins. Infections, tissue healing, exercise, and other factors that affect the client's metabolic rate have implications for the total nutritional status. Change and additional stresses must be factored into the TPN formula for meeting nutritional needs. Maintain TPN at prescribed rates without interruption.
2. Assess skin condition of pressure sites according to physical status. Immobile clients need close observation to prevent pressure sores, especially if the client is emaciated or receiving less than total caloric and protein needs.

NURSING DIAGNOSIS 3

High risk for fluid volume excess, related to the risk of runaway TPN infusion, IV infusions, and client's physical condition.

NURSING INTERVENTIONS AND RATIONALE

For a fluid volume excess with TPN therapy interventions are similar to those with fluid volume excess with other parenteral therapies. Interventions addressed here are specific to TPN and central venous catheters.

1. Observe for signs and symptoms of fluid overload with TPN infusion (cough, dyspnea, engorged neck veins, chest rales, weight gain) that reflect a fluid shift from the cellular to the vascular system (a complication of hyperosmolar solutions) or occur as the result of a misplaced central venous catheter.
2. Monitor solutions and fluid volume closely. Verify all solutions with orders. Maintain a consistent flow rate as calculated. Catch-up or slowdown with TPN volumes is contraindicated and dangerous. Infusion pumps are frequently used to maintain accurate flow rates. Medications are not to be added to or mixed with TPN infusions. Document hanging and completion times. Do not interrupt TPN solutions. Mark containers to monitor hourly infusion expectations.

NURSING DIAGNOSIS 4

Comfort altered, related to parenteral therapy using central venous lines.

NURSING INTERVENTIONS AND RATIONALE

1. Identify type and severity of discomfort. Complaints of pain, numbness, or tingling of the fingers, arm, and neck on the side of the central venous line may indicate thrombus formation. Report these symptoms to the physician. Chest pain and/or respiratory difficulty may indicate a pulmonary embolus resulting from lipid infusions or a dislodged thrombus. This pain indicates an emergency situation.

2. Assess client's physical status. Note for signs and symptoms of infection that may promote discomfort (elevated temperature, labored/rapid breathing). Note changes in condition of infusion site. Observe client for reactions to solutions and additives or symptoms of overhydration. Clients are often apprehensive about infusions through central venous lines.

3. Observe for signs and symptoms of reactions to lipid solutions. Signs and symptoms of immediate reactions include elevated temperature, flushing, sweating, pressure sensation over eyes, nausea/vomiting, headache, chest pain, back pain, dyspnea, and cyanosis, while signs and symptoms of delayed reactions include hepatomegaly, thrombocytopenia, splenomegaly, hyperlipidemia, hepatic damage, and jaundice.

NURSING DIAGNOSIS 5

Gas exchange: impaired, related to air embolism when inserting or removing the central venous line, when changing the central line, and when changing TPN solutions.

NURSING INTERVENTIONS AND RATIONALE

1. Place client on left side with head down and have him or her perform Valsalva maneuver when inserting central lines or changing tubing. Assist client by applying abdominal pressure if necessary. The Valsalva maneuver increases the intra-thoracic pressure and reduces the risk of developing an air embolus.

Other Nursing Diagnoses for which the risks are increased during TPN therapy include:

High risk for fluid volume deficit, related to inadequate fluid intake and osmotic diuresis.
Breathing pattern: ineffective, related to complications of central venous lines and fluid volume excess.
Tissue perfusion (renal, cardiopulmonary, and peripheral): impaired, related to fluid volume deficit and osmotic diuresis.
Knowledge deficit, related to unfamiliarity with TPN therapy and procedures, specific to IV therapy equipment.

NURSING ASSESSMENT FACTORS FOR CLIENTS RECEIVING IV THERAPY

The administration of IV therapy meets five basic purposes: replacement of previous fluid loss, maintenance requirements for fluids and electrolytes, meeting concurrent fluid losses, meeting nutritional needs, and a mechanism for the administration of medications and blood and blood products. An awareness of the specific purpose of the IV therapy is essential to the nurse's assessment. Inherent in the administration of IV infusions are numerous nursing procedural responsibilities and implications for the assessment of risk factors created by IV infusions. The nursing assessment factors and nursing diagnoses discussed in this section are limited to the nursing responsibilities and implications for specific risks associated with IV therapy and fluid balance.

Nursing assessment factors consistent with the nursing responsibilities and risk factors associated with IV therapy include the following:

- Monitor fluid balance. Nursing knowledge of the specific purpose of the prescribed IV therapy along with a basic understanding of the types of IV solutions is essential in promoting fluid balance with IV therapy. While the physician may prescribe the type and amount of IV solution administered, the nurse must coordinate these activities and assess the client for potential risks associated with the prescribed therapy. An accurate record of intake and output, observations for expected and unexpected client responses to IV infusions, close monitoring of laboratory results (electrolytes, hemoglobin and hematocrit, etc.), and keen physical assessment skills focused on the detection of signs and symptoms of dehydration or overhydration are needed to promote early identification of fluid balance problems.

- Monitor equipment used in the administration of IV therapy. IV containers and tubing must be closely observed for leaks. IV therapy requires a closed system, and any leaks or openings provide a medium for microorganisms to invade the system and contaminate the solution. Check the drip size on the IV tubing. Drip size can vary from company to company and has implications for accurately meeting fluid requirements of IV therapy (macrodrips vary from 10 to 20 gtt/mL; microdrips generally equal 60 gtt/mL). Macrodrip chambers should be used when administering amounts of fluid greater than 50 mL per hour. Microdrip chambers should be used if this amount is to be less than 50 mL per hour. Procedures for changing IV tubings and the length of time for their use are usually determined by hospital policy (generally the tubing is changed every 24–48 hours). A single IV container should not be infused over a period longer than 24 hours. Microdrip chambers are suggested to keep the vein open (KVO) with 250–500 mL of fluid running at 10–25 mL per hour.

- Select and observe infusion sites carefully. The selection of the type of needle or catheter and the infusion site are factors that the nurse must assess carefully to promote client comfort and reduce risks associated with IV therapy (see Table 5-2 for specifics related to infusion rates). In order to reduce the risks of phlebitis and dislodged thrombus, the upper extremities are preferred infusion sites. Limbs affected by a stroke, mastectomy, or injury should not be used as an infusion site. Soft restraints and arm boards are helpful in preventing dislodgement of the IV needle. Correct positioning of the tubing prevents kinking or obstruction.

- Continuously assess the flow rate and patency of the infusion system. Calculating flow rates and the regulation of the IV solution are the responsibility of the nurse. Maintenance of the infusion system and the solution flow rate is necessary to meet the fluid and electrolyte needs of the client. Check the rate every 30 minutes to prevent complications and ensure fluid balance. Patency of the system and regulation of the flow rate can be influenced by various factors other than the tubing clamp (height of the solution, repositioning of the extremity, or milking of the tubing can assist in enhancing the flow rate of sluggish IVs). Table 5-5 provides details for adjusting flow rates.

- Assess for problems and complications of IV infusion. Possible complications of IV infusions include infiltration, phlebitis, systemic infections, speed shock, air emboli, pulmonary embolism, pulmonary edema, hematomas, runaway IV fluids, and reactions to additives. Early recognition of the signs and symptoms of these complications is a nursing responsibility.

NURSING DIAGNOSES AND INTERVENTIONS FOR IV THERAPY

NURSING DIAGNOSIS 1

High risk for fluid volume excess, related to runaway IV or volume infused too great for client's physical condition.

NURSING INTERVENTIONS AND RATIONALE

1. Identify source/reason for excessive fluid intake. The nurse must determine whether the fluid overload is accidental in nature or the result of changes in the physiologic status of the client. Report errors in fluid regulation and seek consultation in adjusting fluid volume replacement/maintenance.
2. Assess client's response to fluid overload and risk for medical emergencies (pulmonary edema). Observe for signs and symptoms of fluid overload (see Table 5-5), frequent vital signs, laboratory studies, etc. Notify physician of significant changes in patient's condition.
3. Reduce causative factors. Poor regulation of fluid intake and runaway IV infusion are primary causes of a fluid overload that the nurse can control. Accurately calculate flow rate and monitor the rate every 30 minutes to every 1 hour based on client's physical condition.
4. Use infusion pumps as appropriate to regulate IV intake. Controllers are preferable if available and mandatory when administering specific medications.
5. Monitor blood values. Electrolytes should be monitored every 4 hours in acutely ill clients and prn according to the client's physical condition. Creatinine/BUN ratios and the hemoglobin and hematocrit levels should be evaluated every 8 hours until stable.
6. Monitor weight daily. Report sudden weight gains or losses to determine indications of IV fluid changes related to fluid overload or a fluid deficit.
7. Closely assess physiologic responses to fluid load. Monitor vital signs according to physical condition. Auscultate lungs every 2–4 hours for rales, palpate pedal pulses, test for edema in extremities, and monitor for changes in mental status that may result from electrolyte imbalances. Continuous physical assessment of the client's condition is essential to prevent life-threatening conditions that can result from a fluid overload.

NURSING DIAGNOSIS 2

High risk for fluid volume deficit, related to inadequate fluid intake.

NURSING INTERVENTIONS AND RATIONALE

1. Monitor intake and output. The nurse is responsible for coordinating the factors that control fluid balance for clients. Accurate documentation of intake and output provides essential clues to detecting risks for deficit imbalances. Use an IV controller if available. Accurately calculate fluid rate and monitor rate closely (every $\frac{1}{2}$–1 hour observation).
2. Assess for physiologic signs of dehydration. Check mucous membranes for color and dryness, evaluate skin turgor, assess for orthostatic hypotension when checking vital signs, check vital signs every 1–4 hours according to client's physical condition, and check weight daily. Recognize changes in hydration that indicate a change in status and increase risk for fluid volume overload. Confusion is more common in dehydration than in a fluid overload.

3. Monitor lab studies. Electrolyte imbalances are often the first sign of an increased risk for dehydration. Creatinine/BUN ratios and hemoglobin and hematocrit ratios provide evidence of dehydration. Urine specific gravity can be done every 8 hours (often by the nurse) to assess hydration status. Serum osmolality measurements should be assessed every 24 hours.

NURSING DIAGNOSIS 3

High risk for infection, related to contaminated IV fluids, contaminated equipment, or a break in aseptic technique.

NURSING INTERVENTIONS AND RATIONALE

1. Use sterile technique. When inserting infusion devices, changing IV tubing, changing site dressings, or changing IV containers, sterile techniques are mandatory. IVs are a closed system, and any break in the system provides the potential for bacterial invasion.
2. Assess IV insertion site. Fluid leakage, pain, redness, swelling, or drainage at the insertion site is abnormal. Examination of the insertion site often provides the first clues to infection potential or inadequate function of the system.
3. Change peripheral IV site every 72 hours or according to agency policy. Procedures for the care of IV sites vary with agency policy. A period of 72 hours is generally considered the maximum time for peripheral infusion sites.
4. Change IV tubing and dressing sites every 24–48 hours according to agency procedure. Dressing changes are essential to the prevention of infections. Confirm expiration dates of IV tubing and fluids before hanging to ensure sterility.

Other nursing diagnoses to consider include:

High risk for tissue perfusion (renal, cardiopulmonary, and peripheral): decreased, related to fluid volume deficit and inadequate fluid replacement. This is a collaborative problem. Nursing interventions are similar to those with a fluid volume deficit with special consideration given to the select systems involved.

High risk for knowledge deficit, related to lack of familiarity with IV therapy.

PART II
CLINICAL SITUATIONS

INTRODUCTION

In the clinical setting the nurse provides care for persons experiencing a variety of problems related to fluid and electrolytes. Part II of this book addresses 11 clinical situations. The first 2 situations focus on developmental issues related to the aging adult and infants and children. The remaining chapters focus on gastrointestinal surgery, trauma-acute injury, renal failure with dialysis, burns, cancer, congestive heart failure, cirrhosis, diabetic acidosis, and neurologic conditions. To assess the clients' needs and to provide the appropriate care needed for persons with selected health problems, the nurse must have a working knowledge and understanding of concepts related to fluid and electrolyte balance. Knowledge of these concepts allows the nurse to assess physiologic changes that occur with fluid and electrolyte imbalance and to plan appropriate nursing interventions to assist clients as they adapt to these changes.

In each clinical situation the participant will become acquainted with clients who have fluid and electrolyte imbalances. Clients are presented as part of a clinical situation. Some of the client situations used in this section have already been presented in earlier case study reviews. The participant in this program will gain an understanding of the physiologic changes involved in each clinical situation.

CHAPTER 6

FLUID PROBLEMS OF INFANTS AND CHILDREN

Behavioral Objectives

Upon completion of this chapter, you will be prepared to:

- Identify three physiologic factors that influence infants' and children's responses to changes in fluid and electrolyte balance.
- Compare the total body fluid volume in infants and children to the total body fluid volume in the mature adult.
- Identify normal serum electrolyte values for sodium, potassium, and calcium in infants and children.
- Discuss how the electrolyte values for sodium, potassium, and calcium vary in response to fluid balance changes in infants and children.
- Describe a method to calculate the daily fluid and electrolyte needs of infants and children.
- Describe nursing assessment factors important in determining fluid and electrolyte balance in infants and children.
- Develop nursing diagnoses for infants and children experiencing fluid balance problems.
- Identify nursing interventions specific to selected nursing diagnoses associated with fluid balance problems.

PHYSIOLOGIC FACTORS

The nurse's understanding of the physiologic differences in infants and children that have implications for fluid and electrolyte balance is essential to providing optimal health care. Since these physiologic differences vary significantly throughout infancy and childhood, important regulatory factors are presented from a developmental perspective for infancy and childhood. The nurse should keep in mind that the immature physiologic development in infants and children increases their potential for fluid balance problems. The symptoms of these imbalances in infants and children often occur rapidly and can be very dramatic in their presentation.

Physiologic differences in the infant's total body surface area, immaturity of renal structures, high rate of metabolism, and immaturity of the endocrine system in promoting homeostatic control predispose this age group to various fluid and electrolyte imbalances. The proportionately high ratio of extracellular fluid (ECF) to intracellular fluid (ICF) in the very young predisposes the infant to rapid losses of body fluid. The limited fluid reserve capacity of infants inhibits their adaptation to fluid losses. Additionally the infant's renal structures are not fully developed until the latter half of the second year of life. All of these factors increase the infant's vulnerability to dehydration.

1 The body is composed mostly of water. Body water in the early human embryo represents _____ % of body weight, in the newborn infant _____ %, and in the adult _____ %. (Refer to Chapter 1, Frame 1.)

The low birth weight infant's (premature infant's) body water represents 80–90% of body weight.

97; 77; 60

■ ■ ■

2 Complete the percentage of body weight that is representative of body water in the following:

Early human embryo _____ %

Low birth weight infant _____ %

Newborn infant _____ %

Adult _____ %

97; 80–90; 77; 60

■ ■ ■

3 Infants need proportionately more water than adults. The infant's large body surface area and immature kidney limit the infant's ability to retain water. Their kidneys cannot concentrate urine effectively; thus, urine volume is increased. More water is lost through the infant's skin because of the increased body surface area. Since the infant cannot concentrate urine, water is needed to maintain fluid volume lost through the increased urine output and larger body surface area.

Give two reasons why the infant needs a higher percentage of total body water.

* _____ and

* _____ .

a large body surface (greater amounts of water loss through the skin) and inability to concentrate urine (increased urine output due to immature kidneys)

■ ■ ■

4 Water distribution in an infant is not the same as in an adult. The ECF in the infant is 40% of body weight. Try to recall the percentage of body weight (ECF) in the adult _____ . (Refer to Chapter 1.)

The ICF in the infant is 34% of body weight; whereas in the adult it is _____ . (Refer to Chapter 1.) The proportionately higher ratio of ECF volume in the infant predisposes the infant to (more, less) _____ rapid losses of fluid volume; consequently, _____ develops more rapidly in infants than adults.

20%; 40%; more; dehydration

5   At 1 year, the percentage of the child's total body water is close in amount to the percentage of the adult's (60%) total body water; however, the proportion of ECF and ICF is not the same. It is not until the child is between 3 and 5 years old that the proportion of ECF and ICF volume is similar to the adult's.

The extracellular fluid is composed of _____ and _____ fluid. Another name for intracellular fluid is (cellular/vascular) _____ fluid. (Refer to Chapter 1.)

interstitial and intravascular; cellular

    ■   ■   ■

6   Increased body surface area in the infant causes excess water loss through the _____ . The smaller the infant, the greater the body surface area in proportion to body weight. The infant's kidneys are (mature/immature) _____ ; thus, the urinary volume is (increased/decreased) _____ .

skin; immature; increased

    ■   ■   ■

7   It may take 2 years before the child's kidneys are mature.

The infant's immature kidneys decrease the glomerular filtration rate (GFR); thus, the kidney's ability to concentrate urine is (decreased/increased) _____ , while the urine volume is (decreased/increased) _____ .

Giving too much water could cause (dehydration/overhydration). _____ .

decreased; increased; overhydration

    ■   ■   ■

8   As the child grows, there is muscle growth and cellular growth. More water shifts from the ECF to the ICF compartment.

At ages 3–5 years, when the child's ICF and ECF proportions become similar to the adult's, what do you think could be a contributing factor? *_____

Increased cellular and muscular growth causes water to shift from the ECF space to the ICF space.

    ■   ■   ■

ETIOLOGY

9   The infant has less reserve of body fluid than the adult and is more likely to develop a fluid volume deficit.

   The infant loses one half of his ECF daily; whereas the adult loses only one sixth of his ECF in the same length of time.

   Name two reasons why an infant loses one half of his ECF daily.

a. *_____

b. *_____

   The infant is likely to develop dehydration more rapidly than adults who lose proportionately similar amounts of water. This increased risk for infants is the result of their (increased/decreased) _____ fluid reserve.

a. large body surface area causing water to be lost through the skin (insensible perspiration) and b. increased urinary output (immature kidneys cannot concentrate urine)

decreased

   ■   ■   ■

10   Keeping an infant covered in a stable cool environment (reduces/increases) _____ insensible fluid loss through the body surface.

reduces

   ■   ■   ■

11   Serum electrolytes do not vary greatly between infants and adults. The serum sodium level in a newborn fluctuates at birth. It may be low the first 3–6 hours after birth and then rise slightly (2–6 mEq/L increase) during the first 2 days of life.

   The infant's serum sodium level is 134–150 mEq/L and the child's level is 134–146 mEq/L. What is the normal adult serum sodium level?   *_____

135–146 mEq/L

   ■   ■   ■

12   If a 5-month-old infant consumes cow's milk and commercially prepared baby food, he ingests five times more sodium than a breast-fed infant.

   The name for an elevated serum sodium level is _____ .

hypernatremia (serum sodium excess)

   ■   ■   ■

13 Low birth weight infants tend to develop hypernatremia with a normal to low sodium intake. Their body surface area is (greater/lesser) _____ than an average weight newborn's and their insensible water loss is (increased/decreased) _____ .

  Also, low birth weight infants' kidneys are more immature than the kidneys of average weight infants; therefore, more diluted water is excreted. The loss of water is in excess of the loss of solutes. In low birth weight infants this increases their risk of developing

_____ .

greater; increased; hypernatremia
  ■   ■   ■

14 Hyponatremia can also occur in infants and children. Another name for hyponatremia is
* _____ .

Three causes of hyponatremia are:

a. Overhydration—water overloading
b. Continuous administration of oral or parenteral electrolyte-free solutions
c. Syndrome of inappropriate antidiuretic hormone secretion (SIADHS). This results in an excess secretion of ADH causing excess water reabsorption from the distal tubules. Factors attributing to SIADHS are CNS injuries or illness (head injuries, meningitis), pneumonia, neoplasm, stress, surgery, and drugs (narcotics, barbiturates).

serum sodium deficit
  ■   ■   ■

15 Name three causes of hyponatremia. _____ ,
* _____ , and _____ .

overhydration, continuous administration of electrolyte-free solutions, and SIADH
  ■   ■   ■

16 A rapid decrease in the serum sodium, 120 mEq/L or below, can cause CNS changes such as headache, twitching, confusion, and convulsion.

  The nurse should observe for CNS changes when hyponatremia occurs suddenly. Give three CNS symptoms. _____ , _____ , and

_____ .

headache, twitching, and confusion (also convulsions)
  ■   ■   ■

17 The normal potassium level in the infant is 3.5–5.8 mEq/L. The top level is slightly higher than the adult's and remains in the upper level for the first few months of the infant's life.

Try to recall where the greatest concentration of potassium is found in the body.

_____

cells or ICF (In various institutions, laboratory values vary slightly.)
　　　　　　　　　　■　　　　　　　　　　　■　　　　　　　　　　　■

18 Infants and children may develop hypokalemia (serum potassium deficit) when cellular breakdown occurs from injury, starvation, dehydration, diarrhea, vomiting, diabetic acidosis, and steroids for treating nephrosis. Children do not conserve potassium well. The kidneys continue to excrete body potassium even with little or no potassium intake.

Give at least two signs or symptoms of hypokalemia (Refer to Chapter 3).
_____ , and *_____ .

dizziness, muscular weakness, abdominal distention, decreased peristalsis, and arrhythmia
　　　　　　　　■　　　　　　　　　　■　　　　　　　　　　■

19 Eighty to ninety percent of body potassium loss is excreted in the urine. When oliguria (decreased urine output) occurs, what type of potassium imbalance results? *_____

_____ .

hyperkalemia or serum potassium excess
　　　　　　　■　　　　　　　　　■　　　　　　　　　■

20 The infant's normal serum chloride level is between 96–116 mEq/L. For the first few months of the infant's life the serum sodium range is between *_____ and the serum potassium range is between *_____ . The normal range of the child's serum chloride level is 98–105 mEq/L.

134–150 mEq/L; 3.5–5.8 mEq/L
　　　　　　　■　　　　　　　　　■　　　　　　　　　■

21 The serum calcium level in the cord blood is higher than the maternal serum calcium, however, after birth the infant's serum calcium level decreases to 3.8 mEq/L or 7.7 mg/dL. In low birth weight infants, the serum calcium tends to remain lower for a longer period of time. (A child's normal serum calcium range is 4.5–5.8 mEq/L or 9–11.5 mg/dL.)

Infants do not have calcium stored in the bones as do adults. If the infant is fed cow's milk, the body calcium level may remain low since cow's milk has a higher phosphorus content, which lowers the calcium level.

Breast-fed infants receive more calcium and retain it since breast milk contains less phosphorus.

Which infant retains more body calcium—the infant receiving cow's milk or the breast-fed infant? *_____ . Why?

*_____ .

the breast-fed infant. Breast milk contains more calcium and less phosphorus, which gives the infant more calcium. Thus, reducing phosphorus allows the infant to retain the calcium.

■   ■   ■

22 Newborn infants tend to have a low pH, which is indicative of metabolic acidosis. This is the result of increased acid metabolites that result from the infant's increased metabolic rate and physiologic changes during birth. The pH becomes closer to normal after the first few days or weeks of life. In low birth weight infants, the pH remains low for several weeks.

The low pH of cow's milk combined with the low serum calcium level in infants (does/does not) _____ result in symptoms of tetany.

does not. (Calcium is ionized in an acidotic state regardless of how low it is).

■   ■   ■

23 Calcium is ionized in an acidotic state but not in an alkalotic state. Tetany symptoms occur when hypocalcemia (serum calcium deficit) is present in a normal acid-base balance or in an alkalotic state.

Symptoms of tetany are *_____ and *_____ . (Refer to Chapter 3.)

tingling of fingers and twitching around mouth (also, carpopedal spasm)

■   ■   ■

CLINICAL APPLICATIONS

Table 6-1 suggests a simple method for calculating daily fluid and electrolyte requirements for infants and children. This table is presented only as information for fluid and electrolyte maintenance in children. There are many tables and nomograms used for fluid calculations. Table 6-1 describes only one method used by many pediatricians and hospital personnel.

To calculate the daily fluid and electrolyte needs of infants and children, first calculate the infant's/child's weight in kilograms (kg). Then use this chart to calculate the specific fluid and electrolyte needs according to the body weight in kilograms.

Table 6-1.   FLUID AND ELECTROLYTE DAILY REQUIREMENT FOR INFANTS AND CHILDREN ACCORDING TO THE HOLLEDAY-SENGAR METHOD USING CALORIE EXPENDITURE FROM BODY WEIGHT

Body Weight (kg)	Fluid Requirement (mL/24 h)	Electrolyte Requirement (mEq/L/24 h)
1–10	100 mL/kg	—
11–20	1000 mL +500 mL/kg for each kg above 10	3 mEq of sodium and 1 mEq of chloride and potassium for each 100 mL of water
21 and above	+20 mL/kg for each kg above 20	—

Adapted from Wilmington Medical Center, Pediatric Dept., and H. I. Hochman, et al.: Dehydration, diabetic ketoacidosis and shock in the pediatric patient. *Pediatr Clin of North Am 26*(4):805, November 1979.

This method is not used with neonates less than 14 days old or with conditions of abnormal fluid loss.

24   Using Table 6-1, calculate which of the following are daily fluid requirements for an infant weighing 6 kg:

( ) a. 300 mL
( ) b. 600 mL
( ) c. 900 mL

a. —; b. X; c. —

■   ■   ■

25 Using Table 6-1, calculate which of the following are the daily fluid requirements of a child weighing 5 kg:

( ) a. 1150 mL
( ) b. 1250 mL
( ) c. 1500 mL

The daily sodium requirement according to the fluid requirement for this child is:

( ) d. 15 mEq/L
( ) e. 25.5 mEq/L
( ) f. 37.5 mEq/L

The daily potassium and chloride requirement according to the fluid requirement for this child is:

( ) g. 25 mEq/L
( ) h. 30 mEq/L
( ) i. 35 mEq/L

a. —; b. X; c, —; d. —; e. —; f. X; g. X; h. —; i. —

■   ■   ■

26 Intravenous flow rate should be checked every 15 minutes on an infant and young child and every 30 minutes on an older child (age 6 and above). A microdrip chamber set should be used, and as a safety precaution, only 2 hours of the calculated solution should be in the solution container/set.

Intravenous fluid administered to a 2-year-old child should be checked every _____ minutes.

15

■   ■   ■

NURSING ASSESSMENT

Table 6-2 lists the nursing assessment with rationale for assessing fluid and electrolyte balance in infants and children. This table can be used as an assessment tool in the hospital, clinic, or home. In the nursing assessment column, you would either check or fill in the blanks. The rationale should be eliminated when used as a tool. Study the table and complete the frames related to the nursing assessment. Refer back to the table as needed.

27 The child in the hospital should be assessed for fluid balance every 8 hours; the child with an existing fluid imbalance should be assessed every hour.

The fluid status of a child in fluid imbalance should be closely monitored every

_____ .

hour

Table 6-2. NURSING ASSESSMENT OF FLUID AND ELECTROLYTE IMBALANCE IN INFANTS AND CHILDREN

Observation	Nursing Assessment		Rationale/Interventions
Changes in behavior and general appearance	Irritable	_____	Early symptoms of fluid volume deficit are irritability, purposeless movement, and an unusual high-pitched or whining cry. As dehydration continues, lethargy and unconsciousness may occur. Gray or pallor color indicates a decrease in peripheral circulation from severe fluid loss—shock. Flushed color can indicate sodium excess.
	Unusually quiet	_____	
	Lethargic with	_____	
	hyperirritability on	_____	
	stimulation		
	Purposeless movement	_____	
	Different cry		
	Won't eat	_____	
	Color	_____	
	Pale	_____	
	Gray	_____	
	Flushed		
	Unconsciousness (comatose)		
Neurologic signs	Abdominal distention	_____	Abdominal distention and weakness may indicate a potassium deficit. Tetany symptoms can indicate a calcium and/or magnesium deficit. Serum calcium deficits occur easily in children, since their bones do not readily replace calcium to the blood. Confusion can be due to a potassium deficit and/or fluid volume deficit.
	Diminished reflexes (hypotonia)	_____	
	Weakness/paralysis	_____	
	Tetany tremors (hypertonia)	_____	
	Twitching, cramps	_____	
	Sensorium	_____	
	Confusion	_____	
	Comatose		
	Other		
Weight changes Weight loss	Preillness weight	_____	Weight loss can indicate the degree of dehydration (fluid loss):
	Compared to present weight	_____	Mild—2–5% weight loss
Weight gain	Edema and ascites can occur with fluid imbalances. Fluid overloads can result in hepatomegaly (enlarged liver).		Moderate—6–10% loss Severe—11% and above loss Routine weights should be taken on the same scale and at the same time each day.

Table 6-2. (Continued)

Observation	Nursing Assessment	Rationale/Interventions
Skin (tissue) turgor	Elevated pinched skin (after 2 to 3 s) ⎯⎯⎯ Lack of elasticity ⎯⎯⎯	Skin and subcutanous tissue should be checked together to avoid misinterpretation of dehydration or normal skin turgor. To test skin turgor, pinch the skin over the abdominal and chest wall or the medial aspect of the thigh. Skin turgor on obese infants or children can appear normal even with a fluid deficit. Undernourishment can cause poor tissue turgor with fluid balance. Abdominal distention may mask turgor signs. Poor skin turgor is evidenced with 3% or more weight loss.
Dryness of mucous membrane	Dryness in oral cavity (cheeks and gums) ⎯⎯⎯ Dry tongue with longitudinal wrinkles ⎯⎯⎯	The mucous membranes and tongue are dry with a fluid deficit. Sodium deficit causes the tongue to appear sticky, rough, and red. A dry tongue may also indicate mouth breathing. Some medications and vitamin deficiencies cause dryness of mucous membranes. Dryness in the oral cavity membranes (cheeks and gums) is a better indicator of fluid loss.
Sunken eyeballs and fontanels	Sunken eyeballs ⎯⎯⎯	Sunken eyes and dark skin around them can indicate a severe fluid volume deficit.
Bulging fontanels with soft eyeballs	Sunken fontanels ⎯⎯⎯	Depression of the anterior fontanel is often an indicator of fluid deficit. A fluid excess results in bulging fontanels.

Table 6-2. (Continued)		
Observation	**Nursing Assessment**	**Rationale/Interventions**
Absence of tearing and salivation	Absence of tearing _____ Decrease in saliva _____ Absence of saliva _____	Absence of tearing and salivation are indicators of fluid volume deficit. (Tearing does not begin until approximately 4 months of age). These symptoms occur with moderate dehydration (6–10% body weight loss).

Thirst	Thirst
	  Mild _____
	  Avid _____
		Thirst is an indicator of dehydration (fluid loss). Thirst may be difficult to determine when vomiting is present. If vomiting is present, offer flat carbonated fluid (Coca-Cola or ginger ale). Avid thirst may indicate serum hyperosmolality and cellular dehydration.

Change in urine output	Number of voidings _____
	Amount mL/8 h _____
	     mL/25 h _____
	Weight of saturated urine diaper is used to assess urine output in infants and toddlers (subtract dry diaper weight). _____
	Urine color
	Specific gravity
	  Low (≤1.010)
	  High (1.030)
	Urine pH
	  Acid
	  Alkaline
		Oliguria (decrease in urine output) with very concentrated urine (dark yellow color and ↑ specific gravity) can indicate a fluid volume deficit.
		With severe fluid deficit, the infant may not void for 16–24 h and not show evidence of abdominal distention. Polyuria (increased urine output) with low specific gravity (dilute) can indicate kidney damage, excess fluid intake, extracellular shift from interstitial fluid to plasma, or ↓ ADH. Oliguria can be due to renal insufficiency or extracellular shift from the plasma to the interstitial space. Potassium excess or sodium excess can result.

Table 6-2. (Continued)

Observation	Nursing Assessment		Rationale/Interventions
			Normal Range of Urine Output 6 months: 12 mL/h 1 year: 18–25 mL/h 5 years: 20–30 mL/h 12 years: 25–35 mL/h Adult: 35–50 mL/h *or* Newborn: 50 mL/kg/day All others: 25 mL/kg/day
Stools	Number Consistency Color Amount	_____ _____ _____ _____	The consistency, color, and amount of the stool should be noted. If the stool is of liquid consistency, it should be measured. Frequent, liquid stools can lead to fluid volume deficit, potassium and sodium deficit, and bicarbonate deficit (acidosis).
Vomitus	Number Consistency Color Amount	_____ _____ _____ _____	Vomitus needs to be described according to the amount, color, and consistency. Frequent vomiting of large quantity leads to fluid loss, potassium and sodium loss, and hydrogen and chloride loss (alkalosis). Vital signs should be taken every 15–30 min while the infant or child is seriously ill.
Vital Signs Body temperature changes	Admission temperature Time _____ (1) Time _____ (2)	_____ _____ _____	Fever increases insensible water loss. The child's extremities may feel cold because of hypovolemia (fluid volume deficit), which decreases peripheral circulation. A subnormal temperature may be due to reduced energy output.

Table 6-2.   (Continued)

Observation	Nursing Assessment			Rationale/Interventions

Changes in pulse	Admission pulse
	Pulse rate
	   Time ____
	   Time ____
	   Pattern
		
		(1)
		(2)
		
			____
			
			____
			____
			____
				A weak and rapid pulse rate (↑ 160 infant and ↑ 120 child) may indicate a fluid volume deficit (hypovolemia) and the possibility of shock. Full, bounding, not easily obliterated pulse may indicate a fluid volume excess. Irregular pulse can be due to hypokalemia. A weak, irregular rapid pulse may indicate hypokalemia, while a weak, slow pulse may indicate hypernatremia.

Changes in breathing	Admission rate
	Respiration
	   Time ____
	   Time ____
	   Pattern
		
		(1)
		(2)
		
			____
			
			____
			____
			____
				Note the rate, depth, and pattern of the infant's breathing. Dyspnea and moist rales usually indicate a fluid volume excess.
				Rapid breathing increases insensible fluid loss from the lungs.
				Rapid, deep, vigorous breathing (Kussmaul breathing) frequently indicates metabolic acidosis. Acidosis can be due to poor hydrogen excretion by the kidneys, diarrhea, salicylate poisoning, or diabetes mellitus. Shallow, irregular breathing can be due to respiratory alkalosis.

Blood pressure	Admission BP
	Blood pressure
	   Time ____
	   Time ____
		
		(1)
		(2)
			____
			
			____
			____
				Elasticity of young blood vessels may keep blood pressure stable even when a fluid volume deficit is present. Increased blood pressure may indicate fluid volume excess. Decreased blood pressure may indicate severe fluid volume deficit, extracellular shift from the plasma to the interstitial space, or sodium deficit.

Table 6-2. (Continued)

Observation	Nursing Assessment			Rationale/Interventions
Blood chemistry and hematology changes	*Electrolytes*	*Time*	*Time*	One set of blood chemistry is not sufficient for assessment. Electrolytes should be frequently monitored when they are not in normal range.
	K	⎯⎯	⎯⎯	
	Na	⎯⎯	⎯⎯	
	Cl	⎯⎯	⎯⎯	
	Ca	⎯⎯	⎯⎯	
	Mg	⎯⎯	⎯⎯	
	BUN	⎯⎯	⎯⎯	
	Creatinine	⎯⎯	⎯⎯	
	Hgb	⎯⎯	Hct ⎯⎯	

Norms are
Na: Infant   139–146 mEq/L
     Child   138–145 mEq/L
K: Infant   4.1–5.3 mEq/L
     Child   3.4–4.7 mEq/L
Ca: Infant   4.48–4.92 mEq/L
     Newborn 9.0–10.6 mg/dL
            2.3–2.65 mmol/L
     Child   8.8–10.8 mg/dL
            2.2–2.7 mmol/L
Cl: Infant   96–116 mEq/L
     Child   90–110 mEq/L
Mg: Infant   1.4–1.9 mg/dL
            2–4 days
     Child   1.4–1.7 mg/dL
            2–4 days

BUN if elevated can indicate fluid volume deficit or kidney insufficiency. Creatinine frequently indicates kidney damage.
Norms: BUN 10–25 mg/dL
Creatinine 0.7–1.4 mg/dL
Hgb 11.5–15.5 g/dL
Hct 35–45%
Elevated hemoglobin and hematocrit may indicate hemoconcentration caused by fluid volume deficit. If anemia is present, the hemoglobin and hematocrit may appear falsely normal.

Table 6-2.   (Continued)

Observation	Nursing Assessment		Rationale/Interventions
	Blood gases		Normal range for pH is 7.35–7.45. pH 7.35 and less indicate acidosis. pH 7.45 and higher indicate alkalosis.
	pH	_____	
	Paco$_2$	_____	
	Pao$_2$	_____	Normal range for Paco$_2$ is 35–45 mm Hg.
	HCO$_3$	_____	
	BE	_____	Paco$_2$ ↓ 35 means respiratory alkalosis or compensation (overbreathing-hyperventilating); Paco$_2$ ↑ 45 means respiratory acidosis (lung disorder). Normal range for HCO$_3$ is 24–28 mEq/L and BE −2 to +2. HCO$_3$ ↓ 24 and BE ↓ −2 metabolic acidosis (common in newborns). HCO$_3$ ↑ 28 and BE ↑ +2 metabolic alkalosis (occurs with vomiting—loss of HCl).
GI suction, drainage tubes, and fistula	GI suction		Fluid loss from all sources should be measured. Fluid loss from GI suctioning, drainage tubes, and fistula can contribute to severe fluid and electrolyte imbalances.
	Amount	_____	
	Drainage tube	_____	
	Amount	_____	
	Fistula	_____	
	Color	_____	
	Amount	_____	

■   ■   ■

28   Nursing assessment includes observing changes in behavior and general appearance. Irritability, lethargy, purposeless movement, a high-pitched or whining cry, and pallor or gray color may indicate which of the following:

( ) a. Fluid volume deficit
( ) b. Fluid volume excess
( ) c. Cellular fluid excess

a. X; b. —; c. —

■   ■   ■

29 Neurologic changes may indicate a fluid and electrolyte imbalance. Match the neurologic assessment on the left with the probable imbalance. (Refer to Chapter 3—potassium, calcium, and Chapter 5—dehydration and edema.) Some answers may be used more than once.

_____ 1. Abdominal distention		a. Potassium deficit
_____ 2. Confusion		b. Calcium deficit
_____ 3. Muscle weakness		c. Fluid volume excess
_____ 4. Tetany symptoms		d. Fluid volume deficit

1. a; 2. a, d; 3. a; 4. b. Good.

■   ■   ■

30 A weight loss of 12% is comparable to which of the following degrees of dehydration (fluid loss)?

( ) a. Mild dehydration
( ) b. Moderate dehydration
( ) c. Severe dehydration

a. —; b. —; c. X

■   ■   ■

31 Tissue (skin) turgor can be misleading as an indicator of fluid volume loss. Explain why.

*
_____

_____ .

Subcutaneous fat can give the appearance of normal skin turgor, or abdominal distention may mask poor skin turgor in heavy infants and toddlers.

■   ■   ■

32 Indicate in which areas of the body skin turgor should be checked.

( ) a. Face   ( ) d. Top of thighs
( ) b. Chest wall   ( ) e. Medial aspect of thighs
( ) c. Abdomen

a. —; b. X; c. X; d. —; e. X

■   ■   ■

33   To determine dryness of the mucous membrane, which part of the mouth should be assessed?

( ) a. Cheeks and gums of the oral cavity

( ) b. Teeth

a. X; b. —

■   ■   ■

34   Sunken eyeballs and fontanels frequently do not occur in infants until there is a 10% body weight loss (as fluid loss). Give the type of fluid imbalance that would be present with a 10% fluid loss. *_____ .

moderate to severe dehydration, or the upper range of moderate dehydration

■   ■   ■

35   Thirst and absence of tearing and salivation are indicators of fluid volume

_____ .

deficit

■   ■   ■

36   Normal specific gravity for a young infant is 1.002–1.010 and for a child is 1.005–1.030. If the child's urinary output is decreased and the specific gravity exceeds 1.030, the fluid imbalance is *_____ .

Usually neonates and young infants cannot concentrate urine even when hypovolemia is present.

fluid volume deficit or hypovolemia

■   ■   ■

37   Hyperkalemia (serum potassium excess) can result from (polyuria/oliguria)

_____ .

oliguria (↓ urine output)

■   ■   ■

38 Frequent and increased quantities of vomitus and stools can lead to which of the following:

( ) a. Hypokalemia
( ) b. Hyperkalemia
( ) c. Hyponatremia
( ) d. Hypernatremia
( ) e. Acidosis
( ) f. Alkalosis
( ) g. Dehydration

a. X; b. —; c. X; d. —; e. X (↑ stools due to loss of HCO₃); f. X (↑ vomitus due to loss of HCl); g. X

■   ■   ■

39 Vital signs should be monitored every _____ minutes for the seriously ill infant or child. Check which of the following vital signs can indicate fluid volume loss/deficit.

( ) a. Subnormal temperature
( ) b. Rapid, weak pulse
( ) c. Rapid respiration (Kussmaul)
( ) d. Fever
( ) e. Shallow breathing
( ) f. Systolic pressure below 80

15–30; a. — (in some cases it can indicate loss); b. X; c. X; d. X; e. —; f. X

■   ■   ■

40 An irregular pulse (dysrhythmia) can be caused by a (potassium deficit/potassium excess) *_____ .

A full bounding pulse can mean *_____ .

Why are blood pressure readings in infants and young children a poor indicator of fluid imbalance? *_____ .

potassium deficit; fluid volume excess
Firm elasticity of young blood vessels keeps blood pressure stable.

■   ■   ■

41 An elevated BUN (blood urea nitrogen) can indicate *_____
_____ , whereas an elevated serum creatinine indicates
*_____ .

dehydration (fluid volume deficit) or kidney insufficiency (renal damage); kidney damage

■   ■   ■

42 Arterial blood gases (ABGs) should be part of the assessment tool for assessing acid-base balance.

a. pH of 7.27 indicates *_____.

b. pH of 7.48 indicates *_____.

c. $Paco_2$ of 28 indicates *_____.

d. $Paco_2$ of 60 indicates *_____.

e. HCO_3 of 34 and BE of +8 indicates *_____.

f. HCO_3 of 18 and BE of −6 indicates *_____.

a. acidosis; b. alkalosis; c. hyperventilation due to respiratory alkalosis or compensation for metabolic acidosis; d. respiratory acidosis; e. metabolic alkalosis; f. metabolic acidosis

■   ■   ■

43 Name the fluid imbalance that can result from gastrointestinal suction and from secretions from drainage tubes and fistula. _____.

Name the two important electrolytes that are lost from gastrointestinal suctioning.
_____ and _____.

dehydration (fluid volume deficit); potassium and sodium (important electrolytes), also hydrogen, chloride, bicarbonate, and magnesium

■   ■   ■

44 From the following list of observations and nursing assessments, check the ones that indicate fluid volume deficit (hypovolemia or dehydration).

( ) a. BUN elevated

( ) b. Hemoglobin and hematocrit elevated

( ) c. Increased secretions from GI suction

( ) d. Increased blood pressure

( ) e. Irritability, high-pitched cry

( ) f. Confusion, disorientation

( ) g. Weight gain

( ) h. Decreased, concentrated urine

( ) i. Avid thirst

( ) j. Poor skin turgor

( ) k. Absence of tearing and salivation

( ) l. Sunken eyeballs and anterior fontanel

( ) m. Increased number and quantity of vomitus and stools

( ) n. Temperature 98.2° F or 36.8°C

( ) o. Rapid, weak pulse

( ) p. Rapid breathing

a. X; b. X; c. X; d. —; e. X; f. X; g —; h. X; i. X; j. X; k. X; l. X; m. X; n. —; o. X; p. X

45 Diarrheal dehydration is the number one cause of fluid and electrolyte imbalance in children. When vomiting with diarrhea occurs, fluid and electrolyte loss is more severe.

Other clinical problems causing fluid and electrolyte imbalance are surgery, pyloric stenosis, renal disease, diabetic ketoacidosis, gastroenteritis, and syndrome of inappropriate ADH (SIADH).

The most common cause of fluid and electrolyte imbalance is *_____ .

diarrheal dehydration

■　　　　　　　　　■　　　　　　　　　■

Table 6-3 gives the three degree categories of dehydration: mild, moderate, and severe, with clinical assessment factors. The table should help you identify the degree of dehydration according to clinical symptoms.

Table 6-3. DEGREES OF DEHYDRATION		
Degree	**Dehydration (%)**	**Clinical Observation**
Mild	5.6	Heart rate (10–15% above baseline) Slightly dry mucous membranes Concentrated urine Poor tear production*
Moderate	7.8	Increased severity of above Decreased skin turgor Oliguria Sunken eyeballs* Sunken anterior fontanels*
Severe	>9	Marked severity of above signs Decreased blood pressure Delayed capillary refill Acidosis (large base deficit)

* These signs may be less sensitive indicators of dehydration.
Source: From *The Harriet Lane Handbook: A Manual for Pediatric House Officers,* 12th ed. (p. 272) by M. G. Green, 1991, Baltimore: Mosby-Year Book, Inc. Copyright 1991 by Mosby-Year Book, Inc. Adapted by permission.

■　　　　　　　　　■　　　　　　　　　■

46 The degree of body fluid loss can be determined by the weight loss. However, the weight before illness must be known. Parents should be encouraged to keep an accurate record of the child's weight. Body weight loss in excess of 1% per day represents loss of body water.

To determine the degree of dehydration:

a. Convert pounds to kilograms (2.2 lb = 1 kg).
b. Subtract the present weight from the preillness (wellness) weight.
c. Divide the weight loss by the wellness weight.

Example: Mary weighed 30 pounds or 13.6 kg before she became ill. Now she weighs 26 pounds or 11.8 kg. She has lost 4 pounds or 1.8 kg.

$$1.8 \text{ kg} \div 13.6 \text{ kg} = 0.13 \text{ or } 13\%$$

The percentage of weight loss is _____ %. The degree of dehydration is (mild/moderate/severe) _____ .

(Refer to Table 6-2.)

13; severe

■   ■   ■

47 Indicate which symptoms are present during mild dehydration (1–6% in infants and children):

( ) a. Increased heart rate
( ) b. Decreased tear production
( ) c. Sunken eyeballs
( ) d. Confusion
( ) e. Increased concentration of urine
( ) f. Elevated specific gravity

a. X; b. X; c. —; d. —; e. X; f. X

■   ■   ■

48 Indicate which symptoms are present during moderate dehydration (7–8%) to severe dehydration (>9%) in infants and children.

( ) a. Increased heart rate
( ) b. Decreased tears
( ) c. Sunken fontanels
( ) d. Increased specific gravity
( ) e. Sunken eyeballs
( ) f. Decreased blood pressure
( ) g. Decreased skin turgor
( ) h. Oliguria
( ) i. Acidosis

All of the above.

■   ■   ■

49 With severe dehydration, ECF and ICF are lost. With a slow, progressive fluid loss, the ICF loss is equal to the ECF loss. As ECF loss occurs, ICF shifts into the ECF compartment (vessels and tissue spaces). What do you think occurs when dehydration develops rapidly?

*_____ .

ECF loss is greater than ICF loss. ICF cannot quickly replace ECF loss.

■   ■   ■

Table 6-4 estimates the percentage of ECF and ICF loss caused by a slow to rapid onset of dehydration. ECF is lost first. The ICF attempts to replace this loss. Once the onset and severity of fluid loss has been determined, you can calculate the percentage of fluid loss from the ECF and ICF compartments with the use of this table. Refer back to it as needed.

Table 6-4. EXTRACELLULAR AND INTRACELLULAR FLUID LOSS		
Onset of Dehydration	**ECF loss (%)**	**ICF loss (%)**
<3 days	44	25
3–7 days	60	40
>7 days	·50	50

50 When a child develops dehydration over a period of 5 days, the percentage of ECF loss is _____ and the percentage of ICF loss is _____ .

When dehydration occurs over a period of 2 weeks, the percentage of ECF loss is _____ and the percentage of ICF loss is _____ .

60%; 40%; 50%; 50%

■   ■   ■

51 Dehydration is classified according to the serum concentration of solutes (osmolality). Sodium is the primary contributor to the serum osmolality. Dehydration has three classifications in relation to osmolality and sodium concentration: (a) iso-osmolar dehydration (isonatremic dehydration); (b) hyperosmolar dehydration (hypernatremic dehydration); and (c) hypo-osmolar dehydration (hyponatremic dehydration).

Which type of dehydration has the highest osmolality (concentration)?

_____ .

hyperosmolar or hypernatremic dehydration

■   ■   ■

52 All degrees of dehydration are frequently associated with iso-osmolality or isonatremic dehydration. This is the most common type of dehydration, which results in proportionate losses of fluid and sodium.

   Hypernatremic dehydration and hyponatremic dehydration indicate involvement of the electrolyte _____ .

sodium

■   ■   ■

TYPES OF DEHYDRATION

Table 6-5 lists the three types of dehydration: isonatremic, hypernatremic, and hyponatremic. For each of the dehydrations, the water and sodium loss, serum sodium level, ECF and ICF loss, causes, symptoms, and treatments are described. Study the table carefully, and refer to it as needed.

53 With isonatremic dehydration, there is a proportionate loss of the ions _____ and _____ . The serum sodium level is between _____ and _____ . The ECF volume is (increased/decreased) _____ .

sodium and water; 130 and 150 mEq/L; decreased

■   ■   ■

54 Two common causes of isonatremic dehydration are _____ and _____ .

   With severe dehydration, shock symptoms are common. Give three shock symptoms.

   * _____ ,   * _____ , and * _____

diarrhea and vomiting, also malnutrition
rapid pulse rate, rapid respiration, and decreasing systolic blood pressure (others could be: gray skin color, lethargy)

■   ■   ■

55 With hypernatremic dehydration, which is lost to a greater degree: (water/sodium)? _____ . The serum sodium level is _____ mEq/L. ECF and ICF volumes are decreased. Which body fluid compartment has the largest fluid loss: (ECF/ICF)? _____ .

water; 150 ↑; ICF

■   ■   ■

Table 6-5. TYPES OF DEHYDRATION: ISONATREMIC, HYPERNATREMIC, AND HYPONATREMIC

Types of Dehydration	Water and Sodium Loss	Serum Sodium Level	ECF and ICF Loss	Causes	Symptoms	Treatment
Isonatremic dehydration (iso-osmolar or isotonic dehydration)	Proportionately equal loss of water and sodium	130–150 mEq/L	Extracellular fluid volume is markedly decreased (severe hypovolemia). Since sodium and water loss are approximately the same, there is no osmotic pull from ICF to ECF. The plasma volume is significantly reduced and shock occurs from decreased circulating blood volume. ICF volume remains virtually constant.	Diarrhea, vomiting, and malnutrition (decrease in fluid and food intake) are the most common causes.	With severe fluid loss, symptoms are characteristic of hypovolemic shock: rapid pulse rate, rapid respiration; and later, a decreasing systolic blood pressure. Other symptoms are weight loss, irritability, lethargy, pale or gray skin color, dry mucous membranes, reduced skin turgor, sunken eyeballs, sunken fontanels, absence of tearing and salivation, and decreased urine output.	Fluid should be restored rapidly to correct hypovolemic shock. Iso-osmolar solutions, i.e., Ringer's lactate and 5% dextrose in 0.2% NaCl or 0.3% NaCl are some of the choices. Replacement should be calculated over 24 h; if dehydration is severe, half the amount of solution should be given the first 8 h and the remaining half over the next 16 h.
Hypernatremic dehydration (hyperosmolar or hypertonic dehydration) (second leading type of dehydration in children)	Water loss is greater than sodium loss; sodium excess	↑ 150 mEq/L	ECF and ICF volumes are both decreased. Increased ECF osmolality (solutes) results in a shift of fluid from the ICF to the ECF causing severe cellular dehydration. ECF depletion may not be as severe as	Severe diarrhea (water is lost in excess to solutes) and high solute intake with decreased water intake are the two most common causes. Others include fever, poor renal function, rapid breathing, or any	Shock is less apparent since ECF loss is not as severe. Symptoms include weight loss, avid thirst, confusion, convulsions, tremors, thickened and firm skin turgor, sunken eyeballs and fontanels, absence	The goal is to increase the ICF and ECF volumes without causing water intoxication. Giving excessive hypo-osmolar solutions or only 5% dextrose in water would dilute ECF, causing water to shift to the ICF and water intoxication (ICF volume excess) to occur. A gradual

Table 6-5. (Continued)

Types of Dehydration	Water and Sodium Loss	Serum Sodium Level	ECF and ICF Loss	Causes	Symptoms	Treatment
			ICF depletion. Loss of hypo-osmolar fluid raises the osmolality of ECF.	combination of these conditions.	of tearing, moderately rapid pulse, moderately rapid respirations, frequently normal blood pressure, normal to decreased urine output, and intracranial hemorrhage.	reduction over 48 h of solution is safest. Dextrose 5% with 0.2% NaCl may be ordered and later lactated Ringer's solution. With normal urinary flow, potassium can be added to the solution (2–3 mEq/kg).
Hyponatremic dehydration (hypo-osmolar or hypotonic dehydration)	Sodium loss is greater than water loss; excess water	↓ 130 mEq/L	ECF is severely decreased, and ICF is increased. The osmolality of ECF is lower than the osmolality of ICF. Water shifts from the ECF to the ICF (lesser to the greater concentration). The cerebral cells are frequently affected first as the excess water interferes with brain cell activity.	Severe diarrhea (sodium is lost in excess of water), excessive water intake, electrolyte-free fluid infusions (5% dextrose in water), sodium-losing nephropathy, and diuretic therapy.	Thirst, weight loss, lethargy, comatose, poor skin turgor, clammy skin, sunken and soft eyeballs, absence of tearing, shock symptoms (rapid pulse rate, rapid respirations, and low systolic blood pressure), and decreased urine output.	Ringer's lactate or 5% dextrose in 0.45% NaCl (½ NSS) can help to correct the serum sodium level (125–135 mEq/L). For serum sodium of 15 mEq/L, normal saline can be used. For a serum sodium of 15 mEq/L or less, 3% saline may be indicated. Rapid fluid correction with electrolytes can cause an excessive shift of cellular fluid into the plasma. The result can be overhydration and congestive heart failure.

56 Give two causes of hypernatremic dehydration. *_____ , and
*_____ .

   Shock symptoms (are/are not) _____ common with this type of
dehydration.
   Check the symptoms found with hypernatremic dehydration:

( ) a. Avid thirst   ( ) d. Skin turgor firm and thickened
( ) b. Convulsions   ( ) e. Absence of tearing
( ) c. Tremors   ( ) f. Excess urine output

severe diarrhea and high solute intake; are not

a. X; b. X; c. X; d. X; e. X; f. —

                ■   ■   ■

57 With hyponatremic dehydration, the loss of _____ is greater than the loss of
_____ . The serum sodium level is _____ mEq/L. ECF is
(increased/decreased) _____ and ICF is (increased/decreased)
_____ .

sodium; water; 130; decreased; increased

                ■   ■   ■

58 Give three causes of hyponatremic dehydration. *_____ ,
*_____ , and *_____ .

   Check the symptoms found with hyponatremic dehydration:

( ) a. Thirst   ( ) e. Sunken, soft eyeballs
( ) b. Weight gain   ( ) f. Rapid pulse rate
( ) c. Poor skin turgor   ( ) g. Rapid respiration
( ) d. Clammy skin   ( ) h. Low systolic blood pressure

severe diarrhea, excessive water intake, and electrolyte-free fluid infusions
(others—sodium-losing nephropathy and diuretic therapy)

a. X; b. —;   c. X; d. X;   e. X; f. X; g. X; h. X

                ■   ■   ■

59 With hypovolemic shock, fluids should be restored (slowly/rapidly) _____ .
Replacement of fluids should be calculated over 24 hours, and if dehydration is severe, half is frequently administered in _____ hours and the second half in _____ hours.

What type of fluid imbalance can occur if intravenous fluids are given too rapidly?
*_____ .

rapidly; 8; 16; overhydration or pulmonary edema (CHF)

∎   ∎   ∎

60 The goal for correcting hypernatremic dehydration is to avoid causing what major type of fluid imbalance? *_____ .

What electrolytes should be replaced when correcting hypernatremic dehydration?
_____ and *_____ .

If the serum sodium level is below 115 mEq/L, what type of intravenous fluid may be indicated? *_____ .

water intoxication; calcium and later potassium with normal kidney function; 3% saline

∎   ∎   ∎

Oral rehydration is often the treatment of choice for children with mild to moderate dehydration. Examples of oral solutions used for rehydration include WHO solution, Hydra-Lyte, Rehydralyte, Pedialyte, Lytren, Resol, and Infalyte. These solutions contain similar concentrations of glucose, sodium, potassium, chloride, and bicarbonate or citrate.

Oral rehydration solutions are given in small amounts of 5–10 mL every 5–10 minutes and increased as tolerated. Administering these solutions with a teaspoon or an oral syringe may help to monitor the amounts more accurately. If the child is vomiting, then the amount given should be decreased. With severe vomiting, the solution should be discontinued.

Initially, severe dehydration is treated by intravenous replacement therapy. Oral replacement is initiated again, after the child's condition is stabilized.

Once the child is able to retain the solution, the child's diet is advanced and a maintenance schedule for replacement therapy is prescribed. Breast-fed infants are given 100 mL/kg of rehydration solution to supplement their breast milk feedings. Formula-fed infants are usually started on half-strength formula. The amount of formula given is 100–150 mL/kg over a 24-hour period. Formula is alternated with equal volumes of a rehydration solution.

When children are advanced to a regular diet, 100 mL/kg of a rehydration solution is given as a supplement to the diet. While rehydration solutions are being given, fluids high in carbohydrates or sodium content should be avoided. If children continue to have diarrhea, 4–8 ounces of a rehydration solution should be given for each diarrhea stool.

61 The treatment of choice for many children with mild to moderate dehydration is
*_____ . Identify five solutions that might be used for oral rehydration.

*_____ , _____ , _____ ,

_____ , and _____ .

These solutions contain similar concentrations of glucose and important electrolytes such as

_____ , _____ , _____ , and

*_____ .

oral rehydration
WHO solution, Hydra-Lyte, Rehydralyte, Lytren, Resol, and Infalyte
sodium, potassium, chloride, and bicarbonate of soda

■   ■   ■

62 While severe dehydration is treated with *_____ , after the fluid imbalance and
electrolytes have stabilized, *_____ is initiated.

intravenous therapy; oral replacement therapy

■   ■   ■

63 While children are being given rehydration therapy, fluids high in _____
should be avoided.

carbohydrates

■   ■   ■

64 Breast-fed infants on rehydration therapy are usually given *_____ of
rehydration solution to supplement breast milk feedings.

Formula fed-infants on rehydration therapy are usually given *_____
formula in the amount of *_____ over a 24-hour period. Formula is
_____ with _____ volumes of an *_____
solution such as *_____ .

100 mL/kg; half-strength; 100–150 mL/kg; alternated; equal; oral rehydration
WHO solution, Hydra-Lyte, Rehydralyte, Lytren, Resol, Pedialyte, or Infalyte

■   ■   ■

CASE STUDY REVIEW

Susan, age 4, has had diarrhea and anorexia for 3 days. She has taken only sips of fruit juices for
the last 3 days. She weighed 38 pounds or 17.3 kg preillness and now weighs 35 pounds or 15.9
kg. Her cheeks and gums are dry and her skin turgor is reduced. She is irritable. Susan has voided
once in the last 24 hours. Vital signs: temperature 99°F or 37.2°C, pulse rate 110, respirations 32,
BP 90/60. Blood was drawn for serum electrolytes and BUN.

1. Because of diarrhea, anorexia, decreased fluid intake, and weight loss, the nurse would assume the fluid imbalance to be which of the following:
   ( ) a. Intracellular fluid volume excess (water intoxication)
   ( ) b. Extracellular fluid volume excess (edema or overhydration)
   ( ) c. Extracellular fluid volume deficit (dehydration)

2. In kilograms, Susan has lost _____ kg. What degree of dehydration is present? _____ . (Refer to Table 6-3 if needed.) The severity of her dehydration is (mild/moderate/severe) _____ .

3. The onset of fluid loss (dehydration) has been _____ days. Give the percentage of fluid loss from the ECF _____ and the ICF _____ . (Refer to Table 6-4 if needed.)

4. List Susan's signs and symptoms of dehydration from your nursing assessment.
   * _____ , * _____ ,
   _____ , * _____ ,
   and * _____ .

5. Is Susan's blood pressure indicative of shock? _____ .
   Explain. * _____ .

6. The ranges of serum electrolytes for children are:
   a. K   * _____
   b. Na * _____
   c. Cl * _____
   d. Ca * _____
   (Refer to Frames 11, 17, 20, 21, or to Table 6-2.)

7. The nurse would expect Susan's serum potassium to be (increased/decreased) _____ , serum sodium to be (increased/decreased) _____ , serum chloride to be (increased/decreased) _____ , and serum calcium to be (increased/decreased) _____ .

8. Give some signs and symptoms of hypokalemia. * _____
   _____ .

9. With a serum calcium level of 8.4 mg/dL, the nurse should be observing for symptoms of _____ . Give two of the symptoms. (Refer to Frame 23 if needed.)
   * _____ and * _____ .

10. Susan's BUN is (increased/decreased) _____ . The most likely cause of her BUN is _____ . Explain. * _____ .

11. Susan's preillness weight is 38 pounds or 17.3 kg. Calculate Susan's daily fluid requirements. _____ mL per 24 hours. (Refer to Table 6-1 if needed.)
    Her daily sodium requirement is _____ mEq/L and her daily potassium requirement is _____ mEq/L. (Refer to Table 6-1 as needed.)

12. Susan's type of dehydration according to her serum sodium level is (isonatremic/hypernatremic/hyponatremic). _____ . Why? * _____
    _____ .

13. For the type of dehydration in question 12, fluids should be replaced (slowly/rapidly) _____ .

14. Name three shock symptoms that can occur.
    * _____ , * _____ , and * _____

15. Identify Susan's vital signs that are indicative of impending shock due to hypovolemia (fluid volume loss). *_____ and *_____ .

16. With moderate dehydration, the changes in the urine output and concentration are (refer to Table 6-3 if needed):

Urine volume _____

Urine osmolality _____ mOsm/L

Urine specific gravity _____

■   ■   ■

1. c
2. 1.4; 8%; moderate
3. 3; 60%; 40%
4. cheeks and gums dry, reduced skin turgor, irritable, voided once (decreased urine output), and pulse rate and respiration increased
5. No. Blood pressure for that age group is normal; however, a baseline blood pressure from an office visit would be helpful.
6. a. 3.4–4.7 mEq/L; b. 138–145 mEq/L; c. 90–110 mEq/L; d. 2.2–2.7 mmol/L or 8.8–10.8 mg/dL
7. decreased; decreased; decreased; decreased
8. dizziness, soft muscles, abdominal distention, decreased peristalsis, dysrhythmia, and decreased BP
9. tetany; tingling of fingers and twitching of mouth (others—tremors and carpopedal spasms)
10. increased; dehydration
    With a decreased urine output, there is an increase in serum solutes such as urea (due to hemoconcentration).
11. 1365; 40.8 or 41; 27.2 or 27
12. isonatremic
    The serum sodium level for isonatremic is 130–150 mEq/L.
13. rapidly
14. rapid pulse rate, rapid respiration, and decreasing blood pressure (others—clammy skin, pale or gray color)
15. P 110 (rapid pulse rate) and R 32 (rapid respiration). Baseline vital signs would be helpful.
16. oliguria or decreased; 800; 1.030+

NURSING ASSESSMENT FACTORS

- Early detection of pertinent symptoms and prompt therapeutic management of fluid and electrolyte disturbances are critical in the care of infants and children. Fluid balance in infants and children is so precarious that life-threatening changes can occur rapidly with little symptomatic warning. Conditions that promote fluid imbalances in infants and children include vomiting, diarrhea, sweating, fever, burns, injury, and diseases such as diabetes, renal disease, and cardiac anomalies. A thorough nursing assessment integrates the infant's/child's health history obtained from the parents with data from the physical examination and laboratory tests.

- Knowledge requirements and basic assessment techniques vary for infants and children. Understanding the implications of variations in laboratory studies, total body fluid volume, and developmental differences that influence the responses of infants and children to fluid problems provides the nurse with a basis for data comparison. Assessment begins with observations of the infant's/child's general appearance and behavioral changes. Knowing baseline data from the infant's/child's health history is important to the nursing assessment and interpretation of the findings.
- Monitor vital signs according to the severity of the illness. A baseline reading of the infant's or child's vital signs is important to the interpretation of changes. Seriously ill infants and children need their vital signs monitored every 15 minutes. An elevated temperature can occur with early fluid depletion and can indicate a fluid deficit. An elevated or a subnormal temperature can indicate dehydration. Blood pressure is not a reliable sign of fluid imbalance in young children. A rapid, weak, thready pulse is a symptom of shock. A bounding, not easily obliterated pulse occurs with fluid volume excess when the interstitial fluid shifts to the plasma. A bounding, easily obliterated pulse may indicate an impending circulatory collapse and a sodium deficit. The overall cardiac status reflects changes in levels of important electrolytes. A potassium imbalance is life threatening in a child.
- Dyspnea and moist rales can occur with a fluid volume excess. Respiratory stridor may indicate a calcium deficit. Assess skin and mucous membranes; the skin is usually pale during a fluid deficit and flushed during a fluid excess. The extremities often become cold and mottled with the presence of a fever and a severe fluid volume deficit. Skin elasticity can be assessed by pinching the skin on the abdomen or inner thigh (dent test). In fluid depletion the skin remains raised for several seconds. The skin may feel dry or cold and clammy in sodium deficits (hypotonic dehydration). Fluid deficits cause the mucous membranes of the mouth to become dry. The tongue is observed to have longitudinal wrinkles. A sodium excess (hyperosmolar dehydration) causes a sticky, rough, red, dry tongue.
- Tears and salivation are decreased to absent in fluid volume deficits of infants and children. Fluid volume deficits cause the fontanels and eyeballs to appear soft and sunken. Contrarily, in fluid excess the fontanels bulge and feel taut.
- Tingling fingers and toes, abdominal cramps, muscle cramps, lightheadedness, nausea, and thirst are important symptoms of electrolyte imbalances in infants and children. Other sensory and neurologic signs may include hypotonia and flaccid paralysis indicative of a potassium deficit. Hypertonia is evidenced as a positive Chvostek sign, tremors, cramps, or tetany, which are indicative of a calcium deficit. A magnesium deficit causes twitching.
- Knowing the variations in serum electrolyte ranges for infants and children can help prevent complications of electrolyte imbalances of sodium, potassium, chloride, calcium, and magnesium (see Table 6-2 for serum electrolyte norms).
- Even small weight changes are crucial in fluid balance problems of infants and children. Rapid loss or gain in weight indicates fluid deficits and fluid excesses in the fluid regulation process.
- The normal output for an infant is 2 mL/kg per hour and for the child it is 1–2 mL/kg per hour. Immature kidneys limit the child's ability to concentrate urine. Urine should be monitored for specific gravity and acidity. A specific gravity of less than 1.010 is low and indicates a fluid excess. A specific gravity of 1.030 is high and may indicate a fluid deficit with a sodium excess. An elevated specific gravity is usually accompanied by glycosuria and proteinuria. The specific gravity of infants and children can be used to monitor their hydration level. Fixed low specific gravity readings indicate renal disease.

NURSING DIAGNOSIS 1

Fluid volume deficit, related to decreased fluid reserve.

NURSING INTERVENTIONS AND RATIONALE

1. Identify source of fluid deficit. Fluid deficits result from a decreased fluid intake or an abnormal fluid loss in conditions such as diabetes insipidus, adrenocortical insufficiency, vomiting, diarrhea, hemorrhage, burns, and diabetes mellitus. Fluid deficits in infants and children are accentuated by three factors associated with their immaturity: (a) their proportionately high body surface area; (b) their high rate of metabolism; and (c) their immature renal structures. All of these factors limit the infant's ability to conserve fluid and compensate for fluid deficits.
2. Monitor laboratory values for selected electrolytes (Na, Cl, K, Ca). Recognize differences between the normal values of infants and children and the normal values of adults (see Table 6-2). Report even small changes in laboratory values. The increased vulnerability of infants and children to fluid deficits are not easily detected in observable signs and symptoms. Recognize specific symptoms of electrolyte deficits or excess as outlined in Table 6-2.
3. Closely assess changes in general appearance and neurologic and behavioral signs. Lethargy with hyperirritability on stimulation is an early sign of fluid volume deficits (see Table 6-2). Dry mucous membranes are often the first symptom of fluid deficits. Sunken fontanels are an indication of a fluid volume deficit in an infant.
4. Monitor weight daily. Amount of weight loss is a key assessment factor for determining the severity of the fluid deficit. Knowledge of weight in kilograms is essential to determine the degree of dehydration and calculate the fluid replacement needs (see Table 6-1) of infants and children.
5. Monitor vital signs. A baseline value of the infant or child's normal vital signs is important in determining the degree of the fluid deficit and assessing for hypovolemic shock (see Table 6-2). Check physician's records or ask the parents for the normal values of the child or infant.
6. Measure intake and output. The immature development of the renal structures in infants and children limits the kidney's ability to concentrate urine and increases the infant's risk for dehydration. A balance in intake and output is important in restoring fluid balance.
7. Integrate observations to determine the type (iso-osmolar, hypo-osmolar, or hyperosmolar) and degree of dehydration (mild, moderate, or severe; see Table 6-3). Knowledge of the type and degree of dehydration assists the nurse in identifying the ratio of ICF volume and ECF volume. This information is important in the proper selection of fluids and the regulation of the rate and volume of fluid replacement (see Table 6-5).

NURSING DIAGNOSIS 2

Fluid volume excess, related to inadequate excretion of fluid or alteration of fluid volume regulation.

NURSING INTERVENTIONS

1. Monitor intake and output. The ingestion or infusion of excessive amounts of fluid in infants can result in reduced sodium levels and CNS symptoms. Specific gravity measurements are used to assess urine concentration (see Table 6-2). The kidney's reduced ability to concentrate urine results in an excessive, diluted urine output. The child's urine output should be at least 1–2 mL/kg per hour (as outlined in Table 6-2).

2. Assess neurologic symptoms. Neurologic symptoms of a fluid overload include lethargy, irritability, headache, and/or generalized seizures. These symptoms result because water moves into the brain more rapidly than sodium moves out.
3. Identify source of fluid overload. Sources of fluid overload in infants and children include overload from rapid infusion of IV fluids, excessive fluid replacement with hypotonic solutions, excessive oral replacement after hypotonic fluids (over diluted formulas, too much water), rapid dialysis, tap water enemas, or a rapid reduction of the glucose level often observed in ketoacidosis.
4. Assess for edema. Infants and young children who look well hydrated may have edema. In the very young edema may be localized to a small or large area. Immaturity of the kidneys and inadequate hormone production may predispose infants and children to fluid imbalances that can result in edema.

NURSING DIAGNOSIS 3

Bowel elimination: altered (diarrhea), related to irritable bowel.

NURSING INTERVENTIONS

1. Identify causative factors. Compare and contrast dietary intake 24 hours prior to diarrhea with normal dietary patterns. Assess for the possibility of allergies, contaminated foods, dietary indiscretions, bacterial or viral infections, or malabsorption problems. Often the cause is unknown; whenever possible, eliminate causative factors.
2. Reduce diarrhea. Often the best treatment is providing an opportunity for the bowel to rest. In infants and young children this may mean discontinuing solid foods, formula, and/or milk products. Switching to clear or less irritating fluids may provide the relief the bowel needs. In severe cases, fluids may be completely eliminated until the bowel recovers. Rendering an infant or child NPO requires alternate methods of fluid replacement to maintain fluid and electrolyte balance.
3. Assess stools for frequency and consistency. Liquid/diarrhea-like stools contain significant fluid content and must be measured in infants and children to determine their fluid balance status. Compare frequency and consistency of bowel movements to the infant's normal stooling pattern.
4. Monitor vital signs and weight changes. Determine extent of fluid and electrolyte imbalance based on changes in these assessment factors.
5. Educate parents about signs and symptoms of fluid imbalance. Early treatment of fluid problems is essential to prevent life-threatening complications. Parental knowledge of symptoms allows for early treatment.
6. Educate parents regarding nutritional treatment regimes for diarrhea. The sequence of clear liquids, liquids, and soft food is essential to providing the bowel with the period of rest often needed for restoration of normal bowel functions and fluid and electrolyte balance.

NURSING DIAGNOSIS 4

Nutrition: altered, less than body requirements, related to anorexia secondary to (altered level of consciousness, vomiting, diarrhea, and nausea).

NURSING INTERVENTIONS

1. Identify cause of nutritional deficit. Diarrhea and vomiting are the most common causes of fluid and electrolyte problems in infants and children. These conditions prevent the absorption of adequate nutrients and threaten the precarious fluid balance of infants and young children.
2. Initiate oral nutrition as soon as appropriate. Solid foods and milk products are irritating to the bowel and should be avoided with the initial return to food. Foods containing fiber often cause the bowel to expand and stimulate peristalsis. These foods should also be avoided. The reintroduction of foods usually begins with soft foods. A BRAT (bananas, rice, applesauce, toast) diet is usually recommended for children recovering from diarrhea. Knowledge of the nutritional requirements of various age groups is essential to adequate nutritional replacement. Changes in metabolic needs are affected by physical status and pathophysiologic conditions.
3. Monitor weight. Weight gains or losses are indicative of nutritional status and fluid balance. Small gains or losses are significant in infants and children.

NURSING DIAGNOSIS 5

Tissue integrity: impaired, related to the effects of chemical destruction or tissue deficits, secondary to fluid and electrolyte imbalances (diarrhea, edema).

NURSING INTERVENTIONS

1. Identify risk factors for threats to tissue integrity. Tissue destruction can occur from chemical irritants or mechanical destruction. Conditions such as diarrhea, excessive or unusual secretions, urinary incontinence and edema increase the tissue's vulnerability to destruction. Proper identification and treatment of risk factors reduces the infant's vulnerability to these risks. Since maturity factors in infants and children reduce their ability to adapt, early identification and treatment of risk factors can prevent major complications.
2. Eliminate or reduce causative factors. Diarrhea and edema are symptoms that require early interventions to reduce the risk of tissue destruction.
3. Assess nutritional status. Nutritional status affects the tissue's vulnerability to breakdown. Inadequate protein consumption reduces healing power and increases tissue vulnerability. Vitamins and minerals are also important to the health of body tissues. In fluid imbalance conditions, one's nutritional state is often compromised.
4. Promote mobility as tolerated. Many fluid imbalance problems promote lethargy and immobility. Since adequate circulation is essential to tissue nutrition and oxygenation, frequent position changes and movement promote circulation and reduce the risk of tissue breakdown. Reposition infants carefully to reduce risks related to mechanical destruction of tissues.

NURSING DIAGNOSIS 6

Skin integrity: altered, related to immobility, pressure, friction, or maceration.

NURSING INTERVENTIONS

1. Nursing interventions for skin integrity are much the same as interventions for tissue integrity (see interventions for tissue integrity).

2. Keep skin clean and dry. The child with poor skin turgor related to a fluid deficit is managed in the same manner as a child with edema. Mild (petroleum-based) creams or ointments may be applied to improve comfort on movement and reduce destruction from friction. Gentle massage increases circulation and prevents breakdown.

Other nursing diagnoses and selected nursing interventions to consider when assessing fluid balance problems in infants and children include the following:

1. Oral mucous membranes altered, related to fluid deficit (dehydration):

- Apply a thin layer of a water-soluble ointment to the lips to prevent cracking (glycerin and lemon swabs have a drying effect and should be avoided).
- Rinse mouth with water or warm saline (do not allow swallowing if oral fluids are restricted).
- Clean teeth and gums with a soft sponge. Dryness may cause inflammation, bleeding, or lesions that need interventions to promote comfort and reduce complications.
- Instruct parents to provide these interventions in situations when child is too young or unable to care for self. Maintenance of moist, adequately perfused mucous membranes is important in fluid balance problems.

2. Urinary elimination: altered patterns related to kidney function is considered a collaborative problem addressed by the nurse and the physician to determine appropriate treatment:

- Monitor intake and output. Toilet-trained children and independent older children may not understand the importance of measuring intake and urinary output. This independence may pose a threat to accurate monitoring of intake and output. Altered urine output may indicate dysfunctions such as inadequate blood volume regulatory mechanisms of aldosterone and ADH; excessive fluid intake, or marked fluid loss (hemorrhage, GI bleeding). Monitor urine for presence of protein or glucose and measure its pH level. The preferred method of measuring urine output in diapered infants and children is simply to compare the dry and wet weight of the diaper. (Weight in grams corresponds to volume voided.) Urine can be aspirated from cloth diapers to obtain urine for specific gravity measurements.
- Monitor kidney function for early signs of renal insufficiency. The specific gravity of urine, sufficient amounts of output (30 mL per hour), BUN, serum creatinine, potassium, phosphorus, ammonia, and creatinine clearance times are important in the diagnosis of renal insufficiency.

3. Sensory-perceptual alterations related to metabolic changes secondary to fluid and electrolyte imbalance (acidosis):

- Identify sensory-perceptual alterations. Children can experience different sensory-perceptual alterations depending upon the type of fluid and electrolyte imbalance. Fluid deficits promote irritability and lethargy while fluid shifts that cause cerebral edema may cause irritability and restlessness. Complaints of headaches and nausea with episodes of vomiting are not uncommon. Severe cerebral edema can cause convulsions. Selected electrolyte imbalances result in dizziness, muscle cramping or twitching, and tingling of the fingers and toes.
- Monitor blood values. To identify electrolyte imbalances, an elevated BUN or serum creatinine can alter sensory-perceptual experiences.
- Maintain a cool, quiet environment. To reduce unnecessary stimulation, interventions should be organized in a manner that allows for uninterrupted rest periods. The nurse must prevent unnecessary interruptions during these quiet times.

4. Knowledge deficit (parental) related to detection, care, and treatment of fluid and electrolyte imbalance:

- Teach parents basic fluid balance principles. Knowledge of basic principles of fluid and electrolyte balance can alert parents to symptoms of fluid overload and fluid deficits for early detection of potential complications.
- Involve parents in the infant's/child's care as much as possible. Promoting trust by involving parents enhances treatment and reduces unnecessary anxiety of parents during the infant's/child's illness.
- Teach basic fluid replacement strategies. Many hospitalizations or complications from fluid problems can be prevented by early detection and appropriate fluid replacement strategies initiated at home by alert parents.

CHAPTER 7

FLUID PROBLEMS OF THE AGING ADULT

Behavioral Objectives

Upon completion of this chapter, you will be prepared to:

- Describe structural and functional changes that occur with normal aging of the respiratory, renal, cardiac, integumentary, and gastrointestinal system.
- Discuss the effects of normal aging (on the respiratory, renal, cardiac, integumentary, and gastrointestinal system) that have implications for fluid and electrolyte balance.
- List risk factors, especially chronic diseases, which may cause fluid and electrolyte problems for the older adult.
- Identify six common body fluid problems experienced by the aging adult.
- Assess normal physiologic changes in the aging client as they relate to the signs and symptoms of fluid problems in the aging adult.
- Identify appropriate nursing interventions for aging clients experiencing fluid and electrolyte imbalances.

PHYSIOLOGIC CHANGES

Structural and functional changes which occur as a result of the aging process are usually measured in terms of the body's ability to adapt. Additional risk factors such as chronic diseases increase the debilitating effects of normal functional changes in all of the body's systems and further inhibit the aging client's ability to maintain fluid and electrolyte balance. Nursing assessments provide information about age-related changes and additional factors which may place older adults at risk for fluid and electrolyte imbalances. Miller (1990) proposed the Functional Consequences Model of Gerontological Nursing (Figure 7-1) to show how age-related changes and risk factors may combine to cause negative functional consequences. Appropriate nursing interventions, however, can foster positive functional consequences and decrease the debilitating effects of risk factors.

Table 7-1 lists (a) age-related structural and functional changes in five major body systems, (b) additional risk factors for fluid and electrolyte imbalance, (c) functional changes resulting from age-related changes and additional risk factors, and (d) nursing interventions to foster positive functional outcomes. Study the table and be able to state the specific changes, risk factors, and nursing interventions for changes in each system. Refer to the table as needed.

Figure 7-1. Functional consequences model of gerontological nursing. (Adapted by permission from C. Miller. (1990). *Nursing care of older adults*. Philadelphia, Pa: J. B. Lippincott Co., p. 53).

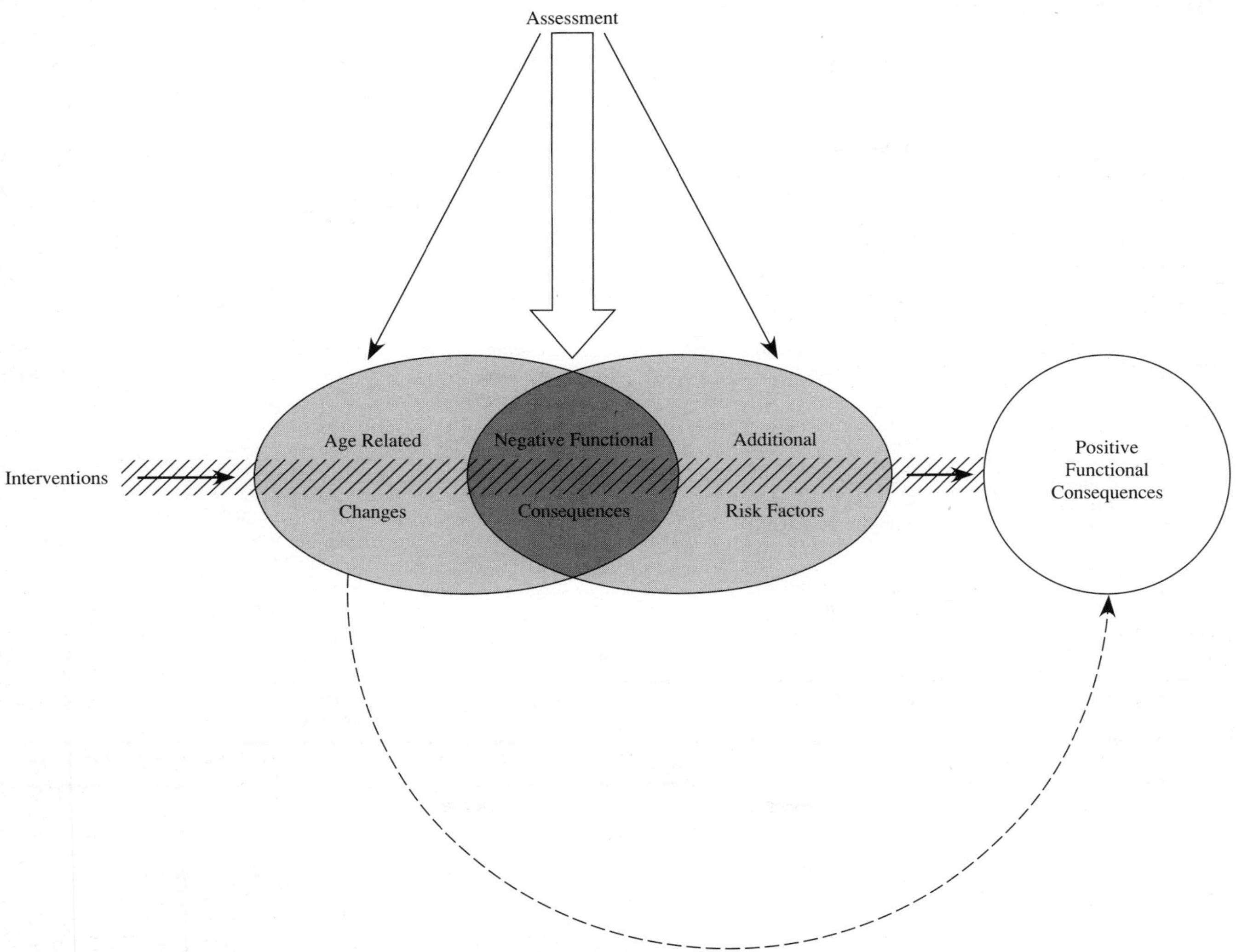

Table 7-1. MAJOR STRUCTURAL CHANGES, RISK FACTORS, AND FUNCTIONAL OUTCOMES IN OLDER ADULTS

Body System	Structural Changes	Additional Risk Factors	Functional Outcomes	Nursing Interventions
Pulmonary function decreased	Loss of elasticity of parenchymal lung tissue Increased rigidity of chest wall Fewer alveoli Decreased strength of expiratory muscles	Chronic diseases Emphysema Asthma Chronic bronchitis Bronchiectasis Tobacco smoking Exposure to air pollutants Occupational exposure to toxic substances	Defective alveolar ventilation Accumulation of bronchial secretions Increased CO_2 retention Increased difficulty in regulating pH	Increase breathing capacity to enhance the elimination of CO_2 by: 1. Breathing exercises with prolonged expiration 2. Coughing after a few deep breaths 3. Frequent position changes 4. Chest clapping 5. Intermittent positive pressure breathing (IPPB)
Renal function decreased	Persistent renal vasoconstriction resulting from arteriosclerotic changes Decrease in number of functioning nephrons (begins by age 40) 30–50% less by age 70	Medications (e.g., diuretics) Genitourinary diseases (e.g., infections, obstructions)	Reduced glomerular filtration Impaired ability to excrete water and solutes causing: 1. A decrease in H^+ excretion; thus metabolic acidosis can occur 2. Reduced ability to concentrate urine 3. Increased accumulation of waste products in body 4. Decreased ability to excrete drugs	Assess adaptive capacity and maintain optimal renal function by: 1. Checking fluid intake and output balance 2. Encouraging fluid intake as appropriate 3. Checking acid-base balance according to serum CO_2 or HCO_3 4. Testing specific gravity to determine kidneys' ability to concentrate urine 5. Noting drugs that may be toxic to renal function 6. Observing for side effects from drug accumulation 7. Observing for desired effects of drugs

Circulation and cardiac function decreased	Increased rigidity of arterial walls (arteriosclerosis) Decreased elasticity of blood vessels Diminished strength of cardiac contractions Decreased cardiac output and stroke volume	Obesity Cigarette smoking dietary habits that contribute to hyperlipidemia Inactivity	Increased blood pressure Stasis of blood causing back pressure on capillaries, which in turn, causes fluid to move into tissue areas causing edema Decreased cardiac output and decreased blood flow Decreased cardiac reserve (capacity of heart to respond to increased burden) slows the adaptive functions as evidenced by: 1. Heart rate same as young adults except under stress takes longer to return to normal 2. Increased incidence of edema and congestive heart failure	Assess adaptive capacity of heart and maintain circulation and cardiac function by: 1. Checking blood pressure for elevations resulting from arteriosclerotic changes 2. Determining blood flow by checking peripheral pulses 3. Checking lungs and dependent extremities for edema from increased capillary pressure 4. Checking pulse rates (apical and radial) and character to determine heart contraction, cardiac output, and pulse deficit 5. Noting changes in heart rate following activity 6. Assessing chest sounds for moist rales
Gastrointestinal function decreased	Atrophy of gastric mucosa Muscular atrophy and loss of supportive structures in small and large intestines Decreased volume of saliva	Alcohol or medications Psychosocial factors (e.g., isolation, depression) Factors that interfere with ability to obtain, prepare, consume, or enjoy food and fluids (e.g., immobility, mental impairment)	Decrease in gastric secretions, especially HCl Metabolic alkalosis related to decreased HCl Atrophic gastritis due to decreased HCl Weakened intestinal wall causing diverticuli Decreased motility (peristalsis) of gastrointestinal tract, causing constipation* Decreased calcium absorption Note: Constipation is not a result of normal aging.	Assess for adaptive changes and maintain gastrointestinal function by: 1. Discussing client preferences for foods 2. Suggesting dietary alterations according to physiologic changes, individual preferences, and nutritional needs, may need increased calcium and vitamin D 3. Encouraging fluid intake 4. Checking frequency, consistency, and stool color in bowel elimination 5. Assessing bowel sounds and level of peristalsis

Table 7-1. (Continued)

Body System	Structural Changes	Additional Risk Factors	Functional Outcomes	Nursing Interventions
Liver function and endocrine gland function decreased	Liver cell decrease in size and character Hormonal cells decrease in size and character, and outputs dwindle	Liver or endocrine diseases Medications (e.g., steroids, cardiac medications, antibiotics) Alcohol consumption	Liver: 1. Decreased hepatic capacity to detoxify drugs 2. Decreased synthesis of cholesterol and enzyme activity Hormonal: 1. Decreased overall metabolic capacity 2. Decreased endocrine gland function to react to adverse drug action	Assess adaptive liver and endocrine gland functioning by: 1. Noting drugs client is taking that may be toxic to liver 2. Observing for toxic effects of drug buildup 3. Observing for desired effects of drugs 4. Assessing alcohol consumption and teaching accordingly 5. Assessing for jaundice
Skin function decreased	Epidermis—thinner Dermis—thinning and loss of elasticity and strength Blood flow—decreased Sebaceous gland—decreased production Sweat gland—decreased production	Exposure to ultraviolet rays (sunlight) Adverse medication effects Personal hygiene habits (e.g., too frequent bathing) Immobility Friction Chemical Mechanical injury Temperature—too high or low Pressure	Dryer, coarser skin Increased threshold level to pain and temperature sensitivity Decreased ability to produce sweat Impaired ability to maintain body temperature	Maintain skin integrity and function by: 1. Maintaining hydration 2. Maintaining optimal skin temperature 3. Maintaining mobility to enhance circulation 4. Turning patient and elevating extremities when necessary to minimize edema and skin breakdown 5. Educating elderly about decreased sensitivity to pain and temperature 6. Providing special mattress or sheepskins for those at risk

1   The aged person adapts more slowly and thus has more difficulty maintaining homeostasis necessary for fluid and electrolyte balance. This factor is complicated by diminished pulmonary, renal, cardiac, gastrointestinal, and integumentary functions.

The changes occurring in the aged are _____ and _____ .

With diminished pulmonary, renal, cardiac, integumentary, and gastrointestinal functions, the aged person is prone to _____ and *_____ .

functional and structural; fluid and electrolyte imbalance
    ■   ■   ■

2   The aging process (increases/decreases) _____ pulmonary function.

The maximal breathing capacity is reduced due to *_____ and
*_____ .

decreases; loss of elasticity of the parenchymal lung tissue and increased rigidity of the chest wall (also fewer alveoli)
    ■   ■   ■

3   Poor diffusion of respiratory gases is related to *_____ and *_____
_____ .

Reduced ventilation can cause which of the following:

( ) a. CO_2 retention
( ) b. CO_2 excretion
( ) c. respiratory alkalosis
( ) d. respiratory acidosis

Name four clinical diseases that cause a decrease in breathing capacity, poor diffusion, and reduced ventilation. _____ , _____ ,
*_____ , and _____ .

defective alveolar ventilation and accumulation of bronchial secretions
a. X; b. —; c. —; d. X
emphysema, asthma, chronic bronchitis, and bronchiectasis
    ■   ■   ■

4   Name five nursing interventions that can increase breathing capacity and facilitate the elimination of CO_2. *_____ , *_____ ,
*_____ , *_____ , and *_____ .

breathing exercises with prolonged expiration, coughing and deep breathing, changing positions, chest clapping, and Intermittent positive pressure breathing (IPPB) treatments
    ■   ■   ■

5   The renal function in the aged is (increased/decreased) _____ .

  The persistent renal vasoconstriction and a decrease in number of functioning nephrons resulting from arteriosclerotic changes causes *_____ and *_____ .

  decreased; a reduced glomerular filtration rate and impaired ability to excrete water and solutes

■   ■   ■

6   Aged kidneys show evidence of a reduction in their ability to *_____ water and solutes.

  The kidneys' ability to excrete hydrogen (increases/decreases) _____ with age. The resulting acid-base imbalance is *_____ .

  retain or excrete; decreases; metabolic acidosis

■   ■   ■

7   The aged kidneys' ability to concentrate urine is _____ , resulting in *_____ .

  reduced/decreased; a buildup (accumulation) of waste products in the body

■   ■   ■

8   Decreased renal function may result in (decreased/increased) _____ drug excretion and (increased/decreased) _____ accumulation of drug in the body.

  decreased; increased

■   ■   ■

9   Name at least four nursing interventions for assessing and maintaining renal functions: *_____ , *_____ , *_____ , and *_____ .

  checking fluid intake and output, encouraging fluid intake, testing urine specific gravity, and noting drugs that may be toxic to renal function, also, observing lab results for signs of acid-base imbalance (according to the serum CO_2 or HCO_3)

■   ■   ■

10 In the aging process, circulation and cardiac function are (increased/decreased)

_____ .

The increased rigidity and decrease in elasticity of the arterial walls due to arteriosclerotic changes cause *_____ and *_____ .

decreased; an increased blood pressure and stasis of the blood
        ■   ■   ■

11 Stasis of blood in the veins can cause back pressure on the capillaries, increasing *_____ . The result of increased capillary pressure is _____ .

capillary pressure/permeability; edema
        ■   ■   ■

12 The diminished strength of heart contractions can cause a decrease in *_____ and *_____ .

cardiac output and blood flow
        ■   ■   ■

13 The aged person has a decrease in cardiac reserve. What is cardiac reserve? *_____

_____ .

Under stress, the heart rate increases both in the young adult and in the elderly. After stress, what happens to the heart rate in the young adult? *_____

_____ . In the elderly? *_____ .

the capacity of the heart to respond to increased burden; quickly returns to normal; takes longer to return to normal
        ■   ■   ■

14 Name at least five nursing interventions for assessing and maintaining circulation and cardiac function.

*_____

*_____

*_____

*_____

*_____ .

checking blood pressure for elevation or hypertension, determining blood flow in lower extremities by checking pulses (peripheral), checking for edema, checking apical and radial pulse rates for pulse deficit, and noting changes in heart rate following activities, also, assessing chest sounds for moist rales
        ■   ■   ■

15   Gastrointestinal functions are (increased/decreased) _____ in the aged.

   Atrophy of the gastric mucosa occurs with aging, causing a reduction in the important gastric secretion of _____ .

   The resulting acid-base imbalance is *_____ .

   decreased; HCl; metabolic alkalosis
   ■   ■   ■

16   Muscular atrophy in the small and large intestines occurs in aging. The gastrointestinal motility (peristalsis) is (increased/decreased) _____ .

   decreased
   ■   ■   ■

17   The aging adult frequently has a reduced ability to detect stimulation for a bowel movement. This type of bowel problem can result in _____ .

   constipation
   ■   ■   ■

18   The supportive structures in the intestinal wall (villae) are (strengthened/weakened) _____ and can cause diverticuli as a result of normal aging. Describe diverticuli.   *_____ .

   weakened; outpouches in the intestinal wall due to a weakened structural area
   ■   ■   ■

19   Name at least five nursing interventions for assessing and maintaining gastrointestinal function.

   * _____
   * _____
   * _____
   * _____
   * _____ .

   discussing with clients their food preference, suggesting diet to meet nutritional needs, encouraging fluid intake, noting color and consistency of bowel movements, and checking frequency of bowel elimination, also, assessing bowel sounds
   ■   ■   ■

20 Aging skin is (more/less) _____ prone to injury and (slower/faster) _____ to heal. This occurs because of the skin's tendency toward (thinning/thickening) _____ of the epidermis and a (thinning/thickening) _____ of the dermis in the aging adult. These changes result in (decreased/increased) _____ elasticity and strength of the skin which may be tested in fluid and electrolyte imbalances that cause either _____ or _____ which makes the skin more vulnerable to injury.

more; slower; thickening; thinning; decreased; overhydration; edema
■ ■ ■

21 Fluid imbalances causing dehydration promote drying of the skin and make it more fragile to handling. Fluid imbalances causing overhydration and edema stretch the skin and make it thinner and more vulnerable to injury. Identify five factors that the nurse should consider to decrease the client's risk for skin injury. _____ , * _____ , * _____ , _____ , and _____ .

friction, chemical injury, mechanical injury, temperature, and pressure
■ ■ ■

22 Identify four to five nursing interventions aimed at maintaining optimal skin integrity.
* _____ , * _____ , * _____ , * _____ , and * _____ .

maintain hydration, maintain optimal skin temperature, increase mobility (turn frequently), elevate edematous extremities, and encourage use of loose or nonrestrictive clothing
■ ■ ■

NURSING ASSESSMENT FACTORS

The normal structural and functional losses that occur as a result of the aging process have important implications for nursing assessments. The physiologic changes that alter the structure and function of the respiratory, renal, cardiac, gastrointestinal, and integumentary systems reduce the aging client's ability to adapt to changes that affect fluid and electrolyte balance. Many of these age-related changes predispose clients to chronic diseases which further decrease the client's ability to adapt to fluid and electrolyte changes.

By recognizing the changes due to normal aging and additional risk factors such as chronic diseases, the nurse can often prevent fluid and electrolyte problems or detect them before major complications have occurred. A critical assessment in clients at risk for fluid imbalances is accurate measurement of fluid intake and output. The magnitude of fluid problems in older adults is often evidenced by discrepancies between their fluid intake and output. Laboratory determinations of electrolytes and clinical assessments such as skin turgor, edema, and chest sounds provide additional information for nursing diagnoses and for planning and implementing nursing care.

23 The total body water in the healthy adult is _____ %. In normal aging the total body water decreases to approximately 54%. Changes include a slight (increase/decrease) _____ in extracellular fluid and a(n) (increase/decrease) _____ in intracellular fluid.

60; increase; decrease
■   ■   ■

24 Hypokalemia is a common deficit experienced by the aged. Potassium is not conserved well at any age. Many aged people receive diuretics (potassium wasting) and steroids which tend to (increase/decrease) _____ the serum potassium level. (Review Chapter 3, potassium with drug relationship, if needed.)

decrease
■   ■   ■

25 The aged person's ECF is (increased/decreased) *_____ , and the ICF is (increased/decreased) _____ .

The total body water in the aged is approximately _____ %.

slightly increased; decreased; 54
■   ■   ■

The six potential body fluid problems commonly experienced by the aged include dehydration, edema, water intoxications, constipation, diarrhea, and diaphoresis. Table 7-2 lists these six fluid problems with their related causes and suggested nursing interventions.

Table 7-2.   BODY FLUID PROBLEMS IN THE AGED

Problems	Etiology	Nursing Interventions
Fluid volume deficit: dehydration	1. Insufficient water intake 2. Increased urinary output 3. Decreased thirst mechanism 4. Diminished response to ADH (antidiuretic hormone) 5. Reduced ability to concentrate urine	1. Measure fluid intake and output to assess fluid balance 2. Encourage adequate oral fluid intake 3. Assess osmolality of IV fluid intake 4. Assess for clinical signs and symptoms of hypovolemia (dehydration) 5. Monitor other types of fluid therapy, e.g., IV clysis and tube feeding. Adjust rate of IV fluid according to age and physiologic state

Table 7-2. (Continued)

Problems	Etiology	Nursing Interventions
Fluid volume excess	1. Slightly elevated ECF	1. Measure fluid intake and output to assess fluid balance
A. Edema	2. Overhydration from IV therapy 3. Increased capillary pressure 4. Cardiac insufficiency	2. Adjust IV flow rate to prevent overhydration 3. Assess for peripheral edema in morning 4. Assess chest sounds for moist rales 5. Observe for signs and symptoms of hypervolemia—overhydration
B. Water intoxication	1. Hypo-osmolar solutions with copious amounts of drinking water	1. Assess types of IV fluids, e.g., 5% dextrose in water replacement to prevent complications 2. Observe for signs and symptoms of water intoxication 3. Check laboratory results for osmolar effects (Hgb, Hct, electrolytes, BUN)
Alternate bowel elimination: constipation	1. Decrease in water intake 2. Muscular atrophy of small and large intestines with decrease in GI motility 3. Perceptual loss of bowel stimulation	1. Encourage fluid intake 2. Assess bowel sounds for peristalsis 3. Administer mild laxative, and teach dangers of abuse 4. Have patient eat at regular times 5. Offer bedside commode 6. Increase roughage in diet as tolerated 7. Observe color, consistency, and frequency of stools
Alternate bowel elimination: diarrhea	1. Tube feedings with too much carbohydrate 2. Constipation—with small amount of liquid stools 3. Partially digested nutrients 4. Viral or bacterial infection	1. Assess for problem causing diarrhea 2. Administer drug(s), e.g., Lomotil, Kaopectate, to decrease motility of bowel 3. Observe color, frequency, and consistency of stool

Diaphoresis	1. Excessive perspiration
	  a. Fever
	  b. High environmental temperature and/or humidity
		1. Identify cause of problem

26 The thirst mechanism in the elderly is frequently (decreased/increased)
_____ , resulting in a decreased fluid intake.

Name two factors that can result in dehydration for the elderly. *_____ , and
*_____ .

decreased; insufficient water intake and increased urinary output

      ■   ■   ■

27 Name four nursing interventions to correct dehydration in the older person.

*_____

*_____

*_____

*_____ .

measure fluid intake and output for balance, encourage taking fluids orally, assess signs and symptoms of dehydration (hypovolemia), and assess intravenous fluid (type and rate), also, adjust replacement fluid rate according to age and condition of the client.

      ■   ■   ■

28 Overloading the vascular system with fluids (hypervolemia) can result in congestive heart failure (CHF). The type of edema occurring in CHF is *_____ .

pulmonary edema from overhydration

29 Peripheral edema can result from dependent or refractory edema. When the feet and ankles are edematous in the morning, the type of edema present is called _____ edema. This type of edema results from *_____ and may also be called (dependent/nondependent/independent) _____ edema.

refractory; cardiac-renal impairment or insufficiency and with little to no diuretic effect; nondependent (since edema is present in the morning and is not necessarily due to gravity)

      ■   ■   ■

30 Identify selected nursing interventions for correcting edema in the aged by marking the correct answers and adjusting the incorrect answers.

( ) a. Measure fluid intake and output to assess fluid balance.
( ) b. Adjust intravenous flow rate according to age and patient condition.
( ) c. Assess for peripheral edema in the evening for refractory or nondependent edema.
( ) d. Assess bowel sounds.
( ) e. Observe for signs and symptoms of hypovolemia.

a. X; b. X; c. —, in the morning; d. —, chest sounds; e. —, of hypervolemia (overhydration)

  ■   ■   ■

31 Explain why 5% dextrose in water might be considered a hypo-osmolar solution. *_____

_____

_____ .

Dextrose 5% in water (D_5W) is an iso-osmolar solution; however, if it is given without other solutes, the dextrose is metabolized by the body, leaving only water; it becomes a hypo-osmolar solution.

  ■   ■   ■

32 Identify appropriate nursing interventions related to constipation and correct the incorrect answers:

( ) a. Encourage fluid intake.
( ) b. Assess bowel sounds for peristalsis.
( ) c. Administer harsh cathartics.
( ) d. Offer bedside commode.
( ) e. Have meals at regular times.

a. X; b. X; c. —, mild laxatives or stool softeners; d. X; e. X

  ■   ■   ■

33 Name four causes of diarrhea in the aged. *_____ , *_____ ,
*_____ , and *_____ .

  What is the most important nursing intervention for correcting diarrhea? *_____

_____ .

tube feedings with too much carbohydrate, constipation with small liquid stools, partially digested nutrients, and viral or bacterial infections; identification of the problem causing diarrhea

  ■   ■   ■

34 The sixth fluid problem occurring with the aged is _____ , or excessive perspiration. What are the two causes of excessive perspiration? _____ and
* _____ .

diaphoresis; fever and high environmental temperature and high humidity
    ■   ■   ■

CASE STUDY REVIEW A

Mrs. Palmer, age 89, is a resident in a nursing home. She has been hypoventilating and says that she has some difficulty with breathing. A nursing assessment further reveals an elevated blood pressure (168/100), an increased pulse rate (104), edema in the extremities, a urinary output of 500 mL per day, and a recent weight gain of 10 pounds.

1. As an aged person, Mrs. Palmer's body systems most prone to changes are
   _____ , _____ , _____ ,
   _____ , and _____ .
2. Mrs. Palmer's reduced breathing capacity may be due to
   a. * _____ .
   b. * _____ .
3. Hypoventilation can result in _____ retention, which may cause an acid-base imbalance called * _____ .
4. Identify at least three nursing interventions that can improve Mrs. Palmer's pulmonary function.
   * _____ , * _____ , and * _____ .
5. Mrs. Palmer's blood pressure is elevated due to * _____
   _____
   _____ .
6. The physiologic reason for edema in her lower extremities is * _____
   _____
7. Identify three nursing interventions regarding Mrs. Palmer's blood pressure and edema.
   a. * _____ .
   b. * _____ .
   c. * _____ .
8. Urine output should be _____ mL per hour or _____ mL per 24 hours to maintain adequate renal function. Mrs. Palmer's urine output was 500 mL in 24 hours, which is (adequate/inadequate) _____ . Identify two possible reasons for her poor urinary output.
   a. * _____
   b. * _____
9. Identify at least three nursing interventions in regard to Mrs. Palmer's renal function.
   * _____ , * _____ , and * _____ .
10. What two physiologic factors can cause Mrs. Palmer's constipation? * _____
    and * _____ .

11. Two nursing interventions for alleviating constipation are *_____ and
    *_____ .

1. *pulmonary, renal, cardiac, gastrointestinal, integumentary, and endocrine*
2. *a. loss of elasticity of the parenchymal lung tissue and b. increased rigidity of the chest wall*
3. CO_2; *respiratory acidosis*
4. *breathing exercise with prolonged expiration, coughing after a few deep breaths, and changing positions, also, chest clapping*
5. *increased rigidity of the arterial walls due to arteriosclerotic changes*
6. *increased capillary pressure forcing fluid into the tissues (nondependent edema)*
7. *a. check blood pressure, b. determine blood flow in lower extremities by checking pulses, and c. check for edema in the morning to determine if it is dependent or nondependent edema*
8. *25; 600; inadequate*
   a. inadequate fluid intake
   b. kidneys unable to excrete water and solute (you could have answered: reduced glomerular filtration rate and decrease in number of functioning nephrons)
9. *check intake and output, encourage fluid intake, and check acid-base balance, also, test specific gravity*
10. *reduced motility of the gastrointestinal tract and loss of perception for bowel elimination*
11. *Suggest diet (foods) to meet nutritional needs and maintain bowel function and encourage fluid intake. Other answers may include check frequency of bowel elimination and determine the presence of peristalsis (bowel sounds).*

CASE STUDY REVIEW B

Tom Fellows is a 67-year-old single Caucasian man who until recently lived alone in his own house. He now lives in an intermediate care unit of a continuing care facility where his meals are provided. He is independent in activities of daily living but requires help with shopping and money management. He was a financial analyst who led an active social life which included almost nightly "happy hours" with work associates until his retirement 5 years ago. After his retirement he started to drink alone. He quit going to the dining room for his meals and gradually stopped drinking fluids other than his beer and wine. The nurse on the day shift recorded his vital signs as temperature 99 °F, pulse 104, and respirations 28. His laboratory studies revealed an elevated hemoglobin and hematocrit. Other laboratory studies revealed serum potassium, 3.4 mEq/L; serum Na, 147; and Cl, 105 mEq/L (review Chapter 3 for normal electrolyte ranges). His skin and mucous membranes were very dry. He complained of constipation.

1. From this history, identify three fluid problems. _____ ,
   _____ , and _____ .
2. What is the clinical source of Mr. Fellows' dehydration?
   *_____
   _____ .

3. Identify four clinical signs and symptoms of dehydration experienced by Mr. Fellows:
   a. *_____
   b. *_____
   c. *_____
   d. *_____

4. Is it possible to have dehydration and edema at the same time? _____ .
   Explain why. *_____
   _____ .

Mr. Fellows was given intravenous fluids for several days and then later given tube feedings daily.

5. While Mr. Fellows was receiving intravenous fluids, identify at least two nursing interventions aimed at maintaining an appropriate fluid balance for clients receiving intravenous fluids.
   *_____ and *_____ .

6. If Mr. Fellows receives continuous intravenous replacements with 5% dextrose in water, what type of fluid problem might result? *_____ .

7. If the intravenous fluids were administered too rapidly, what type of fluid imbalance is Mr. Fellows most likely to develop? *_____ . Identify three symptoms of this imbalance. *_____ , *_____ , and _____ .

8. Tube feedings high in carbohydrate can cause what type of a fluid problem?
   _____ .

9. The normal potassium level in the aged is *_____ , and therefore fluid balances often result in a potassium (deficit/excess) _____ called
   _____ .

10. Fluid imbalances can cause Mr. Fellows to be at an (increased/decreased) _____ risk for skin breakdown.

1. *dehydration, edema, and constipation*
2. *insufficient water intake (you might have answered that a decreased thirst mechanism was present)*
3. *a. vital signs: temperature slightly elevated, pulse and respirations elevated*
   b. Hgb, Hct, and BUN elevated
   c. serum sodium elevated
   d. skin and mucous membranes very dry
4. *Yes. Frequently a person can have edema and be dehydrated due to hypovolemia in the vascular system with increased fluids in the interstitial space.*
5. *assess the intravenous fluid according to the type ordered and its osmolality and adjust the rate of intravenous fluids according to client's age and physiologic state. The nurse should also assess fluid intake and output balance.*
6. *water intoxication or ICFVE*
7. *hypervolemia or overhydration (pulmonary edema)*
   constant, irritating cough, engorged veins (neck and hand), and dyspnea
8. *diarrhea*
9. *poorly conserved; deficit; hypokalemia*
10. *increased*

NURSING DIAGNOSIS AND RELATED INTERVENTIONS

The purpose of assessing clients such as Mrs. Palmer and Mr. Fellows is to form nursing diagnoses based on the assessment data. Nursing interventions are selected to foster positive functional outcomes. Review the Functional Consequences Model of Gerontological Nursing in Figure 7-1 to review age-related changes and additional risk factors to be considered when forming nursing diagnoses and planning nursing interventions for older adults. Then answer the following study questions for Mrs. Palmer and Mr. Fellows:

1. What are the major body systems affected by the client's health problems?
2. What are the client's age-related structural changes related to fluid and electrolyte balance?
3. What are the client's additional risk factors for fluid and electrolyte imbalances?
4. What are the functional changes related to the client's structural changes and additional risk factors?
5. What are the most important nursing diagnoses related to fluid and electrolyte balance for these clients?
6. What negative functional consequences do you wish to prevent?
7. What nursing interventions can help these clients prevent negative functional consequences?

Use Table 7-3 to organize your replies to the study questions. Refer to Tables 7-1 and 7-2 as needed.

Table 7-3. MRS. PALMER

Body System Affected	Structural Changes	Risk Factors	Functional Changes	Nursing Diagnoses	Nursing Interventions	Rationale
Cardiac	Arteriosclerosis Increased capillary pressure Decreased effectiveness of cardiac contractions	Recent weight gain of 10 pounds Low protein intake	High blood pressure Edema Decreased cardiac output Increased heart rate	Fluid volume excess: edema, related to decreased cardiac output as evidenced by taut, shiny skin	1. Monitor intake and output, body weight, vital signs, and neck veins for distension	Checking for overhydration is important to measure the effectiveness for medical treatment and nursing interventions
					2. Monitor hemoglobin and hematocrit	Hemoglobin and hematocrit concentration are important to assess fluid balance changes
					3. Administer diuretics as ordered by physician	A ↓ Hgb and Hct levels can indicate fluid overload
					4. If on diuretics, monitor K+	Diuretics increase fluid loss and decrease edema. Many diuretics cause potassium loss
Respiratory	Loss of elasticity of the parenchymal lung tissue Increased rigidity of the chest wall	Immobility Exertion Hypoventilation	CO_2 retention Respiratory acidosis *and* Reduced breathing capacity	High risk for respiratory insufficiency Impaired gas exchange Ineffective breathing patterns	1. Monitor chest for adventitious sounds	To assess for fluid overload
					2. Observe for cough which may indicate pulmonary edema	Cough is an early sign of fluid overload
					3. Breathing exercises—prolonged expiration	Assists clients to remove excess CO_2

System	Structural Changes	Related Factors	Nursing Diagnosis	Interventions	Rationale
				4. Coughing after a few deep breaths	To enhance gas exchange (O_2 + CO_2)
				5. Change position frequently	Assist in lung expansion
				6. Chest clapping	Loosens mucus
Renal	Persistent renal vasoconstriction from arteriosclerotic changes and decreased number of functioning nephrons	Medications	Fluid volume deficit, related to decreased fluid intake	1. Assess intake and output	To determine amount of excess fluid loss
	Reduced glomerular filtration rate and ability to excrete water and solute	Genitourinary obstructions		2. Encourage oral fluids as tolerated	Assist with fluid replacement
				3. Assess acid-base balance	To observe for metabolic changes
				4. Assess urine specific gravity (SG)	Increased urine SG indicates inadequate fluid intake or decreased renal function
Gastrointestinal	Atrophy of gastric mucosa	Immobility	High risk for constipation, related to decreased fluid volume, age-related changes, and immobility	1. Encourage fluids as tolerated	To assist with proper bowel elimination
	Loss of supportive structure of small and large bowel	Medications		2. Increase mobility as tolerated	Physical mobility enhances GI mobility
	Decreased mobility of GI tract			3. Encourage proper diet to ensure elimination	A balanced diet with fiber enhances bowel elimination
	Loss of perception of signs for bowel elimination			4. Assess bowel sounds	To determine functional status of the GI system
				5. Check frequency of bowel elimination and consistency of stools	To determine risk of bowel complications

Table 7-3. (Continued)

Body System Affected	Structural Changes	Risk Factors	Functional Changes	Nursing Diagnoses	Nursing Interventions	Rationale
Liver N/A						
Integumentary	Loss of elasticity and strength of skin	Edema Immobility	Taut, shiny skin reduces protective function	Skin integrity: impaired, related to edema and immobility	1. Avoid friction, prolonged pressure, chemical irritation, mechanical injury, excessive temperature variations	To reduce possible skin breakdown due to edema and/or immobility
	Decreased blood flow, sebaceous and sweat gland production				2. Encourage mobility to enhance circulation	Good circulation improves skin repair
					3. Raise extremities	To improve circulation and reduce edema
					4. Implement nursing interventions for fluid volume excess and pulmonary congestion (PC) respiratory insufficiency	Fluid balance reduces risks to integumentary system

Now fill in Table 7-4 as you answer the study questions for Mr. Fellows.

Table 7-4. MR. FELLOWS

Body System Affected	Structural Changes	Risk Factors	Functional Changes	Nursing Diagnoses	Nursing Interventions	Rationale
Cardiac*						
Respiratory*						
Renal	Persistent renal vasoconstriction Decreased number of functioning nephrons	Obstructions Disease Medications	Decreased thirst mechanism Reduced glomerular filtration rate Decreased ability to excrete water and solute	Fluid volume deficit related to decreased desire to drink fluids secondary to high alcohol intake and social isolation as evidenced by dry lips, furrowed tongue, and decreased skin turgor	1. Observe for decreased skin turgor, decreased urine output 2. Measure intake and output 3. Check specific gravity of urine 4. Observe lab results for increased red blood cell count, hematocrit, and hemoglobin	Decreased skin turgor is a sign of dehydration. Decreased urine output may be due to dehydration or renal dysfunction To determine fluid balance To assess renal function Provide clues to extent of fluid deficit
Gastrointestinal	Muscular atrophy and loss of supportive structure of small and large intestine Atrophy of gastric mucosa	Alcohol intake Poor diet Immobility Decreased motivation to drink fluids other than alcohol Social isolation	Decreased GI secretions Decreased motility Constipation	Potential complication: gastrointestinal bleeding Colonic constipation related to inadequate intake of food and fluids and lack of exercise as evidenced by infrequent bowel movements, small, hard stools	1. Increase fluid intake of water and fluids 2. Assess fluid balance 3. Encourage a balanced diet with increased roughage 4. Assess bowel sounds 5. Observe color and consistency of stools 6. Hemoccult stools	To enhance bowel elimination and soften stools Fluid balance reduces risk for constipation Balanced diet with fiber stimulates bowel elimination To assess for constipation and/or bleeding Observe for GI bleeding to assess GI motility
Liver	Atrophy of liver cells	Heavy alcohol use Aspirin Social isolation		Potential complication: gastrointestinal bleeding	1. Observe for accumulation of fluids in third spaces	Liver damage can cause fluid shift, e.g., ascites
Integumentary*						

*Not applicable.

Chapter 8

Gastrointestinal Surgery

Larry Purnell, R.N., Ph.D.

Behavioral Objectives

Upon completion of this chapter, you will be prepared to:

- Identify five major electrolytes that may be affected by gastrointestinal (GI) surgery.
- Discuss the physiologic implications of sodium, potassium, and chloride imbalances associated with major GI surgery.
- Discuss the effects of gastric intubation in fluid and electrolyte balance.
- Describe the physiologic implications of hydrogen and bicarbonate balance with alterations in the GI system.
- Describe the fluid management of clients experiencing alterations in the GI system.
- Identify important nursing assessment factors associated with fluid and electrolyte balance that may occur with major GI surgery.
- Identify selected nursing diagnoses and interventions related to fluid and electrolyte balance associated with major GI surgery.

Introduction

The main functions of the gastrointestinal (GI) tract are the ingestion, absorption, and transportation of fluids and nutrients. Diseases and illnesses that interrupt these daily functions place the client at risk for developing fluid and electrolyte imbalances. Diagnostic testing and preparation for gastrointestinal surgery may further increase the client's risk for fluid and electrolyte imbalance. Postoperatively, the client may be NPO, have gastrointestinal drainage tubes, and delayed peristalsis. Preexisting cardiopulmonary, endocrine, and renal conditions in conjunction with diuretics, glucocorticoids, mineralocorticoids, and insulin requirements place the client undergoing major surgery at risk for fluid and electrolyte imbalances. Alterations in fluid volume status can occur rapidly; astute nursing assessment skills and timely interventions may prevent or decrease potential complications.

1   Three of the main functions of the GI tract are _____ ,
     _____ , and _____ of fluids and electrolytes.

ingestion, absorption, and transportation

∎   ∎   ∎

2 Diseases and illnesses that interrupt the normal functions of the GI tract place the client at risk for _____ and _____ imbalances.

fluid and electrolyte

■   ■   ■

3 Postoperative treatment modalities that increase the client's risk for fluid and electrolyte imbalance include _____ , * _____ , and * _____ .

NPO, drainage tubes, and decreased peristalsis

■   ■   ■

4 Name at least three preexisting conditions that increase the surgical client's risk for fluid and electrolyte imbalances.

a. *_____

b. *_____

c. *_____

a. cardiopulmonary disorders (congestive heart failure); b. endocrine disorders (diabetes mellitus, glucocorticoid disorders (Cushing's disease), mineralocorticoid disorders (Addison's disease); c. renal disease (renal impairment or kidney failure). You may have included other conditions as well as the ones mentioned.

■   ■   ■

FLUID AND ELECTROLYTE ALTERATIONS

5 Clients undergoing minor surgery usually experience little or no fluid and electrolyte alterations.

   In major surgery, sodium and water may be retained and potassium may be lost. Before potassium is administered, it is necessary to make certain that:

( ) a. The person can tolerate food
( ) b. Renal function is adequate

a. —; b. X

■   ■   ■

6 After major surgery, there is a tendency for sodium _____ , water _____ , and potassium _____ .

retention; retention; loss

■   ■   ■

7 Many clients undergoing gastrointestinal surgery experience fluid and electrolyte imbalances prior to surgery. Treatment of these imbalances must be considered prior to surgery in conjunction with concurrent fluid losses. Replacement of fluid losses is necessary before, during, and following surgery.

Frequently, these clients have a fluid deficit and will need additional fluids to reestablish renal function. Which type of intravenous solution is indicated to reestablish renal function:

( ) a. Hydrating solutions
( ) b. Plasma expanders
( ) c. Replacement solutions with potassium replacement

a. X; b. —; c. —

■   ■   ■

8 Some clients undergoing gastrointestinal surgery may require fluid and electrolyte replacement therapy for which of the following:

( ) a. Before surgery
( ) b. During surgery
( ) c. After surgery

a. X; b. X; c. X

■   ■   ■

9 Gastric or intestinal intubation (tube passed into the stomach or intestines) for suctioning purposes may be inserted before surgery. This alleviates vomiting due to an obstruction in the gastrointestinal tract or decompresses the stomach or bowel, or both, before and after an operation.

For gastric intubation, a Levine tube or Salem sump is inserted via the nose into the stomach. For an intestinal intubation, a Miller-Abbott tube or Cantor tube is inserted via the nose and stomach into the intestines. The intestinal tubes are longer than the gastric tube and they contain a small balloon filled with air or mercury on the end which helps the tube pass into the lower intestines. A gastric or an intestinal tube is frequently used following abdominal surgery in order to remove secretions until peristalsis returns and to relieve abdominal distention.

Gastric or intestinal intubation before abdominal surgery is used to *_____

_____ .

Gastric or intestinal intubation after abdominal surgery is used to   * _____

_____

and to   * _____ .

alleviate vomiting and decompress the bowel or stomach; remove secretions until peristalsis returns; relieve abdominal distention

■   ■   ■

Table 8-1 lists the electrolytes that are in the stomach and intestines. Note which electrolytes are more concentrated in gastric and intestinal fluids. The client experiencing vomiting, diarrhea, or intubation (gastric or intestinal) loses fluid and electrolytes. Study the table and be able to state which electrolytes are lost.

Table 8-1. CONCENTRATION OF ELECTROLYTES IN THE STOMACH AND INTESTINE (mEq/L)					
Area	**Body Fluid**	**Na$^+$**	**K$^+$**	**Cl$^-$**	**HCO$_3$$^-$**
Stomach	Gastric juice	60.4	9.2*	84*	0–14 H$^+$*
Small intestine	Intestinal juice	111.3*	4.6	104.2*	31*

* Electrolytes that are highly concentrated in these areas.

10 Identify three highly concentrated electrolytes that are lost with vomiting and gastric intubation. _____ , _____ , and _____ .
Name other electrolytes that are lost from the stomach. _____ and

_____ .

potassium, chloride, and hydrogen; sodium and bicarbonate (chloride is in high concentration in the stomach and the intestines)

■   ■   ■

11 What are the major electrolytes lost by clients with diarrhea or intestinal intubation?
_____ , _____ , and _____ . Another
electrolyte lost from the intestines is _____ .

sodium, chloride, and bicarbonate; potassium

■   ■   ■

12 Sodium ions are more plentiful in the (stomach/intestines) _____ .
   Potassium ions are more plentiful in the (stomach/intestines) _____ .

intestines; stomach

■   ■   ■

13 Bicarbonate ions are more plentiful in the (stomach/intestines) _____ .

What type of acid-base imbalance results when a large amount of bicarbonate is lost?
* _____ .

intestines; metabolic acidosis

■ ■ ■

14 Hydrogen is more plentiful in the (stomach/intestines) _____ .

What type of acid-base imbalance results when hydrogen is lost? * _____ .

stomach; metabolic alkalosis

■ ■ ■

15 Name the electrolyte-acid-base imbalances that can occur if potassium, chloride, and hydrogen are lost from the stomach. * _____ .

hypokalemia alkalosis

■ ■ ■

CLINICAL APPLICATIONS

Mr. Drum was admitted to the hospital complaining of severe, persistent hiccups and abdominal pain. The client noticed a mass in the lower left quadrant of his abdomen for approximately 5–6 days before admission. Mr. Drum experienced several episodes of this left groin mass that could be reduced manually.

Mr. Drum stated he had not had a bowel movement for the past 3 days and he was not able to "keep anything down" over the past 3 days. His skin was warm and dry with poor turgor. He was very weak.

16 Which of the following signs and symptoms might indicate that Mr. Drum had a fluid volume deficit:

( ) a. Vomiting—unable to retain food for 3 days
( ) b. Skin warm, dry, and lacking elasticity
( ) c. Not having a bowel movement for 3 days
( ) d. Weakness
( ) e. Hernia could be manually reduced
( ) f. Severe abdominal pain in left lower quadrant

a. X; b. X; c. —; d. X; e. —; f. —

■ ■ ■

Table 8-2 gives the laboratory studies for Mr. Drum and shows how his results changed from the norm at the time of his illness. Memorize the "normal" laboratory ranges as given in Table 8-2 in the left-hand column. Use the values throughout the chapter. Refer to Table 8-2 as needed.

Table 8-2.   LABORATORY STUDIES OF MR. DRUM

Laboratory Tests	On Admission	First Day	Second Day	Third Day	Fourth Day
Hematology					
Hemoglobin (12.9–17.0 g)	21.2	18.4	13.1	13.2	
(Hematocrit (40–46%)	58	54	38	39	
WBC (white blood count) (5000–10,000/mm³)	10,700				
Biochemistry					
BUN (blood urea nitrogen) (10–25 mg/dL)*	85	68	68	19	19
Plasma/serum† CO₂					
50–70 vol%	52	61	—	39	50
22–32 mEq/L	24	28	—	18	22
Plasma/serum chloride (98–108 mEq/L)	73	78	73	91	97
Plasma/serum sodium (135–146 mEq/L)	122	128	122	132	145
Plasma/serum potassium (3.5–5.3 mEq/L)	5.2	4.0	4.0	4.2	4.1

*mg/100 mL = mg/dL.
† *Plasma* and *serum* are used interchangeably.

17 The "normal" ranges from hemoglobin, hematocrit, and white blood count are

*_____ , _____ , and _____ , respectively.

12.9–17.0 g, 40–46%, and 5000–10,000/mm³
▪   ▪   ▪

18 BUN is the abbreviation for blood urea nitrogen. Explain how urea is formed. *_____

_____ .

How is it excreted? *_____ .

What is the "normal" BUN range? *_____ .

by-product of protein metabolism; through the kidney; 10–25 mg/dL
▪   ▪   ▪

19 The "normal" serum CO_2 range is _____ vol % or _____ mEq/L.

Would a client with a serum CO_2 of 18 mEq/L be in metabolic (acidosis/alkalosis)? _____ . Refer to Chapter 4 for further clarification.

50–70; 22–32; acidosis

■   ■   ■

20 The "normal" range of the serum chloride is 95–108 mEq/L. Identify the "normal" range of the serum potassium and serum sodium: Serum potassium: * _____ mEq/L, and serum sodium: * _____ mEq/L. Refer to Chapter 3 for further clarification.

K, 3.5–5.3; Na, 135–146

■   ■   ■

21 Which of Mr. Drum's admission laboratory results indicate a fluid and electrolyte imbalance:

( ) a. Hemoglobin 21.2 g
( ) b. Hematocrit 58%
( ) c. Serum CO_2 52%
( ) d. Serum CO_2 24 mEq/L
( ) e. Serum chloride 73 mEq/L
( ) f. Serum sodium 122 mEq/L
( ) g. Serum potassium 5.2 mEq/L

a. X; b. X; c. —; d. —; e. X; f. X; g. —

■   ■   ■

22 Mr. Drum's elevated hemoglobin and hematocrit on admission and the first day postoperatively indicate * _____ .

fluid volume deficit (If you answered hemoconcentration or dehydration, OK.)

■   ■   ■

23 A high BUN is indicative of renal impairment or dehydration or both. Mr. Drum's elevated BUN indicates which of the following:

( ) a. An increased urine output
( ) b. A retention of urea, the by-product of protein metabolism, in the circulating blood
( ) c. An abnormal excretion of urea, the by-product of protein metabolism

a. —; b. X; c. —

■   ■   ■

24 The third day postoperatively, Mr. Drum's plasma CO_2 decreased. This indicates which of the following:

( ) a. An increased bicarbonate ion in the plasma
( ) b. A decreased bicarbonate ion in the plasma
( ) c. Metabolic acidosis
( ) d. Metabolic alkalosis

a. —; b. X; c. X; d. —
∎   ∎   ∎

25 Below are some of Mr. Drum's laboratory results. Use the following symbols to label the imbalance that they might indicate:

D for dehydration
K for kidney dysfunction
E for electrolyte imbalance
M for metabolic acidosis
O for normal range or for those that do not pertain to the above four

Some results may be associated with more than one imbalance.

___ a. Hematocrit 38%
___ b. Hemoglobin 21.2 g
___ c. BUN 68 mEq/L
___ d. BUN 19 mEq/L
___ e. Serum potassium 4.0 mEq/L
___ f. Serum sodium 122 mEq/L
___ g. Serum CO_2 18 mEq/L
___ h. Serum CO_2 28 mEq/L
___ i. Serum chloride 73 mEq/L

a. O; b. D; c. K, D; d. O; e. O; f. E; g. M; h. O; i. E
∎   ∎   ∎

CLINICAL MANAGEMENT—PREOPERATIVE

The preoperative management for Mr. Drum should include:

1. Hydrate rapidly utilizing 4–5 liters over the next 6–8 hours.
2. Insert a Levine tube and connect to low intermittent suction.
3. Prepare for OR for a left inguinal herniorrhaphy as soon as he is hydrated.
4. Monitor renal function—urine output.

Solution for hydration: 4500 cc 5% D/½ NS (dextrose in ½ normal saline or 0.45%)

26 Which of the following conditions resulted from Mr. Drum's vomiting?

( ) a. Severe fluid volume deficit
( ) b. Water intoxication
( ) c. A loss of sodium and chloride
( ) d. A low serum bicarbonate level
( ) e. A low serum potassium level

a. X; b. —; c. X; d. X; e. —

■   ■   ■

27 He was hydrated (before/after) _____ the herniorrhaphy. A gastric tube was inserted to do which of the following:

( ) a. Relieve distention
( ) b. Remove secretions from the stomach
( ) c. Lessen vomiting
( ) d. Provide nutrition

before. On admission his potassium was high normal, probably because of the severe fluid volume deficit that caused hemoconcentration.
a. X; b. X; c. X; d. —

■   ■   ■

CLINICAL MANAGEMENT—POSTOPERATIVE

28 The postoperative fluid and electrolyte management for Mr. Drum should include the following:

1. Connect gastric tube to low suction and check drainage hourly.
2. Monitor parenteral therapy:
   1000 cc 5% D/½ NS
   1000 cc 5% D/NS
   1000 cc 5% lactated Ringer's
3. A 1-ampule (50-mEq) sodium bicarbonate IV push.
4. Check urine output hourly and test for specific gravity and pH.
5. Assess serum electrolyte findings.
6. Administer antibiotic as prescribed for febrile condition.
7. Encourage client to cough and deep breathe every 30 minutes for the first 4 hours.

Mr. Drum received gastric intubation following surgery to *_____ and
*_____ .

relieve abdominal distention and remove gastric secretions

■   ■   ■

29 Gastrointestinal secretions contain solid particles that may accumulate and obstruct the tube. Irrigating the tube will assure patency and proper drainage.

Frequent irrigations, using large amounts of water, should be avoided to prevent the loss of fluid and electrolytes.

Irrigation of Mr. Drum's tube will assure * _____ .

Name the "major" electrolytes lost through frequent gastric irrigation with large quantities of water. _____ , _____ , and _____ .

patency for proper drainage; potassium, hydrogen, and chloride

  ▪   ▪   ▪

30 The gastric tube should be irrigated at specific intervals with small amounts of saline to keep it patent.

A change in the client's position helps to alleviate tube obstruction.

The use of small amounts of air to check the patency of the tube may be ordered instead of irrigating the tube to help prevent the loss of fluids and electrolytes. Listen with the stethoscope over the stomach for a "whoosh" sound when air is injected into the tube.

Three methods to maintain the patency of Mr. Drum's gastric tube are
* _____ , * _____ , and * _____
_____ .

irrigate at specific intervals with small amounts of saline, change the client's position, and introduce small amounts of air and listen with a stethoscope for a "whoosh" sound

  ▪   ▪   ▪

31 Mr. Drum was allowed sips of water to alleviate the dryness in his mouth and lessen irritation in his throat.

Special attention should be taken to limit the amount of water by mouth, because water dilutes the electrolytes in the stomach and the suction then removes them.

What might happen to Mr. Drum's electrolytes if he drinks a lot of water during gastric intubation? * _____
_____ .

The electrolytes in the stomach would be diluted, and suction would remove them.

  ▪   ▪   ▪

32 After Mr. Drum's gastric tube is removed, the nurse should observe for:

1. A feeling of fullness
2. Vomiting
3. Abdominal distention
4. Diminished bowel sounds

These symptoms indicate that Mr. Drum's gastrointestinal tract (is/is not)
_____ functioning.

The signs and symptoms that indicate Mr. Drum's peristalsis has not returned to normal are
* _____ , _____ , * _____ , and
* _____ .

is not; a feeling of fullness, vomiting, abdominal distention, and diminished bowel sounds
　　　　　■　　　　　　　　　■　　　　　　　　　■

33 Frequently, the tube is clamped for a period of time and then unclamped. The amount of residual gastric fluid is measured. A large residual of gastric fluid released when the tube is unclamped indicates that peristalsis has not returned.

A feeling of fullness, vomiting, and abdominal distention are signs and symptoms that indicate that peristalsis (has/has not) _____ returned.

Using the clamping and unclamping method, how would the nurse know if peristalsis has returned? * _____ .

has not; a small amount of fluid return indicates peristalsis has returned
　　　　　■　　　　　　　　　■　　　　　　　　　■

34 Since suction removes fluids and electrolytes, oral fluid intake is restricted and parenteral therapy is initiated.

Mr. Drum received intravenous fluids containing dextrose, saline, and lactated Ringer's to do which of the following:

( ) a. Replace sodium and chloride loss
( ) b. Maintain nutritional needs
( ) c. Maintain electrolyte balance
( ) d. Replace and maintain the fluid volume

a. X; b. X; c. X; d. X
　　　　　■　　　　　　　　　■　　　　　　　　　■

35 If Mr. Drum received 3–4 (or more) liters of 5% dextrose in water (D_5W) with no other solutes, what type of fluid imbalance could occur?

( ) a. Dehydration
( ) b. Overhydration
( ) c. Water intoxication

Why? *_____

_____ .

a. —; b. — (maybe); c. X.
The diluted fluid in the vessels (vascular) shifts to the cells due to the process of osmosis.
Osmosis causes fluid to diffuse from the lesser to the greater concentration.

■   ■   ■

36 Mr. Drum received an ampule of sodium bicarbonate IV push. This would do which of the following:

( ) a. Increase the plasma CO_2 or bicarbonate
( ) b. Decrease the plasma CO_2 or bicarbonate
( ) c. Reduce his metabolic acidotic state
( ) d. Reduce his metabolic alkalotic state

a. X; b. —; c. X; d. —

■   ■   ■

37 Mr. Drum should be encouraged to cough and deep breathe to help keep the lungs inflated and promote effective gas exchange. Inadequate ventilation due to pain, narcotics, and anesthesia causes CO_2 retention and respiratory acidosis.

In respiratory acidosis, Mr. Drum would (hypoventilate/hyperventilate)

_____ .

Indicate the type of breathing associated with CO_2 retention (respiratory acidosis). (Refer to Chapter 4 if needed.)

( ) a. Deep, rapid, vigorous breathing
( ) b. Dyspnea—difficult or labored breathing
( ) c. Overbreathing

hypoventilate
a. —; b. X; c. —

■   ■   ■

CASE STUDY REVIEW

Preoperatively the nurse should assess Mr. Drum's fluid and electrolytes and kidney function. To assess the fluid balance, the nurse checks all laboratory findings.

1. Mr. Drum's elevated hemoglobin and hematocrit on admission and the first day postoperatively is indicative of _____ .

2. His elevated BUN is also indicative of _____ and possibly of
   * _____ .

3. Mr. Drum's serum sodium and chloride were low due to fluid loss. His serum potassium was 5.2 mEq/L on admission. Explain why Mr. Drum's serum potassium is a high normal with vomiting and dehydration. * _____
   _____
   _____ .

4. What happened to Mr. Drum's serum potassium level when he was hydrated?
   * _____ .

5. Mr. Drum's decreased serum CO_2 may indicate * _____
   _____ .

6. What type of fluid imbalance may occur when rapidly hydrating a debilitated individual with 4–5 liters of fluid intravenously? * _____
   _____ .

7. If Mr. Drum were hydrated with 4–5 liters of 5% dextrose in water, what type of fluid imbalance might occur? * _____ .
   Explain why. * _____
   _____ .

8. Mr. Drum received intravenous fluids containing dextrose, saline, and lactated Ringer's for:
   a. Replacing _____ and _____ loss
   b. Maintaining _____ needs
   c. Maintaining _____ balance
   d. Replacing and maintaining * _____

9. Frequent irrigations of the gastric tube with a large quantity of water might have what effect?
   * _____
   _____ .

10. The three methods that the nurse used to maintain the patency of Mr. Drum's gastric tube are
    * _____ , * _____ , and * _____ .

11. Why is it important for the nurse to assess Mr. Drum's urine output pre- and postoperatively?
    * _____
    _____
    _____ .

12. Why is it important for Mr. Drum to cough and deep breathe after surgery?
    * _____
    _____ .

1. *dehydration*
2. *dehydration; renal impairment*
3. *With dehydration, potassium is lost from cells and accumulates in ECF. If urine volume is low, the serum potassium level could increase.*
4. *serum potassium level decreased, with hydration*
5. *metabolic acidosis*
6. *hypervolemia or overhydration*
7. *water intoxication. Dextrose is metabolized rapidly by the body, leaving water or hypo-osmolar, fluid which passes into cells.*
8. a. *sodium; chloride*
   b. *nutritional*
   c. *electrolyte*
   d. *fluid volume*
9. *depletion of electrolytes in the GI tract*
10. *irrigating with small amounts of saline, changing the client's position, and introducing a small amount of air and listening with a stethoscope for a "whoosh" sound*
11. *to determine kidney function. Also, it can be an indication of overhydration. When fluids—orally and parenterally—are being pushed and urine output is low, overhydration can occur.*
12. *to inflate the lungs and promote effective gas (O_2 and CO_2) exchange*

NURSING ASSESSMENT FACTORS

- Clients undergoing gastrointestinal surgery are at an increased risk for fluid and electrolyte disturbances. Preexisting health status and medications further increase the potential risk for fluid and electrolyte disturbances. Clients with preexisting cardiac, pulmonary, endocrine, and renal disease who have gastrointestinal surgery add further challenges for the nurse. Uncorrected preoperative hypovolemia and anemia may increase the risk of fluid and electrolyte disturbances postoperatively.
- Astute assessments and early interventions improve the client's recovery rate and decrease postoperative complications. Fluid and electrolyte imbalances may have deleterious effects on cardiac conductivity, contractility, and rhythm. Pulmonary gas exchange and renal tissue perfusion are also affected by fluid and electrolyte imbalances. Gastrointestinal intubation tubes are used postoperatively to decompress the stomach and intestines to prevent abdominal distension and prevent or relieve nausea and vomiting. The amount of GI drainage must be considered when assessing fluid and electrolyte balance.
- To reduce the client's risk for postoperative complications, the nurse should assess vital signs with close attention to blood pressure and pulse rate, rhythm, and volume. Decreased fluid volume causes hypotension, orthostatic hypotension, decreased pulse pressure, and reflex tachycardia. Potassium disturbances may cause cardiac conduction and rhythm disturbances. Assess peripheral pulses for presence and quality. Hypovolemic states may decrease peripheral pulse quality and may ultimately lead to peripheral thrombosis in extreme states.
- Auscultate cardiac sounds for presence or worsening of an S_4, which may indicate an overstretched myocardium from a fluid volume excess. Check respirations every 2 hours or more frequently if indicated. Hypoventilation may occur as a result of the decreased rate and depth of respirations due to pain from the abdominal incision and the side effects of anesthesia and pain

medications. Auscultate lungs for rales or crackles, which indicate retention of fluid in the alveoli. Frequent coughing and deep breathing will expand the lung alveoli, help prevent the occurrence and buildup of pulmonary secretions, and prevent atelectasis.

- Measure intake and output hourly in the acute stage and every 8 hours for clients who have stabilized. Careful monitoring of intake and output is essential to ascertain the client's ongoing fluid volume status. Daily weights are essential for monitoring the overall fluid volume status. Urinary output relative to specific gravity also helps determine the adequacy of the client's renal perfusion.
- Assess skin turgor at least every 8 hours: Hot, dry, scaly skin with poor turgor indicates a fluid volume deficit. Sacral and/or peripheral edema may indicate a fluid volume excess. Assess serum electrolytes daily and more frequently according to the client's overall health status. Low potassium (hypokalemia) levels may indicate excess diuresis, inadequate replacement, or postoperative excess antidiuretic hormone release. High potassium levels (hyperkalemia) may indicate excess potassium administration or impaired renal tubule function even when the total output is adequate in volume. Monitor creatinine/BUN and hemoglobin-hematocrit ratios as an indicator of fluid volume status as well as impaired renal functioning. Creatinine/BUN ratios greater than 1 : 20 indicate a fluid volume deficit. Hemoglobin-hematocrit ratios greater than 1 : 3 also indicate a fluid volume deficit.
- Ascertain current and preoperative medication regimes. Potassium-wasting diuretics such as HydroDiuril may further aggravate low potassium levels. Potassium-sparing diuretics such as aldactone may precipitate or further aggravate high potassium levels. Clients receiving steroids also need close monitoring of potassium. Steroids may cause or aggravate hypokalemia and hypernatremia as well as increase fluid retention.
- Assess client's bowel sounds. Oral fluids and foods are not introduced postoperatively until bowel sounds are returned. Be sure to turn off the suction to GI intubation tubes before auscultation of the abdomen.
- Maintain patency of GI tubes to ensure proper functioning. Irrigating GI tubes with normal saline or air every 2 hours will help ensure their patency. Proper location of gastric tubes may be determined by auscultating the stomach for a "whoosh" sound while injecting air into the tube. Changing the client's position frequently helps to prevent the tube lumen from lodging against the gastric mucosa.
- Assess the client's mental status pre- and postoperatively. Changes in mental status reflecting irritability and confusion may be a primary indicator of a fluid volume excess or deficit. Left untreated, the client's condition may deteriorate to the point of seizures or coma.
- Assess blood glucose for clients with preexisting hyperadrenal secretions and diabetes mellitus. Uncontrolled hyperglycemia will cause osmotic diuresis and fluid volume deficit.

NURSING DIAGNOSIS 1

High risk for ineffective airway clearance, related to pain, ineffective coughing, deep breathing, and viscous mucous secretions.

NURSING INTERVENTIONS AND RATIONALE

1. Elevate head of bed 45°–90° and change every 2 hours to promote lung expansion and take advantage of gravity decreasing diaphragmatic pressure.
2. Encourage coughing and deep breathing hourly while awake, and wake every 2–4 during sleeping hours, to improve alveolar expansion, mobilize secretions, and prevent atelectasis.

3. Splint abdominal incision to decrease pain and maximize effects of coughing and deep breathing exercises.
4. Suction orally and/or nasotracheally to clear airway.
5. Auscultate lung fields for rales (crackles) and respiratory movement.
6. Observe for signs of respiratory distress—tachypnea, restlessness, anxiety, moistness of mucous membranes, and use of accessory muscles of breathing.
7. Maintain adequate hydration to liquify and mobilize pulmonary secretions.
8. Provide opportunities for rest to prevent fatigue and facilitate coughing and deep breathing.

NURSING DIAGNOSIS 2

Fluid volume deficit, related to GI loss, decreased fluid intake, and fluid volume shift.

NURSING INTERVENTIONS AND RATIONALE

1. Monitor intake and output at least every 8 hours and weigh daily to determine changes in fluid volume. In normovolemic clients, intake should be approximately 500 mL more than output in a 24-hour period. For hypovolemic clients intake should be greater than 500 mL for the total output in 24 hours. Hypervolemic clients should have an output equal to or greater than their intake.
2. Take blood pressure and pulse (include orthostatics) every 4 hours or more frequently if client is unstable. Hypovolemic clients will have reflex tachycardia and hypotension. A blood pressure decrease of more than 20 mm Hg systolic or a pulse increase of more than 10 beats per minute with position changes indicate hypovolemia.
3. Check mucous membranes and skin turgor. Poor skin turgor with dry scaly skin and dry mucous membranes indicates a fluid volume deficit.
4. Check temperature every 4 hours. Body water acts as a coolant and temperature increases as body water decreases.
5. Monitor for peripheral and sacral edema to determine fluid shifts from ECF to ICF volume.
6. Palpate peripheral pulses every 4 hours for presence and volume. Hypovolemia decreases the volume of peripheral pulses.
7. Assess creatinine/BUN and Hgb-Hct ratios for hemoconcentration which indicates hypovolemia versus renal failure.
8. Assess serum potassium and sodium to determine changes. Hyperkalemia and hypernatremia may be early indicators of decreased body waters.
9. Measure urine specific gravity every 8 hours as the fluid volume decreases, unless there is renal failure.
10. Note medications that can alter fluid status and electrolyte alterations such as diuretics, insulin, and steroids.

NURSING DIAGNOSIS 3

Pain, related to trauma of abdominal surgery, decreased or absent bowel sounds, and decreased GI motility.

NURSING INTERVENTIONS AND RATIONALE

1. Ascertain cause of pain and treat accordingly. Medicate for surgical wound pain. Ascertain and maintain the correct functioning of GI tubes to decrease distention, nausea, and vomiting.

2. Evaluate client's response and attitude to pain. Determine pain characteristics and degree of pain; use a 0–10 scale. Observe verbal and nonverbal cues. Explore cultural aspects of pain and methods of control.
3. Medicate for pain to enhance effectiveness of ambulation, coughing, and deep breathing exercises.
4. Use diversional activities to increase pain threshold, e.g., visitors, television, calm environment, relaxation exercises, and reading.

Behavioral Objectives

Upon completion of this chapter, you will be prepared to:

• Discuss the physiologic changes in fluids and electrolytes that occur as the result of traumatic injuries and shock.

• Describe the clinical manifestations associated with traumatic injuries and shock.

• Discuss the nursing assessment guide for fluids, electrolyte, and acid-base imbalances in the traumatically injured client.

• Identify the four types of shock and the physiologic basis for specific clinical symptoms.

• Discuss the clinical management of traumatic injuries related to the four types of shock.

• Identify the nursing assessment factors for evaluating shock and trauma clients.

• Develop nursing diagnoses and interventions with rationale appropriate in the clinical treatment of trauma and shock clients.

Introduction

This chapter is divided into two sections relating to fluid and electrolyte changes: trauma and shock.

TRAUMA

Fluid, electrolyte, and acid-base changes occur rapidly in the acutely traumatized patient. Quick medical and nursing assessments and actions are needed for survival.

In trauma (acute injury), the sodium shifts into cells, potassium shifts, and the fluid shifts from the vascular to the interstitial spaces and cells. These shifts can result in severe fluid and electrolyte imbalances.

1   The two electrolytes that change spaces during trauma are _____ and

_____ .

      Explain the fluid shifts during trauma.   *_____

_____ .

potassium and sodium
Fluid shifts from the vascular to the interstitial spaces and cells.

■   ■   ■

PATHOPHYSIOLOGY

Following a severe traumatic injury, there is cellular breakdown due to cell damage and hypoxia. The physiologic changes that occur during trauma are described in Table 9-1. Be familiar with these physiologic changes and their causative factors. The information in this table will help you to accurately assess traumatic injuries.

Table 9-1. PHYSIOLOGIC CHANGES ASSOCIATED WITH TRAUMA	
Physiologic Changes	**Causative Factors**
Potassium, sodium, chloride, bicarbonate	Potassium is lost from cells due to catabolism (cellular breakdown). As potassium leaves, sodium and chloride with water shift into the cells. The sodium pump does not function properly (see Chapter 3).
Fluid changes	Fluids along with sodium shift into cells and to the third space (interstitial space—at the injured site). The increased cellular and third-space fluids cause a vascular fluid deficit (dehydration) and hyponatremia.
	Serum osmolality may be normal or increased due to the fluid deficit and excess solutes other than sodium, such as potassium and urea. Remember, sodium influences the osmolality of plasma. (see Chapter 1).
	The volume and composition of extracellular fluid (ECF) fluctuates depending on the number of cells injured and the body's ability to restore balance. Two to 3 days following injury, fluid shifts from the third space at the injured site back into the vascular space.
Protein changes	Trauma results in nitrogen loss due to increased protein catabolism, decreased protein anabolism, and/or a protein shift with water to the interstitial space. The colloid osmotic pressure is decreased in the vascular fluid and increased in the interstitial fluid (tissues), which causes fluid volume deficit (vascular) and edema.
Capillary permeability	Increased capillary permeability causes water to flow into and out of the cells and into tissue spaces. This contributes to hypovolemia (fluid volume deficit).
Hormonal influence	ADH and aldosterone help to restore the ECF. A vascular fluid deficit and/or increased serum osmolality stimulates ADH secretion, which causes water reabsorption from the distal tubules of the kidneys. In certain traumatic situations (surgery, trauma, pain), SIADH (syndrome of inappropriate ADH) occurs and causes excess water reabsorption from the kidneys.
	Aldosterone is secreted from the adrenal cortex due to hyponatremia and stress. Aldosterone promotes sodium reabsorption from the renal tubules and is reabsorbed with water. Potassium is excreted.

Table 9-1. (Continued)	
Physiologic Changes	**Causative Factors**
Kidney influence	Kidney activity is altered during and after a severe traumatic injury. Sodium, chloride, and water shift to the injured site, which causes hypovolemia. Decreased circulatory flow can decrease renal arterial flow, which can cause temporary or permanent kidney damage. Decreased kidney function results in hyperkalemia.
Acid-base changes	With cellular breakdown nonvolatile acids (acid metabolites), e.g., lactic acid, increase in the vascular fluid, causing metabolic acidosis.
	Kidneys conserve or excrete the hydrogen ion to maintain the acid-base balance. Decreased kidney function can cause hydrogen retention and acidosis.
	The lungs try to compensate for the acidotic state by blowing off excess CO_2—hyperventilation. Blowing off CO_2 decreases the formation of carbonic acid.

2   Explain what happens to the following electrolytes and water:

   a. Potassium *_____ .
   b. Sodium *_____ .
   c. Chloride *_____ .
   d. Water *_____ .

a. potassium is lost from the cells; b. sodium shifts into the cells; c. chloride shifts into the cells; d. water shifts into the cells

    ■   ■   ■

3   The sodium pump is necessary for cellular activity (see Table 3-12).

   Explain the sodium pump action. *_____

_____ .

To maintain cellular activity, sodium shifts into the cells and potassium shifts out of the cells. Or, sodium shifts into the cell and depolarization occurs, and then potassium shifts back into the cell and repolarization occurs.

    ■   ■   ■

4   During and after an acute injury, fluids shift to _____ and

*_____ .

Do you know what is meant by fluids shifting to the third space? *_____

_____ .

cells and injured site(s) or cells and interstitial (third) space
Fluids shift to the interstitial space at the injured site. Fluid in the third space is considered
physiologically useless or nonfunctional fluid.

■   ■   ■

5   With vascular fluid deficit (loss), the serum osmolality is (increased/decreased)

_____ .

What happens to the permeability of capillaries as a result of injury?

*_____ .

increased; increase or *increased capillary permeability*

■   ■   ■

6   Explain how ADH and aldosterone restore water balance.

ADH   *_____ .

Aldosterone   *_____ .

ADH promotes water absorption from the distal tubules of the kidneys due to hypovolemia
and/or the increased serum osmolality.
Aldosterone causes sodium to be reabsorbed from the distal tubules of the kidney when
hyponatremia or stress is present.

■   ■   ■

7   The syndrome of inappropriate antidiuretic hormone secretions (SIADH) frequently occurs
following surgery, trauma, stress, pain, and CNS depressants (narcotics). The water
reabsorption can be continuous for several days.

The nurse should assess for what type of fluid imbalance:

( ) a. Overhydration (hypervolemia)
( ) b. Dehydration (hypovolemia)

a. X; b. —

■   ■   ■

8 Kidneys are the chief regulators of sodium and water balance. Kidneys conserve sodium when there is a sodium deficit. The hormone that is responsible for sodium reabsorption is _____ . This hormone also causes potassium (excretion/retention). _____ .

aldosterone; excretion
■ ■ ■

9 A decrease in circulation from trauma, stress, or shock can cause a decrease in renal arterial blood flow. What effect does this have on the kidney?
* _____

For circulating blood to perfuse the kidneys, the systolic blood pressure should be _____ mm Hg or greater. (Refer to Chapter 2, ECFV deficit, if needed.).

temporary or permanent kidney damage; 60
■ ■ ■

10 Severe trauma releases nonvolatile acids (acid metabolites), such as lactic acid, from cells. What type of acid-base imbalance can occur? *_____ .
How do the lungs compensate for this imbalance? *_____ .

metabolic acidosis; by blowing off CO_2 (reducing carbonic acid)
■ ■ ■

11 From the following list of fluid, electrolyte, and acid-base changes, check those that are affected by trauma, and correct the incorrect responses.

( ) a. Cellular loss of potassium
( ) b. Sodium shifts into cells
( ) c. Hypervolemia or overhydration
( ) d. Fluid shifts to the cells and injured site(s)
( ) e. Protein loss
( ) f. Decreased capillary permeability
( ) g. ADH secretion promoting reabsorption of water from the kidneys

a. X; b. X; c. —; d. X; e. X; f. —; g. X
Corrections: c. hypovolemia or dehydration; f. increased capillary permeability
■ ■ ■

CLINICAL MANIFESTATIONS

The physician assesses the injured sites, orders fluid replacements, and performs medical or surgical interventions as needed.

The nurse's responsibility is to assess and report fluid, electrolyte, and acid-base imbalances as they occur.

12   The three imbalances that the nurse should assess are _____ , _____ , and _____ .

fluids, electrolytes, and acid-base

■   ■   ■

The clinical manifestations that frequently occur in traumatic injuries depend upon the type of imbalance (fluid, electrolyte, or acid-base) and include changes in vital signs, behavioral changes, cardiac conduction changes, venous changes, renal changes, neuromuscular changes, integumentary changes, and laboratory findings. Table 9-2 lists the signs and symptoms that may occur as the result of trauma. For further clarification of these changes and rationale, refer to Table 9-3 on assessment.

13   Indicate the effects of trauma on the vital signs:

   a. Pulse   *_____ .
   b. Blood pressure   *_____ .
   c. Respiration   *_____ .
   d. Temperature   *_____ .

   a. *tachycardia, irregular pulse rate, or full-bounding pulse*
   b. *slightly decreased blood pressure, narrow pulse pressure*
   c. *tachypnea, dyspnea, or deep vigorous breathing*
   d. *slightly elevated temperature (body fluid loss)*

■   ■   ■

14   Behavioral changes are frequently observed with fluid and electrolyte imbalances.

   Name two behavioral changes that can occur following severe trauma.
   _____ and _____ .

irritability and confusion (also restlessness, disorientation)

■   ■   ■

15   Trauma usually results in loss of body fluid. When elevated above the heart level the hand veins become (engorged/flat) _____ .

flat

■   ■   ■

Clinical Manifestations	Signs and Symptoms

Table 9-2.   CLINICAL MANIFESTATIONS RELATED TO TRAUMA

Vital Signs

Pulse — Increased pulse rate (tachycardia) / Irregular pulse rate / Full-bounding pulse

Blood pressure — Blood pressure slightly depressed unless severe fluid loss occurs / Pulse pressure narrows

Respiration — Increased breathing (tachypnea) / Dyspnea / Deep, vigorous breathing (Kussmaul breathing)

Temperature — Slightly elevated temperature unless infection is present

Behavioral changes — Irritability, restlessness, and confusion

Cardiac conduction changes — ECG: T-wave changes (inverted or peaked), ST-segment changes

Venous changes — Neck and hand vein engorgement / No vein engorgement

Renal changes — Hourly urine output decreases

Neuromuscular changes — Muscular weakness / Abdominal distention / Tetany symptoms

Integumentary changes — Poor skin turgor / Dry mucous membrane / Edema / Diaphoresis / Draining wound, exudate

Laboratory Findings

Electrolytes ↓ or ↑ — Serum potassium, sodium, magnesia, chloride may be decreased or increased

Serum CO_2 — Decreased CO_2 indicates metabolic acidosis; increased CO_2 indicates metabolic alkalosis

BUN ↑ — Increased BUN: fluid loss or decreased renal function

Serum creatinine ↑ — Increased serum creatinine indicates decreased renal function

Arterial blood gases: pH, $Paco_2$, HCO_3 — Decreased pH and HCO_3 indicate metabolic acidosis

16 Urine output following trauma may be _____ .

Following trauma, urine output should be checked (every hour/every 8 hours/once a day) _____ .

decreased; every hour

■   ■   ■

17 Integumentary changes may not be noted immediately following severe trauma with fluid losses. However, after several hours or a day, the skin turgor can be affected and mucous membranes become (dry/wet) _____ .

These signs indicate (hypovolemia/hypervolemia) _____ .

dry; hypovolemia

■   ■   ■

18 Many abnormal laboratory results occur in severe trauma.

Cellular breakdown and poor urine output (increase/decrease) _____ the serum potassium level.

Poor renal function causes the BUN and serum creatinine to (increase/decrease) _____ .

Frequently, metabolic acidosis results following severe trauma due to cellular breakdown and poor tissue perfusion. Which arterial blood gas changes are indicative of metabolic acidosis?

( ) a. pH decreased
( ) b. $Paco_2$ increased
( ) c. HCO_3 decreased

increase; increase; a. X; b. —; c. X

■   ■   ■

CLINICAL APPLICATIONS

Nursing assessment is vitally important when planning and implementing nursing care. Table 9-3 is a guide that the nurse may use when assessing the client for fluid, electrolyte, and acid-base imbalances. The table includes key observations, nursing assessment factors, and rationale/comments. To understand the significance of the nursing assessment, the rationale helps to identify the type of imbalance that is present. Use this table in clinical assessments.

Table 9-3. NURSING ASSESSMENT OF FLUID, ELECTROLYTE, AND ACID-BASE IMBALANCES IN THE TRAUMATICALLY INJURED CLIENT

Observation	Nursing Assessment		Rationale/Comments
1. Vital signs: Pulse	Pulse rate Volume Pattern	_____ _____ _____	Changes in vital signs (VSs) are indicators of client's physiologic status. Several VSs should be taken and the first reading acts as the baseline for comparison. Pulse rate and pattern should be monitored frequently. Pulse rate > 120 may indicate hypovolemia and the possibility of shock. Full, bounding pulse can mean hypervolemia and an irregular pulse can mean hypokalemia.
Blood pressure	Admission BP Time Time	 _____ _____	Changes in BP (systolic and diastolic) may not occur until several hours after the injury. Several BP readings should be taken, and the first BP reading acts as the baseline and for comparison. A drop in systolic pressure can indicate hypovolemia. Pulse pressure (systolic minus diastolic) of <20 can indicate shock.
Respiration	Respiration Pattern	_____ _____	Note changes in rate, depth, and pattern. A rate >32 can indicate hypovolemia. Deep, rapid, vigorous breathing can indicate acidosis as a result of cellular damage and shock. Hyperventilating (fast, shallow breathing) can be due to anxiety or hypoxia.
Temperature	Temperature on admission Date/Time	_____ _____	Changes in temperature do not occur immediately after an injury. If there is a slight elevation several hours or days later, it can indicate hypovolemia or impending shock.
2. Behavioral changes	Irritable Apprehensive Restless Confused Delirious Lethargic	_____ _____ _____ _____ _____ _____	Irritability, apprehension, restlessness, and confusion are indicators of hypoxia and later of fluid and electrolyte imbalances (hypovolemia, water intoxication, and potassium imbalance).

3. Neurologic and neuromuscular signs	Sensorium
	  Confused
	  Semiconscious
	  Comatose
	Muscle weakness
	Abdominal distention
	Pupil dilation
	Tetany
	  Tremors
	  Twitching
	Others
		
		_____
		_____
		_____
		_____
		_____
		
		_____
		_____
		_____
			Changes in sensorium can be indicative of fluid imbalance. Muscle weakness and abdominal distention may be due to a potassium deficit (may not occur for hours or days later). Symptoms of tetany can indicate a calcium and magnesium deficit.

4. Fluid loss	Wound(s)
	Urine
	  Number of voidings
	  Amount
	    mL/h
	    mL/8 h
	    mL/24 h
	  Color
	  Specific gravity
		_____
		
		_____
		_____
		_____
		_____
		_____
		_____
		_____
			Note the presence of an open draining wound. Kidneys regulate fluids and electrolytes. Monitoring the urine output hourly is most important. Oliguria can indicate a lack of fluid intake or renal insufficiency due to decreased circulation/circulatory collapse or hypovolemia.

Table 9-3. (Continued)

Observation	Nursing Assessment		Rationale/Comments

	Vomitus
	  Number
	  Consistency
	  Amount
		_____
		_____
		_____
			Frequent vomiting in large quantities leads to fluid, electrolyte (potassium, sodium, chloride), and hydrogen losses. Metabolic alkalosis can occur.

	Nasogastric tube
	  Amount—mL/8h
	  Amount—mL/24 h
		_____
		_____
			Gastrointestinal secretions should be measured. Large quantity losses of GI secretions can cause hypovolemia.

	Drain(s)
	  Number
	  Amount
		_____
		_____
			Excess drainage could contribute to fluid loss and should be measured if possible.

5. Skin and mucous membrane	Skin color
	  Pale
	  Gray
	  Flushed
		_____
		_____
			Pale and/or gray-colored skin can indicate hypovolemia or shock. Flushed skin can be due to hypernatremia or metabolic acidosis.

	Skin turgor
	  Normal
	  Poor
		_____
		_____
			Poor skin turgor can result from hypovolemia/dehydration. This may not occur until 1–3 days after the injury.

	Edema—pitting peripheral
	  Feet
	  Legs
		_____
		_____
			Edema indicates sodium and water retention. Sodium, chloride, and water shift into the cells and to the injury site(s) (interstitial or third space).

	Dry mucous membranes Sticky secretions	_____ _____	Dry, tenacious (sticky) secretions and dry membranes are indicative of dehydration or fluid loss. This may not occur until 1–3 days after the injury.
	Diaphoresis	_____	Increased insensible fluid loss can result from diaphoresis (excess perspiration). Amount of fluid loss from skin can double.
6. Chest sounds and vein engorgement	Chest rales	_____	The chest should be checked for rales due to overhydration (pulmonary edema).
	Neck vein engorgement Hand vein engorgement	_____ _____	Neck and hand vein engorgements are indicators of fluid excess. Rales and vein engorgements can occur from excess IV fluids or rapid IV administration.

7. ECG (EKG)	T wave
	  Flat
	  Inverted
	  Peaked
		_____
		_____
			Flat and inverted T waves indicate cardiac ischemia and/or a potassium deficit. Peaked T waves indicate a potassium excess.

8. Fluid intake	Oral fluid intake
	  Amount
	    mL/8 h
	    mL/24 h
		_____
		_____
			Oral fluids should not be given until the injury(s) can be assessed. If surgery is indicated, the client should be NPO.

	Types of IV fluids
	  Crystalloids
	  Colloids
	  Blood
	  Amount
	    mL/8 h
	    mL/24 h
	    mL/h
		_____
		_____
		_____
		
		_____
		_____
		_____
			Crystalloids, i.e., 5% dextrose in water, normal saline, lactated Ringer's, are normally ordered first to restore fluid loss, correct shocklike symptoms, restore or increase urine output, and serve as a lifeline to administer IV drugs.
			
			Five percent dextrose in water given continuously can cause water intoxication (ICF volume excess).

Table 9-3. (Continued)

Observation	Nursing Assessment		Rationale/Comments
9. Previous drug regime	Diuretics Digitalis Cortisone Antibiotics	_____ _____ _____ _____	A drug history should be taken and reported to the physician. Potassium-wasting diuretics taken with a digitalis preparation can cause digitalis toxicity. Cortisone causes sodium retention and potassium excretion. Antibiotics cause sodium retention.
10. Chemistry, hematology, and arterial blood gas changes	Electrolytes *Serum* K _____ Na _____ Cl _____ Ca _____ Mg _____	*Urine/24 h* K _____ Na _____ Cl _____	Electrolytes should be drawn immediately after a severe injury and used as a baseline for future electrolyte results. (See Chapter 3 for normal values.) Urine electrolytes are compared to serum electrolytes. Normal range for urine electrolytes are: K 25–120 mEq/24 h Na 40–220 mEq/24 h Cl 150–250 mEq/24 h
	Serum CO$_2$	_____	Serum CO$_2$ >32 mEq/L indicates metabolic alkalosis and <22 mEq/L indicates metabolic acidosis.

	Osmolality
	  Serum
	  Urine
		_____
		_____
			Serum osmolality >295 mOsm/kg indicates hypovolemia/dehydration and <280 mOsm/kg indicates hypervolemia. Urine osmolality can be 100–1200 mOsm/kg with a normal range of 200–600 mOsm/kg.

	BUN
	Creatinine
		_____
		_____
			An elevated BUN can indicate fluid volume deficit or kidney insufficiency. Elevated creatinine indicates kidney damage.
			
			Normal range:
			  BUN 10–25 mg/dL
			  Creatinine 0.7–1.4 mg/dL

	Blood glucose	_____	Blood sugar increases during stress (up to 180 mg/dL)
	Hbg _____	Hct _____	Elevated hemoglobin and hematocrit can indicate hemoconcentration caused by fluid volume deficit (hypovolemia).

	Arterial blood gases
	(ABGs)
	  pH
	  Pa$_{CO_2}$
	  HCO$_3$
	  BE
		
		_____
		_____
		_____
		_____
			pH: <7.35 indicates acidosis and >7.45 indicates alkalosis.
			
			Pa$_{CO_2}$ (respiratory component):
			  Norms 35–45 mm Hg
			Respiratory acidosis (↓ pH, ↑ Pa$_{CO_2}$) may occur due to inadequate gas exchange. A ↑ pH and ↓ Pa$_{CO_2}$ indicate respiratory alkalosis from hyperventilating due to anxiety and apprehension.
			
			HCO$_3$ (renal component):
			  Norms 24–28 mEq/L
			A ↓ HCO$_3$ and ↓ pH means metabolic acidosis, which is the most common acid-base imbalance following injury. Cellular catabolism occurs. (See Table 9-1.)
			
			A ↑ HCO$_3$ and ↑ pH means metabolic alkalosis.
			
			BE (base excess)
			  Norms +2 to −2. Same as bicarbonate.

19 Vital signs should be constantly monitored during an acute injury. Tachycardia or pulse rate greater than 120 can indicate _____ and should be reported.

hypovolemia or fluid volume deficit

    ■   ■   ■

20 Blood pressure does not immediately fall after an injury. With a fluid volume deficit, the pulse rate increases first, and later the blood pressure drops if fluid loss is not replaced.

    A pulse pressure of less than 20 can indicate _____ .

shock

    ■   ■   ■

21 A respiratory rate greater than 32 can indicate _____ .

    Deep, rapid, vigorous breathing occurring after cellular damage or shock due to acute injury can indicate (metabolic acidosis/metabolic alkalosis). *_____ Why?

*_____ .

hypovolemia or fluid volume deficit; metabolic acidosis
Acid metabolites, such as lactic acid, are released from cells due to cellular breakdown.

    ■   ■   ■

22 Temperature changes frequently do not occur immediately after injury. When there is a slight temperature elevation, this can indicate _____ .

    If a high temperature elevation occurs 3–5 days after the injury, what might it indicate?

_____ .

hypovolemia or a fluid volume deficit or dehydration; infection

    ■   ■   ■

23 Irritability, apprehension, restlessness, and confusion are usually the result of hypoxia and of fluid and electrolyte imbalances. Name two fluid and one electrolyte imbalance associated with the stated behavioral changes.

Fluid imbalances: *_____ and *_____

_____ .

Electrolyte imbalance: _____ .

hypovolemia or fluid volume deficit; water intoxication; hypokalemia

    ■   ■   ■

24 Match the neurologic and neuromuscular signs on the left with fluid and electrolyte imbalances on the right:

___ 1. Decreased sensorium
___ 2. Muscle weakness
___ 3. Abdominal distention
___ 4. Tetany—tremors and twitching

a. Hypokalemia
b. Hypovolemia
c. Hypocalcemia

1. b; 2. a; 3. a; 4. c
■   ■   ■

25 Oliguria is not uncommon following an acute injury. Decreased urine output can be due to
* _____ .

Do you recall what elevated specific gravity (>1.030) indicates?   *_____ .

hypovolemia, circulatory collapse, or a lack of fluid intake; dehydration/hypovolemia or lack of fluid intake
■   ■   ■

26 Vomitus, nasogastric tubes, and diarrhea can cause what type of fluid imbalance?
_____ .

Indicate which acid-base imbalance listed on the right occurs with the causes of fluid loss listed on the left:

___ 1. Vomiting
___ 2. Nasogastric tubes (loss of stomach secretions)
___ 3. Diarrhea

a. Metabolic alkalosis
b. Metabolic acidosis

hypovolemia; 1. a; 2. a; 3. b
■   ■   ■

27 Pale or gray-colored skin can indicate _____ .

Poor skin turgor, dry mucous membranes, and tenacious or sticky mucous secretions are indicative of _____ .

hypovolemia or shock; dehydration or fluid loss
■   ■   ■

28 When the client is receiving IV therapy at an increased flow rate to correct fluid loss, the client should be assessed for potential signs of overhydration.

Excess and/or rapidly administered IV fluids can cause what type of fluid imbalance? _____ .

Name two symptoms associated with this imbalance. (Refer to Chapter 2, section on ECFVE.) * _____ and * _____ .

overhydration or ECFV excess (extracellular cellular fluid volume excess)
chest rales and neck or hand vein engorgement (also constant irritating cough or dyspnea)
■ ■ ■

29 A flat or inverted T wave can indicate _____ , and a peaked T wave can indicate _____ .

hypokalemia or potassium deficit or cardiac ischemia; hyperkalemia or potassium excess
■ ■ ■

30 Immediately after an acute injury, oral fluids (should/should not) _____ be given. Why? * _____ .

should not
The patient may need surgery and would be NPO (nothing by mouth).
■ ■ ■

31 Indicate which of the following are crystalloids used in IV therapy.

( ) a. Dextrose 5% in water (D_5W)
( ) b. Dextran 40, 6%
( ) c. Plasmanate
( ) d. Normal saline (0.9% NaCl)
( ) e. Lactated Ringer's

Give two reasons for using crystalloids. * _____ and
* _____ .

What type of fluid imbalance occurs when using 5% dextrose in water for several days?
* _____ .

a. X; b. —; c. —; d. X; e. X
to restore fluid loss and correct shocklike symptoms (correction may be temporary) (also, increase urine output)
water intoxication (ICFV excess). In early shock/trauma massive infusions of D_5W can cause hyperglycemia and increased diuresis.
Dextrose 5% in water may not be the choice crystalloid.

           ■   ■   ■

32 Identify the drugs that cause sodium retention.

    ( ) a. Diuretics   ( ) c. Cortisone
    ( ) b. Digitalis   ( ) d. Antibiotics

Which of the following drugs cause potassium excretion?

    ( ) e. Diuretics (potassium wasting) ( ) g. Cortisone
    ( ) f. Digitalis   ( ) h. Antibiotics

a. —; b. —; c. X; d. X; e. X; f. —; g. X; h.—

           ■   ■   ■

33 After a severe injury, the serum potassium level may be (increased/decreased) _____ even with a normal urine output.

    Which type of sodium imbalance may be present? _____ . If lactic acid is released from the cells due to cellular breakdown, would the serum CO_2 be (increased/decreased)? _____ . Serum CO_2 is a bicarbonate determinant.

decreased (can be in normal range when there is severe cell damage—excess release of potassium. If urine output is poor, serum K would be increased.)
hyponatremia; decreased

           ■   ■   ■

34 A serum osmolality greater than 295 mOsm/kg indicates (hypovolemia/hypervolemia). _____ .

    A serum osmolality less than 280 mOsm/kg indicates (hypovolemia/hypervolemia). _____ . Why? *_____

_____ .

hypovolemia; hypervolemia
It is caused from overhydration or hemodilution (excess water in proportion to solutes).

           ■   ■   ■

35 An elevated BUN can indicate *_____ or *_____ .

   After hydration, if the BUN does not return to normal, the elevated BUN indicates

   *_____ .

   An elevated hemoglobin and hematocrit level can indicate hemoconcentration caused by

   _____ .

   fluid volume deficit; renal insufficiency; renal insufficiency; hypovolemia or fluid volume deficit

   ■   ■   ■

36 What type of acid-base imbalance is present if the client's arterial blood gases are: pH 7.25; $Paco_2$ 35 mm Hg; and HCO_3 18 mEq/L? *_____ .

   metabolic acidosis

   ■   ■   ■

37 From the following list of observations and nursing assessments, mark the ones that indicate fluid volume deficit (hypovolemia).

   ( ) a. Pulse 76
   ( ) b. Blood pressure 86/68
   ( ) c. Irritability, restlessness, confusion
   ( ) d. Specific gravity 1.034
   ( ) e. Excess GI drainage (>2 liters)
   ( ) f. Dry mucuous membrane and dry, tenacious mucous secretions
   ( ) g. Chest rales
   ( ) h. Peaked T waves
   ( ) i. Elevated BUN and Hgb

   a. —; b. X; c. X; d. X; e. X; f. X; g. —; h. —; i. X

   ■   ■   ■

CASE STUDY REVIEW

Marjorie Rockland, age 58, was in an automobile accident and was taken by ambulance to the emergency room of a large medical center. Her vital signs on admission are blood pressure 134/88, pulse rate 106, respiration 30, temperature 98.8°F (37.1°C). She complained of pain in her abdomen and leg. A liter of 5% dextrose in water is started. Blood chemistry and x-rays (leg and abdomen) are ordered. Abdominal area appears distended, and there are diminished bowel sounds. A nasogastric tube is inserted and attached to intermittent suction.

1. Ms. Rockland's pulse rate indicates tachycardia (mild to moderate) and can be indicative of
   *_____ .

2. Her blood pressure is (normal/high/low) _____ and may mean
   *_____ .

3. Name the solution category for 5% dextrose in water. *_____ .
4. A distended abdomen and decreased peristalsis can indicate *_____

_____ .
5. The purpose for the nasogastric tube connected to suction would be *_____

_____ .

   The x-rays showed a fractured right femur and possible abdominal fluid. Vital signs 2 hours later were blood pressure 106/86, pulse rate 128, respiration 34. Ms. Rockland was apprehensive and restless and had periods of confusion. Blood chemistry results were K 3.7 mEq/L, Na 134 mEq/L, Cl 99 mEq/L, serum CO_2 24 mEq/L. A Foley catheter was inserted, and 350 mL of urine was obtained. The secretions from GI suction were "bloody."

6. Changes in the vital signs indicate:
   a. Pulse *_____ .
   b. Blood Pressure *_____ .
   c. Respiration *_____ .
7. Indicate whether the results from the blood chemistry are normal (N), low (L), or high (H).
   ( ) a. Potassium
   ( ) b. Sodium
   ( ) c. Chloride
   ( ) d. Serum CO_2
8. Why is a Foley catheter inserted? *_____ .
   Was the amount of urine obtained (adequate/inadequate)? _____ .
9. Bloody GI secretions can indicate *_____ .
10. Ms. Rockland's apprehension, restlessness, and bouts of confusion can indicate

   _____ .

   Four hours after admission, Ms. Rockland's vital signs are blood pressure 84/66, pulse rate 136, respiration 36. Her skin color is gray and she is diaphoretic. Urine output is averaging 15–20 mL per hour. Blood chemistry, type, and cross-match and blood gases are ordered. A second liter of 5% dextrose in water to run for 4 hours is ordered.

11. Vital signs are indicative of *_____ .
12. Explain why there is a fluid volume deficit. *_____

_____ .
13. Is the hourly urine output adequate? _____ . Why? *_____

_____ .

14. Is 5% dextrose in water an appropriate IV solution to be used continuously?
    _____ . Why? *_____

_____ .

   An hour later, she is scheduled for the OR. The second laboratory results are K 5.0 mEq/L, Na 130 mEq.L, Cl 94 mEq/L, serum CO_2 18 mEq/L, blood sugar 166 mg/dL, BUN 32 mg/dL, ABG—pH 7.32, $Paco_2$ 35 mm Hg, HCO_3 19 mEq/L.

15. Her lab results indicate:
    a. Potassium _____
    b. Sodium _____
    c. Chloride _____
    d. Serum CO_2 * _____
    e. Blood sugar _____
    f. BUN _____
    g. pH _____
    h. Pa_{CO_2} _____
    i. HCO_3 * _____

1. fluid loss or hypovolemia or impending shock
2. normal; heart rate (pulse) was compensating for fluid loss and in response to injury. Later, if heart rate does not compensate, blood pressure would fall.
3. crystalloids. This group of solutions increases fluid volume and acts as a lifeline for emergency IV drugs.
4. loss of bowel tone, fluid shift to the abdominal area (most likely a traumatized or injured area)
5. to remove accumulated stomach and intestinal fluid (secretions) that resulted from an abdominal injury
6. a. tachycardia from fluid volume deficit (hypovolemia); b. drop in BP and pulse pressure 20 indicate hypovolemia and shock (impending); c. tachypnea from hypovolemia and stress
7. a. N; b. L; c. N; d. N
8. to monitor urine output (This is common practice following a traumatic injury.); adequate
9. GI injury or abdominal injury
10. hypovolemia and/or hypoxemia
11. hypovolemia (severe) and shock
12. Fluid shifts from the vascular fluid to the cells and to the injured sites (third spaces—abdominal area and injured leg tissue area). Fluids are also lost from GI suction and from diaphoresis.
13. No. It is less than 25 mL per hour.
14. No. Dextrose 5% in water (D_5W) would not correct hyponatremia and can cause water intoxication if used continuously.
15. a. normal; b. hyponatremia; c. hypochloremia; d. metabolic acidosis; e. stress; f. hypovolemia/dehydration; g. acidosis; h. low normal; i. metabolic acidosis

SHOCK

INTRODUCTION

The state of circulatory callapse, known as *shock*, occurs when the hemostatic circulatory mechanism, which regulates circulation, fails to maintain adequate circulation. With shock, the cardiac output is insufficient to provide vital organs and tissues with blood. There are four categories of shock: (1) hypovolemic, which includes hematogenic from hemorrhage; (2) cardiogenic; (3) septic; and (4) neurogenic. Most shock-induced conditions are associated with trauma.

38 Shock is a state of *_____ .

    Shock occurs when the hemostatic circulatory mechanism fails to

*_____ .

circulatory collapse; maintain adequate circulation or provide adequate blood to vital organs and tissues

        ■   ■   ■

39 A common feature of shock, regardless of the cause, is a low circulating blood volume in relation to the vascular capacity. There is a loss of blood, not necessarily from hemorrhaging, but from "pooling" in body areas so that adequate blood does not circulate. This causes inadequate tissue perfusion.

    A low blood volume is known as _____ .

    A disproportion between the volume of blood and the capacity (size) of the vascular chamber is the essential feature of _____ .

hypovolemia; shock or circulatory collapse

        ■   ■   ■

40 A common feature of shock is *_____

    With shock, is hypovolemia always due to hemorrhaging? _____ .

    Explain. *_____ .

a low circulating blood volume or loss of blood
No! It can be due to pooling of blood in body areas.

        ■   ■   ■

PATHOPHYSIOLOGY

    The physiologic changes resulting from shock include a decrease in blood pressure, increase in vasoconstriction of the blood vessels, increase in heart rate, a decrease in metabolism (inadequate oxygenation of the blood, electrolyte changes, metabolic acidosis, and decline in liver glycogen), and a decrease in renal function. Table 9-4 describes these physiologic changes. Study the table, noting if there is an increase or decrease in action or function. Refer to the table as needed as you proceed to the frames.

Table 9-4. PHYSIOLOGIC CHANGES RESULTING FROM SHOCK

Physiologic Changes	Rationale
Arterial blood pressure: decreased	Reduced venous return to heart decreases cardiac output and arterial blood pressure (BP).
	Decrease in BP is sensed by pressoreceptors in carotid sinus and aortic arch which leads to immediate reflex increase in systemic vasomotor activity. (This center is found in medulla.) Cardiac acceleration and vasoconstriction occur in order to maintain homeostasis with respect to blood pressure. This may be sufficient for early or impending shock.
Vasoconstriction of blood vessels: increased	Increased sympathetic nerve activity causes vasoconstriction. Vasoconstriction tends to maintain blood pressure and reduce discrepancy between blood volume and vascular capacity (size). Vasoconstriction is greatest in skin, kidneys, and skeletal muscles and not as significant in cerebral vessels. Coronary arteries actually dilate with a decrease in blood volume. This provides sufficient blood to the heart muscle (myocardium) for heart function.
Heart rate: increased	Heart rate is increased to overcome poor cardiac output and to increase circulation. Rapid, thready pulse is one of first identifiable signs of shock.
Metabolism: decreased	Fall in plasma hydrostatic pressure reduces urinary filtration. Unopposed plasma colloidal osmotic pressure draws interstitial fluid into vascular bed. Blood loss results in loss of serum potassium, phosphate, and bicarbonate. Inadequate oxygenation of cells prevents their normal metabolism and leads to formation of nonvolatile acids (acid metabolites), thus lowering serum pH values. With a fall in serum pH and a decrease in HCO_3, metabolic acidosis results. A rise in blood sugar is first seen due to release of epinephrine; later, blood sugar falls due to a decline in liver glycogen.
Kidney function: decreased	Low blood pressure causes inadequate circulation of blood to the kidneys. Renal ischemia is the result of a lack of O_2 to the kidneys. Renal insufficiency follows prolonged hypotension. Systolic blood pressure must be 60 mm Hg and above to maintain kidney function.
	One of the body's compensatory mechanisms in shock is to shunt blood around kidney to maintain intravascular fluid. Deficient blood supply makes tubule cells of kidneys more susceptible to injury.
	Urine output of less than 25 mL per hour may be indicative of shock and/or decrease in renal function.

41 Place I for increase and D for decrease beside the physiologic factors as they occur with shock.

    ____ a. Arterial blood pressure

    ____ b. Kidney function

    ____ c. Heart rate

    ____ d. Metabolic changes

    ____ e. Vasoconstriction

a. D; b. D; c. I; d. D; e. I

    ■   ■   ■

42 When there is a low blood pressure, the pressoreceptors in the carotid sinus and aortic arch cause an increase in the systemic vasomotor activity that leads to what two activities in order to maintain homeostasis? _____ and *_____ .

    Increased systemic vasomotor activity occurs in order to maintain _____ .

vasoconstriction and cardiac acceleration; homeostasis

    ■   ■   ■

43 Increased sympathetic activity results in (vasoconstriction/vasodilation)

_____ .

    Vasoconstriction is greatest in what three parts of the body? _____ ,

_____ , and *_____ .

    The coronary arteries (dilate/constrict) _____ with a decrease in blood volume.

vasoconstriction; skin, kidneys, and skeletal muscles; dilate

    ■   ■   ■

44 Heart rate in shock is (increased/decreased) _____ to overcome poor cardiac output and to increase circulation.

    The pulse rate is _____ and _____ .

    A person with a pulse rate above 120 has (bradycardia/tachycardia) _____ .

increased; rapid and thready; tachycardia

    ■   ■   ■

45 The following metabolic changes occur with shock:

Fluid is drawn from the interstitial space into the vascular space due to what kind of pressure? *_____ .

Inadequate oxygenation of cells leads to the formation of nonvolatile acids (acid metabolites), causing the pH to (rise/fall) _____ .

A fall in pH and HCO_3 leads to (metabolic acidosis/metabolic alkalosis) *_____ .

In shock, there is a release of epinephrine, which causes the blood sugar to (rise/fall) _____ . Later, there is a (rise/fall) _____ in blood sugar due to a decline in liver glycogen.

colloidal osmotic pressure; fall; metabolic acidosis; rise; fall

■   ■   ■

46 In shock, the compensatory mechanisms shunt the blood around the kidney in order to maintain the volume of *_____ . This results in a lack of oxygen in the kidneys known as *_____ , causing a decrease in kidney function.

The systolic blood pressure for kidney function must be at least *_____ .

An indication of shock related to kidney dysfunction is a urine output of less than *_____ .

intravascular fluid; renal ischemia; 60 mm Hg; 25 mL per hour

■   ■   ■

47 Extracellular fluid volume shifts occur during shock. In *early* shock, fluid is shifted from the interstitial space to the intravascular space to compensate for the fluid deficit in the vascular system. More fluid in the vascular system increases the venous return to the heart; thus it increases cardiac output.

As the interstitial fluid becomes depleted, tissue (dehydration/edema) _____ occurs.

dehydration

■   ■   ■

48 In *late* shock, fluid is forced from the intravascular space (blood vessels) back into the interstitial space (tissues).

In early shock, fluid is shifted from the *_____ to the
*_____ . Why? *_____ .

interstitial space; intravascular space
This shift compensates for fluid deficit in the vascular system.

■   ■   ■

ETIOLOGY

The clinical symptoms and related physiologic basis for each of the four types of shock—hypovolemic, cardiogenic, septic (also known as endotoxic or vasogenic), and neurogenic—are presented. Table 9-5 describes the four types of shock, the clinical causes, and the rationale and physiologic changes that occur with each type.

Study the table carefully, noting the causes (etiology) for each type of shock. Refer to the glossary for unfamiliar terms and refer to the table as needed.

49 The four types of shock are _____ , _____ ,
_____ , and _____ .

hypovolemic, cardiogenic, septic, and neurogenic

■   ■   ■

50 Match the following types of shock with the appropriate clinical causes.

a. Hypovolemic shock
b. Cardiogenic shock
c. Septic shock
d. Neurogenic shock

____ 1. High spinal anesthesia, emotional factors, or trauma from an extensive operative procedure

____ 2. Hemorrhaging from surgery or injury, burns, or GI bleeding

____ 3. Severe bacterial infection, immunosuppressant therapy

____ 4. Myocardial infarction, cardiac failure, and cardiac tamponade

1. d; 2. a; 3. c; 4. b

■   ■   ■

Table 9-5. TYPES AND CLINICAL CAUSES OF SHOCK		
Type of Shock	**Clinical Causes**	**Rationale and Physiologic Results**
Hypovolemic: Hematogenic (from hemorrhage)	Severe vomiting or diarrhea—acute dehydration. Burns, intestinal obstruction, fluid shift to third space. Hemorrhage that results from internal or external blood loss	Blood, plasma, and fluid loss from decreased circulating blood volume. *Physiologic Results* 1. Decreased circulation 2. Decreased venous return 3. Reduced cardiac output 4. Increased afterload 5. Decreased preload 6. Decreased tissue perfusion
Cardiogenic	Myocardial infarction. Severe arrhythmias. Congestive heart. Cardiac tamponade. Pulmonary embolism	Because of these clinical problems, the pumping action of the heart is inadequate to maintain circulation. (Pump failure of myocardium.) *Physiologic Results* 1. Decreased circulation 2. Decreased stroke volume 3. Decreased cardiac output 4. Increased preload 5. Increased afterload 6. Increased venous pressure 7. Decreased venous return 8. Decreased tissue perfusion
Septic: Endotoxic Vasogenic	Severe systemic infections. Septic abortion. Peritonitis. Debilitated conditions. Immunosuppressant therapy	Septic shock is characterized by increased capillary permeability that permits blood, plasma, and fluid to pass into surrounding tissue. Usually caused by a gram-negative organism. *Physiologic Results* 1. Vasodilatation and peripheral pooling of blood 2. Decreased circulation 3. Decreased preload, early shock and increased preload, late shock 4. Decreased afterload, early shock and increased afterload, late shock 5. Decreased tissue perfusion

Table 9-5. (Continued)		
Type of Shock	**Clinical Causes**	**Rationale and Physiologic Results**

Neurogenic	Mild to moderate neurogenic shock:
	    Emotional stress
	    Acute pain
	    Drugs: narcotics, barbiturates, phenothiazines
	    High spinal anesthesia
	    Acute gastric dilatation
	Severe neurogenic shock:
	    Spinal cord injury
	Trauma:
	    Extensive operative procedure
		Neurogenic shock is caused by loss of vascular tone.
		
		Physiologic Results
		1. Decreased circulation
		2. Vasodilatation and peripheral pooling of blood
		3. Decreased cardiac output
		4. Decreased venous return
		5. Decreased tissue perfusion

51 Match the following types of shock with the appropriate rationale.

a. Hypovolemic shock

b. Cardiogenic shock

c. Septic shock

d. Neurogenic shock

____ 1. Failure of the myocardium causes a decrease in the circulating blood volume

____ 2. Loss of vascular tone with vasodilation

____ 3. Decrease in blood volume due to loss of blood and plasma

____ 4. Increase in capillary permeability resulting from an infection

a. b; 2. d; 3. a; 4. c

•   •   •

52 Match the following types of shock with the physiologic results. Your response may be used more than once.

a. Hypovolemic shock
b. Cardiogenic shock
c. Septic shock
d. Neurogenic shock

—, —, —, — 1. Decreased circulation

—, —, — 2. Decreased cardiac output

—, — 3. Vasodilatation

—, —, — 4. Decreased venous return

—, —, —, — 5. Decreased tissue perfusion

1. a, b, c, d; 2. a, b, d; 3. c, d; 4. a, b, d; 5. a, b, c, d

■   ■   ■

CLINICAL MANIFESTATIONS

The clinical manifestations of shock are listed in Table 9-6 with the types of shock and rationale that are related to the signs and symptoms. Immediate medical action needs to be taken when shock occurs so that it can be reversed. Therefore, the nurse should frequently check for signs and symptoms of shock when impending shock is present.

Study the table carefully and be able to explain the signs and symptoms that frequently occur in shock.

Table 9-6. CLINICAL MANIFESTATIONS OF SHOCK

Signs and Symptoms	Types of Shock	Rationale
Skin: pallid and/or cold and moist	Hypovolemic Cardiogenic Neurogenic Septic (late)	Pale, cold, and/or moist skin results from increased sympathetic action. Peripheral vasoconstriction occurs and blood is shunted to vital organs. Skin is warm and flushed in early septic shock.
Tachycardia (pulse fast and thready)	Hypovolemic Cardiogenic Septic	Increased pulse rate is frequently one of the early signs, except in neurogenic shock, in which the pulse is often slower than normal. Norepinephrine and epinephrine, released by the adrenal medulla, increase the cardiac rate and myocardial contractibility. Tachycardia, pulse >100, occurs before arterial blood pressure falls.
Apprehension, restlessness	Hypovolemic Cardiogenic Septic	Apprehension and restlessness, early signs of shock, result from cerebral hypoxia. As the state of shock progresses disorientation and confusion occur.

Table 9-6.   (Continued)

Signs and Symptoms	Types of Shock	Rationale
Muscle weakness, fatigue	Hypovolemic Cardiogenic Septic Neurogenic	Muscle weakness and fatigue, which occur early in shock, are the result of a buildup of acid metabolites.
Arterial blood pressure: early, a rise in or normal BP; late, a fall in BP	Hypovolemic Cardiogenic Septic Neurogenic	In early shock blood pressure rises or is normal as a result of increased heart rate. As shock progresses, blood pressure falls because of a lack of cardiac and peripheral vasoconstriction compensation.
Pulse pressure: narrowed, <20 mm Hg		Narrowing of pulse rate occurs because the systolic BP falls more rapidly than the diastolic BP.
Pressures: CVP, PAP, PCWP—decreased in hypovolemic, septic, neurogenic; increased in cardiogenic	Hypovolemic Cardiogenic Septic Neurogenic	Normal values: 1. Central venous pressure (CVP): 5–12 cm H_2O. With decreased blood volume CVP < 5 cm H_2O. 2. Pulmonary artery pressure (PAP): 20–30 mm Hg systolic, 10–15 mm Hg diastolic. With blood volume depletion or pooling of blood PAP in hypovolemic <10 mm Hg, septic <10 mm Hg, neurogenic <10 mm Hg. In cardiogenic shock PAP > 30 mm Hg. 3. Pulmonary capillary wedge pressure (PCWP): 4–12 mm Hg. With blood volume depletion or peripheral pooling the PCWP in hypovolemic, septic, and neurogenic < 10 mm Hg and in cardiogenic > 20 mm Hg.
Respiration: increased rate and depth (tachypnea)	Hypovolemic Cardiogenic Septic Neurogenic	Increased hydrogen ion concentration in the body stimulates the respiratory centers in the medulla, thus increasing the respiratory rate. Acid metabolites, e.g., lactic acid from metabolic catabolism, increases the rate and depth of respiration. Rapid respiration acts as a compensatory mechanism to decrease metabolic acidosis.
Temperature: subnormal	Hypovolemic Cardiogenic Neurogenic	Body temperature is subnormal in shock because of decreased circulation and decreased cellular function. In septic shock the temperature is elevated.
Urinary output: decreased	Hypovolemic Cardiogenic Septic Neurogenic	Oliguria (decreased urine output) occurs in shock because of decreased renal blood flow caused by renal vasoconstriction. Blood is shunted to the heart and brain. Urine output should be >25 mL/h.

53 Two early mental changes occurring in shock are _____ and

_____ .

    They generally result from *_____ .

apprehension and restlessness; cerebral hypoxia
                ■   ■   ■

54 The central venous pressure (CVP), pulmonary artery pressure (PAP), and pulmonary capillary wedge pressure (PCWP) are decreased in which types of shock?

( ) a. Hypovolemic
( ) b. Cardiogenic
( ) c. Septic
( ) d. Neurogenic

a. X; b. —; c. X; d. X
                ■   ■   ■

55 Increased rate and depth of respirations are present in shock. Why? *_____

_____ .

Increased hydrogen ion concentration stimulates the respiratory center in the medulla; OR nonvolatile acids (acid metabolites) from cellular catabolism increase respiratory rate and depth.
Note: The purpose of increased rate and depth of respiration is to decrease the acidotic state.
                ■   ■   ■

56 Frequently the urinary output is decreased in all types of shock. Why? *_____

_____ .

Decreased urinary output is the result of decreased renal blood flow caused by renal vasoconstriction.
                ■   ■   ■

57 In shock, tachycardia is frequently seen before the arterial blood pressure begins to fall.

    The heart beats faster to (increase/decrease) _____ the circulating blood volume. This is an early compensatory mechanism to overcome shock.

    With shock, what happens to the arterial blood pressure? *_____

_____ .

increase; it will first rise and then fall
                ■   ■   ■

58 Below are some signs and symptoms. Check the ones that are true about shock. Correct the false ones.

( ) a. Arterial blood pressure low
( ) b. Bradycardia
( ) c. Respiration slow and deep
( ) d. Apprehension, restlessness
( ) e. Temperature low in all types of shock
( ) f. Urine output increased
( ) g. Central venous pressure high in cardiac shock and in hypovolemic shock
( ) h. Skin pallid and hot

a. *Arterial blood pressure rises, then falls*
b. *Tachycardia*
c. *Fast and deep*
d. *X*

e. *Not in early septic shock*
f. *Decreased output*
g. *It is low in hypovolemic (hematogenic) shock*
h. *Pallid or cold and moist, or both*

■   ■   ■

CLINICAL APPLICATIONS

59 Normal blood pressure is the usual level of blood pressure in a person and varies to some extent from person to person.

A systolic blood pressure of less than 90 mm Hg is significant of shock in most people.

A systolic pressure of 60–70 mm Hg is necessary to maintain the coronary circulation and renal function (urinary output). A person with a systolic pressure of 50–60 mm Hg is said to be in _____ .

shock

■   ■   ■

60 A low pulse pressure, which is the difference between the systolic and diastolic pressures, is indicative of shock. The systolic blood pressure usually decreases before the diastolic.

To maintain coronary circulation and renal function, the systolic pressure should be at least *_____ .

A pulse pressure of 20 mm Hg is indicative of _____ .

60–70 mm Hg; shock

■   ■   ■

61 Blood supply to the organs most susceptible to acute anoxia (absence or lack of oxygen), i.e., the brain and the heart, is maintained as long as possible at the expense of the less vital organs and tissues.

The two organs most susceptible to anoxia are the _____ and _____ .

The brain can survive 4 minutes in an anoxic state before cerebral damage occurs.

heart and brain

■   ■   ■

62 Which of the following physiologic symptoms indicate shock?

( ) a. Arterial blood pressure less than 90
( ) b. Pulse pressure of 55 mm Hg
( ) c. Pulse pressure of 20 mm Hg

Which two organs are most susceptible to acute anoxia?

( ) a. Heart
( ) b. Brain
( ) c. Intestines

The organ that cannot survive anoxia longer than 4 minutes without permanent damage is the _____ .

a. X; b. —; c. X
a. X; b. X; c. —
brain

■   ■   ■

CLINICAL MANAGEMENT

To maintain body fluid volume and particularly the intravascular fluid, fluid resuscitation must begin immediately for clients who are in shock or impending shock. Improvement of blood volume is needed to maintain tissue perfusion and oxygen delivery. The types of solutions for fluid replacement include crystalloids or balanced salt solutions and colloid solutions.

CRYSTALLOIDS

Crystalloids expand the volume of the ECF (intravascular and interstitial spaces). The two common types of crystalloids used for fluid replacement are normal saline solution (0.9% sodium chloride) and lactated Ringer's solution. Lactated Ringer's solution contains the electrolytes sodium, potassium, calcium, and chloride with their milliequivalents which are similar to the plasma values. Other commercially prepared crystalloids may be used for fluid replacement, such as Normosol R and Plasma-lyte R. These solutions contain magnesium plus many of the same electrolytes as lactated Ringer's.

Table 9-7 lists examples of crystalloids that can be used for fluid replacement.

Table 9-7. CRYSTALLOIDS FOR FLUID REPLACEMENT							
	mEq/L						
Crystalloids	Na	K	Ca	Mg	Cl	Lactate	Gluconate
0.9% NaCl (NSS)	154	—	—	—	154	—	—
lactated Ringer's	130	4	3	—	109	28	—
Normosol R	140	5	—	3	98	—	23
Plasma-lyte R	140	10	5	3	103	—	23

63 Name two commonly prescribed crystalloids that are used for fluid resuscitation.
    *_____ and *_____ .

   0.9% NaCl (normal saline solution) and lactated Ringer's solution
                        ■   ■   ■

64 Normal saline solution (0.9% NaCl) is a popular IV solution used for fluid resuscitation because it is iso-osmolar (approximately the same milliosomoles as plasma). Excess use of normal saline can increase the serum sodium level and can cause (hypochloremia/hyperchloremia) _____ .

   If metabolic acidosis is present, the chloride level can (increase/decrease) _____ the acidotic state.

   hyperchloremia; increase
                        ■   ■   ■

65 The lactate of the lactated Ringer's solution acts as a buffer to increase the pH, thus decreasing the acidotic state. Large quantities of lactated Ringer's solution might cause metabolic (acidosis/alkalosis) _____ .

   alkalosis
                        ■   ■   ■

66 If the client has a liver disorder, the lactate is not metabolized into bicarbonate; therefore lactic acid can result.

If large quantities of lactated Ringer's solution are administered to a client with a liver disorder, the metabolic acidotic state can be (intensified/lessened) _____ .

Alternating the crystalloid solutions, such as normal saline solution and lactated Ringer's solution, usually (maintains/disturbs) _____ the electrolyte and acid-base balance.

intensified; maintains

■   ■   ■

67 Intravenous solutions containing calcium should NOT be administered with blood transfusions. The calcium in the solution precipitates when it comes in contact with blood.

Indicate which of the following solutions can be administered through the same IV line with blood.

( ) a. 0.9% NaCl (normal saline solution)
( ) b. Lactated Ringer's solution
( ) c. Normosol R
( ) d. Plasma-lyte R

a. X; b. —; c. X; d. — (see Table 5-1, Chapter 5 or Table 9-7, Chapter 9)

■   ■   ■

68 Which of the following crystalloids do you think is the most expensive?

( ) a. 0.9% NaCl
( ) b. Plasma-lyte R
( ) c. Lactated Ringer's solution

a. —; b. X; c. —

■   ■   ■

69 The crystalloid 5% dextrose in water (D_5W) is seldom ordered for total fluid replacement during shock. A liter of D_5W may be initially used and then the IV therapy is switched to a balanced salt solution.

Dextrose 5% in water is an iso-osmolar solution, but if it is used continuously, it becomes a (hypo-osmolar/hyperosmolar) _____ solution. Why? *_____

_____ .

hypo-osmolar
The dextrose is rapidly metabolized, leaving water, a hypo-osmolar solution. Continuous use of D_5W can lead to intracellular fluid volume excess (water intoxication) or cellular swelling.

■   ■   ■

COLLOIDS

Colloids are substances that have a higher molecular weight than crystalloids and therefore cannot pass through the vascular membrane. Colloids increase the intravascular fluid volume. When colloid therapy is used, less fluid is needed to reestablish the fluid volume in the vascular space.

Table 9-8 lists the colloids that may be used for fluid replacement.

Table 9-8. COLLOIDS FOR FLUID REPLACEMENT		
Colloids*	**Brand Names**	**Comments**
Albumin, 5% or 25%	Albuminar Plasbumin	Not used in acute shock. 1–4 mL/minute.
Plasma protein fraction, 5%	Plasmanate	Rapid infusion rate can decrease blood pressure.
Hetastarch	Hespan	Synthetic starch similar to human glycogen. Very expensive
Dextran 40 Dextran 70 in 0.9% NaCl or D$_5$W	Dextran, Gentran, Macrodex	Low-molecular-weight dextran 40 may prolong bleeding time. High-molecular-weight dextran 70 increases blood viscosity. Interference with type and cross-match (T&C) may occur if drawn *after* dextran is infused.

* Colloid therapy is more expensive than crystalloid therapy.

70 In comparison with crystalloids, colloids are (more/less) _____ expensive. Colloid therapy requires (more/less) _____ solution replacement than needed with crystalloid solutions for fluid replacement.

more; less

■ ■ ■

71 Colloid solutions are useful in replacing fluid losses from which of the following:

( ) a. Intravascular space (blood vessels)
( ) b. Interstitial space (tissue area)
( ) c. Cellular space (cells)

a. X; b. —; c. —

■ ■ ■

72 Blood typing takes 5 minutes, but cross-matching takes at least 45 minutes. Until blood typing and cross-matching has been completed, what two groups of IV solutions can be used? _____ and _____ .

crystalloids and colloids

■ ■ ■

73 There has been much controversy as to whether crystalloids or colloids should be used for a client in shock. The central venous pressure (CVP) and the pulmonary capillary wedge pressure (PCWP) should be monitored during fluid resuscitation.

From which group of fluids might the physician select for a client with a traumatic injury and heart disease (CHF), (crystalloids/colloids)? _____ .

Why?   *_____

_____ .

colloids
Massive amounts of crystalloids are needed to increase the fluid volume loss. This can result in overhydration for a client with a heart disorder.

　　　　　　　　■　　　　　　　　　■　　　　　　　　　■

74 The colloids albumin 5%, plasma protein fraction (Plasmanate), and hetastarch increase the vascular volume to approximately the same amount that is infused. With the low molecular weight dextran (40), the vascular fluid is expanded by one to two times the amount that is infused. With albumin 25%, the vascular volume is expanded four times the amount that is infused.

To increase the vascular volume more than the amount of colloid that is infused, which of the following colloid solutions might be used?

( ) a. Albumin 5%
( ) b. Albumin 25%
( ) c. Plasmanate
( ) d. Dextran 40
( ) e. Hetastarch

a. —; b. X; c. —; d. X; e. —

　　　　　　　　■　　　　　　　　　■　　　　　　　　　■

Crystalloids are usually the first choice for treating hypovolemic shock. Crystalloids can restore fluid volume in the vascular and interstitial spaces and improve renal function; however large quantities of crystalloids are needed. Excessive infusions of crystalloids might cause fluid overload in clients who are elderly or who have heart disease. Frequently, a combination of crystalloids and colloids is used for fluid replacement. If severe blood loss occurs, whole blood transfusion may be necessary after infusion of 1–2 liters of crystalloids. Each fluid replacement situation differs and each individual situation must be evaluated separately.

There are many suggested formulas for restoring fluid loss, especially for clients in hypovolemic shock who have lost massive amounts of blood and/or body fluid. Examples of formulas for fluid volume replacement include minimal trauma (4 mL/kg per hour); moderate trauma (6 mL/kg per hour); and severe trauma (8 mL/kg per hour). Table 9-9 outlines the calculation of blood loss and fluid replacement for three states of hypovolemic shock from hemorrhage.

Table 9-9.   CALCULATION OF BLOOD LOSS AND FLUID REPLACEMENT FOR THREE STATES OF HYPOVOLEMIC SHOCK FROM HEMORRHAGE

State of Hypovolemic Shock	Systolic Blood Pressure (mm Hg)	Estimated Blood Volume Loss (%)	Replacement Needed for Blood Volume Loss in Person Weighing 70 kg (mL)
Mild	90–95	15–20	750–1100
Moderate	75–90	20–30	1100–1700
Severe	Below 75	30–50	2000–3000 and up

Note: When blood is not available, large amounts of balanced salt solution, 100–150 mL/kg of body weight, are given. There should be 50 mL replacement for each percentage of blood volume loss in a 70-kg person or as determined by physician.

75   If a client is in *mild* hypovolemic shock, her blood volume loss is *_____ %, and her systolic blood pressure is probably _____ mm Hg. The replacement needed for this blood volume loss is *_____ mL.

If a client is in *moderate* hypovolemic shock, her blood volume loss is *_____ %, and her systolic blood pressure is probably *_____ mm Hg. The replacement needed for this blood volume loss is *_____ mL.

Of if a client is in *severe* hypovolemic shock, her blood volume loss is *_____ %, and her systolic blood pressure is probably *_____ mm Hg. The replacement needed for this blood volume loss is *_____ mL.

15–20; 90–95; 750–1100
20–30; 75–90; 1100–1700
30–50; below 75; 2000–3000

■   ■   ■

76   There should be _____ mL replacement for each percentage blood volume loss in a man of average height, 150 pounds (70 kg).

50

■   ■   ■

77 Place the word Mild, Moderate, or Severe in the space provided as it relates to:

_____ Systolic blood pressure below 75 mm Hg

_____ Systolic blood pressure of 86 mm Hg

_____ Systolic pressure of 92 mm Hg

_____ 50% blood volume loss

_____ 15–20% blood volume loss

_____ 20–30% blood volume loss

_____ 1100–1700 mL replacement needed

_____ 2000–3000 mL replacement needed

_____ 750–1100 mL replacement needed

Severe; Moderate; Mild; Severe; Mild; Moderate; Moderate; Severe; Mild
  ▪   ▪   ▪

Table 9-10 outlines the clinical management for alleviating four types of clinical shock: hypovolemic, cardiogenic, septic, and neurogenic. Many years ago the first and foremost treatment of shock was to administer a vasopressor drug. The drug constricts the dilated blood vessels which occur with shock and raises the blood pressure. Vasopressors act as a temporary treatment for shock, and the shock continues to increase if the cause is not alleviated or removed. Today vasopressors are used for severe shock and types of shock nonresponsive to treatment. Note that vasopressors are *not* effective in the treatment of hypovolemic shock, since constricting blood vessels does not aid in the circulation of blood when the cause is most obvious—a lack of blood, causing hypovolemia. Replacing blood volume loss should correct this type of shock. Remember, removal of the cause is first and foremost in alleviating various types of shock.

Study this table carefully and be able to explain the treatments for each type of shock.

78 What is shock? *_____ .

What is a common feature of shock? *_____

_____ .

a state of circulatory collapse
low circulating blood volume or hypovolemia. This can be due to loss of blood from the body or "pooling" of blood in selected areas.
  ▪   ▪   ▪

Table 9-10. CLINICAL MANAGEMENT FOR ALLEVIATING VARIOUS TYPES OF CLINICAL SHOCK

Hypovolemic Shock	Cardiogenic Shock	Septic Shock	Neurogenic Shock

1. IV fluids, such as
  a. Lactated Ringer's
  b. Normal saline
  c. Whole blood
  d. Plasma or plasmanate
  e. Dextran
	1. IV therapy is limited when edema is present and venous pressure is elevated. Close monitoring CVP and PCWP	1. Blood culture first and then IV fluids (salt solutions, plasma, dextran)	1. IV therapy for severe shock

2. No vasopressors	*2. Vasopressors, if severe (dopamine)	*2. Vasopressors for nonresponsiveness	*2. Vasopressors, if severe
3. Electrolyte replacement	3. Lidocaine (to abort ventricular dysrhythmias) Sodium nitroprusside/ Nipride/ Nitropress; nitroglycerin/NTG; and prazosin/ Minipress (decrease preload and decrease afterload). Digitalis Sedatives Diuretics	3. Antibiotics via IV fluids Steroids, e.g., hydrocortisone	3. Sedation for emotional shock
4. ABGs 5. O$_2$	4. O$_2$		

* Examples of vasopressors are (1) levarterenol bitartrate/Levophed, (2) metaraminol bitartrate/Aramine, (3) dopamine hydrochloride/Intropin, and (4) dobutamine/Dobutrex (primary for cardiogenic shock).

79 The clinical management for *hypovolemic shock* may consist of which of the following:

( ) a. Dextran IV solution
( ) b. Whole blood
( ) c. Digitalization
( ) d. Vasopressors
( ) e. Oxygen
( ) f. Lactated Ringer's solution
( ) g. Normal saline
( ) h. Electrolyte replacement
( ) i. Lidocaine

a. X; b. X; c. —; d. —; e. —; f. X; g. X; h. X; i. —

■   ■   ■

80 When administering crystalloids, such as normal saline or lactated Ringer's solution, for hypovolemic shock, these IV solutions may be given rapidly at first to decrease the symptoms of shock and prevent fluid shift into the interstitial space at the injured site. Later, the flow rate should be slowed.

What type of fluid imbalance can occur if massive quantities of crystalloids are rapidly administered intravenously? _____ .

overhydration (hypervolemia). This occurs most likely with the older adult, child, or debilitated person.

■   ■   ■

81 Clinical management for *cardiogenic shock* may consist of which of the following:

( ) a. Limited IV therapy
( ) b. No vasopressors
( ) c. Antibiotics
( ) d. Oxygen
( ) e. Digitalis product
( ) f. Sedation
( ) g. Sodium nitroprusside/Nipride

a. X; b. —; c. —; d. X; e. X; f. X; g. X

■   ■   ■

82 Clinical management for *septic shock* may consist of which of the following:

( ) a. Blood culture
( ) b. Antibiotics in IV fluids
( ) c. Hydrocortisone
( ) d. Vasopressors
( ) e. Digitalization
( ) f. Massive IV therapy with whole blood

a. X; b. X; c. X; d. X; e. —; f. —

■ ■ ■

83 Antibiotics and pain medications should be given intravenously if the client is in shock. Since circulation is poor, medications given intramuscularly (IM) are not fully absorbed. If given IM, after circulation is restored, the accumulated drug in the tissue spaces can be toxic.

Do you think the same dosage prescribed for IM should be given intravenously?

* _____ .

Not always. Please check with the physician. Frequently, large doses are given diluted in 50–100 mL of IV solution. IV morphine is given slowly (approximately 5 minutes). In some cases, one half of the IM dose is given IV.

■ ■ ■

84 Clinical management for *neurogenic shock* may consist of which of the following:

( ) a. Blood culture
( ) b. Vasopressors
( ) c. IV therapy as needed
( ) d. Massive IV therapy
( ) e. Sedation

a. —; b. X; c. X; d. —; e. X

■ ■ ■

85 Explain the action of vasopressors (see introduction to Table 9-10, if necessary).

* _____ .

The four vasopressors listed at the bottom of Table 9-10 are *_____ ,
*_____ , *_____ , and *_____ .

Vasopressors constrict blood vessels in hopes of improving circulation.

levarterenol bitartrate/Levophed, metaraminol bitartrate/Aramine, dopamine HCl/Intropin, and dobutamine/Dobutrex

■ ■ ■

86 Vasopressors should be used with care; however, they are helpful at the right time and with the right clinical problem.

When vasopressors are used, it is best to keep the systolic pressure no higher than 90 mm Hg to prevent cardiac dysrhythmias.

Levophed (levarterenol bitartrate), a strong vasopressor, is norepinephrine, which increases blood pressure and cardiac output by constricting blood vessels.

Maintaining the blood pressure higher than 90 mm Hg with Levophed can cause
*_____ .

cardiac dysrhythmias

■   ■   ■

87 Aramine (metaraminol bitartrate) triggers the body to release norepinephrine from storage sites to the blood vessels and heart. When discontinuing Aramine, the drug should not be completely stopped, but tapered gradually to prevent relapse into shock. The use of Aramine for a long period of time may deplete the body's norepinephrine, especially after an abrupt stop.

What vasopressor do you think the physician might switch to for replacing the hormone norepinephrine when stopping Aramine? _____

Levophed

■   ■   ■

88 Aramine does not tend to cause cardiac dysrhythmias.

Levophed is a (strong/weak) _____ vasopressor and can cause cardiac dysrhythmias if the systolic blood pressure is maintained above _____ mm Hg.

Vasopressors are titrated according to the blood pressure and should be checked every 2–5 minutes.

strong; 90

■   ■   ■

89 Dopamine HCl (Intropin) is a catecholamine precursor of norepinephrine. It increases blood pressure and cardiac output. It also dilates renal vessels, thus increasing renal blood flow and the glomerular filtration rate.

Levophed and Aramine cause vasoconstriction, which affects the renal arteries and can decrease kidney function. The vasopressor that increases blood pressure, cardiac output, and urinary output is *_____ .

dopamine HCl

■   ■   ■

90 Dopamine is helpful in the treatment of cardiogenic shock, but not when severe hypotension exists.

What two vasopressors can be used in severe shock? _____ and _____ .

Aramine and Levophed

■   ■   ■

91 Dobutamine/Dobutrex is an adrenergic drug that increases blood pressure moderately and raises heart rate and cardiac output. Dobutamine is effective in increasing myocardial contractility without arrhythmias. It is frequently used with sodium nitroprusside.

Explain why dobutamine is not used to treat severe hypotension. *_____
_____ .

Dobutamine has only a moderate effect on increasing blood pressure.

■   ■   ■

92 Identify the treatments listed below that may be used in various types of shock by placing:

H for hypovolemic shock
C for cardiogenic shock
S for septic shock
N for neurogenic shock

Some treatments may be used for more than one type of shock.

_____	a. IV therapy: lactated Ringer's, normal saline, dextran
_____	b. Digitalis products
_____	c. Electrolyte replacement
_____ , _____	d. Sedatives
____ , ____ , ____	e. Vasopressors
_____	f. Oxygen
_____ , _____	g. Limited IV therapy
_____	h. Antibiotics in IV fluids
_____	i. Hydrocortisone
_____	j. Lidocaine

a. H	*f. C*
b. C	*g. C, N*
c. H	*h. S*
d. C, N	*i. S*
e. C, S, N	*j. C*

■   ■   ■

CASE STUDY REVIEW

Mr. Martz, age 58, had diverticulitis. The diverticulum ruptured, causing peritonitis and systemic septicemia. His vital signs are temperature 104°F (40°C), pulse 126 rapid and thready, respirations 32, and blood pressure 65/45. His urinary output is 25 mL per hour. His skin is warm and dry. He is markedly apprehensive and restless. He is diagnosed as being in septic shock.

1. Shock occurs when the hemostatic circulatory mechanism fails to maintain adequate
   * _____ .

2. Septic shock is characterized by * _____
   _____ .

3. Identify four of Mr. Martz's clinical signs and symptoms of shock. * _____ ,
   * _____ , * _____ ,
   and * _____ .

4. Mr. Martz's temperature was elevated due to _____
   _____ .

5. His pulse pressure was 20 mm Hg (65 minus 45), which is indicative of _____
   _____ .

6. His urine output is _____ mL for 24 hours, which is in the low "normal" range. If his urine output goes below 25 mL per hour, what may this indicate?
   * _____ .

7. If Mr. Martz's systolic blood pressure drops below 60 mm Hg, what can occur to his renal function? * _____
   _____ .

8. In shock, which frequently occurs first, blood pressure decrease or pulse rate increase?
   * _____
   Why? * _____ .

9. Based on Mr. Martz's blood pressure, the state of shock is (mild/moderate/severe)
   _____ .

10. Name the four methods for managing septic shock. * _____ ,
    * _____ , * _____ ,
    and * _____ .

11. If vasopressors were used for Mr. Martz, which two would be indicated?
    _____ or _____ .

12. What advantage does dopamine hydrochloride have on kidney function that other vasopressors do not have? * _____
    _____ .

1. *circulation or blood volume*
2. *capillary permeability, permitting blood and plasma to pass into the surrounding tissues*
3. *pulse 126, respiration 32, blood pressure 65/45 and low pulse pressure, and apprehension and restlessness*
4. *septicemia (bacterial infection)*
5. *shock*
6. *600; kidney dysfunction or insufficiency*
7. *decreased renal function and output. It can lead to renal failure if prolonged.*
8. *pulse rate increase. Heart beats faster to maintain circulating blood volume. Increased pulse rate is an early compensatory mechanism to overcome shock.*

9. *severe*
10. *blood culture, antibiotics in IV fluids, vasopressors as needed, and steroids, e.g., hydrocortisone*
11. *Aramine; Levophed*
12. *It dilates the renal arteries and increases blood flow and urine output.*

NURSING ASSESSMENT FACTORS

- Check vital signs and report signs and symptoms that may indicate hypovolemia and shock: tachycardia, narrowing of the pulse pressure [difference between systolic and diastolic (less than 20 mm Hg is an indicator of shock)], tachypnea (rapid breathing), and skin cool and clammy.
- Obtain a drug history of the injured client. Report if the client is regularly taking potassium-wasting diuretics, digitalis, cortisone preparation, or antibiotics.
- Relate acute clinical problem with the signs and symptoms of hypovolemia and shock.
- Assess the behavioral and neurologic status of the injured client and/or the client in shock. Irritability, apprehension, restlessness, and confusion are symptoms of fluid volume deficit. Apprehension and restlessness are early symptoms of shock.
- Check urinary output. Less than 25 mL per hour or 200 mL per 8 hours can indicate fluid volume deficit or renal insufficiency. In severe shock, severe oliguria or anuria might occur.
- Check laboratory results, especially serum electrolytes and BUN and serum creatinine. Report abnormal laboratory results immediately.

NURSING DIAGNOSIS 1

Fluid volume deficit, related to traumatic injury and/or shock.

NURSING INTERVENTIONS AND RATIONALE

1. Monitor vital signs. Compare the vital signs with those taken on admission, and report abnormalities immediately. Significant vital sign changes that could be due to fluid loss or shock include rapid, thready pulse rate, drop in blood pressure, and narrowing of the pulse pressure (<20 mm Hg).
2. Check skin color and turgor. Note changes. Pallor, gray, cold, clammy skin, and poor skin turgor are symptoms of shock and fluid volume deficit.
3. Record amounts of vomitus, diarrhea, stools, secretions from nasogastric suction, and drains that contribute to fluid losses.
4. Check the mucous membranes for dryness. Observe for dry tenacious secretions.
5. Monitor IV therapy. Crystalloids are usually rapidly administered initially to hydrate the client and to increase urine output. Normal saline solution and/or lactated Ringer's solution are the choice crystalloids for fluid replacement. Colloids may be used in combination with crystalloids for the aged client with cardiac problem (fluid excess should be avoided).
6. Monitor central venous pressure (CVP) and pulmonary capillary (arterial) wedge pressure (PCWP) which is needed to adjust fluid balance. Norm for CVP is 5–12 cm/H_2O and for PCWP it is 4–12 mm Hg. Keeping PCWP between 12 and 15 mm Hg in shock conditions provides the filling pressure required for adequate stroke volume and cardiac output. If PCWP drops below 10 mm Hg, administration of fluids is usually needed. If PCWP is greater than 18 mm Hg, fluid restriction may be necessary.

7. Draw blood chemistry, hematology, and arterial blood gases as ordered. Report abnormal findings immediately to the physician.
8. Monitor laboratory results, especially the serum electrolytes. The serum potassium (K) levels can vary after trauma. The low K serum level can be due to excess urine output. The serum K level may be normal even though there is a cellular potassium deficit. Hyperkalemia can occur due to excessive cellular breakdown and oliguria (decreased urine output). The serum potassium level should be known before administering potassium in IV fluids.
9. Monitor ECG readings and report flat, inverted, or peaked T waves, which are indicative of a potassium imbalance.

NURSING DIAGNOSIS 2

Fluid volume excess, related to massive infusions of crystalloids.

NURSING INTERVENTIONS AND RATIONALE

1. Monitor IV fluid therapy. Regulate flow rate to prevent overhydration (hypervolemia). Report to physician if the patient is receiving 5% dextrose in water continuously without any other solutes such as saline.
2. Auscultate the lungs for rales. Overhydration from excess fluids and rapid administration of IV fluids can cause pulmonary edema. Heart failure can be another result.
3. Instruct the client to cough and breathe deeply to expand the lungs and provide effective ventilation.
4. Check for neck vein engorgement and/or hand vein engorgement when overhydration is suspected. Check jugular vein at a 45° angle and hand veins by raising hand above heart level. Look for hand engorgement after 10 seconds.
5. Check for pitting edema in the feet and legs. Weigh client to determine if there is fluid retention.

NURSING DIAGNOSIS 3

Urinary retention, related to fluid volume deficit and shock.

NURSING INTERVENTIONS AND RATIONALE

1. Monitor urine output. Hourly urine should be measured and, if less than 25 mL per hour, the IV fluid rate should be increased. Don't forget to check for overhydration when pushing fluids—IV or orally. Renal artery vasoconstriction occurs in shock, which causes a decrease in kidney perfusion.
2. Report systolic blood pressure of 60 mm Hg or less immediately. Kidney damage can occur if systolic blood pressure is below 60 mm Hg for several hours.
3. Check the BUN and creatinine. If both are highly elevated, it could be due to renal insufficiency. If they are slightly elevated and return to normal when the patient is hydrated, it could be due to the fluid volume deficit.

NURSING DIAGNOSIS 4

Tissue perfusion: altered: renal, cardiopulmonary, cerebral, and peripheral, related to decreased blood volume and circulation secondary to hypovolemia and shock.

NURSING INTERVENTIONS AND RATIONALE

1. Monitor blood pressure when administering vasopressors in IV fluids. The flow rate should be adjusted to keep the systolic pressure between 90 and 110 mm Hg. If the vasopressor is Levophed, the systolic pressure should be approximately 90 mm Hg to avoid cardiac dysrhythmias. If urine output is poor, the vasopressor of choice may be dopamine.

2. Monitor arterial blood gases (ABGs). Metabolic acidosis frequently results from cellular damage due to severe hypovolemia and shock. In acidosis, the pH is below 7.35, HCO_3 is below 24 mEq/L, and base excess (BE) is less than -2. Signs of Kussmaul breathing (rapid, vigorous breathing) may be present. Respiratory acidosis may also result due to the lungs' inability to excrete carbon dioxide. The ABGs that indicate respiratory acidosis include: $pH < 7.35$ and $Paco_2 > 45$ mm Hg. Dyspnea may be present.

Behavioral Objectives

Upon completion of this chapter, you will be prepared to:

- Identify the physiologic changes associated with congestive heart failure (CHF).
- Explain the clinical manifestations related to CHF.
- Identify abnormal laboratory results associated with CHF.
- Differentiate between left-sided heart failure and right-sided heart failure and pulmonary edema and peripheral edema.
- Explain the three major treatment modalities for correcting CHF.
- Identify selected nursing diagnoses and interventions with rationales for CHF.

Introduction

Heart failure is the inability of the heart to pump an adequate supply of blood (pump failure) to meet the body's metabolic needs. It is the result of increased stress on the heart and is secondary to major disease entities, i.e., arteriosclerotic heart disease, hypertension, pulmonary diseases, kidney diseases, and hyperthyroidism.

Congestive heart failure (CHF) is circulatory congestion related to pump failure. Acute heart failure develops quickly; shock, cardiac arrest, or sudden death can occur. Chronic heart failure develops more slowly, begins with milder symptoms, and usually does not become severe until compensatory mechanisms fail.

1   With CHF, there is circulatory congestion related to the heart's inability to pump   *_____

_____ .

     CHF is referred to as pump _____ .

an adequate supply of blood; failure

           ▪   ▪   ▪

2   Congestive heart failure is frequently (primary/secondary) _____ to major disease entities.

secondary

           ▪   ▪   ▪

PATHOPHYSIOLOGY

Table 10-1 lists the pathophysiologic factors associated with CHF and the compensatory mechanisms to prevent heart failure. Left-sided and right-sided heart failure present different symptoms. Each type is included as a part of the pathophysiologic factors. Study the table and refer to it as necessary.

Table 10-1. PHYSIOLOGIC CHANGES ASSOCIATED WITH CHF	
Physiologic Changes	**Rationale**
Cardiac reserve (decreased) ↓	Decreased cardiac reserve is the inability of heart to respond to increased burden, e.g., fever, exercise, or excitement.
Cardiac compensation	The heart, in early heart failure, compensates for loss of cardiac reserve. The heart increases its cardiac output through ventricular dilatation, ventricular hypertrophy, and tachycardia.
Ventricular dilatation	Muscle fibers of myocardium increase in length and the ventricle enlarges to augment its output. Heart muscle stretches to a certain point and then ceases to increase heart contractility. A dilated heart needs more oxygen than a "normal" heart; however, the decreased coronary blood flow limits the O_2 supply to the heart muscle.
Ventricular hypertrophy	There is increased thickening of ventricular wall, which increases the weight of the heart. Ventricular hypertrophy mostly follows dilatation, and hypertrophy aids in heart contractility. A hypertrophied heart works harder than a normal heart and has a greater O_2 need.
Tachycardia	The increased heart rate is the least effective of three compensatory mechanisms. The heart rate increases to a point that the ventricles are unable to fill adequately. As the heart rate increases, diastole time is reduced. The stroke volume first decreases, causing the cardiac output to increase, and later decreases as the heart rate greatly increases and diastole time shortens.
Cardiac decompensation	Occurs when the three compensatory mechanisms fail to maintain heart function and adequate circulation. Symptoms develop with normal activity.
Left-sided heart failure	Generally results from left ventricular damage to the myocardium. The heart at first is unable to eject the full blood volume from the ventricle. Three compensatory mechanisms come into play. With compensatory mechanism failure, residual blood remains in the dilated ventricle. The left atrium dilates and atrial hypertrophy results. When the atrium is unable to receive blood from pulmonary veins, pulmonary congestion or pulmonary edema occurs.

Table 10-1. (Continued)	
Physiologic Changes	**Rationale**
Left-sided heart failure (Continued)	Etiologic factors include hypertension, myocardial infarction (heart attack), rheumatic fever affecting aortic valve, or syphilis. Symptoms of left-sided heart failure are similar to symptoms of overhydration (Chapter 2), i.e., irritated cough, dizziness, engorged neck veins, moist rales.
Right-sided heart failure	Generally results from increased pressure in the pulmonary vascular system. The right ventricle tries to pump blood into the congested lungs, thus meeting resistance. Blood and fluids are "backed up" in the venous circulation, causing congestion in the GI tract, liver, and kidneys. Peripheral edema also occurs. Right-sided heart failure generally follows left-sided heart failure; however, occasionally, it is independent of left-sided failure. Symptoms of right-sided heart failure include liver congestion and enlargement, fullness in abdomen, and peripheral edema of lower extremities, mostly refractory and pitting.

3   With CHF, there is a(n) (increase/decrease) _____ in cardiac reserve.

   What is cardiac reserve? *_____ .

decrease; ability of the heart to respond to increased burden

■   ■   ■

4   In early heart failure, the heart compensates in order to meet oxygen and circulatory needs. The three methods by which the heart compensates are *_____ ,
   *_____ , and _____ .

ventricular dilatation, ventricular hypertrophy, and tachycardia

■   ■   ■

5   Physiologically, how does ventricular dilatation occur? *_____

   _____ .

   With ventricular dilatation, does the heart need (more/less) _____ oxygen?

the muscle fibers of the myocardium increase in length and so the ventricle enlarges to increase output and circulation; more

■   ■   ■

6 Explain the rationale for ventricular hypertrophy in CHF. *_____
_____.

There is an increased thickening of the ventricle wall, which increases heart contractility.
       ■   ■   ■

7 Tachycardia is *_____.
Tachycardia increases in rate until the ventricles are *_____.

a fast heart beat or fast pulse rate (frequently over 100); unable to fill adequately
       ■   ■   ■

8 What is cardiac decompensation? *_____
_____.

It is the failure of the three compensatory mechanisms to maintain heart function.
       ■   ■   ■

9 Left-sided heart failure generally results from *_____.
When the compensatory mechanisms fail with left-sided failure, what happens to the ventricle and to the atrium? *_____
_____.

left ventricle damage
The ventricle remains dilated with residual blood. The atrium dilates and atrial hypertrophy results.
       ■   ■   ■

10 What type of edema occurs from left-sided heart failure? _____.
Name four symptoms of left-sided heart failure (overhydration). *_____,
_____, *_____, and *_____.

pulmonary; constant, irritating cough, dyspnea, engorged veins, and moist rales
       ■   ■   ■

11   Right-sided heart failure generally results from   * _____

_____ .

What occurs when the right ventricle fails to adequately pump blood to the lungs?

* _____

_____

_____ .

increased pressure in the pulmonary vascular system
Blood and fluids are "backed up" in the venous circulation, increasing venous pressure and causing GI, liver, and kidney congestion. Peripheral edema in the lower extremities also results.

■   ■   ■

12   Explain the occurrence of right-sided heart failure in relation to left-sided heart failure.

* _____ .

What type of peripheral edema occurs?   * _____ . Should it be assessed in the morning or in the evening?   * _____ .

Right-sided heart failure generally follows left-sided heart failure.
refractory or nondependent edema, also pitting edema; in the morning

■   ■   ■

CLINICAL MANIFESTATIONS

The heart compensates for inadequate blood flow by increasing the heart rate. Table 10-2 lists the common clinical manifestations and rationale associated with CHF. Study the table carefully, noting the reasons for the signs and symptoms related to CHF.

13   Vital sign changes associated with CHF are:

a. Pulse rate is _____ .
b. Respiratory rate is _____ .
c. Blood pressure may be _____ .

a. increased; b. increased; c. increased

■   ■   ■

Table 10-2. CLINICAL MANIFESTATIONS ASSOCIATED WITH CHF	
Clinical Manifestations	**Rationale**
Vital Signs (VSs) Increased pulse rate (tachycardia)	Increased heart rate is a compensatory mechanism to improve circulation of the blood.
Increased respiration (tachypnea)	Respirations increase to increase oxygen intake for tissue oxygenation.
Increased blood pressure (hypertension)	When hypertension occurs, it is usually because of atherosclerosis. Noncirculating vascular fluid can also increase blood pressure.
Edema Pulmonary	Caused by left-sided heart failure. Because of pump failure, fluid is "backed up" in the pulmonary system, causing fluid congestion in the lung tissues. The fluid inhibits adequate gas exchange (O_2 and CO_2). Signs and symptoms of pulmonary edema are similar to the signs and symptoms of overhydration.
Peripheral	May result from right-sided heart failure. Fluids accumulate in the extremities due to the fluid backed up in the venous circulation.
Cyanosis	Cyanosis is a sign of hypoxia due to inadequate blood flow to body tissues.
Laboratory Results Plasma/serum sodium: increased (hypernatremia) or normal	Usually sodium retention in the extracellular fluid (ECF) occurs even when the serum sodium is within normal range. This is mostly due to hemodilution.
Plasma/serum potassium: normal or decreased (hypokalemia)	The serum potassium level can be decreased with the use of potassium-wasting diuretics and due to hemodilution from fluid volume excess.
Plasma/serum magnesium: normal or decreased (hypomagnesemia)	Long-term use of potassium-wasting diuretics can cause both hypomagnesemia and hypokalemia.

14   When the pulse rate is greater than 100, it is known as _____ .

The reason for an increase in heart rate is (increase/decrease) _____ in blood circulation to body tissues.

tachycardia; increase

■   ■   ■

15 A rapid increase in respirations is known as _____ .

   A high blood pressure reading is called _____ .

   tachypnea; hypertension
   ▪   ▪   ▪

16 The reason for an increased respiratory rate is to increase *_____ . More (oxygen/carbon dioxide) _____ intake occurs.

   gas exchange; oxygen
   ▪   ▪   ▪

17 The two types of edema associated with CHF are _____ and _____ .

   Initially, left-sided heart failure causes what type of edema? _____ .

   Right-sided heart failure is associated with what type of edema? _____ .

   pulmonary and peripheral; pulmonary; peripheral
   ▪   ▪   ▪

18 Indicate which of the serum electrolyte results are related to CHF.

   ( ) a. Hypernatremia
   ( ) b. Hyperkalemia
   ( ) c. Hypermagnesemia
   ( ) d. Normal serum sodium level
   ( ) e. Hypokalemia
   ( ) f. Hypomagnesemia

   a. X; b. —; c. —; d. X; e. X; f. X
   ▪   ▪   ▪

CLINICAL APPLICATIONS

Mrs. Allen, age 68, was admitted to the hospital with CHF. She has shortness of breath when walking up a flight of stairs. The nurse assessed Mrs. Allen's physiologic status and noted an irritating cough, dyspnea on exertion, moist rales in the lungs, hand vein engorgement in upward position after 30 seconds, and swelling in the ankles and feet. Her blood pressure is 154/96 and pulse was 110. Her ECG showed ventricular hypertophy.

19 Mrs. Allen has two compensatory physiologic changes present for maintaining cardiac function, which are _____ and *_____ .

Are these compensatory mechanisms effective? _____ Explain why.

*_____

_____ .

tachycardia and ventricular hypertrophy
No. Most likely, ventricular dilatation is present; symptoms of congestive heart failure are present.

■　　　　　　■　　　　　　■

20 According to Mrs. Allen's symptoms, which type(s) of heart failure is (are) present?

( ) a. Left-sided heart failure
( ) b. Right-sided heart failure

a. X; b. X

■　　　　　　■　　　　　　■

21 The nursing assessment of Mrs. Allen to determine pulmonary congestion includes:

a. *_____
b. _____
c. *_____
d. *_____

a. irritating cough; b. dyspnea; c. moist rales; d. hand vein engorgement

■　　　　　　■　　　　　　■

22 Swelling in the feet and ankles is indicative of _____ -sided heart failure.

right

■　　　　　　■　　　　　　■

Table 10-3 gives the laboratory results for Mrs. Allen on the day of admission and the second and fourth days. Be able to state which laboratory results are normal and which are not. Explain the abnormal laboratory findings.

23 Mrs. Allen's serum sodium is _____ . Sodium retention can cause Mrs. Allen's extracellular fluid volume to (rise/decrease) _____ .

What type of fluid imbalance was present? _____ .

elevated or increased; rise; edema or ECFVE

■　　　　　　■　　　　　　■

Table 10-3. LABORATORY STUDIES OF MRS. ALLEN			
Laboratory Tests	**On Admission**	**Day 1**	**Day 4**
Hematology			
Hemoglobin (12.9–17.0 g)	12.5		
Hematocrit (40–46%)	40		
WBC (white blood count)	8200		
Biochemistry			
BUN (blood urea nitrogen) (10–25 mg/dL)*	28	24	18
Plasma/serum CO_2†	22	24	24
Plasma/serum chloride (95–108 mEq/L)	107	106	107
Plasma/serum sodium (135–146 mEq/L)	151	148	143
Plasma/serum potassium (3.5–5.3 mEq/L)	3.6	3.8	4.0

*mg/100 mL = mg/dL.
†*Plasma* and *serum* are used interchangeably.

24 Mrs. Allen's low-average serum potassium may be due to a(n) (increase/decrease) _____ in ECF. Explain why. *_____

_____ .

Give another reason why Mrs. Allen's serum potassium may be low-average. *_____

_____ .

increase
Potassium may be diluted due to an increase of ECF or hemodilution.
There is a lack of food intake containing potassium or cellular breakdown from insufficient circulation. If she were receiving diuretics, this might cause a low serum K.

■ ■ ■

CLINICAL MANAGEMENT

The "three D's" are frequently employed in the management of congestive heart failure. They are:

1. Diet
2. Digitalization
3. Diuretics

The clinical management for CHF in Mrs. Allen's case incorporates the "three D's."

DIET

25 Mrs. Allen was placed on a low-sodium diet and her fluid intake was limited to 1200 mL (300 mL below daily requirement).

Salt and water intake is limited for which of the following reasons:

( ) a. Increase edema
( ) b. Prohibit further increase of edema
( ) c. Decrease water intoxication

a. —; b. X; c. —

■   ■   ■

DIGITALIZATION OR LOADING DOSES

Digitalization is the process of increasing the serum level of digitalis to achieve the desired physiologic effect. It is also referred to as a loading dose or doses.

Digitalis preparations are classified as cardiac glycosides (cardiotonic). The action of digitalis is to slow the ventricular contractions and increase the forcefulness of the contractions. Examples of digitalis preparations are digoxin, digitoxin, gitaligin, deslanoside (Cedilanid), and digitalis leaf. Digoxin is the choice cardiac glycoside for prolonged use in the treatment of CHF.

26 Digitalis is classified as a *_____ .

This drug slows the *_____ and makes the heat beat *_____

_____ .

cardiac glycoside; ventricular contractions (heart rate); more forcefully

■   ■   ■

27 Mrs. Allen was digitalized with digoxin and then placed on a daily maintenance dose of digoxin, 0.25 mg. This (increases/decreases) _____ cardiac output. Blood circulation is then _____ . The urinary output is _____ .

It is important that you remember the toxic effects of digitalis preparations, which include pulse below 60, nausea, vomiting, and anorexia.

increases; improved or increased; increased

■   ■   ■

DIURETICS

(Review Chapter 3, Table 3-8 and the section on diuretics.)

28 Diuretics are used for the excretion of sodium and water. Many diuretics increase the excretion of sodium, water, and chloride, and the valuable electrolyte _____ .

potassium

■   ■   ■

29 Frequently, physicians prescribe a potassium-sparing diuretic with a potassium-wasting diuretic to prevent excessive loss of what ion? _____ .

potassium

■   ■   ■

30 Identify diuretics that are potassium-wasting and potassium-sparing by placing K-W for potassium-wasting diuretics and K-S for potassium-sparing diuretics.

___ a. Hydrochlorothiazide (HydroDIURIL)
___ b. Triamterene (Dyrenium)
___ c. Furosemide (Lasix)
___ d. Mannitol
___ e. Spironolactone (Aldactone)

a. K-W; b. K-S; c. K-W; d. K-W; e. K-S

■   ■   ■

31 Give at least five symptoms of hypokalemia (potassium deficit). (Refer to Chapter 3 if necessary). *_____ , _____ , _____ , *_____ , and *_____ .

muscular weakness; dizziness, arrhythmia, silent ileus (decrease peristalsis), and abdominal distention

■   ■   ■

CASE STUDY REVIEW

Mrs. Allen, age 68, is in congestive heart failure on admission. The clinical assessment of her symptoms and findings are stated under clinical applications.

1. In early heart failure, name the three compensatory mechanisms that assisted Mrs. Allen to maintain her cardiac output to maintain circulation. *_____ , *_____ , and _____ .
2. Is Mrs. Allen in cardiac (compensation/decompensation)? _____ . Explain your answer. *_____
_____ .
3. Does the heart need (more/less) _____ blood when there is ventricular dilatation and hypertrophy?
4. With right-sided heart failure, the venous (hydrostatic) pressure is (increased/decreased) _____ . Explain why. *_____
_____ .

The nurse assessed Mrs. Allen's physiologic status and identified symptoms of left-sided heart failure and right-sided heart failure.

5. Mrs. Allen's symptoms of left-sided heart failure include:
    a. *_____
    b. *_____
    c. *_____
    d. *_____
    e. *_____
    f. *_____
6. The symptoms of left-sided heart failure are similar to symptoms of

    _____ .
7. Mrs. Allen's symptom of right-sided heart failure is *_____

    _____ .
8. Clinical management for Mrs. Allen consisted of the "three D's," which include
    _____ , _____ , and _____ .
9. Mrs. Allen is receiving HydroDIURIL. Is this a (potassium-wasting/potassium-sparing)
    _____ diuretic? The potassium imbalance that can occur is
    (hypokalemia/hyperkalemia) _____ .
10. If Mrs. Allen's serum potassium was below average, what effect does this have on digoxin.
    (Review Chapter 3 if necessary.) *_____

    _____ .
11. Give three symptoms of digitalis intoxication.
    a. *_____
    b. _____
    c. *_____

1. ventricular dilatation, ventricular hypertrophy, and tachycardia
2. decompensation
   The compensatory mechanisms failed to maintain cardiac output, since symptoms were present.
3. more
4. increased
   The blood is backed up in the venous system, causing increased pressure.
5. a. irritating cough; b. dyspnea on exertion; c. moist rales; d. hand vein engorgement;
   e. pulse 110 (tachycardia); f. ventricular hypertrophy
6. overhydration
7. swelling in the ankles and feet
8. diet, digitalization, and diuretics
9. potassium-wasting; hypokalemia
10. Hypokalemia enhances the action of any digitalis preparation, making the digoxin stronger
    (cumulative action can occur).
11. a. bradycardia—pulse ↓ 60 or arrhythmia, or both
    b. anorexia
    c. nausea and vomiting

NURSING ASSESSMENT FACTORS

- Obtain baseline vital signs to determine abnormal changes and for comparison with future vital signs.
- Assess for signs and symptoms of left-sided heart failure (overhydration or pulmonary edema), i.e., constant, irritating cough, dyspnea, neck and/or hand vein engorgement, chest rales.
- Assess for signs and symptoms of right-sided heart failure, i.e., pitting peripheral edema, liver enlargement, fullness of abdomen.
- Check serum electrolyte levels, especially potassium and sodium. Report abnormal findings. Use baseline electrolyte results for comparison with future serum electrolytes.

NURSING DIAGNOSIS 1

Fluid volume excess, related to cardiac decompensation secondary to left-sided and right-sided heart failure.

NURSING INTERVENTIONS AND RATIONALE

1. Auscultate lung areas to detect abnormal breath sounds, such as moist rales due to lung congestion (pulmonary edema).
2. Monitor vein engorgement by checking hand veins for fluid overload. Lower the hand below the heart level until the hand veins are engorged; then raise the hand above the heart level. If the hand veins remain engorged above heart level after 15 seconds, fluid volume excess is most likely present.
3. Check the feet and ankles daily in the early morning before client rises. If edema is present, the reason is probably due to cardiac and/or renal dysfunction.
4. Instruct client not to use table salt to season foods. Salt contains sodium, which can cause water retention. Suggest other ways to enhance flavor of foods.
5. Instruct the client to eat foods rich in potassium (fruits, vegetables) if he or she is taking a potassium-wasting diuretic and digoxin. Hypokalemia can enhance the action of digoxin and can cause digitalis toxicity (slow, irregular pulse, nausea/vomiting).
6. Assess for signs and symptoms of hypokalemia (serum potassium deficit), i.e., dizziness, muscular weakness, abdominal distention, diminished peristalsis, and dysrhythmia, if client has been receiving potassium-wasting diuretics for several months.

NURSING DIAGNOSIS 2

Ineffective breathing patterns, related to fluid in the lung tissues.

NURSING INTERVENTIONS AND RATIONALE

1. Monitor breathing patterns. Report the presence of dyspnea, shortness of breath, rapid breathing, and wheezing.
2. Elevate the head of the bed 30°–75° to lower the diaphragm and increase aveoli spaces for gas exchange. Client may sit upright in a chair or in an orthopneic position to increase available air space.

NURSING DIANGOSIS 3

Tissue integrity impaired, related to fluid accumulation in the extremities and buttocks.

NURSING INTERVENTIONS AND RATIONALE

1. Encourage the client to change positions frequently. Edematous tissue can break down due to hypoxia and constant pressure on skin surface.
2. Provide skin care, especially to edematous areas, at least twice daily.

NURSING DIAGNOSIS 4

Self-care deficit: feeding, bathing, and hygiene, related to fatigue and breathlessness secondary to CHF.

NURSING INTERVENTIONS AND RATIONALE

1. Assist client with activities of daily living such as feeding and bathing. COPD increases body fatigue and the inability to perform small tasks without extreme exhaustion.
2. Encourage family member(s) to participate in meeting client's needs as necessary.
3. Encourage the client to be self-sufficient if he or she is able to perform basic tasks and meet his or her needs, such as dressing, bathing, and hygiene care (brushing teeth).

OTHER POTENTIAL NURSING DIAGNOSIS

Tissue perfusion: altered, related to cardiopulmonary insufficiency.

CHAPTER 11

RENAL FAILURE: HEMODIALYSIS, PERITONEAL DIALYSIS, AND CONTINUOUS RENAL REPLACEMENT THERAPY

MARGARET POPPITI; R.N., M.S., C.N.N.

Behavioral Objectives

Upon completion of this chapter, you will be prepared to:

• Discuss the physiologic changes related to acute and chronic renal failure.

• Identify the etiologic factors associated with acute and chronic renal failure.

• Discuss common fluid, electrolyte, and acid-base imbalances in renal failure.

• Define the three types of clinical management for renal failure.

• Discuss the purposes for continuous renal replacement therapy (CRRT), hemodialysis, and peritoneal dialysis.

• Discuss the important nursing assessment factors associated with the clinical management of renal failure.

• Describe selected complications associated with the clinical management of renal failure.

• List selected nursing diagnoses and corresponding nursing interventions with rationale for clients with renal failure.

Introduction

Renal failure is the inability of the kidneys to excrete the by-products of cell metabolism and normal amounts of body water. Renal failure is classified as acute or chronic. *Acute renal failure (ARF)* results from an acute insult, primarily ischemia, toxicity, or obstruction. *Chronic renal failure (CRF)* frequently results from a disease process that affects the renal parenchyma and eventually causes cessation of renal function.

1 The term that describes the kidneys' inability to excrete waste products and the normal amounts of body water is *_____ .

 renal failure

■ ■ ■

PATHOPHYSIOLOGY

Acute renal failure (ARF) may progress through four phases: initial, oliguric, diuretic, and recovery. The characteristics of these four phases are described in Table 11-1.

Table 11-1. PHASES OF ARF

Phases	Characteristics
Initial	This phase begins when the insult occurs and continues until signs of azotemia and/or oliguria appear.
Oliguric	Urine output is less than 400 mL per day. BUN and creatinine are markedly elevated. Dialysis is initiated in this phase.
Diuretic	It starts with a sudden increase in urine output, 1.5 liters (1500 mL) or more per day. Nephrons do not concentrate urine sufficiently to conserve electrolytes and water. Risk of dehydration and death are high. This phase can continue for days to weeks.
Recovery	This phase is noted by a decrease in azotemia with kidneys showing an ability to concentrate urine. It may last from weeks to months.

2   When the urinary volume is less than 400 mL per day and azotemia is present, the client is in the _____ phase.

   If a sudden increase in urine output occurs (1.5 liters or more per day), the client is in the _____ phase. In the diuretic phase the greatest risk is _____ .

oliguric; diuretic; dehydration (if you answered electrolyte loss, true, but the greatest risk is ECFV deficit or dehydration)

■   ■   ■

3   The phase of ARF in which the kidneys can concentrate urine and azotemia is less apparent is called the *_____ .

recovery phase

■   ■   ■

   Chronic renal failure (CRF) is defined as insidious, progressive loss of renal function that is irreversible. The three stages of CRF are (1) decreased renal reserve, (2) renal insufficiency, and (3) end-stage renal disease (ESRD). Table 11-2 lists the three stages and the pathophysiologic factors associated with these stages.

4   The three stages of chronic renal failure are *_____ , *_____ , and *_____ .

decreased renal reserve, renal insufficiency, and end-stage renal disease

■   ■   ■

Table 11-2. STAGES OF CRF

Stages	Pathophysiologic Factors
Stage I: decreased renal reserve	Residual renal function is 40–70% of the normal kidney function. Excretory and regulatory renal functions are intact. Renal laboratory studies are asymptomatic (BUN and serum creatinine are normal). At least a 50–60% loss of renal function is required before signs of renal failure are evident. No symptoms are evident until there is a loss of at least 80% renal function.
Stage II: renal insufficiency	Residual renal function is 20–40% of the normal kidney function. There is a decrease in the glomerular filtration rate (GFR), solute clearance, ability to concentrate urine, and hormone secretion. Renal laboratory studies reveal a rising BUN and serum creatinine, mild azotemia, polyuria, nocturia, and anemia. Signs and symptoms become more severe if the kidneys are stressed, i.e., fluid volume depletion or exposure to a nephrotic substance.
Stage III: end-stage renal disease (ESRD)	Residual renal function is <15% of the normal kidney function. Excretory, regulatory, and hormonal renal functions are severely impaired and unable to maintain homeostasis. Renal laboratory studies and physical symptoms reveal markedly elevated BUN and serum creatinine levels. Anemia, hyperphosphatemia, hypocalcemia, metabolic acidosis, hyperuricemia, hyperkalemia, fluid overload, usually oliguric, and urine osmolality similar to serum osmolality. A uremic syndrome develops and all body systems are affected by renal failure. Mortality rate is 100% if peritoneal dialysis, hemodialysis, or renal transplant is not implemented.

5   In stage I, renal function is _____ % of normal; in stage II, renal function is _____ % of normal; and in stage III, renal function is _____ % of normal.

40–70; 20–40; <15

■   ■   ■

6 Indicate the blood urea nitrogen (BUN) and serum creatinine response to the three stages of CRF:

a. Stage I: BUN _____ , creatinine _____

b. Stage II: BUN _____ , creatinine _____

c. Stage III: BUN *_____ , creatinine *_____

a. *normal; normal*

b. *increased; increased*

c. *markedly elevated; markedly elevated*

■   ■   ■

7 Hyperkalemia, hyperphosphatemia, hypocalcemia, and metabolic acidosis occur frequently with which stage of CRF? _____ .

stage III

■   ■   ■

ETIOLOGY

The causes of ARF are listed in three categories: ischemia, toxicity, and obstruction. Table 11-3 lists examples of the causes, with contributing problems.

Table 11-3. CAUSES OF ARF		
Ischemia	**Toxicity**	**Obstruction**
Dehydration	Antibiotics:	Prerenal:
Shock:	Aminoglycosides	Arterial emboli
Distributive/sepsis	Penicillins	Aneurysm
Hypovolemic/hemorrhagic	Cephalosporins	Postrenal:
Cardiogenic	Nonsteroidal anti-inflammatory drugs	Ureteral obstruction
	Organic compounds:	Bladder obstruction
	Carbon tetrachloride	Catheter obstruction
	Methyl alcohol	
	Miscellaneous:	
	Myoglobin, transfusion reactions	

8 Acute renal failure usually results from insult to the kidney causing a rapid deterioration of renal function. The three major categories of the causes of ARF are _____ , _____ , and _____ .

ischemia, toxicity, and obstruction

■   ■   ■

9   Give examples of the following major causes of ARF:

Ischemia: _____

Toxicity: _____

Obstruction: * _____

shock

antibiotics, e.g., aminoglycosides

arterial emboli (prerenal) or ureteral obstruction (postrenal)

Causes of CRF are listed in Table 11-4.

Table 11-4. CAUSES OF CRF	
Etiology	**Examples**
Congenital/developmental disorders	Bilateral renal hypoplasia Fused kidney Ectopic or displaced kidney Bilateral renal dysplasia
Cystic disorders	Polycystic kidney disease Medullary cystic kidney disease
Tubular disorders	Renal tubular acidosis (RTA) Fanconi's syndrome
Glomerular disorder	Glomerulonephritis (major cause of ESRD)
Neoplasms	Benign tumor Malignant tumor Wilm's tumor
Infectious diseases	Pyelonephritis Renal tuberculosis
Obstructive disorders	Nephrolithiasis Retroperitoneal fibrosis
Systemic diseases	Diabetes mellitus (DM): approximately 25% of ESRD clients with DM. Approximately 50% of Type I DM (juvenile onset) develop ESRD within 20 years of onset of DM. Diabetes insipidus Systemic lupus erythematosus (SLE) Hepatorenal syndrome Hypertensive nephropathy Amyloidosis Scleroderma Primary hyperparathyroidism Goodpasture's syndrome Henoch-Schoenlein purpura

10 An example of an infectious disease causing CRF is _____ . A major cause of end-stage renal failure (ESRF) is _____ .

pyelonephritis; glomerulonephritis

■   ■   ■

11 Approximately 25% of the clients with ESRD have the systemic chronic disease
*_____ .

diabetes mellitus

■   ■   ■

12 Name five systemic diseases that can lead to ESRD. *_____ ,
*_____ , *_____ , *_____ , and
*_____ .

diabetes mellitus, diabetes insipidus, hepatorenal syndrome, hypertensive nephropathy, and systemic lupus erythematosus (others: scleroderma, amyloidosis)

■   ■   ■

13 Urine output in renal failure varies. No urine output is labeled *anuria*. In ARF the cause of anuria may be prerenal or postrenal obstruction. In CRF anuria indicates total loss of parenchymal function.

ARF means *_____ .
CRF means *_____ .
    Anuria, which is *_____ , differs in ARF and CRF. In ARF anuria may be the result of *_____
_____ , and in CRF anuria may cause
*_____ .

acute renal failure; chronic renal failure
no urine output
prerenal or postrenal obstruction; total loss of parenchymal function

■   ■   ■

14   Normal urine output exceeds 30 mL per hour. Urine output of less than 400–500 mL per 24 hours is *oliguria*. No urine output is called _____ .

In ARF ischemia and nephrotoxicity are the causes of oliguria, whereas in CRF oliguria indicates a decline in parenchymal function.

anuria

       ■   ■   ■

15   Symptoms of ARF and CRF appear when renal function decreases to at least 20%. When renal function decreases to less than 15%, death results if dialysis treatment is not initiated.

Indicate which of the following problems contribute to acute and chronic renal failure by using ARF for acute renal failure and CRF for chronic renal failure.

_____ a. Severe dehydration (hypovolemia)
_____ b. Diabetes mellitus
_____ c. Bladder obstruction
_____ d. Glomerulonephritis
_____ e. Hypertension nephropathy
_____ f. Severe fluid volume deficit
_____ g. Systemic lupus erythematosus
_____ h. Aminoglycoside therapy
_____ i. Pyelonephritis
_____ j. Nephrosclerosis
_____ k. Carbon tetrachloride
_____ l. Sepsis

a. ARF; b. CRF; c. ARF; d. CRF; e. CRF; f. ARF; g. CRF; h. ARF; i. CRF; j. CRF; k. ARF; l. ARF

       ■   ■   ■

CLINICAL MANIFESTATIONS

16   Two measurements of nitrogenous waste products, by-products of protein metabolism, are BUN and creatinine. A rise in the level of BUN and creatinine is known as azotemia.

The two by-products of protein metabolism or nitrogenous waste products are _____ and _____ . Azotemia occurs when *_____

_____ .

BUN and creatinine; BUN and creatinine levels rise

       ■   ■   ■

17 In ARF, the earliest sign after the insult is a rise in the BUN and serum creatinine accompanied by oliguria or nonoliguria.

The two renal laboratory results that can indicate an early sign of ARF are

*_____ and *_____ .

increased BUN and increased serum creatinine
■   ■   ■

The earliest manifestations of the disease that may lead to CRF are hematuria and proteinuria. At least 50–60% loss of renal tissue is required before signs are evident. If undetected, renal disease progresses, renal function degenerates, and azotemia ensues. No symptoms are evident until loss of renal tissue is at least 80%.

18 In ARF oliguria is usually caused by _____ and _____ . In CRF oliguria indicates *_____ .

In CRF two early manifestations of renal disease are _____ , and

_____ .

ischemia and nephrotoxicity; a decline in parenchymal function; hematuria and proteinuria
■   ■   ■

FLUID, ELECTROLYTE, AND ACID-BASE IMBALANCES

Table 11-5 outlines the fluid, electrolyte, and acid-base changes that occur in renal failure and lists the rationale for the signs and symptoms. Study the table carefully, noting the changes that occur.

Table 11-5. FLUID, ELECTROLYTE, AND ACID-BASE IMBALANCES IN RENAL FAILURE		
Imbalances	**Rationale**	**Signs and Symptoms**
Fluid Overload Decreased urine output	Inability of the kidneys to concentrate, dilute, and excrete urine with normal or excessive intake of fluid. When creatinine clearance is less than 4–5 mL/min, volume overload is usually the major problem.	Noninvasive: elevated jugular venous pressure Pitting edema: preorbital, hands, feet, sacral, anasarca.
Sodium retention	Increased tubular reabsorption of sodium due to reduced renal perfusion and/or increased renin-angiotensin-aldosterone secretion. Occurs in ischemia and malignant hypertension.	Increased blood pressure Weight gain Moist rales Dyspnea Pulmonary edema

Table 11-5.   (Continued)

Imbalances	Rationale	Signs and Symptoms
Reduced oncotic pressure	Loss of intravascular protein through damaged glomeruli leads to decreased intravascular volume. ADH secretion increases water retention to maintain intravascular volume. Continued protein loss decreases oncotic pressure in capillaries and causes water to move into the interstitial space. Seen in nephrotic syndrome, glomerular diseases, and liver ascites.	Invasive: increased central venous pressure Elevated pulmonary artery and wedge pressure
Potassium Excess Potassium retention	*Hyperkalemia* Inability of the kidneys to excrete potassium in severe oliguric and anuric states.	Noninvasive: weakness, parathesia, Nausea, vomiting ECG: elevated T wave Tachycardia Cardiac arrest
Cellular injury	Massive tissue injury, acidosis, and protein catabolism cause potassium to leave cells.	Invasive: serum K >5.3mEq/L Decreased pH (arterial blood) Decreased serum CO_2 and arterial HCO_3
Potassium Deficit Potassium loss	*Hypokalemia* Excessive loss of GI secretions or excessive loss in dialysis.	Noninvasive: muscle weakness Abdominal distention Arrhythmia
Diuretic phase of ARF	Excessive loss of electrolytes and water due to the kidneys' inability to concentrate urine.	Anorexia, N/V ECG: flat or inverted T wave, prominent U wave, and AV block
Renal tubular acidosis	Nonoliguric azotemia causes excretion of K^+. Present in Fanconi's syndrome, nephrotic syndrome, multiple myeloma, cirrhosis, and some drug toxicities.	Invasive: serum K <3.5 mEq/L

Table 11-5.   (Continued)

Imbalances	Rationale	Signs and Symptoms
Sodium Excess Increased tubular sodium absorption	*Hypernatremia* With decreased intravascular volume, aldosterone secretion increases sodium retention to improve intravascular volume. May be seen in nephrotic syndrome and liver ascites.	Noninvasive: edema Dry tongue Tachycardia Thirst Weight gain Increased BP
Dietary sodium ingestion	Increased dietary ingestion of sodium, especially in anuric states.	Invasive: serum Na >145 mEq/L
Sodium Deficit Sodium loss	*Hyponatremia* Excessive loss of gastrointestinal secretion through suction, vomiting, and diarrhea.	Noninvasive: decreased skin turgor Decreased BP
Diuretic phase of ARF	Excessive loss of electrolytes and water because of the kidneys' inability to concentrate urine.	Rapid pulse Dry mucous membrane Muscle weakness Invasive: serum Na <130 mEq/L
Excessive fluid intake	Increased fluid intake with oliguria or anuria present dilutes the serum sodium level.	
Metabolic acidosis	Sodium shifts into cells as potassium shifts to plasma during acidosis.	
Phosphorus Excess Phosphorus (phosphate) retention	*Hyperphosphatemia* Occurs because of decreased renal phosphate excretion, which increases metabolic acidosis. Phosphorus affects serum calcium level by altering the balance of their reciprocal relationships. Parathyroid hormone (PTH) (parathormone) enhances phosphorus or phosphate excretion in the urine.	Noninvasive: nausea and diarrhea Tachycardia Tetany with low Ca Hyperreflexia Muscle weakness Flaccid paralysis Invasive: serum P >4.5 mg/dL or >2.6 mEq/L

Table 11-5. (Continued)

Imbalances	Rationale	Signs and Symptoms
Calcium Deficit Increased phosphorus retention	*Hypocalcemia* Decreases the balance between calcium and phosphorus. PTH demineralizes the bone to increase serum calcium. Untreated hypocalcemia and hyperphosphatemia lead to renal osteodystrophy and metastatic calcification (deposits of calcium phosphate crystals in soft tissues). The goal is to maintain serum Ca-P product of approximately 40 mg/mL.	Noninvasive: tetany Muscle twitching Tingling Carpopedal spasm Laryngeal spasm Abdominal cramps Muscle cramps Decreased clotting Cardiac dysrhythmias Positive Chvostek sign Positive Trousseau sign
Decreased absorption of calcium from intestines	Impaired vitamin D activity from renal impairment causes reduced calcium absorption.	Invasive: serum Ca <9 mg/dL or <4.5 mEq/L PTH >375 pg Eq/mL Ca-P product >70 mg/dL
Metabolic Acidosis Hydrogen ion retention	Inability of kidneys to excrete daily hydrogen ion load.	Noninvasive: weakness Lassitude; Increased respiration (rate and depth)
Reduced buffering mechanisms in tubules	Refer to Chapter 4, on renal regulatory mechanisms.	Restlessness Flushed skin
Ammonia	Reduced nephron function inhibits conversion of ammonia and HCl to NH_4Cl for excretion.	Invasive: pH <7.35 HCO_3 <24 mEq/L anion gap >16 mEq/L
Phosphate salts	Reduced nephron function inhibits the combination of hydrogen ion with $NaHPO_4$ to form NaH_2PO_4 for excretion.	
Bicarbonate (HCO_3)	With damaged nephrons, less HCO_3 is regenerated and reabsorbed in the tubules.	
Retention of metabolic acids	Inability of the kidneys to excrete uric, sulfuric, phosphate, and other acids of metabolism.	
Lactic acid formation	Occurs from tissue hypoxemia from an ischemic insult.	

Table 11-5. (Continued)		
Imbalances	**Rationale**	**Signs and Symptoms**
Increased fat breakdown	Malnutrition from decreased nutritional intake causes accumulation of ketone acids.	
Urine Sodium and Osmolality Urine sodium	Ischemic state increases ADH and aldosterone secretions. Renal efforts to conserve sodium show fewer Na ions in urine, <20 mEq. However, damaged nephrons cannot filter sufficiently; therefore it is possible that urine sodium level >20 mEq.	
Urine osmolality	Ischemic state increases renal filtration; thus urine osmolality >500 mOsm/kg/H$_2$O. Injured nephrons with impaired filtration have urine osmolality similar to plasma, 290 mOsm/kg/H$_2$O.	

19 In renal failure fluid overload can occur from the following pathologic response:

a. *_____

b. *_____

c. *_____

a. *decreased urine output;* b. *sodium retention;* c. *reduced oncotic pressure*
∎ ∎ ∎

20 Name six symptoms of fluid overload (noninvasive and invasive). *_____ ,
*_____ , *_____ , *_____ ,
_____ , and *_____ .

elevated jugular venous pressure, pitting edema, weight gain, increased blood pressure, dyspnea, and increased central venous pressure (others: moist rales, pulmonary edema, elevated pulmonary artery, and wedge pressures)
∎ ∎ ∎

21 A potassium excess occurs primarily with which urinary symptoms? *_____ .

A potassium excess can cause cardiac muscle to exhibit which two symptoms?
*_____ , and *_____ .

severe oligura and anuria; ventricular tachycardia and cardiac arrest

■ ■ ■

22 Name the conditions that may cause potassium deficits.

a. *_____
b. *_____
c. *_____

a. loss of GI secretions or from dialysis; b. diuretic phase of ARF; c. renal tubular acidosis

■ ■ ■

23 Name the conditions that may cause sodium excess.

a. *_____
b. *_____

a. increased tubular absorption; b. dietary ingestion

■ ■ ■

24 Name the conditions that may cause sodium deficits.

a. *_____
b. *_____
c. *_____
d. *_____

a. loss of GI secretions; b. diuretic phase of ARF; c. excessive fluid intake; d. metabolic acidosis

■ ■ ■

25 An excess serum phosphorus/phosphate level in renal failure is caused by
*_____ . The retention of phosphorus/phosphate alters the balance between calcium and phosphorus. The result of the calcium imbalance is _____ .

decreased excretion of phosphate; hypocalcemia or calcium loss (deficit)

■ ■ ■

26 Calcium deficit results in symptoms of tetany, three of which are *_____ ,
_____ , and *_____ .

In which acid-base imbalance are the symptoms of tetany decreased? *_____ .

muscle twitching, tingling, and laryngeal spasms (also carpopedal spasm and positive Chvostek and Trousseau's signs); metabolic acidosis

■   ■   ■

27 Calcium deficits enhance the toxic effect of a high serum potassium by increasing cardiac muscle irritability.

When a low serum calcium exists, the serum potassium must be monitored to prevent
*_____ .

cardiac muscle irritability

■   ■   ■

28 Name the metabolic changes associated with renal failure that cause metabolic acidosis.

a. *_____
b. *_____
c. *_____
d. *_____
e. *_____

a. hydrogen ion retention; b. reduction of buffering mechanisms; c. retention of metabolic acids; d. lactic acid formation; e. increased breakdown of fats

■   ■   ■

29 What respiratory symptom occurs in metabolic acidosis? *_____ .

an increased respiratory rate and depth or Kussmaul breathing

■   ■   ■

30 Two urinary tests for assessing damaged nephrons are *_____ and
*_____ .

urine sodium and urine osmolality

■   ■   ■

31 A low urine sodium indicates increased ADH and aldosterone secretions. Nephrons damaged by ischemia or toxins cannot filter sufficiently and the urine sodium can be

_____ .

increased

■   ■   ■

32 The urine osmolality measures the kidneys' ability to dilute and concentrate urine. Damaged nephrons impair filtration and decrease the kidneys' ability to concentrate urine. As a result of damaged nephrons, the urine is (diluted/concentrated) _____ .

diluted

■　　　　　　　■　　　　　　　■

Table 11-6 explains the effects of renal failure on body systems. Refer to the table as needed to answer the following frames.

Table 11-6. SYSTEMIC EFFECTS OF RENAL FAILURE	
Body Systems	**Rationale**
Neurologic	Uremic waste products cause slow neural conduction. Changes in personality, thought processes, levels of consciousness, and seizures can occur.
Cardiovascular	Fluid retention causes fluid overload, hypertension, and cardiac hypertrophy. Electrolyte imbalance causes arrhythmias. Uremic waste products can irritate the pericardium and lead to pericarditis and cardiac tamponade.
Respiratory	Fluid retention causes pulmonary edema. Thick bronchial secretions and impaired immune response increase susceptibility to bacterial infections.
Gastrointestinal	Ulcerations can develop anywhere in the mucosa of the GI tract from the breakdown of urea to ammonia. Metallic taste in mouth, hiccups, indigestion, nausea, and urine smell to breath from buildup of uremic waste products are added effects.
Hematologic	Failure of the kidneys to secrete erythropoietin results in decreased red cell production and anemia. Platelet survival is diminished and bleeding tendencies are increased. Immune deficiency develops from uremic waste products.
Musculoskeletal	Brittle bones and metastatic calcification result from bone demineralization in response to phosphorus and calcium imbalance.
Endocrine	Secondary hyperparathyroidism can develop from phosphorus and calcium imbalances. Sexual and menstrual dysfunctions are the result. Growth and mental retardation occur in children and carbohydrate and lipoprotein metabolism are altered.
Integumentary	Uremic waste products cause pruritis and dryness. Retained pigments and anemia give the skin a bronze cast.

33 Which of the following body systems are affected by renal failure?

( ) a. Cardiovascular
( ) b. Respiratory
( ) c. Eye
( ) d. Neurologic
( ) e. Gastrointestinal
( ) f. Integumentary
( ) g. Musculoskeletal
( ) h. Endocrine
( ) i. Hematologic

a. X; b. X; c. —; d. X; e. X; f. X; g. X; h. X; i. X
                ■   ■   ■

CLINICAL MANAGEMENT: DIALYSIS—CONTINUOUS RENAL REPLACEMENT THERAPY (CRRT), HEMODIALYSIS, AND PERITONEAL DIALYSIS

Dialysis is the process of filtrating uremic waste products and excess body fluid through a semipermeable membrane to restore body homeostasis.

Diffusion is the movement of molecules/solutes in a solution. In diffusion the rate of movement across the permeable membrane is greater from the areas of higher concentration to the areas of lower concentration.

Osmosis is the movement of water molecules across a semipermeable membrane from an area of higher water concentration to an area of lower water concentration.

Ultrafiltration is the pressure gradient that enhances the movement of water molecules across the semipermeable membrane.

34 The movement of molecules across a semipermeable membrane from an area of higher concentration to an area of lower concentration is _____ .

The pressure gradient that enhances the movement of water molecules is called

_____ .

The movement of water molecules across a semipermeable membrane from an area of higher water concentration to one of lower water concentration is called _____ .

diffusion; ultrafiltration; osmosis
                   ■   ■   ■

35 Types of dialysis therapy are continuous renal replacement therapy (CRRT), hemodialysis, and peritoneal dialysis.

The objectives for all these types are to restore electrolyte balance, to remove uremic waste products, and to restore the patient's dry weight. *Dry weight* is normal body weight without excess fluid.

Name two goals of dialysis. *_____ , and *_____ .

to restore electrolyte balance and to remove uremic waste products (also to restore client's dry weight)

■   ■   ■

CONTINUOUS RENAL REPLACEMENT THERAPY

36 The type of dialysis most effective in the treatment of ARF is continuous renal replacement therapy (CRRT). In CRRT, an extracorporeal circuit is created with arterial to venous blood flow using the client's mean arterial pressure (MAP) as the primary driving force. This acute treatment is administered in the ICU setting.

For CRRT, the client's *_____ is used as the primary driving force for creating the arterial to venous blood flow.

MAP

■   ■   ■

37 CRRT uses a hemofilter which is a very porous blood filter with a semipermeable membrane that is positioned in an extracorporeal circuit with arterial outflow to venous return access.

A very porous blood filter with a semipermeable membrane used in CRRT is called a

_____ .

hemofilter

■   ■   ■

38 Unlike hemodialysis, CRRT requires cannulation of both an artery and a vein for extracorporeal blood flow.

Types of CRRT are (1) slow continuous ultrafiltration (SCUF), (2) continuous arteriovenous hemofiltration (CAVH), and (3) continuous arteriovenous hemodialysis (CAVHD).

CRRT requires cannulation in both an _____ and a

_____ .

artery; vein

■   ■   ■

39 The three types of CRRT are *_____ , *_____ , and
*_____ .

*slow continuous ultrafiltration, continuous arteriovenous hemofiltration, and continuous
arteriovenous hemodialysis*
■   ■   ■

Indications for CRRT in the ICU setting include:

1. Clients with *CRF* with a preexisting vascular access who are clinically unable to tolerate routine
   hemodialysis procedures, such as with acute pulmonary edema, CHF, recent gastrointestinal
   bleeding, and/or cardiogenic shock.
2. Clients with *ARF* who are too hemodynamically unstable for aggressive hemodialysis and for
   whom peritoneal dialysis is contraindicated. Examples include postoperative cardiac bypass
   surgery, recent myocardial infarction, sepsis, ARDS, and postoperative vascular bypass surgery.
3. Clients with *ARF* who are very catabolic and require daily clearance of uremic toxins and
   electrolyte and bicarbonate replacements.
4. Clients with oliguria who require large quantities of IV fluids either as medication or
   hyperalimentation.

40 Indicate which clients with the following clinical health problems might be candidates for
CRRT:

( ) a. Has CRF and cardiogenic shock occurs
( ) b. Has ARF and has an acute myocardial infarction
( ) c. Has an early stage of pyelonephritis
( ) d. Has ARF and has blood uremic toxins
( ) e. Has oliguria and requires large amounts IV therapy
( ) f. Has polyuria and does not receive sufficient fluids

a. X; b. X; c. —; d. X; e. X; f. —
■   ■   ■

41 Hemodialysis and peritoneal dialysis are similar in the following ways: Both use dialysate,
which is a solution that contains electrolytes approximating normal plasma, and both use a
semipermeable membrane.

List two ways in which hemodialysis and peritoneal dialysis are similar.
*_____ , and *_____ .

*They both use dialysate similar in composition to normal plasma, and they both use a
semipermeable membrane.*
■   ■   ■

HEMODIALYSIS

42 In hemodialysis the artificial kidney (AK) is a semipermeable membrane made of a cellophanelike material through which only molecules of a particular size can diffuse.

The semipermeable membrane of the artificial kidney is a membrane through which only molecules of a *_____ .

particular size can diffuse

■   ■   ■

43 The dialysate solution is prepared in the delivery system, where it is mixed to the correct concentration, heated, and pumped into the artificial kidney.

List the functions of the delivery system:

a. *_____
b. *_____
c. *_____

a. mixes dialysate in the correct concentration; b. heats dialysate; c. pumps dialysate

■   ■   ■

44 Dialysate for hemodialysis contains five basic components: calcium chloride, magnesium chloride, potassium chloride, sodium chloride, and sodium acetate or bicarbonate. The concentration of these iso-osmolar/isotonic components resembles low plasma concentrations, but it can be prepared to correct an electrolyte or acid-base imbalance.

If a client has a potassium excess, the dialysate can be prepared with low potassium. If a client has metabolic acidosis, acetate or bicarbonate in dialysate can be used.

Dialysate can be individualized for correcting imbalances of _____ and _____ .

electrolytes or potassium; acid-base or acidosis

■   ■   ■

45 There are no uremic waste products in the dialysate. Therefore urea, creatinine, and other metabolic waste products diffuse rapidly from the blood across the membrane into the dialysate.

Uremic waste products rapidly diffuse from the _____ into the _____ .

blood; dialysate

■   ■   ■

46 Vascular access to the client's bloodstream must be obtained to initiate hemodialysis. This access is surgically created or obtained by catheterizing a large vein.

To initiate hemodialysis, vascular access to the _____ must be obtained.

bloodstream

■   ■   ■

47 During hemodialysis blood is pumped through tubing to the membranes of the AK. Two common types of AK design are the flat plate and hollow fiber. The flat plate is a stack of plastic plates with two membranes between each plate. Blood flows between these membranes. The hollow fiber has thousands of tiny hairlike fibers through which blood flows.

By using the flat-plate AK blood flows *_____ .

With the hollow-fiber AK blood flows *_____ .

between the membranes; through the tiny hairlike fibers

■   ■   ■

48 A complication of hemodialysis is blood clotting in the blood lines and AK. This can be prevented by administering heparin, an anticoagulant, during the procedure.

Heparin administered during hemodialysis prevents _____ .

clotting

■   ■   ■

49 The delivery system pumps dialysate through the AK and around membranes. A negative pressure gradient, created by the delivery system, pulls excess water from the blood across the semipermeable membrane. A positive pressure gradient that pushes excess water across the membrane can occur. Ultrafiltration results and excess fluid is removed from the client's bloodstream.

A negative pressure gradient results from *_____

_____ . Excess fluid is removed from the client by _____ .

the pull of water across the semipermeable membrane; ultrafiltration

■   ■   ■

50   The goal of ultrafiltration is to obtain the client's dry weight and prevent cardiovascular complications such as hypertension, pulmonary edema, and ventricular hypertrophy.

Dry weight is   *_____ .

Maintaining the client's dry weight prevents _____ complications.

the normal body weight without excess fluid; cardiovascular

■   ■   ■

51   Hemodialysis treatment takes 3–4 hours to complete. The results should be the removal of
*_____ , restoration of   *_____ , and removal of
*_____ .

Hemodialysis is done on a constant basis for client with CRF and intermittently for those in ARF until renal function improves.

uremic waste products; electrolyte balance; excess fluid

■   ■   ■

PERITONEAL DIALYSIS

52   In peritoneal dialysis the peritoneum that surrounds the abdominal cavity is used as the semipermeable membrane.

The semipermeable membrane used in peritoneal dialysis is the _____ .

peritoneum

■   ■   ■

53   The dialysate for peritoneal dialysis is a sterile solution that contains similar levels of sodium, magnesium, calcium, and chloride as the plasma.

The dialysate electrolyte levels of sodium, magnesium, calcium, and chloride are similar to
_____ .

The dialysate solution is _____ .

plasma; sterile

■   ■   ■

54   Potassium is not included in peritoneal dialysate solutions. The physician prescribes the amount of potassium that can be added to the dialysate according to the client's serum potassium level.

Why do you think potassium is not added to the solution?   *_____ .

The client's potassium level may be high. Adding too much potassium to the solution could increase the hyperkalemic state OR similar answer. Very good.

■   ■   ■

55 Acid-base balance is corrected in peritoneal dialysis by adding acetate, a bicarbonate precursor, to the dialysate solution. This buffers metabolic acids.

Acetate can be added to peritoneal dialysate to correct what acid-base disorder?
* _____ .

metabolic acidosis

■   ■   ■

56 Ultrafiltration is accomplished in peritoneal dialysis by creating an osmotic pressure gradient with glucose. The glucose concentration in the dialysate creates a hyperosmolar solution that pulls water across the peritoneal membrane.

Glucose in peritoneal dialysate creates an * _____ gradient. The dialysate solution in peritoneal dialysis is _____ .

osmotic pressure; hyperosmolar

■   ■   ■

57 Peritoneal dialysate has four concentrations of glucose: 1.5, 2.5, 3.5, and 4.5%. The physician prescribes the concentration needed on the basis of the client's state of fluid overload. The higher the glucose concentration, the more hyperosmolar the solution. The result is more ultrafiltration.

More ultrafiltration occurs in peritoneal dialysis when the dialysate has a
* _____ .

high glucose concentration

■   ■   ■

58 Peritoneal dialysis begins by inserting a catheter into the peritoneal cavity. Capillary beds within the layers of peritoneum provide an indirect access to the bloodstream for the dialysate.

Access for peritoneal dialysis is obtained by a _____ .

catheter

■   ■   ■

59 A serious complication of peritoneal dialysis is peritonitis, the result of an infection caused by the peritoneal catheter, e.g., contamination.

Peritonitis is a serious complication of * _____ . It is caused by an
* _____ .

peritoneal dialysis; infection associated with the catheter

■   ■   ■

60 Two liters of dialysate is usually infused by gravity into the peritoneal cavity where it remains (dwells) for a prescribed time. Infusion of fluid by gravity takes approximately 10 minutes for a 2-liter volume. The dwell or equilibration period provides time for diffusion and osmosis to occur. A typical dwell or equilibration time for acute peritoneal dialysis is 30–60 minutes; in chronic peritoneal dialysis, the dwell time is 4–6 hours. The excess fluid, electrolytes, and uremic waste products (ultrafiltrate) move through the peritoneal membrane into the dialysate. The solution is then drained from the abdomen by gravity. The drainage of 2 liters of dialysate and ultrafiltrate takes approximately 10 minutes providing that the catheter is patent.

Dialysate solution is infused by gravity into the   *_____ .

How is the dialysate removed from the abdomen?   *_____ .

peritoneal cavity; by gravity

■   ■   ■

61 The approximate time for infusion or inflow of solution by gravity is _____ minutes.

The time for the dialysate to dwell (equilibrate) in the peritoneal cavity for acute conditions is _____ minutes.

The approximate time for the return of dialysate and ultrafiltrate (excess fluid, electrolytes, and uremic waste products) is _____ minutes.

10; 30–60; 10

■   ■   ■

62 Each infusion of fresh dialysate is referred to as an exchange. The treatment plan prescribed by the nephrologist includes the dialysis regimen, combined with the method of peritoneal dialysis, dialysis solution concentration, the frequency of exchanges, and the infusion volume and prescribed dwell time.

When ordering peritoneal dialysis, four of the treatment plans that the nephrologist must prescribe are *_____ , *_____ , *_____ , and *_____ .

dialysis regimen, method of peritoneal dialysis, dialysis solution concentration, and frequency of exchanges (others: infusion volume and dwell or equilibration time)

■   ■   ■

63 When a peritoneal catheter is first inserted, heparin is added to the dialysate to maintain catheter patency by preventing the obstruction of the peritoneal catheter with fibrin and/or blood.

The purpose of heparin in the dialysate is to *_____ .

maintain catheter patency (prevent fibrin and clot formation)

■ ■ ■

64 The amount of dialysate returned by gravity determines the amount of fluid loss from the body. The return must be accurately measured to maintain fluid balance. If the dialysate return is more than the amount of the infusion fluid being removed, there is a fluid imbalance.

The process by which this exchange occurs is called _____ .

When the amount of dialysate returned is less than the amount infused, fluid is being (retained/excreted) _____ . An accurate record of these differences must be maintained by the nurse.

ultrafiltration; retained

■ ■ ■

65 If 2000 mL of dialysate is infused and 2500 mL is returned, an excess of 500 mL is being _____ .

If 2000 mL of dialysate is infused and 1500 mL is returned, 500 mL is being _____ .

ultrafiltrated or excreted; retained

■ ■ ■

66 Retained dialysate can be reabsorbed and can lead to a fluid overload. Symptoms of fluid overload or overhydration are increased blood pressure, dyspnea, constant irritating cough, neck vein engorgement, chest rales, and edema.

One cause of fluid overload during peritoneal dialysis is the *_____ .

Name four symptoms associated with fluid overload. *_____ , _____ , *_____ , and *_____ .

retention of dialysate fluid; increased blood pressure, dyspnea, neck vein engorgement, and chest rales (also edema and irritated cough)

■ ■ ■

67 Excessive ultrafiltration can result in dehydration. Solutions such as 2.5% (398 mOsm/L) and 4.5% glucose dialysate (486 mOsm) or excessive exchanges can result in dehydration if not properly monitored. Symptoms of dehydration are decreased blood pressure, poor tissue turgor, tachycardia, dry mucous membranes, and hypernatremia.

Dehydration can result from *_____ or *_____ .

Name three symptoms of dehydration and fluid loss. *_____ ,
*_____ , and _____ .

4.5% glucose dialysate; excessive exchanges
decreased blood pressure, poor tissue turgor, and tachycardia (also dry mucous membranes)
■   ■   ■

Table 11-7 compares the three types of dialysis treatment for renal failure. Unlike hemodialysis, CRRT is a continuous form of therapy which achieves a more stable maintenance of the volume and composition of body fluids. Rapid intercompartmental fluid shifts observed in hemodialysis are avoided and blood pressure instability is prevented. The solute concentration changes observed in intermittent therapy are often avoided; thus the physician is able to remove or add electrolytes independent of changes in total body water. CRRT is used only as an acute therapy. This treatment takes place in an ICU (intensive care unit) for a limited period of time until there is a recovery in the client's kidney function or either peritoneal dialysis or hemodialysis is instituted.

68 Enter HD for hemodialysis, PD for peritoneal dialysis, and CRRT for continuous renal replacement therapy for the effect of the appropriate dialysis procedure:

___ a. Removes fluid rapidly
___ b. Removes excess potassium slowly
___ c. Removes waste products quickly
___ d. Needs no direct access to the bloodstream
___ e. Is used in the ICU setting as an acute treatment
___ f. Requires complex equipment and specialized training
___ g. Can be used for hemodynamically unstable clients
___ h. Is poorly tolerated by clients with cardiovascular disease
___ i. Has high cost
___ j. Risk of peritonitis
___ k. Requires small amounts of heparin

a. HD; b. PD; c. HD; d. PD; e. CRRT; f. HD; g. CRRT; h. HD; i. HD; j. PD; k. PD
■   ■   ■

Table 11-7. COMPARISON OF HEMODIALYSIS, PERITONEAL DIALYSIS, AND CRRT

Hemodialysis	Peritoneal	CRRT
Rapid removal of fluid	Fluid removed slowly	Rapid removal of fluid
Potassium lowered quickly	Potassium lowered slowly	Allows for removal or addition of electrolytes independent of changes in total body water
Waste products removed quickly	Waste products removed at a slower rate	
Rapid removal of poisonous drugs	Inefficient for removal of poisonous drugs	
Treatment time 3–4 hours	Usual treatment process includes three to four exchanges per day	A continuous treatment process
Requires complex equipment and specialized training	Uses less complex equipment and less specialized personnel.	Requires the use of a simple filter and ICU personnel
Requires vascular access	Requires no direct access to the bloodstream; causes no blood loss; used for clients with poor vascular access, i.e., children and the elderly	Requires vascular access
Requires large doses of heparin	Requires none or very small amounts of heparin	Requires the use of heparin and close monitoring for clotting in both the filter and tubing
Poorly tolerated by clients with cardiovascular disease	Minimal stress to clients with cardiovascular disease	Minimal stress for patients with cardiovascular disease
Contraindicated for clients in shock or hypotension	Can be used for clients with unstable cardiovascular status	Can be used for clients with unstable cardiovascular status
Can be used for clients with abdominal trauma	Contraindicated for clients with a colostomy, abdominal adhesions, ruptured diaphragm, or recent surgery	Can be used for clients with abdominal trauma or who are hemodynamically unstable
Cost is high	Cost effective	Cost effective
Risk of clotting increased with vascular access	Risk for peritonitis increased	Risk of clotting access increased; Risk of dehydration from inappropriate fluid replacement increased
Treatment prescribed for chronic or acute conditions	Treatment prescribed for chronic or acute conditions	Treatment is prescribed only for acute conditions and is provided only in ICU setting

CLINICAL APPLICATIONS

Mr. Tom Smith, age 36, sustained critical injuries in a motor vehicle accident. Assessment in the emergency room indicated that he suffered from blunt trauma to the chest and abdomen and two fractured femurs. He was also in shock. He went to surgery immediately for an exploratory laparotomy in which a splenectomy, aspiration of a large retroperitoneal hematoma, and repair of a ruptured diaphragm were performed. It was noted that he had bilateral contusion of both kidneys. An open reduction of his fractures was done and he was placed in balanced traction.

His urine after surgery was grossly bloody and the output ranged from 10 to 20 mL per hour. Mr. Smith experienced hypotension after his injury and surgery. He was transfused with eight units of whole blood. Postoperatively, Mr. Smith was sent to the SICU on ventilatory support with a subclavian line for fluids, nutritional support, and hemodynamic monitoring. Laboratory studies were done daily.

69 Because Mr. Smith was hemodynamically acutely unstable due to an abdominal injury, the choice of treatment can be either _____ or _____ .

hemodialysis; CRRT

■   ■   ■

70 The intravascular fluid volume lost from Mr. Smith's injuries can cause increased ADH and aldosterone secretion.

Two days after his accident Mr. Smith's serum sodium increased. Which hormone prevents excretion of sodium? _____ .

aldosterone

■   ■   ■

Table 11-8 lists the lab results, urine output, weight, and urinary sodium for Mr. Smith during admission, surgery, and the first four days of hospitalization. Refer to the table as you respond to the frames.

71 Which factors in Mr. Smith's history contributed to the development of the initial phase of ARF? _____ and *_____ .

hypotension and hemorrhagic shock

■   ■   ■

72 A rise in serum potassium is noted the day after surgery. An increase in potassium in this situation is caused by *_____ .

massive tissue damage

■   ■   ■

Table 11-8. LABORATORY STUDIES I: MR. SMITH

Tests	Admission	Surgery	Day 1	Day 2	Day 3	Day 4
Potassium (serum) (3.5–5.3 mEq/L)	3.6	4.2	6.5	5.1	5.9	6.8
Sodium (serum) (135–146 mEq/L)	138	142	144	143	144	143
Chloride (serum) (95–108 mEq/L)	110	110	110	108	103	104
CO_2 (serum) (22–32 mEq/L)	17	24	27	29	25	21
BUN (10–25 mg/dL)			30	34	57	84
Creatinine (serum) (0.6–1.2 mg/dL)			1.6	4.7	7.2	10.2
Urine output (mL/24 h)			580	440	320	290
Weight (lb)		185	189	191	196	198
Urine sodium (mEq/L)						93

73 Mr. Smith shows signs of oliguric azotemia on the second and third days. What are the two clinical indicators of decreased renal function? *_____ , and *_____ .

urine output less than 400 mL in 24 hours, and elevated BUN and creatinine

    ■   ■   ■

74 The nephrologist who cared for Mr. Smith diagnosed his renal problem as acute renal failure secondary to shock and myoglobinuria. Shock and myoglobinuria are listed under which two causes of renal failure? _____ and _____ .

ischemia and toxicity

    ■   ■   ■

75 On the fourth day Mr. Smith's serum potassium measures 6.8 mEq/L. His ECG showed peaked T waves and signs of cardiac irritability. These are symptoms of (hypokalemia/hyperkalemia) _____ .

hyperkalemia

■   ■   ■

76 Hyperkalemia can be treated temporarily by methods that decrease serum potassium. (Refer to Chapter 3 on potassium if needed.)

List four methods used in the treatment of hyperkalemia:

a. *_____
b. *_____
c. *_____
d. *_____

a. Kayexalate and sorbitol; b. IV sodium bicarbonate; c. 10% calcium gluconate; d. insulin and glucose

■   ■   ■

77 ECG changes indicate a need to rapidly lower Mr. Smith's serum potassium level. Name two methods that can be used to shift potassium back into the cells. *_____ , and *_____ .

sodium bicarbonate, and glucose and insulin

■   ■   ■

78 Another treatment prescribed for Mr. Smith was a Kayexalate retention enema. Kayexalate, a cation exchange resin, is mixed with sorbitol and given orally or rectally to induce an "osmotic diarrhea." The sodium in Kayexalate is exchanged with potassium in the intestines to lower the serum potassium level.

The resin used in excreting potassium from the intestine is _____ .

Kayexalate

■   ■   ■

79 It is noted that Mr. Smith had had a 13-pound weight increase since admission. Edema is evident in his hands, feet, and face. His blood pressure is 160/80 and his central venous pressure (CVP) and pulmonary artery wedge pressure (PAWP) are elevated. Auscultation of lung fields revealed coarse rales bilaterally. These symptoms indicate what type of fluid imbalance? *_____ .

fluid overload OR overhydration

■   ■   ■

80 Mr. Smith's electrolytes for day 4 show a serum Na 143, Cl 104, and CO_2 21. He has an anion gap of 18. An anion gap greater than 16 mEq/L is indicative of what condition? _____ (refer to Chapter 4 on anion gap if necessary).

acidosis. If you answered metabolic acidosis—OK.

■   ■   ■

81 Once the urine is clear of blood, a random urine sodium test is ordered. The result of 93 mEq/L means that the kidneys are unable to concentrate urine. What does this test indicate about the nephrons?   *_____ .

they are damaged

■   ■   ■

82 The decision is made to prescribe CRRT until Mr. Smith regains kidney function or becomes stable enough to tolerate hemodialysis. Explain why CRRT is selected over peritoneal dialysis or hemodialysis.   *_____

_____

_____ .

Mr. Smith is hemodynamically unstable and has abdominal trauma. Peritoneal dialysis is contraindicated after abdominal surgery. CRRT prevents the rapid intercompartmental fluid shifts which occur in hemodialysis and is poorly tolerated in a hemodynamically unstable client.

■   ■   ■

83 Several days later, a decision was made for Mr. Smith to have hemodialysis for 3 hours every day. What type of access is needed for hemodialysis?   *_____ .

vascular access

■   ■   ■

84 During hemodialysis what method is used to remove excess fluid?   _____ .
What can be done in hemodialysis to lower the serum potassium?   *_____ .

ultrafiltration; the use of a low potassium dialysate

■   ■   ■

85 In hemodialysis the rapid shift of fluids and electrolytes can cause central nervous system disturbances such as agitation, twitching, and seizures. This is known as the *disequilibrium syndrome*.

This condition is caused by a   *_____ .

rapid shift of fluids and electrolytes during hemodialysis

        ■   ■   ■

86 The nurse must observe for signs of the disequilibrium syndrome that include _____ , _____ , and _____ .

agitation, twitching, and seizures

        ■   ■   ■

Table 11-9 lists Mr. Smith's test results on days 6, 14, 35, 37, 40, and 47. He is given hemodialysis until day 49. Refer to the table as needed.

87 On day 14 Mr. Smith became anuric. He also developed a severe infection that caused catabolism and increased his BUN, creatinine, and WBC count. Hemodialysis time is increased to 5 hours per day. From Table 11-9 what three problems are controlled with dialysis on day 14? _____ , _____ , and *_____ .

acidosis, hyperkalemia, and fluid overload

        ■   ■   ■

88 Mr. Smith's serum phosphorus is very high (9.7 mg/dL). When the serum calcium and phosphate are multiplied, the Ca $\times$ P product is 83.1. This is an indication of *_____ .

metastatic calcification

        ■   ■   ■

89 The nephrologist ordered a phosphate binding agent to lower the serum phosphorus. This agent contains aluminum, which attracts and binds phosphorus compounds in the intestines for excretion in the stool.

The drug/agent that lowers serum phosphate is   *_____

_____ .

a phosphate binding agent OR an agent that contains aluminum, e.g., Amphojel or Basaljel

        ■   ■   ■

Table 11-9. LABORATORY STUDIES II: MR. SMITH						
Tests	Day 6	Day 14	Day 35	Day 37	Day 40	Day 47
WBCs (5000–10,000 mm^3)		38,000				
Potassium (serum) (3.5–5.3 mEq/L)	5.3	5.2	3.8	3.9	3.8	4.8
Sodium (serum) (135–146 mEq/L)	142	135	134	128	133	147
Calcium (serum) (9–11 mg/dL)		8.5		8.6		
Chloride (serum) (95–108 mEq/L)	102	93	99	90	97	112
Phosphorus (serum) (2.5–4.5 mg/dL)		9.7		4.2		
CO_2 (serum) (22–32 mEq/L)	25	25	21	21	22	17
BUN (10–25 mg/dL)	71	110	86	89	86	140
Creatinine (serum) (0.6–1.2 mg/dL)	9.2	11.1	7.1	6.5	5.8	4.3
Weight (lb)	193	180	171	169	165	164
Intake (mL/24 h)	600	600	600	600	3000	4955
Output (mL/24 h)	170	0	250	550	3000	4650

90 On day 35 Mr. Smith's urine output returned and hemodialysis was decreased to 4 hours per day. By day 37 his urine output increased further and dialysis times were reduced.

Note: Electrolytes stabilize to low normal levels in daily dialysis therapy.

His intake and output were about the _____ . His serum phosphorus was within high normal limits because of the *_____ prescribed.

same; phosphate binding agent (phosphate binders)

■   ■   ■

91 On day 40 Mr. Smith's urinary output increased to 3000 mL per 24 hours. This indicates that he is in the _____ phase of ARF. Identify a potential serious complication of this phase? _____ .

diuretic; dehydration

■   ■   ■

92 By day 47 Mr. Smith's urine output continues to be high, but his serum sodium and BUN are also high. Skin turgor is poor, mucous membranes are dry, and he complains of thirst. His blood pressure is 120/60 and his pulse is 92. These symptoms are indicators of what type of fluid imbalance? _____ .

dehydration

■   ■   ■

93 By day 55 Mr. Smith is no longer azotemic and his urine output and electrolytes are in normal range. This phase of ARF is _____ .

recovery

■   ■   ■

CASE STUDY REVIEW

Mrs. Alice Grady, age 68, has a 3-year history of renal insufficiency from glomerulonephritis and a history of several myocardial infarctions. Mrs. Grady is admitted to the hospital for shortness of breath with no dyspnea. Her laboratory results on admission are Hgb 6.1 g/dL, Hct 19%, BUN 78 mg/dL, creatinine 5.2 mg/dL, serum CO_2 13 mEq/L, serum potassium 5.6 mEq/L, serum sodium 124 mEq/L, serum calcium 8.4 mg/dL, and serum phosphorus 5.2 mg/dL. Physical assessment reveals edema of her face, hands, and lower legs. Lung sounds indicate bilateral coarse rales but no frothy sputum. Blood pressure is 170/98 and her jugular venous pressure is elevated. She notes a weight gain of 5 pounds in the preceding 3 days and her urine output is approximately 500 mL per day. Mrs. Grady complains of thirst.

1. Chronic renal failure usually develops over *_____ . A progressive loss of _____ is the result.
2. What is the cause of Mrs. Grady's chronic renal failure? _____ .
3. Mrs. Grady's low hemoglobin and hematocrit indicate what clinical condition? _____ . Explain why? *_____ _____ .
4. Her BUN and serum creatinine are (elevated/decreased) _____ , which is indicative of _____ .
5. Mrs. Grady's serum CO_2 is (elevated/decreased) _____ , which is indicative of _____ .
6. Her serum potassium is 5.6 mEq/L. The normal range of potassium is *_____ . Identify two reasons why hyperkalemia occurs in renal failure. *_____ and *_____ .

7. Her serum sodium is (elevated/decreased) _____ . Identify two reasons for her hyponatremia. *_____ , and *_____ .

8. Peritoneal dialysis is chosen to treat Mrs. Grady's uremia. Why is peritoneal dialysis the best choice for her? *_____
_____ .

9. What four symptoms indicate signs of fluid overload? *_____ ,
_____ , *_____ , and *_____ .

10. After trocar insertion, the first exchange of peritoneal dialysate is a 4.25% dextrose dialysate with no potassium. The 4.25% dextrose dialysate is _____ . It is used for _____ . Dialysate without potassium increases *_____
_____ .

11. When dialysate infuses into the peritoneum, it can push the diaphragm upward. The nurse must assess the patient for signs of *_____
_____ .

12. Excessive use of 4.25% dextrose dialysate can lead to _____ .

13. An essential intervention during peritoneal dialysis to maintain fluid balance is
*_____ .

14. Retention of dialysate during exchanges can lead to *_____
_____ .

15. On the second day of peritoneal dialysis Mrs. Grady's potassium is 2.8 mEq/L, which indicates _____ . Potassium must be added to the _____ .

16. Mrs. Grady's phosphorus is slightly elevated. The drug given to decrease her serum phosphorus is *_____ .

17. To prevent fluid overload in the future, it is important to determine Mrs. Grady's
*_____ .

1. *periods of time; nephrons*
2. *glomerulonephritis*
3. *Anemia. Kidneys are not producing erythropoietin to stimulate the bone marrow to build red blood cells.*
4. *elevated; azotemia*
5. *decreased; acidosis*
6. *3.5–5.3 mEq/L; potassium retention due to oliguria and massive tissue destruction*
7. *decreased; excessive fluid intake, and metabolic acidosis*
8. *It causes minimal stress to patients with cardiovascular disease; it is frequently used for patients with unstable cardiovascular disease.*
9. *weight gain, edema, increased blood pressure, and bilateral rales (also elevated jugular venous pressure)*
10. *hyperosmolar; ultrafiltration; diffusion of potassium into the dialysate*
11. *respiratory distress*
12. *dehydration*
13. *Strict measurement of dialysate from each exchange*
14. *fluid overload*
15. *hypokalemia; dialysate*
16. *phosphate binding agents, e.g., Amphojel*
17. *dry weight*

NURSING ASSESSMENT FACTORS

- Obtain a client history concerning frequency and amounts of urination, fluid intake, and history of any past renal health problems.
- Obtain baseline vital signs for abnormal findings and for comparison with future vital signs. Obtain client's weight.
- Record the amount of urine output for 8 hours. Report if the urine output amount is not within the desired range (>30 mL per hour).
- Check admitting laboratory results, especially the BUN, serum creatinine, serum electrolytes, and complete blood count (CBC).
- Assess for signs and symptoms that relate to the client's abnormal laboratory values.
- Assess for edema in the extremities. A decrease in urine output in conjunction with edema in the lower extremities can indicate a renal disorder.

NURSING DIAGNOSIS 1

Fluid volume excess, related to fluid retention secondary to renal failure.

NURSING INTERVENTIONS AND RATIONALE

1. Monitor fluid intake and output. Report a decrease in urine output of less than 30 mL per hour.
2. Monitor vital signs. Report abnormal vital signs, such as an increase in pulse rate, an increase or decrease in blood pressure, and difficulty breathing.
3. Check for signs of hypervolemia, i.e., constant irritating cough, neck and hand vein engorgements, dyspnea, and chest rales.
4. Check weights daily before breakfast. Weigh the client with the same clothes and on the same scale. An increase in weight may indicate fluid retention. One liter of fluid weighs approximately 2.2 pounds.
5. Check for edema in the lower extremities early in the morning before the client rises. The presence of feet, ankle, and/or leg edema in the morning frequently indicates a renal or cardiac dysfunction.
6. Check abdominal girth. Monitor for fluid shifts by noting rigidity or girth changes in the abdomen.
7. Encourage clients to follow a restricted sodium diet and fluid limitation as ordered by the physician.

NURSING DIAGNOSIS 2

Fluid volume deficit, related to excess ultrafiltration or diuresis.

NURSING INTERVENTIONS AND RATIONALE

1. Monitor vital signs, especially the pulse rate and blood pressure. An increased pulse rate with a decreased blood pressure may be indicative of a fluid volume deficit.
2. Monitor fluid balance associated with dialysis procedures. Excessive ultrafiltration during hemodialysis causes hypotension. If blood pressure postdialysis is low, it may cause decreased blood flow through the vascular access and result in clotting. Excessive ultrafiltration from peritoneal dialysis can produce hypovolemia and hypernatremia because of the rapid movement of water across the peritoneum.

3. Monitor urinary output in the diuretic phase of ARF. Excessive urine output can deplete the intravascular volume and cause severe dehydration.
4. Replace fluid loss rapidly as prescribed by the physician to increase blood pressure and perfusion to vital organs when hypovolemia is due to the dialysis procedure.

NURSING DIAGNOSIS 3

Tissue perfusion altered: renal, cardiopulmonary, cerebral, related to hypovolemia and decrease in cardiac output secondary to dialysis.

NURSING INTERVENTIONS AND RATIONALE

1. Monitor vital signs and ECG. Report abnormal findings that may indicate poor tissue perfusion.
2. Check for signs of edema. Edema decreases tissue perfusion.
3. Monitor CVP and PAWP for early signs of decreased cardiac output and decreased perfusion.
4. Check specific gravity (SG) to detect changes in the concentration that result from decreased intravascular volume and may lead to decreased renal perfusion.

NURSING DIAGNOSIS 4

Urinary elimination: altered, related to renal disorder.

NURSING INTERVENTIONS AND RATIONALE

1. Check urine output daily at specified times.
2. Instruct clients with renal disorders to monitor their fluid intake and urine output. A decreased output may signify decreased function. Urinary output should be at a minimum of 30 mL per hour. The physician must be notified if the urine output drops.

NURSING DIAGNOSIS 5

High risk for infection, related to dialysis and the care of the vascular access site.

NURSING INTERVENTIONS AND RATIONALE

1. Monitor temperature and white blood cell (WBC) count for elevations, which can indicate an infection.
2. Use aseptic technique in caring for the access site to reduce risk of infection.
3. Check for swelling, redness, and drainage at the access site, which can indicate an infection. Note any discharge from the access sites or wounds. Culture potentially infected sites.
4. Check for the patency of the vascular access site used for hemodialysis. A surgically re-created vascular access should have bruits and pulsation on auscultation. Blood can be aspirated and infused through femoral and subclavian catheters.
5. Check for mechanical factors, such as kinking of the tubing, displacement of the catheter, and lying on the access site, which could cause poor blood flow.
6. Observe the peritoneal catheter site for crusting or redness.
7. Instruct the client on how to care for the access site and maintain asepsis.
8. Teach the client good hygiene, to avoid crowds, and to obtain yearly inoculation for flu viruses as indicated by the physician.

NURSING DIAGNOSIS 6

High risk for injury, related to mechanical equipment and central nervous system dysfunction from fluid and electrolyte imbalances.

NURSING INTERVENTIONS AND RATIONALE

1. Monitor new dialysis clients and catabolic clients in ARF for signs of central nervous system dysfunction that may lead to disequilibrium syndrome. Observe for tremors, irritability, confusion, and seizures that indicate the disequilibrium syndrome.
2. Monitor serum electrolyte values associated with renal disorders and observe for symptoms of electrolyte imbalance. Report the laboratory results that indicate hyperkalemia, hypocalcemia, and hyperphosphatemia immediately to the physician. These results can be life threatening.
3. Monitor the ECG for peaked T waves that can indicate hyperkalemia.
4. Administer phosphate binding agents as ordered to control the serum phosphorus level. A low serum calcium level can be caused by hyperphosphatemia, restricted calcium intake in the diet, and/or alterations in vitamin D metabolism needed for intestinal absorption of calcium. Overuse of aluminum-phosphate binding drugs can cause hypophosphatemia.
5. Check the symptoms of tetany when the serum calcium level is low and acidosis is corrected. Serum calcium deficits can indicate a need for vitamin D supplements.

NURSING DIAGNOSIS 7

Breathing patterns: ineffective, related to peritoneal dialysate infusion.

NURSING INTERVENTIONS AND RATIONALE

1. Monitor respiratory rate. Report signs of dyspnea.
2. Check for dyspnea when administering solutions for peritoneal dialysis. Rapid infusion of dialysate can push the diaphragm upward, thus decreasing the area for lung expansion.

CHAPTER 12

INCREASED INTRACRANIAL PRESSURE

LARRY PURNELL, R.N., PH.D.

Behavioral Objectives

Upon completion of this chapter, you will be prepared to:

- Explain the physiologic changes that are associated with fluid and electrolyte balance in individuals with an increase in intracranial pressure.
- Describe the three types of intracerebral edema.
- Describe the pathophysiologic changes that increase intracranial pressure.
- Identify complications that result from increased intracranial pressure.
- Apply principles of fluid balance in the assessment and nursing care of a client with increasing intracranial pressure.
- Apply principles of fluid balance in the nursing care of a client with increased intracellular fluid (ICF).
- Describe nursing assessment factors, nursing diagnoses, and interventions related to increased intracranial pressure.
- Describe treatment priorities in the clinical management of increased intracranial pressure.

Introduction

Intracranial pressure is that pressure within the intracranial cavity which is exerted by the volume of blood, cerebrospinal fluid, and brain parenchyma contained within the cavity. A small increase or decrease in any of these three components may have deleterious effects on brain structures and function. The nurse has a major responsibility in monitoring the neurologically impaired client for signs and symptoms of increasing intracranial pressure.

Because the brain is enclosed in the rigid cranial vault, a small increase in intracerebral fluid may result in a dramatic increase in intracranial pressure. Therefore, the nurse must closely monitor the neurologically impaired client for early signs of increasing intracranial pressure to help prevent adverse effects.

This chapter discusses the physiology of intracranial pressure, the three types of intracerebral edema, factors that increase and decrease intracranial pressure, and associated complications that may occur with intracerebral hypertension. Signs and symptoms of increasing intracranial pressure along with management priorities and principles of fluid and electrolyte balance in the management of intracerebral hypertension are discussed.

PATHOPHYSIOLOGY

1   Intracranial pressure is determined by the pressure within the intracranial cavity which is
    exerted by the volume of _____ , * _____ , and
    * _____ .

    blood, cerebrospinal fluid, and brain parenchyma

    ■   ■   ■

2   A small increase in intracerebral fluid may result in a dramatic increase in intracranial pressure
    because * _____ .

    the brain is enclosed in a rigid cranial vault

    ■   ■   ■

3   In general, there are three types of cerebral edema: vasogenic, cytogenic, and interstitial. The
    three types of cerebral edema are _____ , _____ , and
    _____ .

    vasogenic, cytogenic, and interstitial

    ■   ■   ■

Vasogenic edema is the most common type of fluid accumulation within the brain. It is essentially
an extracellular edema. Vasogenic edema results from damage to the cerebral blood vessels causing
increased capillary permeability. This allows a transudation of proteins and an influx of water from
the extracellular space into the brain parenchyma. Causes of vasogenic edema include trauma,
tumors, ischemia, and infection or abscess.

4   The most common type of cerebral edema is _____ edema, which results
    from * _____ .

    vasogenic; damage to cerebral blood vessels causing an increase in capillary permeability

    ■   ■   ■

5   Increased capillary permeability results in * _____

    _____ .

    *a transudation of proteins and influx of water from the extracellular space into the brain
    parenchyma*

    ■   ■   ■

Cytogenic edema is intracellular. Increased capillary permeability results in an overall increase in
water content within the brain and an inhibition of the sodium-potassium (Na-K) pump. This
inhibition allows potassium to leave the cell and sodium chloride and water to enter the cell,
causing the brain cells to swell. Clinical causes of cytotoxic edema include hypoxia from trauma or
cerebral hemorrhage and hypo-osmolality.

6 Cytogenic edema is (extracellular/intracellular) _____ .

　Vasogenic edema is (extracellular/intracellular) _____ .

intracellular; extracellular

　　　　　　■　　　　　　　　　■　　　　　　　　■

7 Cytogenic edema inhibits the Na-K pump, resulting in _____ leaving the cell and *_____ and _____ entering the cell.

potassium; sodium chloride and water

　　　　　　■　　　　　　　　■　　　　　　　　■

8 Name three clinical conditions that may cause cytogenic edema. *_____ ,
*_____ , and _____ .

hypoxia from trauma, cerebral hemorrhage, and hypo-osmolality

　　　　　　■　　　　　　　■   ．　　　　　　■

9 Interstitial edema results from obstructive conditions such as hydrocephalus, tumors or infections that predispose the client to an excess of fluid in the brain, and a buildup of cerebrospinal fluid in the ventricles of the brain.

　Three clinical conditions that may cause interstitial edema are _____ , _____ , and _____ .

hydrocephalus, tumors, and infections

　　　　　　■　　　　　　　■　　　　　　　■

10 The three types of cerebral edema are _____ , _____ , and _____ .

vasogenic, cytogenic, and interstitial

　　　　　　■　　　　　　　■　　　　　　　■

11 Regulators of blood flow within the central nervous system include CO_2, O_2, core body temperature, hydrogen ion concentration, and serum osmolality.

　Name five regulators of cerebral blood flow. _____ , _____ , *_____ , *_____ , and
*_____ .

CO_2, O_2, core body temperature, hydrogen ion concentration, and serum osmolality

　　　　　　■　　　　　　　■　　　　　　　■

12 Hypercapnia (an increase in $Paco_2$) causes vasodilation, which results in an increase in intracranial pressure. Hypoxemia (a decrease Pao_2) may also cause an increase in intracranial pressure.

Hypercapnia causes a/an (increase/decrease) _____ in intracranial pressure.

Hypoxemia causes a/an (increase/decrease) _____ in intracranial pressure.

increase; increase

■   ■   ■

An increase in core body temperature increases metabolism and results in an increase in intracranial pressure. A decrease in core body temperature causes a decrease in body metabolism and results in a decrease in intracranial pressure.

13 What effect does an increased core body temperature have on intracranial pressure?
* _____ .

What effect does a decrease in core body temperature have on intracranial pressure?
* _____ .

It increases it.
It decreases it.

■   ■   ■

Prolonged hyperventilation causes excessive elimination of CO_2 and leads to respiratory alkalosis (increased pH and decreased $Paco_2$). This may cause an increase in intracranial pressure.

14 Hyperventilation can cause what clinical condition? * _____ .

Respiratory alkalosis may cause a/an (increase/decrease) _____ in intracranial pressure.

respiratory alkalosis; increase

■   ■   ■

Hypoventilation causes excessive retention of CO_2 and leads to respiratory acidosis (decreased pH and increased $Paco_2$), which is far more dangerous than hyperventilation. Carbon dioxide is the most potent vasodilator known. As vasodilation increases, so does intracranial pressure.

15 Hypoventilation causes what clinical condition? _*_____ . The most potent vasodilator known is _*_____ . Respiratory acidosis causes a/an (increase/decrease) _____ in vasodilation and results in (increased/decreased) _____ intracranial pressure.

respiratory acidosis; carbon dioxide or CO_2; increase; increased

■   ■   ■

Serum osmolality is the number of formed particles in the serum and is an indication of serum concentration. Decreased serum osmolality indicates a fluid overload and may result in an increase in intracranial pressure.

16 A decrease in serum osmolality may cause a/an (increase/decrease) _____ in intracranial pressure.

Five regulators that increase intracranial pressure are _*_____ , _*_____ , _*_____ , _*_____ , and _*_____ .

increase; an increase in Pa_{CO_2}, a decrease in Pa_{O_2}, an increase in body temperature, a change in hydrogen ion concentration, and decreased serum osmolality

■   ■   ■

Hypo-osmolar fluids such as dextrose and water are generally avoided in the neurologically compromised client suspected of having an increase in intracranial pressure. Using intravenous fluids such as 5% dextrose in water (D_5W) results in the dextrose being metabolized, releasing free water which is absorbed by the brain cells, leading to cerebral edema.

17 Hypo-osmolar fluids may cause a/an (increase/decrease) _____ in intracranial pressure.

increase

■   ■   ■

CLINICAL MANIFESTATIONS

Table 12-1 lists the early, progressive, and advanced clinical manifestations of increasing intracranial pressure.

18 Name at least four early signs and symptoms of increased intracranial pressure.

_____ , _____ , _____ , and _____ .

headache, irritability, restlessness, and confusion (others: diplopia, and other visual changes)

■   ■   ■

Table 12-1. CLINICAL MANIFESTATIONS OF INCREASING INTRACRANIAL PRESSURE	
Early signs and symptoms	Headache Irritability Restlessness Confusion Diplopia Other visual changes
Progressive signs and symptoms	Nausea Projectile vomiting Bradycardia Decreased and/or irregular respirations Increased systolic pressure Decreased diastolic pressure Widened pulse pressure (difference between systolic and diastolic pressures) Decreased level of consciousness Pupillary changes
Advanced signs and symptoms	Rhinorrhea Otorrhea Changes in motor/sensory function Posturing, apnea, death

If early signs and symptoms of intracranial pressure are missed or unable to be controlled, progressive clinical manifestations occur.

19 Name the changes that occur with the following parameters related to an increase in intracranial pressure:

a. Mental status *_____

b. Vision *_____

c. Pulse _____

d. Respiration *_____

e. Systolic blood pressure _____

f. Diastolic blood pressure _____

g. Pulse pressure _____

a. irritability, restlessness and confusion, decreased level of consciousness; b. diplopia and/or visual changes; c. decreases; d. decreases and/or irregular; e. increases; f. decreases; g. increases, widens

■   ■   ■

If the progressive clinical manifestations of increasing intracranial pressure are not controlled, more deleterious effects are likely. The symptoms are those of decompensation. Once decompensation occurs, autoregulation (the compensatory alteration in the diameter of the intracranial blood vessels designed to maintain a constant blood flow during changes in cerebral perfusion pressure) is lost with progressively increased intracranial pressure.

20 Name six advanced clinical manifestations of increased intracranial pressure.

* _____ , _____ , _____ ,

_____ , _____ , and _____ .

What is meant by autoregulation of cerebral blood flow? *_____ .

changes in motor sensory function, otorrhea, rhinorrhea, posturing, apnea, and death
the compensatory alteration in the diameter of the intracranial blood vessels designed to
maintain a constant blood flow during changes in cerebral perfusion pressure

■ ■ ■

In addition to the effects on brain metabolism and function, intracerebral hypertension has implications in the dysfunction of other major organ systems. Changes in the cardiopulmonary system include pulmonary rales (crackles), adventitious sounds, S_3, atrial fibrillation, and hypotension. Hypotension drastically worsens cerebral edema because of a resultant decrease in cerebral perfusion pressure and compensatory fluid retention.

21 In addition to changes in brain function and metabolism resulting from intracerebral hypertension, name two other body systems affected. _____ and

_____ .

Name at least five cardiopulmonary complications resulting from intracerebral hypertension.

* _____ , * _____ , _____ ,

* _____ , and _____ .

The development of stress ulcers and gastrointestinal bleeding may occur as a result of medical treatment. Identify two changes in the gastrointestinal system that can occur as a result of the medical treatment of intracerebral hypertension. *_____ and

_____ .

cardiopulmonary and gastrointestinal
pulmonary rales, adventitious sounds, S_3, atrial fibrillation, and hypertension
stress ulcers and bleeding

■ ■ ■

22 Systemic hypotension (increases/decreases) _____ cerebral perfusion pressure and results in a/an (increase/decrease) _____ in intracerebral hypertension.

decreases; increase

■ ■ ■

CLINICAL MANAGEMENT

Clinical management of intracerebral hypertension includes careful administration of fluids and electrolytes, maintaining an airway and adequate ventilation, medication administration, temperature control, and prevention of the Valsalva maneuver, which increases intracranial pressure.

23 Name four major areas for managing increasing intracranial pressure. * _____ , _____ , * _____ , and * _____ .

fluid management, ventilation, medication administration, and prevention of Valsalva maneuver (also temperature control)

■   ■   ■

Careful fluid management in the neurologically impaired client is essential. Hypo-osmolar fluids such as dextrose and water are generally avoided. Dextrose metabolizes and free water is absorbed by brain cells, leading to cerebral edema. Physiological normal saline (0.09% NSS) or Ringer's solution are the preferred iso-osmolar intravenous fluids.

24 Intravenous fluids that should be avoided in the treatment of increased intracranial pressure include * _____ .

Preferred intravenous fluids for treatment of the neurologically impaired client include * _____ and * _____ .

dextrose in water (hypo-osmolar) solutions; physiological saline and Ringer's lactate (iso-osmolar solutions).

■   ■   ■

Extracellular fluid volume is directly dependent upon total body sodium. The principal osmotic electrolyte of extracellular fluid is sodium (Na). Most clients with hyponatremia are hypo-osmolar. The other major cation for fluid balance maintenance is potassium (K). It is essential to maintain normal Na and K levels in order to maintain normal serum osmolality. If the NA and K levels are not maintained within normal limits, the Na-K pump becomes defective. Potassium leaves the cell and Na, Cl, and water enter the cells.

25 The two major cations that regulate serum osmolality and total body water are _____ and _____ .

Clients with hyponatremia generally have serum (hypo-osmolality/hyper-osmolality) _____ .

Explain the role of the Na-K pump in the regulation of intracerebral pressure. * _____ _____ .

sodium and potassium; hypo-osmolality; for maintenance of an appropriate ratio of Na and K ions to maintain a normal serum osmolality level

■   ■   ■

Mannitol and urea are osmotic diuretics capable of relieving elevated intracranial pressure when given intravenously. Mannitol intravenous dosage is 1 mg/kg of body weight administered over 10–30 minutes and can be repeated once or twice every 4–6 hours. Mannitol pulls intracellular fluid into the extracellular plasma and decreases intracranial pressure. Care must be taken to monitor for possible complications of pulmonary edema and water intoxication. An additional complication that can occur with the administration of osmotic diuretics to clients with intracranial hemorrhage is rebleeding. As the brain tissue shrinks from osmotic diuretics, rebleeding may occur.

26 Two osmotic diuretics given intravenously to decrease intracranial pressure are
_____ and _____ .

The dosage and frequency of use for the administration of mannitol in increased cerebral pressure is _____ mg/kg of body weight and may be repeated
*_____ every _____ hours.

Explain the mechanism of how mannitol works to decrease intracranial pressure. It is an _____ diuretic and pulls fluid from *_____ to
*_____ .

Two possible complications with osmotic diuretics are *_____ and
*_____ .

mannitol and urea
1; once or twice; 4–6
osmotic; intracellular tissue; extracellular spaces
pulmonary edema and water intoxication

■   ■   ■

Glycerol, an oral osmotic dehydrating agent, may be used instead of mannitol or urea. The duration of action is longer (approximately 12 hours), and it is given in divided doses every 4–6 hours. Complications such as a rebound increase in intracranial pressure, hyperglycemia, and hemolysis may occur.

27 An oral osmotic diuretic given for increased intracranial pressure is _____ .
Name three complications of glycerol administration. *_____ ,
_____ , and _____ .

glycerol; rebound increasing intracranial pressure, hyperglycemia, and hemolysis

■   ■   ■

Loop diuretics such as furosemide (Lasix) may be administered in conjunction with osmotic diuretics to help eliminate excess fluid from the extracellular space.

28 Furosemide may be given in conjunction with osmotic diuretics to *_____ .

increase diuresis of extracellular fluid

■   ■   ■

Steroids, primarily dexamethasone (Decadron), may be used to treat both acute and chronic cerebral edema. The effects of Decadron are slower in onset than osmotic diuretics and peak in 24 hours. Dexamethasone, additionally, is a potent anti-inflammatory agent and protects cell wall stability. It is especially useful in cytotoxic edema.

29   The steroid used to treat both acute and chronic cerebral edema is _____ .
The disadvantage of dexamethasone on acute intracranial pressure is *_____

_____ .

Dexamethasone is especially helpful in which type of cerebral edema? _____ .

dexamethasone (Decadron); it is slower acting and does not peak for 24 hours; cytotoxic
   ■   ■   ■

Like all steroids, dexamethasone has the long-term complications of decreasing wound healing, electrolyte imbalance, and gastrointestinal bleeding.

30   Name three long-term complications from using dexamethasone in controlling cerebral
pressure. *_____ , *_____ , and *_____ .

decreased wound healing, electrolyte imbalance, and gastrointestinal bleeding
   ■   ■   ■

Hyperventilation with a resultant increase in $Paco_2$ acts immediately to decrease cerebral blood flow and thus reduces intracranial pressure. It is preferable to give rapid ventilation of low volume to help reduce the effects of respiratory alkalosis over an extended period of time. This intervention increases the rate and decreases the volume of each breath. Clients may need long-term mechanical ventilation to prevent respiratory acidosis, which is far more serious than respiratory alkalosis. Increased concentration of $Paco_2$ in respiratory acidosis is a more potent vasodilator than is an increase in Pao_2 resulting from respiratory alkalosis.

31   How does hyperventilation work to help reduce intracranial pressure? *_____

_____ .

Which clinical condition is more serious for the client with increasing intracranial pressure,
respiratory acidosis or respiratory alkalosis? *_____ . Why? *_____

_____ .

hyperventilation reduces $Paco_2$ concentration (a power vasodilator); respiratory acidosis; an
increase in $Paco_2$ is a more powerful vasodilator than an increase in Pao_2
   ■   ■   ■

Further measures to control or decrease intracranial pressure are aimed at preventing the Valsalva maneuver and permitting gravity to help reduce intracranial pressure. Alert and cooperative clients should be encouraged to not cough, bend, stoop, lift, hold their breath, sneeze, or strain at bowel elimination. To prevent a transient increase in intracranial pressure, stool softeners are administered to help prevent straining with bowel movements. The head of the bed should be elevated 30°–45°

to let gravity have its effect on reducing intracranial pressure. The head and neck should be midline with no flexion, extension, or rotation. These maneuvers may result in an increase in intracranial pressure.

32 List six measures that clients should be instructed to avoid in order to prevent a transient increase in intracranial pressure. _____ , _____ , _____ , _____ , * _____ , and _____ . In what position should the client's bed be placed to help prevent intracranial pressure? * _____ . What may occur if the client flexes, extends, or rotates the neck? * _____ . What is the purpose of administering stool softeners to the client with increased intracranial pressure? * _____

_____ .

cough, bend, stoop, lift, hold their breath, and sneeze (also strain at bowel movement)
30°–45° angle
transient increase in intracranial pressure; to help prevent straining with bowel movements

■   ■   ■

Clients with increased intracranial pressure are prone to seizures. Seizures may cause a transient increase in intracranial pressure, create safety issues for the client, or cause further hypoxia and hypercapnia. Preventive measures for seizure control include the administration and careful monitoring of anticonvulsant medications.

33 What are two deleterious effects of seizure activity in the client with increased intracranial pressure? * _____ and * _____ .

transient increase in intracranial pressure and safety issues

■   ■   ■

CASE STUDY REVIEW

Mrs. Foote, age 46, was involved in a multiple vehicle accident. She suffered head trauma of unknown dimension. She was unconscious at the scene of the accident but is now alert and oriented and is admitted to an inpatient unit for observation. She is presently complaining of a headache and blurred vision. Vital signs upon admission are blood pressure, 134/74; pulse, 88 and regular; respirations, 20 per minute and regular and unlabored; temperature, 98.4°F orally. You are to monitor Mrs. Foote for signs and symptoms of increasing intracranial pressure.

1. If Mrs. Foote does develop signs and symptoms of increasing intracranial edema, what type(s) of edema would she have? _____ and _____ .
   Why? * _____ .
2. What symptoms does Mrs. Foote currently have to indicate that she might have increasing cerebral edema? * _____ .
3. The most significant observation of changes in Mrs. Foote's behavior that indicates an increase in intracranial pressure is a change in her * _____ .

The physician places Mrs. Foote on NPO status and initiates an intravenous line. Intravenous orders include normal saline, 1000 mL at 75 mL per hour, and oxygen per nasal canal at 4 liters per minute.

4. Why did the physician order an IV of normal saline solution instead of a dextrose solution?
   * _____ .

5. Mrs. Foote had no difficulty with respiration. Why was oxygen ordered? * _____ .

6. If Mrs. Foote develops an increase in intracranial pressure her respirations will (increase/decrease) _____ .

7. Her pulse rate will (increase/decrease) _____ .

8. Her systolic blood pressure will (increase/decrease) _____ .

9. Her diastolic blood pressure will (increase/decrease) _____ .

10. If Mrs. Foote's blood pressure changes from 134/74 to 145/60, this would indicate an increase in * _____ ?

Two hours after admission, Mrs. Foote's temperature became elevated to 99.8°. Even though she was NPO, she was ordered and received acetaminophen (Tylenol) grains 10 by mouth with a sip of water.

11. Why was the Tylenol prescribed? * _____ .

The nurse elevated the head of Mrs. Foote's bed to 45°, placed a bite block at the bedside, and padded her side rails.

12. The head of the bed was elevated to 45° to help prevent * _____ . The side rails were padded and the bite block was placed at the bedside for * _____ .

Mrs. Foote continued to become more restless and could not remember where she was. Vital signs were taken with the following results: blood pressure, 160/60; pulse, 66; and respirations, 16. Dexamethasone 4 mg IV push and Lasix 40 mg IV push were ordered. The IV fluid rate was decreased to 50 mL per hour.

13. Mrs. Foote is experiencing what phenomena? * _____ .

14. What data in Frame 13 indicate increased intracranial pressure? * _____ .

15. Mrs. Foote's IV rate was decreased in order to * _____

   _____ .

16. Lasix was ordered to * _____ .

17. Dexamethasone was ordered to * _____ .

18. A secondary benefit of dexamethasone for Mrs. Foote is * _____

   _____ .

An endotracheal intubation tray and ventilator were placed on standby at the bedside. ABGs were drawn with the following results: pH 7.48, $Paco_2$ 34, HCO_3 28, and Pao_2 96.

19. The blood gas results suggest * _____ .

20. Why was the ventilator placed on standby? * _____ .

Mrs. Foote's confusion eased. She remained on dexamethasone with stable vital signs. She was permitted out of bed to a chair.

21. What instructions should the nurse give Mrs. Foote to help prevent transient intracerebral edema? *_____

_____.

Additional physician orders include cimetadine, 300 mg IV every 8 hours, and Maalox, 30 mL PO four times a day.

22. Cimetadine and Maalox are ordered because *_____

_____.

1. Vasogenic and cytogenic. Trauma may cause damage to cerebral blood vessels (vasogenic edema). Trauma may also cause hypoxia and/or hemorrhage (cytogenic edema).
2. headache, blurred vision
3. level of consciousness
4. Iso-osmolar fluids such as dextrose and water are metabolized into dextrose free water creating a hypo-osmolar, which may cause the brain to swell.
5. Oxygen was ordered to prevent CO_2 buildup, which is a potent vasodilator that can increase cerebral edema.
6. decrease
7. decrease
8. increase
9. decrease
10. pulse pressure
11. As an antipyretic to reduce core body temperature. An increase in core body temperature increases cerebral metabolism and increases brain edema.
12. cerebral edema; safety measures in case Mrs. Foote developed seizures
13. increasing intracranial pressure
14. restlessness and confusion, systolic blood pressure increasing, diastolic blood pressure decreasing, pulse rate decreasing, respiration decreasing, pulse pressure widening
15. decrease overall fluid intake and thereby decrease intracerebral edema
16. cause a diuresis of extracellular fluid
17. decrease intracranial pressure over a prolonged period of time
18. stabilize cell wall capillary permeability
19. respiratory alkalosis
20. If Mrs. Foote's $Paco_2$ increases, intubation would be considered to improve oxygenation and decrease the $Paco_2$ level.
21. no stooping, bending, lifting, coughing, or straining at stool
22. dexamethasone increases the potential for gastrointestinal bleeding and cimetadine and Maalox may help prevent GI distress

NURSING ASSESSMENT FACTORS

- The most significant change that may indicate an increase in intracranial pressure is a change in the level of consciousness. Subtle changes initially include irritability, restlessness, and visual changes.
- Assess vital signs every 15–30 minutes for bradycardia, slowed and/or irregular respirations, hyperthermia, systolic hypertension, diastolic hypotension, and a widening pulse pressure. Careful

monitoring of fluid balance is essential to help prevent cerebral hypertension. Hourly intake and output, careful monitoring of intravenous fluid rate, and daily weights are important nursing assessment factors.

- Additional parameters to monitor include serum osmolality, arterial blood gases, and electrolytes. Decreased serum osmolality, increased $Paco_2$, increased serum potassium, and decreased serum sodium may indicate an impending increase in intracranial pressure.
- Assess pulmonary sounds for rales, heart sounds for an S_3, and an increase in skin turgor as indications for fluid retention.
- Clients with increased intracranial pressure may develop seizures. The nurse assesses for seizure activities and additional complications of cerebral hypertension such as rhinorrhea, otorrhea, and brain stem herniation.
- Administration and assessment of therapeutic effects of the following medications are essential: loop diuretics, osmotic diuretics, steroids, and anticonvulsants.

NURSING DIAGNOSIS 1

High risk for ineffective breathing pattern, related to cerebral edema and occluded/obstructed venous drainage.

NURSING INTERVENTIONS AND RATIONALE

1. Maintain head of bed elevated 30°–45° and keep body in good alignment in order for gravity to help reduce intracranial pressure.
2. Suction prn for no longer than 15 seconds to maintain clear airway and adequate oxygenation. Suction applied for longer than 15 seconds may cause a transient rise in CO_2 levels, resulting in increased intracranial pressure.
3. Administer oxygen per nasal cannula or face mask to maintain Pao_2 levels and help prevent excessive buildup of CO_2, resulting in vasodilation and increased intracranial pressure.
4. Assess rate, depth, and pattern of respirations, which indicates patency of airway.
5. Assess skin, lips, and nail beds for cyanosis as an indicator for adequate central oxygenation.
6. Monitor arterial blood gases every 4–8 hours and prn. Hypercapnia and acidosis are to be prevented. The most potent vasodilator known is an increase in $Paco_2$ levels.
7. Maintain an ambu bag at the bedside to be used to provide controlled hyperventilation if necessary.

NURSING DIAGNOSIS 2

Tissue perfusion (cerebral): altered, related to increased intracranial pressure associated with trauma and cerebral edema.

NURSING INTERVENTIONS AND RATIONALE

1. Assess for changes in level of consciousness, arousability, irritability, agitation, memory loss, and inability to follow commands. A change in level of consciousness is the earliest and most sensitive clinical evidence of an alteration in cerebral perfusion pressure. Arousability is a reflection of the functioning of the reticular activating system (RAS).
2. Assess for headache, nausea, and vomiting. These may be early, nonspecific signs and symptoms of increasing intracranial pressure.

3. Monitor vital signs every 15–30 minutes to assess for signs and symptoms of increased intracranial pressure. Client responses to increasing intracranial pressure can change rapidly. Observe for widening of pulse pressure.
4. Assess for sensory function: visual changes, hearing changes, touch, and proprioception. This affords an evaluation of the sensory pathways in the parietal lobes.
5. Assess for motor function changes: decerebrate and decorticate posturing, muscle strength and tone, and deep-tendon reflexes. Appropriate motor function reflects total or partial intact motor pathways at the neuromuscular junction.
6. Assess pupillary reaction and ocular movements. Increasing pressure in the midbrain and pons may cause changes in cranial nerve functioning.
7. Implement proper positioning for intracranial pressure reduction: Elevate head of bed 30°–45°, avoid use of pillows, maintain body in midline, maintain head-neck alignment, avoid neck rotation, extension, and flexion, and prevent hip flexion. Head elevation allows for optimal venous drainage. Proper body alignment prevents vein compression or obstruction. Hip flexion may increase intra-abdominal pressure and impede jugular venous cerebral drainage.
8. Instruct client on measures to prevent a transient rise in intracranial pressure: no coughing, sneezing, bending, lifting, or straining with bowel movements. These physical maneuvers cause a transient rise in intracranial pressure.
9. Palpate for bladder distention, auscultate for the presence of bowel sounds, and check for constipation. These conditions may cause abdominal distension resulting in an increase in intra-abdominal pressure.
10. Maintain normal body temperature and prevent shivering. Hyperthermia and shivering may increase cerebral metabolism and result in increased intracranial pressure.

NURSING DIAGNOSIS 3

High risk for fluid-electrolyte imbalance, related to osmotic diuresis and/or fluid retention.

NURSING INTERVENTIONS AND RATIONALE

1. Measure intake and output hourly along with fluid restriction to help decrease extracellular fluid volume that may contribute to cerebral edema. A mild dehydration status is usually maintained.
2. Auscultate for rales, rhonchi, and an S_3 to detect early signs of volume overload.
3. Monitor serum and urine osmolality every 8 hours. Increased serum osmolality helps draw fluid from brain interstitium and reduce cerebral edema.
4. Monitor urine specific gravity every 8 hours. Cerebral trauma predisposes the client to diabetes insipidus.
5. Monitor serum electrolytes, BUN, creatinine, serum proteins, hemoglobin, and hematocrit every 8 hours and prn to detect fluid volume overload or degree of dehydration.
6. Administer corticosteroids (dexamethasone or methylprednisolone) per physician's order. These pharmacologic agents ameliorate cerebral edema.
7. Monitor arterial blood gases every 8 hours and prn. Increased Pa_{CO_2} and decreased Pa_{O_2} may cause vasodilation and result in an increase in cerebral pressure.
8. Administer osmotic diuretics (mannitol/urea) ordered by physician cautiously and assess for therapeutic effect. Osmotic diuretics may have a rebound effect.
9. Monitor for rhinorrhea and otorrhea. These symptoms may indicate brain stem herniation resulting from increased cerebral pressure.

JULIE WATERHOUSE, R.N., M.S.
WITH MARILYN HALSTEAD

Behavioral Objectives

Upon completion of this chapter, you will be prepared to:

• Describe fluid and electrolyte disturbances commonly seen in individuals with uncontrolled cancer cell growth.

• Differentiate the metabolic effects of cachexia associated with cancer.

• Give two examples of fluid and electrolyte disturbances caused by ectopic hormone secretion.

• Explain the effect of tumor lysis syndrome on fluid and electrolyte balance.

• Assess fluid and electrolyte changes in individuals with cancer.

• Describe appropriate nursing interventions for fluid and electrolyte disturbances related to cancer.

PATHOPHYSIOLOGY

1   Cancer is a group of diseases characterized by abnormal and uncontrolled cell growth. Cancer cells are malignant (capable of invading normal tissues and spreading to distant sites).

   Cancer is characterized by   *_____ .
   Cancer cells are considered to be (malignant/benign)   _____ .

   abnormal and uncontrolled cell growth; malignant

                  ▪   ▪   ▪

2   Fluid and electrolyte disturbances occur frequently in individuals with cancer because of the nature of the malignant cell growth and the effects of therapies used to control it.

   Give two reasons why fluid and electrolyte disturbances occur frequently in individuals with cancer.   *_____ and   *_____ .

   the nature of the malignant cell growth and effects of therapies used to control this cell growth

                  ▪   ▪   ▪

3   Cancer may begin as an individual solid tumor (carcinoma or sarcoma) or may arise throughout the body in the blood-forming cells of bone marrow or lymph nodes (leukemia and lymphoma).

Match the following types of cancer with their tissues of origin:

a. Lymphoma
b. Leukemia
c. Carcinoma
d. Sarcoma

_____ , _____   *1. Epithelium or supporting tissue*
 _____   *2. Bone marrow*
 _____   *3. Lymphoid tissue*

1. c, d; 2. b; 3. a

■   ■   ■

4   Malignant cells are more primitive (anaplastic) than normal cells. They may be undifferentiated or may differentiate in abnormal and bizarre ways.

This lack of normal differentiation causes malignant cells to produce unusual proteins, hormones, enzymes, and other chemicals. Because the proteins produced by malignant cells are abnormal, they do not respond to normal regulatory mechanisms such as diet and hormonal and metabolic controls.

Cancer of the colon may produce carcinoembryonic antigen (CEA), a fetal antigen.

Why?   *_____

_____ .

malignant cells lack normal differentiation and thus a more primitive embryonic protein may be produced

■   ■   ■

CLINICAL MANIFESTATIONS

5   One major consequence of these biochemical abnormalities is cachexia, a complex process manifested by anorexia, weight loss, wasting, weakness, anemia, fluid and electrolyte disturbances, and increased basal metabolic rate.

A major problem associated with cancer is _____ . This serious problem is manifested by:

a. _____
b. _____
c. * _____
d. * _____

cachexia

a. anorexia; b. weakness; c. weight loss; d. fluid and electrolyte disturbances (others are wasting, anemia, and increased basal metabolic rate)

■   ■   ■

6   Cachexia involves changes in the metabolism of all the major nutrients. Glucose utilization is higher than in normal cells and anaerobic metabolic pathways are used more often than the aerobic. This produces higher than usual concentrations of lactic acid and may result in lactic acidosis.

Glucose utilization is higher in malignant cells. What specific acid-base imbalance is caused by anaerobic metabolism? * _____ .

lactic acidosis

■   ■   ■

7   Nitrogen transferred from body tissues to the tumor often leaves the client in negative nitrogen balance. Similarly, cancer clients retain sodium, with a total of 120% that of healthy individuals. Sodium, however, is concentrated in the tumor and the serum sodium may be low (hyponatremia).

Often in clients with cancer the nitrogen balance is (positive/negative) _____ . Why? * _____

_____ .

negative; nitrogen is transferred from the body tissues to the tumor, thus causing a negative nitrogen balance

■   ■   ■

8   Does the cancer client (retain/excrete) _____ sodium? Concentration of sodium is in the _____ . Because the sodium is not in the vascular fluid, (hyponatremia/hypernatremia) _____ results.

retain; tumor; hyponatremia

■   ■   ■

9   The client with cancer may also experience malabsorption syndrome, which involves inflammation, ulceration, decreased patency, and decreased secretions of the GI tract. The problems that result in protein and fat absorption may compound fluid and electrolyte disturbances of cachexia.

Malabsorption syndrome may occur in cancer clients. It can involve _____ , _____ , and *_____ .

inflammation, ulceration, and decreased patency OR decreased secretions of the GI tract
■   ■   ■

10   A second major consequence/problem of the primitive biochemical function of malignant cells is the secretion of abnormal hormones (ectopic hormone secretion).

An example is bronchiogenic cancer, which may secrete antidiuretic hormone (ADH), parathyroid hormone (PTH), or adrenocorticotropic hormone (ACTH). The resulting hormonal abnormalities may lead to fluid and electrolyte problems such as water intoxication (ICFVE), hyponatremia, hypokalemia, and hypophosphatemia.

The first major consequence of biochemical abnormalities in progressive cancer is _____ . The second major consequence is *_____ .

cachexia; secretion of abnormal hormones OR ectopic hormone secretion
■   ■   ■

11   Abnormal hormonal secretions may occur in bronchiogenic cancer. Examples are (use abbreviations) _____ , _____ , and _____ .

What four fluid and electrolyte problems can result from these abnormal hormonal secretions? *_____ , _____ , _____ , and _____ .

ADH, PTH, and ACTH
water intoxication, hyponatremia, hypokalemia, and hypophosphatemia
■   ■   ■

12   A third problem which commonly occurs in cancer clients in whom large numbers of malignant and normal cells are destroyed by radiation or chemotherapy is catabolism (breakdown) of purine nucleic acids in cells. The result is an increase in serum uric acid.

Three problems that may result in fluid and electrolyte disturbances in cancer clients are _____ , *_____ , and *_____ .

cachexia, secretion of abnormal hormones (i.e., ADH, PTH, ACTH), and catabolism of purine nucleic acids
■   ■   ■

13 Uric acid is poorly soluble in body fluids and is excreted primarily through the kidneys. Small increases above normal serum concentrations can cause uric acid precipitation in the renal tubules and collecting ducts.

Do you know what could happen if uric acid precipitated in the renal tubules?

*_____ .

renal disorders and possible renal failure

■   ■   ■

FLUID AND ELECTROLYTE DISTURBANCES

Table 13-1 lists the fluid and electrolyte disturbances commonly associated with cancer and cancer therapy. Also given are abnormal serum levels and the rationale for their occurrence.

Table 13-1. FLUID AND ELECTROLYTE DISTURBANCE IN CANCER AND CANCER THERAPY			
Fluid/Electrolyte Disturbance	**Commonly Associated Cancer and Cancer Therapy**	**Defining Characteristics**	**Rationale/Comments**
Hypercalcemia	Breast cancer, multiple myeloma, ovarian cancer, pancreatic cancer, leukemia, lymphoma, lung cancer, bladder cancer, kidney cancer, head and neck cancer, and prostate cancer	Serum calcium >11 mg/dL	Hypercalcemia occurs in 10–20% of all cancer clients and in 40–50% of those with metastatic breast cancer or multiple myeloma. It is caused by bone destruction by metastatic tumors, elevated parathyroid hormone (PTH) levels related to some tumors, and elevated prostaglandin and osteoclast activating factor (OAF). Prolonged immobility is also a causative factor.
Hyponatremia (usually associated with dehydration)	Lung cancer, pancreatic cancer, multiple myeloma, head and neck cancer, stomach cancer, brain cancer, colon cancer, ovarian cancer, and prostate cancer; aggressive diuretic therapy. High-dose cyclophosphamide/Cytoxan therapy; daunorubicin or cytosine chemotherapy (decreases blast cell count)	Serum sodium <135 mEq/L	Hyponatremia is caused by liver, thyroid, and adrenal insufficiencies, renal failure, and congestive heart failure. A condition known as cerebral salt wasting is caused by some intracranial neoplasms. In this condition the brain releases a postulated natriuretic factor or the neural innervation to the brain is altered. The result is the kidneys' inability to conserve sodium.
Syndrome of inappropriate antidiuretic hormone (SIADH)	Lung cancer, pancreatic cancer, brain cancer, ovarian cancer, colon cancer, sarcoma, leukemia, prostate cancer, Hodgkin's disease, and other lymphomas; vincristine, cyclophosphamide chemotherapy	Serum sodium <130 mEq/L, serum osmolality <280 mOsm/kg	SIADH occurs because of increased release of ADH from posterior pituitary or ectopically from neoplastic tumors. The posterior pituitary then becomes impervious to the usual feedback control mechanism.

Table 13-1. (Continued)

Fluid/Electrolyte Disturbance	Commonly Associated Cancer and Cancer Therapy	Defining Characteristics	Rationale/Comments
Hyperuricemia	Leukemias, lymphomas, multiple myeloma, any cancer treated aggressively with chemotherapy or radiation	Serum uric acid >7.0 mg/dL, uric acid crystals in urine	Breakdown of large numbers of cells causes release of uric acid into the bloodstream (tumor lysis syndrome). Precipitation of uric acid in the kidneys results in gouty nephropathy, acute hyperuricemic nephropathy, and eventual renal failure. First signs of hyperuricemic renal failure may be nausea, vomiting, and lethargy. This type of renal failure may or may not be reversible. Symptoms of hyperuricemia include hematuria, flank pain, nausea, vomiting, and symptoms of renal failure.
Hypokalemia	Colon cancer, multiple myeloma, Hodgkin's disease, pancreatic cancer, stomach cancer, thyroid cancer, adrenal adenoma, adrenal hyperplasia tumors, and cancers that secrete adrenocorticotropic hormone (ACTH) ectopically	Serum potassium <3.5 mEq/L	Dietary intake of potassium is deficient when the client is anorexic, vomiting, or NPO. Excessive diarrhea that leads to rapid potassium depletion occurs with many GI tumors, chemotherapy, radiation therapy to the lower abdomen, and antibiotic therapy. Excessive urinary excretion may be caused by diuretics, hypercalcemia, hypomagnesemia, antibiotic therapy, ectopic ACTH secretion, nephrotoxicity due to chemotherapy or radiation, and renal tubular necrosis due to Hodgkin's disease, multiple myeloma, and acute blast crisis. Ileostomy, colostomy, fistulas, and the diuretic phase of renal failure also contribute to hypokalemia.
Hypomagnesemia	Lung cancer, especially oat cell, ovarian cancer, and testicular cancer; total parenteral nutrition (TPN), cis-platinum chemotherapy	Serum magnesium <1.5 mEq/L	Low magnesium level occurs most often in clients with severe diarrhea, vomiting, malabsorption syndrome, cachexia, ADH secretion, or renal disease. The cis-platinum and nephrotoxic antibiotics also contribute to hypomagnesemia.
Lactic acidosis	Hodgkin's disease, lymphoma, leukemia, lymphosarcoma, and lung cancer (especially oat cell with liver metastasis)	Arterial blood pH <7.35, HCO_3 <24 mEq/L, serum CO_2 <22 mEq/L	Lactic acidosis (metabolic acidosis) occurs because rapidly growing malignant cells utilize large amounts of glucose. When the glucose is metabolized by the anaerobic pathway (glycolysis), pyruvic acid is the end product. When hypoxia exists, pyruvate is converted to lactic acid. Elevated serum lactic acid concentrations may exceed the liver's ability to metabolize and the kidneys' to excrete.

Table 13-1.   (Continued)

Fluid/Electrolyte Disturbance	Commonly Associated Cancer and Cancer Therapy	Defining Characteristics	Rationale/Comments
Hyperkalemia	Hodgkins' disease, lymphoma, leukemia, lung cancer (especially oat cell), and liver metastasis; aggressive chemotherapy	Serum potassium >5.3 mEq/L	Intracellular-extracellular redistribution occurs during respiratory and metabolic acidosis (including lactic acidosis). Extracellular hydrogen ions shift into the cell in an attempt to raise serum pH. Intracellular potassium ions then shift out of the cell to compensate. Lysis of large numbers of malignant and normal cells during radiation and chemotherapy causes the release of massive amounts of potassium from destroyed cells (tumor lysis syndrome). Renal failure and hypoaldosteronism can cause renal retention of potassium.
Hypophosphatemia	Leukemia, multiple myeloma, PTH-secreting tumors; total parenteral nutrition (TPN) (hyperalimentation)	Serum phosphorus <2.5 mg/dL	Hypophosphatemia occurs with cancers that contain and secrete PTH (PTH normally regulates the rate of phosphorus reabsorption by the kidneys). Aggressive hyperalimentation/parenteral nutrition often induces hypophosphatemia because the phosphorus influx into cells is accelerated during carbohydrate metabolism. Malabsorption, sepsis, diuretics, corticosteroids, and thrombocytopenia are other contributing factors. Symptoms of hypophosphatemia are fatigue, weakness, anorexia, irritability, paresthesia, seizures, and coma.
Decreased vascular volume (shift to the third space)	Liver cancer, including liver metastasis, stomach cancer, pancreatic cancer, colon cancer, and head and neck cancer	Serum albumin <3/2 g/dL, decreased BP, increased H & H, increased BUN	Decreased vascular volume occurs when serum protein is decreased, when tumor cells exude fluids, or when vascular permeability is increased by infection. Protein depletion occurs with anorexia/cachexia, nausea, and vomiting due to disease or therapy or to decreased protein synthesis in cancer clients. Some individuals with cancer have increased loss of protein via the GI tract; elevated basal metabolic rate due to disease or infection results in accelerated protein loss. Decreased serum protein leads to decreased blood volume and a drop in blood pressure. The client may have ample or excess extracellular fluid but is unable to retain it within the vascular space. Without treatment, cardiovascular failure and death result.

Fluid/Electrolyte Disturbance	Commonly Associated Cancer and Cancer Therapy	Defining Characteristics	Rationale/Comments
Hypocalcemia/ hyperphosphatemia	Leukemia, lymphoma, and multiple myeloma; aggressive chemotherapy and radiation	Serum calcium <9 mg/dL, serum phosphorus >4.5 mg/dL	Rapid cell lysis causes the release of large amounts of phosphate. Immature blast cells contain up to four times more phosphate than mature lymphocytes. The rise in serum phosphorus then causes a drop in serum calcium. Renal failure may result from precipitation of calcium phosphate in the kidneys. Symptoms include oliguria, anuria, azotemia, and tetany.

14 Bone destruction that results from metastatic tumors causes what type of calcium imbalance? _____ . The serum level would be _____ mg/dL.

hypercalcemia or calcium excess; >11

■   ■   ■

15 Can hyponatremia be associated with cancer? _____ .

Explain how? * _____

_____ .

Can hypernatremia be associated with cancer? _____ .

Yes. Liver, thyroid, and adrenal insufficiencies are followed by a loss of sodium. Also intracranial neoplasms could result in cerebral salt wasting and the inability of the kidneys to conserve sodium.
Not usually.

■   ■   ■

16 The syndrome of inappropriate antidiuretic hormone (SIADH) can be associated with cancer. As a result, more water is (reabsorbed/excreted) _____ by the kidneys.

The two drug therapies that contribute to SIADH are _____ and

_____ .

reabsorbed; vincristine and cyclophosphamide

■   ■   ■

17 Hyperuricemia can occur in any cancer treated aggressively with _____ and
_____ .

   Explain the effect of a high-serum uric acid on kidney function. *_____
_____ .

chemotherapy and radiation
It could cause renal failure by precipitation of uric acid crystals in the kidneys.
   ■   ■   ■

18 Name three symptoms of hyperuricemia. _____ , *_____ ,
and *_____ .

hematuria, flank pain, and nausea and vomiting (also symptoms of renal failure)
   ■   ■   ■

19 Can hypokalemia occur as the result of cancer? _____ .

   Give three reasons why there may be a low potassium level. *_____ ,
*_____ , and *_____ .

   The serum potassium level is _____ mEq/L.

Yes.
poor dietary intake of potassium, excessive diarrhea, and excessive urinary secretion (also
vomiting, colostomy, and excess adrenal gland secretion from tumor)
<3.5
   ■   ■   ■

20 Can hyperkalemia be induced by cancer? _____ .

   Explain why? *_____
_____ .

   The serum potassium level is _____ mEq/L.

Yes.
The breakdown of malignant and normal cells causes potassium to shift from cells to vascular
fluid.
>5.3
   ■   ■   ■

21   Why does hypomagnesemia develop?   *_____
_____ .

because of vomiting, malabsorption syndrome, severe diarrhea, cachexia, and total parenteral nutrition (TPN)

∎   ∎   ∎

22   Hypophosphatemia is usually associated with cancer in   *_____   and
*_____ .

PTH secreting tumors; total parenteral nutrition (TPN)

∎   ∎   ∎

23   A large amount of glucose is utilized by rapidly growing malignant cells. Pyruvic acid is the end product of anaerobic metabolism of glucose. When hypoxia exists, pyruvate is converted to lactic acid. The specific acid-base imbalance is   *_____ .

The arterial blood pH is   _____ .

The arterial bicarbonate is   _____   mEq/L.

lactic acidosis; <7.35; <24

∎   ∎   ∎

24   Calcium and phosphorus imbalance may be present in leukemia, lymphoma, multiple myeloma, and aggressive chemotherapy and radiation.

Identify the imbalances that occur together:

( ) a. Hypocalcemia
( ) b. Hypercalcemia
( ) c. Hypophosphatemia
( ) d. Hyperphosphatemia

a. X; b. —; c. —; d. X

∎   ∎   ∎

25 When protein depletion occurs because of anorexia/cachexia and nausea/vomiting, what type of fluid imbalance may result? *_____ .

Explain why. *_____

_____

_____ .

decreased vascular volume or ECFV deficit (vascular)
Protein loss decreases osmotic pressure and less fluid is held in the vascular space. When protein shifts to an injured or damaged site and permeability is increased, fluid shifts to the third space (to the injured or damaged site).

■ ■ ■

26 Indicate which of the following electrolyte imbalances are frequently associated with cancer and cancer therapy:

( ) a. Hypercalcemia
( ) b. Hypernatremia
( ) c. Hypokalemia
( ) d. Hyperkalemia
( ) e. Hypomagnesemia
( ) f. Hypermagnesemia
( ) g. Hypophosphatemia
( ) h. Hypocalcemia/hyperphosphatemia

a. X; b. —; c. X; d. X; e. X; f. —; g. X; h. X

■ ■ ■

CLINICAL APPLICATIONS

The fluid and electrolyte disturbances listed in Table 13-1 can develop in almost any individual with cancer at any time during diagnosis, treatment, recovery, or terminal stages of the disease.

Fluid and electrolyte problems are *most common*, however, with the following clinical conditions:

1. *Cachexia.* Severe anorexia, nausea, vomiting, and/or diarrhea are present.
2. *Tumor lysis syndrome.* Large numbers of cells are destroyed by chemotherapy radiation.
3. *Uncontrolled cell growth.* Rapid, widespread cell growth with multiple metastasis or multiple organ infiltration.
4. *Ectopic hormone production.* Ectopic hormones are secreted by the tumor(s).

CACHEXIA

Cachexia may occur because of the effects of the malignancy itself and/or be caused by radiation and chemotherapy. Contributing problems include anorexia, nausea, vomiting, diarrhea, draining wounds, and fistulas. The most frequently encountered fluid and electrolyte disturbances are hypomagnesemia, hypokalemia, and decreased vascular volume.

27   Name the two electrolytes that are most commonly lost due to cachexia.

_____ and _____ .

Do you recall the methods/routes for replacing potassium and magnesium? See Chapter 3 on potassium and magnesium replacement.

Potassium: _____ and _____

Magnesium: _____ , _____ , and _____

potassium and magnesium
intravenously and orally
intravenously, intramuscularly, and orally

■   ■   ■

28   Anorexia, nausea, and vomiting decrease protein intake; diarrhea, malabsorption syndrome, and wound drainage increase protein loss in the cancer client.

Decreased vascular volume occurs in cachexic clients because of *_____ (see Table 13-1).

Protein synthesis is (increased/decreased) _____ in many cancer clients. Metabolic changes and infections accelerate *_____ .

protein depletion or loss; decreased; protein loss

■   ■   ■

29   The basic goal of therapy in cancer clients with decreased vascular volume is to maintain blood pressure. Whole blood, packed red blood cells (RBCs), or albumin may be given to increase plasma oncotic pressure (colloid osmotic pressure) to restore fluid balance in the vascular space. Whole blood, packed RBCs, and albumin restore the fluid balance in the vessels by

*_____ .

increasing plasma oncotic pressure OR increasing colloid osmotic pressure in vascular space

■   ■   ■

30 Carefully prescribed and monitored hyperalimentation (TPN) can correct hypokalemia and hypomagnesemia and improve vascular volume.

What happens to the serum phosphorus level when TPN is aggressively administered?

* _____

_____ (Refer to Table 13-1).

Prolonged parenteral nutrition without magnesium supplement can cause

_____ .

Hypophosphatemia occurs because of phosphorus influx into cells during carbohydrate metabolism.
hypomagnesemia

■   ■   ■

TUMOR LYSIS SYNDROME

Following the destruction of large numbers of cells by chemotherapy, usually in leukemia or lymphoma, vast numbers of intracellular electrolytes enter the bloodstream. The cancer client can develop hyperuricemia, hyperkalemia, hyperphosphatemia, and/or hypocalcemia. Renal failure or cardiac arrest may result.

31 When a large number of cells in the body is destroyed by chemotherapy what two life-threatening situations can result? *_____ and *_____ .

Identify the imbalances that occur during massive cell destruction:

( ) a. Hypokalemia
( ) b. Hyperkalemia
( ) c. Hypocalcemia
( ) d. Hypercalcemia
( ) e. Hyperphosphatemia
( ) f. Hyperuricemia

renal failure and cardiac arrest
a. —; b. X; c. X; d. —; e. X; f. X

■   ■   ■

32   The purpose of therapy for cancer clients who are undergoing the destruction of large numbers of cells is the prevention of renal failure and   *_____ .

   Management includes aggressive hydration (3000 mL/day) to increase urinary volume and excretion of   *_____ ,   _____ , and   _____ .

electrolyte imbalance. If your answer was cardiac arrest, true, but that usually results from severe electrolyte imbalance.
uric acid, potassium, and phosphorus (phosphate)
   ▪   ▪   ▪

33   Drugs used for the management of fluid and electrolytes include

   Potent diuretics such as furosemide/Lasix when there is fluid retention;
   Allopurinol to decrease uric acid;
   Calcium gluconate IV infusion if hypocalcemia develops;
   Sodium bicarbonate to alkalinize the urine if hyperuricemia occurs (uric acid is less soluble in acid urine).

   Four imbalances found with massive cell destruction are   _____ ,
   _____ ,   _____ , and   _____ .

hyperkalemia, hyperphosphatemia, hyperuricemia, and hypocalcemia
   ▪   ▪   ▪

UNCONTROLLED CELL GROWTH

Individuals with cancer may experience severe electrolyte disturbances whenever rapid and widespread malignant cell growth occurs. This uncontrolled cell growth is marked by multiple metastatic lesions (metastatic carcinoma or sarcoma) or by multiple organ infiltration (leukemias and lymphomas).

34   Hypercalcemia is usually present when   *_____
_____ (refer to Table 13-1).

   Hypercalcemia in individuals with cancer develops more rapidly and becomes more severe than hypercalcemia from other causes. When acute hypercalcemia crisis occurs, the mortality rate is extremely high (up to 50%).

metastatic tumors cause bone destruction OR metastatic cell growth or infiltration destroys bone
   ▪   ▪   ▪

35 Management of mild and moderate hypercalcemia involves IV normal saline (NaCl 0.9%) to achieve adequate hydration and promote calcium excretion.

For severe hypercalcemia the following drugs are indicated:

Furosemide/Lasix to decrease tubular reabsorption of calcium.
Steroids to increase calcium excretion.
Calcitonin to inhibit bone resorption.
Mithramycin to inhibit bone resorption.
Biphosphonates to inhibit calcium release from bone.
Gallium nitrate to make calcium dissolution more difficult.
IV inorganic phosphates (severe side effects could be calcium precipitation in lung, kidney, or heart tissues).

With mild and moderate hypercalcemia effective management includes
*_____ .

Two drugs frequently prescribed for severe hypercalcemia are _____ and _____ . A diuretic that promotes kidney excretion of calcium is

_____ .

IV normal saline; mithramycin and calcitonin; furosemide

■   ■   ■

36 Lactic acidosis and hyperkalemia may occur during periods of uncontrolled malignant cell growth.

Lactic acidosis is the result of *_____

_____ (refer to Table 13-1).

What is the cause of hyperkalemia? *_____

_____ (refer to Table 13-1).

rapidly growing malignant cells that utilize excess glucose with anaerobic metabolism and cause lactic acid as a by-product
Acidosis causes a compensatory shift of extracellular hydrogen ions and intracellular potassium.

■   ■   ■

ECTOPIC HORMONE PRODUCTION

Abnormal hormones may be secreted by any malignant cells. The most commonly involved cancers and hormones are those listed in Table 13-2. Study the contents in the table and refer back to it as needed.

Table 13-2. HORMONES COMMONLY SECRETED ECTOPICALLY BY MALIGNANT CELLS		
Hormones	**Type of Cancer**	**Common Associated Problems**
Antidiuretic hormone (ADH)	Lung (oat cell) Pancreas Hodgkin's disease Prostate gland Sarcoma	SIADH Hyponatremia Hypomagnesemia
Parathyroid hormone (PTH)	Lung Leukemia Multiple myeloma Breast	Hypercalcemia Hypophosphatemia Hypomagnesemia
Adrenocorticotropic hormone (ACTH)	Lung (oat cell and non-oat cell)	Hypokalemia
Osteoclast activating factor (OAF)	Multiple myeloma Lymphoma	Hypercalcemia
Prostaglandins (E series)	Breast Kidney Pancreas	Hypercalcemia

37 Name three ectopic hormones that can be secreted by malignant cells.

_____ , _____ , and _____ .

Ectopic hormone secretions occur most commonly with what type of cancer?

_____ .

ADH or antidiuretic hormone; PTH or parathyroid hormone; and ACTH or adrenocorticotropic hormone
lung

■　　　　　　■　　　　　　■

38 Acute complications caused by ectopic hormone secretions in cancer patients include fluid and electrolyte imbalances. If the imbalances are severe, cardiac arrest may occur.

According to Table 13-2, four common electrolyte imbalances that result from ectopic hormone secretions are _____ , _____ , _____ , and _____ .

hypercalcemia, hypomagnesemia, hyponatremia, and hyperphosphatemia (also hypokalemia)

■　　　　　　■　　　　　　■

39 The primary goal of therapy in cancer clients with ectopic hormone secretion is the eradication or reduction of the hormone-secreting tumor. If surgery, radiation, and/or chemotherapy do not eliminate the tumor and control the symptoms, long-term pharmacologic therapy may be ordered.

What are the three methods that can be used to reduce or eradicate the hormone-secreting tumor?   *_____ , _____ , and _____ .

surgery, radiation, and chemotherapy

■   ■   ■

40 Treatment of SIADH varies with the severity of the symptoms.

Mild SIADH: Restriction of water and fluid intake to 500–1000 mL per day.
Severe SIADH: 3–5% saline infusion to restore serum sodium; furosemide (Lasix) to increase water excretion; demeclocycline or lithium carbonate to interfere with the action of ADH on renal tubules.

Extreme care should be taken when hyperosmolar saline is administered (3–5% saline solution) because it could raise the serum sodium level too rapidly and cause shrinkage of CNS neurons and neurologic dysfunction.

SIADH is the abbreviation for   *_____ .

Treatment for mild SIADH is   *_____ .

secretion (syndrome) of inappropriate antidiuretic hormone; restriction of fluid to 500–1000 mL daily.

■   ■   ■

41 Indicate which of the following treatments may be used for managing severe SIADH:

( ) a. 0.9% saline (normal saline solution)
( ) b. 3–5% saline infusion
( ) c. Radiation to tumor
( ) d. Chemotherapy to tumor
( ) e. Surgical removal of ADH-secreting tumor
( ) f. Lithium carbonate
( ) g. Ampicillin
( ) h. Demeclocycline

a. —; b. X; c. X; d. X; e. X; f. X; g. —; h. X

■   ■   ■

42 What can happen if excessive amounts of 3–5% saline are administered to correct SIADH?

* _____

_____ .

An elevated serum sodium level (hypernatremia) causes shrinkage of CNS neurons and neurologic dysfunction.

■   ■   ■

43 Name the four major problems found in cancer clients that are commonly associated with fluid and electrolyte disorders. _____ , * _____ ,

* _____ , and * _____ .

cachexia, tumor lysis syndrome, uncontrolled cell growth, and ectopic hormone production

■   ■   ■

CLINICAL APPLICATIONS: CASE STUDY I

Ralph Peterson, a 53-year-old auto mechanic, complained to his doctor of progressive dyspnea, a persistent, productive cough, fatigue, anorexia, and weight loss.

A chest x-ray, sputum cytology, and bronchoscopy were performed and Mr. Peterson was diagnosed as having stage II squamous-cell lung cancer. The primary tumor was removed by lobectomy and radiation therapy was given a month later to reduce the risk of metastasis.

Fourteen months after his surgery Mr. Peterson was readmitted because of severe weight loss (30 pounds in 3 months), fatigue, and dyspnea. CT scans revealed that Mr. Peterson had a large metastatic lesion in the liver and two smaller tumors in the right lung.

Laboratory studies were ordered for Mr. Peterson on admission, on day 3, on day 10, on day 11, and a month later. The results of his laboratory tests are given in Table 13-3. Complete the frames related to his laboratory studies by following the table.

Laboratory Tests	On Admission	Day 3	Day 10	Day 11	One Month
Table 13-3. LABORATORY STUDIES: MR. PETERSON					
Hematology					
Hemoglobin (Hgb) (Male: 13.5–18 g)	18.5	14			
Hematocrit (Hct) (Male: 40–54%)	54	46			
Biochemistry					
BUN (10–25 mg/dL)	34	21			
Creatinine (Cr) (0.6–1.2 mg/dL)	2.1	1.5			
Uric acid (Male: 3.5–7 mg/dL)	7.8				
Lactate (serum) (6–16 mg/dL)	17				
Albumin (serum) (3.5–5.0 g/dL)	2.8	4.3			
Potassium (K) (3.5–5.3 mEq/L)	3.1	4.2	3.0		
Sodium (Na) (135–145 mEq/L)	118	135			
Chloride (Cl) (95–108 mEq/L)	103	102			
Calcium (Ca) (9–11 mg/dL)	8.8	8.8	14.4	13.4	16.6
Phosphorus (P) (2.5–4.5 mg/dL)	3.1		2.2		
Magnesium (Mg) (1.5–2.5 mEq/L)			1.3		

44 On admission, Mr. Peterson's lab tests suggested that he had decreased vascular volume, also called ECFV deficit or dehydration. (Refer to Chapter 2 on dehydration if needed.)

Which of his following laboratory results are indicative of decreased vascular volume?

( ) a. Hemoglobin 18.5 g
( ) b. Hematocrit 54%
( ) c. BUN 34 mg/dL
( ) d. Serum albumin 2.8 g/dL
( ) e. Serum potassium 3.1 mEq/L (hypokalemia)
( ) f. Serum sodium 118 mEq/L (hyponatremia)
( ) g. Serum chloride 103 mEq/L
( ) h. Serum calcium 8.8 mg/dL
( ) i. Serum phosphorus 3.1 mg/dL
( ) j. Serum lactate 17 mg/dL
( ) k. Serum uric acid 7.8 mg/dL

a. X; b. X (very high normal); c. X; d. X; e. X (possible); f. X (possible); g. —; h. —; i. —; j. —; k. —

■   ■   ■

45 Hemoglobin and BUN may be elevated because of (hemodilution/hemoconcentration) _____ .

Protein, sodium, and potassium are shifted to the tumor site, thus (increasing/decreasing) _____ oncotic pressure/colloid osmotic pressure. Will this have an effect on vascular fluid balance? _____ . Explain *_____ .

hemoconcentration; decreasing
Yes. Decreased oncotic pressure in the vascular space causes fluid loss or dehydration.

■   ■   ■

46 On admission, Mr. Peterson's vital signs were temperature (T) 100°F, pulse rate (P) 124, respiration (R) 28, and blood pressure (BP) 96/60.

Which of his vital signs are indicative of fluid volume deficit (vascular fluid):

( ) a. T 100°F
( ) b. P 124
( ) c. R 28
( ) d. BP 96/60

a. X; b. X; c. X (possible); d. X

■   ■   ■

47 IV albumin and packed RBCs were given to raise the serum oncotic pressure and to maintain vascular fluid and adequate blood pressure. He was started on hyperalimentation (TPN) to improve his overall nutritional status prior to chemotherapy. His anorexia, nausea, and fatigue gradually lessened and his BP stabilized at 116/74—110/70.

The purpose of IV albumin and packed RBC administration is to *_____ ,
*_____ , and *_____ .

raise the serum oncotic pressure; maintain vascular fluid; maintain adequate blood pressure
  ∎   ∎   ∎

48 Were Mr. Peterson's laboratory results 3 days after admission of normal values?
_____ . Please explain. *_____
_____ .

Yes. Creatinine is slightly elevated and serum sodium is low normal.
                ∎   ∎   ∎

49 Ten days after he was admitted Mr. Peterson's condition had greatly improved and chemotherapy was scheduled to begin the next day. However, he became restless and irritable and by evening was disoriented and combative. He also became increasingly weak and vomited several times.

On his tenth day after admission his serum electrolytes were not within normal values.

Name four electrolyte imbalances present. _____ , _____ ,
_____ , and _____ .

hypokalemia, hypercalcemia, hypomagnesemia, and hypophosphatemia
              ∎   ∎   ∎

50 His immediate treatment consisted of the following:

1. Calcitonin 100 MRC units subcutaneously every 12 hours
2. Furosemide 20 mg IV push every 6 hours
3. Sodium phosphate ($Na_2 HPO_4$) 15 mL PO three times daily
4. Potassium and magnesium increased in TPN
5. IV rate increased to 150 mL per hour

On the eleventh day the calcitonin dose was changed:

1. Calcitonin 300 MRC units subcutaneously every 12 hours
2. Mithramycin 1 mg IV push

Why was calcitonin administered? *_____ .
Why were mithramycin and calcitonin given on the eleventh day? *_____

_____ .

to decrease the high serum calcium level
The serum calcium level was still high and both hypocalcemic agents decreased the serum level.

■   ■   ■

51 To determine the cause of Mr. Peterson's hypercalcemia, a bone scan and PTH level was done. The bone scan was negative. This indicates *_____ .
His PTH level of 455 pg Eq/mL (norm: 163–375 pg Eq/mL) indicated that the metastatic tumors in his lung were secreting PTH ectopically. This increased PTH secretion causes the two electrolyte imbalances. _____ and _____ .

that hypercalcemia was not due to bone destruction; hypercalcemia and hypophosphatemia (also hypomagnesemia)

■   ■   ■

52 Mr. Peterson was started on a combination of chemotherapeutics (Cisplatin, cyclophosphamide/Cytoxan, and Doxorubicin HCl) to shrink the tumors and decrease the PTH secretion.

After 5 days of chemotherapy his serum calcium was 9 mg/dL. Is this in normal range? Explain *_____ . He was alert, oriented, and eating and drinking well; soon he was discharged.

yes, on the lower normal side

■   ■   ■

53 A month later he was readmitted with a serum calcium level of 16.6 mg/dL. The type of imbalance present is _____ .

A similar drug regime was followed, and after his serum calcium level returned to normal, he was discharged on daily calcitonin injections.

hypercalcemia

■   ■   ■

CLINICAL APPLICATIONS: CASE STUDY II

Steven Blackman, 15 years old, was rushed to the local emergency room by his parents when he awakened feeling weak and short of breath. His parents told the physician that he had complained of feeling tired for 2 or 3 weeks and had a sore throat and swollen glands and two nosebleeds the week before. Steven's lungs were not congested, but the physician noted moderate lymphadenopathy and an enlarged liver and spleen. He was admitted to the adolescent unit with a suspected diagnosis of acute leukemia.

Vital signs were as follows:

T 101°F, P 124, R 30, BP 100/66

Steven Blackman's laboratory results on admission, day 1, and day 6 are given in Table 13-4. Refer to the table as needed as you proceed with this clinical example.

54 On admission, Steven's hemoglobin and hematocrit were decreased because his bone marrow had been infiltrated by leukemic cells which led to decreased RBC production. This could be the reason for his _____ .

His platelet count was (high/low) _____ , a possible reason for his

_____ .

His elevated WBCs are indicative of a serious problem.

weakness or fatigue; low; nosebleeds. Good.
■ ■ ■

55 His ABGs indicate what acid-base disorder? *_____
(refer to Chapter 4 if needed).

At his elevated serum lactate level the specific acid-base imbalance would be

*_____ .

metabolic acidosis (his pH and HCO₃ are low)
lactic acidosis. This is the result of an abnormal carbohydrate metabolism in the blast cells (immature WBCs).
■ ■ ■

56 Steven's elevated BUN and creatinine could be caused by *_____
because his uric acid, in particular, is elevated.

renal insufficiency. Remember, if the BUN were slightly elevated and the creatinine in normal range, this insufficiency could be due to ECFV deficit or dehydration. Renal insufficiency reduces the body's ability to excrete the excess lactic acid.
■ ■ ■

Laboratory Tests	On Admission	Day 1	Day 6
Table 13-4. LABORATORY STUDIES: STEVEN BLACKMAN			
Hematology			
Hemoglobin (Hgb) (12.5–18 g/dL)	7		
Hematocrit (Hct) (36–54%)	18		
Platelets (150,000–400,000 mm^3)	56,000		
White blood cells (WBC) (5000–10,000 mm^3)	31,000		
Differential			
Blasts (0–5%)	46%		
Biochemistry			
BUN (10–25 mg/dL)	30	28	41
Creatinine (Cr) (0.6–1.2 mg/dL)	1.8	1.7	2.6
Uric acid (3.5–7 mg/dL)	8.6		19
Lactate (serum) (6–16 mg/dL)	17		
Potassium (serum) (3.5–5.3 mEq/L)	5.7	4.1	5.9
Sodium (serum) (135–145 mEq/L)	140		
Calcium (serum) (9–11 mg/dL)	9.0		7.6
Magnesium (serum) (1.5–2.5 mEq/L)	2.0		
Chloride (Cl) (95–108 mEq/L)	103		
Phosphorus (serum) (2.5–4.5 mEq/L)	3.8		8.0
Arterial Blood Gases (ABGs)			
pH (7.35–7.45)	7.28	7.38	
Pao$_2$ (70–90%)	90	92	
Paco$_2$ (35–45 mm Hg)	34	38	
HCO$_3$ (24–28 mEq/L)	22	26	

57 His potassium level indicated _____ . This could be cellular breakdown and acidotic state.

hyperkalemia

      ■   ■   ■

58 Steven received $NaHCO_3$ in D_5W to correct acidosis. His serum potassium had to be carefully monitored while the acidotic state was being corrected. Why? *_____

_____ .

As the pH rises, potassium will shift back into the cells and too much $NaHCO_3$ could cause alkalosis and hypokalemia.

      ■   ■   ■

59 A bone marrow biopsy showed that the marrow had been almost entirely replaced by immature myeloblasts. This confirmed Steven's diagnosis of acute myelogenous leukemia (AML).

    Steven was started on a chemotherapeutic regimen in an attempt to induce remission (absence of all leukemic cells).

    High doses of chemotherapy result in the lysis of large numbers of malignant cells; therefore Steven was monitored for signs and symptoms of *_____ .

tumor lysis syndrome

      ■   ■   ■

60 On day 6 he complained of flank pain and his urinary output decreased sharply. Laboratory values were indicative of tumor lysis syndrome.

    Name four imbalances that are significant of this disorder. _____ ,

_____ , _____ , and _____ .

hyperuricemia, hyperkalemia, hypocalcemia, and hyperphosphatemia

      ■   ■   ■

61 Two other laboratory values that were indicative of his decreased urine output were *_____ and *_____ .

elevated BUN and elevated creatinine

      ■   ■   ■

62 His uric acid was corrected with increased IV fluids and allopurinol (to promote uric acid excretion).

His nurses monitored his intake and output carefully and checked for edema, chest rales, and level of consciousness (LOC). Explain why? *_____

_____ .

Decreased urinary output and increased IV fluids could result in fluid overload or ECFV excess.

■   ■   ■

NURSING ASSESSMENT FACTORS

Assessment for and recognition of fluid and electrolyte imbalance in clients with cancer are especially difficult because the symptoms (e.g., anorexia, vomiting, fatigue, diarrhea, and muscle weakness) mimic those of chemotherapy, radiation, or general deterioration in advanced cancer.

Many fluid and electrolyte conditions in cancer clients can be reversed or controlled. It is essential that nurses assess them. Table 13-5 gives the nursing assessment for fluid and electrolyte imbalance in cancer clients. This table can be used in hospitals and clinics or at home. To use it as an assessment tool, check the blanks in the nursing assessment column. For additional information or clarification use the comment column.

Table 13-5.   NURSING ASSESSMENT OF FLUID AND ELECTROLYTE IMBALANCE
TYPE OF PRIMARY CANCER: _____
STAGE: _____ LIVER METASTASIS: _____ BONE METASTASIS: _____

Observation	Nursing Assessment		Comments
Vital signs	Temperature	_____	
	Pulse	_____	
	Respiration	_____	
	Blood pressure	_____	
		_____	
	Heart sounds	_____	
	Peripheral pulses	_____	
Intake	PO	_____	
	IV infusions	_____	
	Amounts	_____	
Output	Amounts	_____	
	Specific gravity	_____	
	Urine osmolality	_____	
	Polyuria	_____	
	Oliguria	_____	
	Anuria	_____	

Table 13-5. (Continued)

Observation	Nursing Assessment	Comments
Weight and skin changes	Daily weight	
	Skin turgor	
	Skin temperature	
	Edema	
	Ascites	
GI changes	Anorexia	
	Nausea	
	Vomiting	
	Diarrhea	
	Constipation	
	Bowel sounds	
	Abdominal distention	
	Abdominal cramps	
	Fistula	
	GI suction	
	Draining tube	
Respiratory changes	Dyspnea	
	Hyperpnea	
	Chest rales	
	Others	
Neurologic changes	Headache	
	LOC changes	
	Irritability	
	Disorientation	
	Confusion	
	Paresthesia	
	Altered perception	
	Seizures	
	Coma	
State of being	Alert	
	Fatigue	
	Lethargic	
Muscular changes	Muscle weakness	
	Hyporeflexia	
	Hyperreflexia	
	Muscle cramps	
	Twitching	
	Tetany signs	

Table 13-5. (Continued)

Observation	Nursing Assessment	Comments
Body chemistry and hematology changes	Hemoglobin	
	Hematocrit	
	Platelets	
	WBCs	
	Differential	
	Electrolytes:	
	Potassium	
	Sodium	
	Calcium	
	Magnesium	
	Chloride	
	Phosphorus	
	Serum osmolality	
	Protein	
	Albumin	
	BUN	
	Creatinine	
	Uric acid	
	Lactate	
	ABGs:	
	pH	
	Pa_{O_2}	
	Pa_{CO_2}	
	HCO_3	
Chemotherapy	Drug	
	Dose, route	
	Side effects	
Radiation therapy	Dose	
	Times	
	Target area	

63 Which of the following laboratory tests should be monitored?

( ) a. Hemoglobin   ( ) g. Lactate
( ) b. Hematocrit   ( ) h. Uric acid
( ) c. Electrolytes   ( ) i. Lipoproteins
( ) d. Hormones, e.g., PTH ( ) j. BUN
( ) e. Phenylketonuria   ( ) k. Creatinine
( ) f. Protein and albumin ( ) l. ABGs

a. X; b. X; c. X; d. X; e. —; f. X; g. X; h. X; i. —; j. X; k. X; l. X
   ■   ■   ■

CASE STUDY REVIEW

1. The three problems associated with primitive biochemical function of malignant cells are
   _____ , * _____ , and * _____ .
2. Give the names of electrolyte imbalances associated with cancer and cancer therapy:
   a. Calcium _____
   b. Calcium _____
      and phosphorus _____
   c. Sodium _____
   d. Potassium _____
      _____
   e. Phosphorus _____
3. Hyperuricemia is a serious condition that results from massive cell destruction by radiation or
   chemotherapy. What is its effect on the renal tubules? * _____ . What could
   happen to the body? * _____
   _____ .
4. Three symptoms of hyperuricemia are _____ , * _____ , and
   * _____ .
5. Hypercalcemia is a serious condition. It is generally caused by * _____
   _____ or * _____ .
   A very high calcium level can cause _____ and * _____ .
6. SIADH is another serious condition. Why? * _____
   _____ .
7. Give three reasons why hypokalemia may occur. * _____ ,
   * _____ , and * _____ .
8. What type of acid-base imbalance is caused by anaerobic metabolism of glucose? * _____
   _____ .
   Explain how. * _____
   _____ .

9. Name the four most common causes of fluid and electrolyte imbalance in cancer clients.
_____ , *_____ , *_____ , and
*_____ .

Mr. Peterson had been diagnosed 14 months before as having lung cancer. He was readmitted to the hospital because of severe weight loss, fatigue, and dyspnea.

10. Mr. Peterson's hemoglobin and hematocrit were elevated. This may be the result of
_____ .

11. His BUN and creatinine were slightly elevated. This may be caused by _____
or _____ .

12. What effects do low serum protein and albumin levels have on the vascular fluid?
*_____ . Why? *_____
_____ .

On day 10 after admission Mr. Peterson's calcium level was high. He was restless, irritable, disoriented, combative, weak, and vomiting.

13. Two drugs Mr. Peterson received to decrease his serum calcium level were
_____ and _____ .

Steven Blackman, 15 years old, was diagnosed as having acute leukemia. The results of his hematology on admission indicated a low hemoglobin, hematocrit, and platelet count and an elevated WBC.

14. Steven's pH and HCO_3 were low and his serum lactate was slightly elevated. What acid-base disorder do you suspect? *_____ .

15. His serum potassium level was 5.7 mEq/L. What potassium imbalance is present?
_____ . Why? *_____
_____ .

16. When correcting acidosis with $NaHCO_3$ name the imbalance that may occur.
*_____ .

17. Steven was given chemotherapy in massive doses to destroy the large numbers of malignant cells. His uric acid was 19 mg/dL. What disorder frequently results from elevated uric acid?
*_____ .
What imbalance did he have? _____ .

18. Steven was given increased amounts of IV fluids, allopurinol, and $NaHCO_3$ (which alkalinizes the urine) to correct what imbalance? *_____ .

1. *cachexia, abnormal (redundant) hormone secretion, and increased uric acid or breakdown of purine nucleic acids*
2. a. *hypercalcemia*
   b. *hypocalcemia; hyperphosphatemia*
   c. *hyponatremia*
   d. *hypokalemia; hyperkalemia*
   e. *hypophosphatemia*

3. uric acid precipitates in the renal tubules and collecting ducts; a small increased level can cause renal disorder and possible renal failure
4. hematuria, flank pain, and nausea and vomiting (also symptoms of renal failure)
5. bone destruction which results from metastasis or elevated PTH
   confusion, disorientation, and cardiac arrest (also brittle bones)
6. ADH may be secreted ectopically from neoplastic tumors, e.g., lung tumor. SIADH can cause severe water intoxication, hyponatremia, headaches, and behavioral changes.
7. decreased dietary intake, vomiting/diarrhea, and excessive urinary output due to diuretics (also ileostomy, colostomy, and fistulas)
8. Lactic acidosis (metabolic acidosis). Anaerobic metabolism of glucose produces pyruvic acid, which is converted during hypoxia to lactic acid.
9. cachexia, tumor lysis syndrome, uncontrolled cell growth, and ectopic hormone production
10. dehydration, fluid loss, or hemoconcentration
11. dehydration; renal insufficiency
    If the BUN returns to normal after hydration the problem is dehydration.
12. Decreased vascular volume. Protein shifts to tumor site, thus decreasing oncotic pressure.
13. Calcintonin and mithramycin
14. lactic acidosis (if the results were based on ABGs, metabolic acidosis)
15. hyperkalemia; cellular breakdown and acidotic state
16. hypokalemic alkalosis (potassium shifts back into cells)
17. tumor lysis syndrome; hyperuricemia
18. high uric acid or hyperuricemia

NURSING ASSESSMENT FACTORS

- Fluid and electrolyte balance must be monitored carefully in clients with any type of cancer and at all stages of diagnosis and treatment. Assessment is particularly important in clients during and after treatment with chemotherapy, radiation, surgery, biologic response modifiers, and/or bone marrow transplantation. In addition, fluid and electrolyte problems are particularly common in clients dying from cancer.
- Assess for anorexia, nausea, vomiting, diarrhea, edema, weight loss or gain, neurologic status, fatigue, and activity levels. Laboratory values of sodium, calcium, potassium, magnesium, and phosphorus should be checked and reported frequently. Arterial blood pH, serum albumin, and serum uric acid should also be assessed as indicated.
- Assessment of fluid and electrolyte disturbances is particularly difficult in individuals with cancer because symptoms of these disturbances mimic symptoms often related to other causes, such as chemotherapy, systemic effects of tumor growth, and psychological responses to cancer.

NURSING DIAGNOSIS 1

Fluid volume deficit, related to decreased serum protein, excessive sodium excretion, and/or decreased concentrating ability of renal tubules.

NURSING INTERVENTIONS AND RATIONALE

1. Check frequently for signs and symptoms of dehydration. Signs such as rapid pulse and dry mucous membranes may be the first indication of fluid volume deficit.
2. Check BP in supine and standing positions. Report to the physician a fall of more than 15 mm Hg systolic or more than 10 mm Hg diastolic. A drop of this extent may signal marked dehydration.
3. Monitor intake and output, weight, pulse rate, serum electrolytes, and serum protein. These signs may be early indicators of fluid volume deficit.
4. Maintain adequate hydration, with oral fluids if appropriate or with IV fluids as ordered by the physician. Fluids are necessary to replace or maintain the serum volume.
5. Administer albumin, packed cells, whole blood, or other blood products as ordered. Albumin helps to maintain the colloid osmotic pressure of the blood and increase plasma volume. Administration of blood products helps to raise blood pressure and improve renal flow.
6. Maintain optimal nutritional status, especially protein intake. An adequate protein intake is essential to maintain normal colloidal pressure and retain fluid in the vascular space.

NURSING DIAGNOSIS 2

Nutrition: altered: less than body requirements, related to anorexia, vomiting, diarrhea, wound drainage, and/or malabsorption.

NURSING INTERVENTIONS AND RATIONALE

1. Assess current and normal height and weight, diet history, caloric intake, anthropometric measurements, and physiologic factors such as difficulty swallowing or anorexia. This assessment facilitates identification of individuals with existing nutritional abnormalities or at high risk for nutritional problems. These data are also required to plan and monitor nutritional interventions.
2. Monitor serum albumin, creatinine, lymphocyte count, and nitrogen balance. These values are the most likely to be affected in malnutrition related to cancer.
3. Enhance oral nutrition by encouraging a high-protein, high-calorie diet fortified with commercial supplements. If adequate nutrition can be obtained orally, this route is safer and easier for the client.
4. Encourage small, frequent feedings of calorie-dense and nonacidic foods. Cancer patients often experience an early sensation of fullness, so feedings should be small and spaced apart and should avoid empty calories.
5. Administer medications to control or reduce nausea, vomiting, mouth pain, and diarrhea as needed. Medications that reduce these symptoms increase the client's potential intake and absorption of nutrients.
6. If oral nutrition is inadequate, administer tube feedings through nasogastric, gastrostomy, or jejunostomy tube. The enteral route for provision of nutrition is preferable to the parenteral route.

7. Assist in administration and monitoring of total parenteral nutrition if needed. The parenteral route for administering nutritional support is the least preferable due to the risk of complications, expense, and potential difficulties.

NURSING DIAGNOSIS 3

Fluid volume excess, related to dilutional hyponatremia and increased levels of ADH.

NURSING INTERVENTIONS AND RATIONALE

1. Monitor intake and output, urine specific gravity, breath sounds, heart sounds, peripheral pulses, edema, nausea, vomiting, anorexia, weakness, and fatigue. Congestive heart failure, weakness, nausea, and vomiting can occur due to hyponatremia and water toxicity.
2. Monitor serum electrolytes and notify physician of Na < 120 mEq/L, K < 3.5 mEq/L, Ca < 8.5 mg/dL, or serum osmolality < 280 mOsm/kg. Symptoms of hyponatremia and water toxicity begin near these levels.
3. Monitor and report changes in LOC. Irritability, restlessness, confusion, convulsions, and unresponsiveness can occur.
4. Report weight gain of greater than 2 kg per day. Sudden weight gain may indicate fluid retention.
5. Restrict fluid intake as ordered by physician. Mild cases of SIADH may be controlled simply by restricting fluid intake.
6. Administer 3% saline IV and drugs (furosemide, demeclocycline, or lithium carbonate) as ordered by the physician. IV saline raises serum sodium, and diuretics prevent circulatory overload.
7. Decrease or discontinue the dosage of vincristine and cyclophosphamide chemotherapy, which can induce SIADH per physician's order.

NURSING DIAGNOSIS 4

High risk for injury, related to bone demineralization or alterations in potassium balance.

NURSING INTERVENTIONS AND RATIONALE

1. Check for fatigue, apathy, depression, confusion, and weakness. These are neuromuscular symptoms of hypercalcemia and hypokalemia.
2. Institute safety precautions to prevent accidental falls. Fractures are more likely because of bone demineralization and mental changes.
3. Report new or worsening metastasis, especially bone metastasis. Hypercalcemia is more likely in the presence of bony metastasis. Hypokalemia can be caused by vomiting, diarrhea, nephrotoxicity, and hypercalcemia.
4. Monitor serum calcium levels and notify physician of calcium levels above 11 mg/dL. Elevated serum calcium can lead to pathologic fractures and cardiac arrest.

NURSING DIAGNOSIS 5

Cardiac output (decreased): altered, related to increased serum potassium.

NURSING INTERVENTIONS AND RATIONALE

1. Monitor potassium levels frequently, especially during and after aggressive radiation or chemotherapy. Hyperkalemia is particularly likely following the destruction of large numbers of cells.
2. Notify physician or potassium levels above 5.3 mEq/L. Cardiac dysrhythmias become more common as serum potassium increases above this level.
3. Carefully monitor cardiac rhythm and EKG pattern and report abnormalities. Peaked T waves are an early sign of hyperkalemia. Tachycardia, bradycardia, heart block, and cardiac arrest may follow.
4. Administer Kayexalate in sorbitol PO or by enema to correct hyperkalemia. These agents cause a sodium-potassium ion exchange resulting in the excretion of excess potassium.

NURSING DIAGNOSIS 6

Thought processes: altered, related to altered electrolyte balance.

NURSING INTERVENTIONS AND RATIONALE

1. Assess fluid and electrolyte balance frequently, particularly during periods of uncontrolled cell growth, tumor lysis, cachexia, ectopic hormone secretion, chemotherapy, and radiation. Fluid and electrolyte disturbances are most likely in cancer patients at these times, and many of these abnormalities (hypercalcemia, hypokalemia, hyponatremia, hypomagnesemia, etc.) can influence neuromuscular function.
2. Administer agents to correct acidosis and/or electrolyte imbalance. Medicate for nausea, vomiting, diarrhea, or cardiac arrhythmias as ordered. Control of these processes is necessary to prevent progression of neurological problems.
3. Monitor serum potassium levels frequently. Administer potassium in IV solution as ordered. If potassium is excreted by the kidneys or shifts back into the cells hypokalemia may occur.
4. Reorient to time, place, and person if confusion or disorientation is apparent. Impairment of thought processes can cause increased anxiety for the client and family.
5. Check LOC, respiratory status, cardiac rhythm, renal function, and blood gases and report changes to physician. Changes in these parameters may signal worsening of the fluid and electrolyte disturbance.

NURSING DIAGNOSIS 7

Urinary elimination: altered, related to cell lysis and buildup of uric acid in the nephron.

NURSING INTERVENTIONS AND RATIONALE

1. Monitor urinary output and urine color, clarity, hematuria, and specific gravity. It is particularly important to monitor these factors during and after chemotherapy, particularly in leukemia and lymphoma.
2. Check for flank pain and medicate appropriately. Uric acid renal stones may cause acute, severe pain.
3. Report signs of renal failure. Obstruction of urine flow by renal calculi can cause kidney damage and eventual renal failure.

4. Report to physician serum uric acid > 7.0 mg/dL, urinary output < 30 mL per hour, BUN > 25 mg/dL, creatinine > 1.2 mg/dL, or sudden weight gain with elevated BP, lung congestion, or edema.
5. Administer allopurinol and increase IV fluid rate as ordered before chemotherapy or radiation. Allopurinol reduces uric acid concentration, and increased IV fluids help to maintain hydration and adequate renal function.
6. Teach the client and family dietary modifications to increase the alkalinity of the urine. Uric acid is more likely to precipitate in acidic urine.

Behavioral Objectives

Upon completion of this chapter, you will be prepared to:

- Identify the pathophysiologic changes associated with diabetic ketoacidosis (DKA).
- Explain the clinical manifestations related to DKA.
- Identify abnormal laboratory results associated with DKA.
- Discuss the treatment modalities suggested for correcting DKA.
- Identify potential nursing diagnoses associated with DKA.
- Discuss nursing interventions and rationale for nursing diagnoses associated with DKA.

Introduction

The inability of the body to utilize glucose due to a lack of insulin secretion results in an increased concentration of sugar in the blood. The main cause of excess blood sugar is diabetes mellitus (DM). There are two common types of DM: insulin-dependent (IDDM), or Type I, and non-insulin-dependent (NIDDM), or Type II. With NIDDM, some insulin secretion occurs.

Diabetic ketoacidosis (DKA) is associated with IDDM, or Type I diabetes, and results from a severe or complete deficit of insulin secretion. DKA is characterized by a blood sugar exceeding 300 mg/dL, ketosis, a blood pH below 7.30, and a HCO_3 level under 14 mEq/L. Hyperglycemic hyperosmolar nonketotic (HHNK) is associated with NIDDM, or Type II diabetes. With HHNK, ketosis seldom occurs. HHNK is characterized by a blood sugar above 500 mg/dL, dehydration, and a serum osmolality above 300 mOsm/kg.

1   A cessation or deficit of insulin secretions (increases/decreases) _____ the body's utilization of glucose.

decreases

        ■   ■   ■

2   Diabetic ketoacidosis (DKA) is more likely to occur with which type of diabetes mellitus? (IDDM/NIDDM) _____ .

IDDM

        ■   ■   ■

3   Characteristics of DKA are:

    a. Blood sugar _____ mg/dL

    b. pH _____

    c. HCO_3 _____ mEq/L

    d. (Ketosis/nonketosis) _____

    >300; <7.30; <14; ketosis
    ■   ■   ■

4   Characteristics of HHNK are:

    a. Blood sugar _____ mg/dL

    b. Serum osmolality _____ mOsm/L

    c. (Overhydration/dehydration) _____

    a. >500; b. >300; c. dehydration
    ■   ■   ■

PATHOPHYSIOLOGY

With an insulin deficit, glucose utilization is reduced and the cells are starved of important nutrients. Fat and protein catabolism (breakdown) occurs to provide the body with needed energy. Fatty acids are released from the breakdown of adipose (fat) tissue. Acids are further broken down into ketonic acids (ketones) and acetoacetate (acetone). Since the liver cannot oxidize the excess ketones, these ketone bodies accumulate in the blood. The acetone is excreted by the lungs.

5   Failure to metabolize glucose leads to a(n) (increase/decrease) _____ in fat catabolism. Ketosis occurs, which results in a(n) (deficit/excess) _____ of ketone bodies (ketonic acids) in the blood.

    increase; excess
    ■   ■   ■

6   With an increase in bicarbonate ion excreted by the kidneys due to osmotic diuresis, more hydrogen ions are reabsorbed into the circulation. Cellular breakdown causes lactic acid to be released from the cells. The increase in ketone bodies, hydrogen ions, and lactic acid increases the (acidotic/alkalotic) _____ state of the body.

    acidotic
    ■   ■   ■

7 Failure of glucose metabolism can cause which of the following:

( ) a. Glucose utilization for energy
( ) b. fat catabolism which releases excessive amounts of ketone bodies

An excessive number of ketone bodies in the body is known as _____ .

Ketosis leads to diabetic _____ .

a. —; b. X
ketosis; ketoacidosis

■   ■   ■

8 An elevation of the blood sugar level, >180 mg/dL, increases the glucose concentration in the glomeruli of the kidneys. When the concentration of glucose in the glomeruli exceeds the renal threshold for tubular reabsorption, glycosuria results. Increased glucose concentration acts as an osmotic diuretic which causes diuresis.

What does *glycosuria* mean? *_____ .

What does *diuresis* mean? *_____ .

sugar in the urine; excess urine excretion

■   ■   ■

9 An elevated blood sugar also increases the hyperosmolality of the extracellular fluid.

The hyperosmolality of the extracellular fluid leads to a withdrawal of fluid from the cells. Thus the ECF space is increased.

The fluid from the cells dilutes the extracellular sodium concentration, producing (hypernatremia/hyponatremia) _____ .

The migration of intracellular fluid into the extracellular fluid results in which of the following:

( ) a. Cellular dehydration
( ) b. Cellular hydration

hyponatremia
a. X; b. —

■   ■   ■

10 In renal excretion, the ketones (strong acids) combine with the cation sodium, causing sodium depletion. Ketone bodies (ketones) are excreted as ketonuria. The additional solute load of ketones in the glomeruli results in which of the following:

( ) a. A decreased loss of water in the formation of ketonuria
( ) b. An increased loss of water in the formation of ketonuria

a. —; b. X

■   ■   ■

11 Polyuria can result from which of the following:

( ) a. Glycosuria
( ) b. Anuria
( ) c. Ketonuria

With the loss of water, the solute concentration of the blood (increases/decreases) _____ and the blood volume (increases/decreases) _____ .

a. X; b. —; c. X
increases; decreases

■   ■   ■

12 As a result of DKA, nausea and vomiting occur, causing a severe fluid and electrolyte imbalance.

There is an increase in water loss by way of the lungs due to Kussmaul breathing (rapid vigorous breathing).

Dehydration occurs from which of the following:

( ) a. Nausea and vomiting
( ) b. Kussmaul breathing
( ) c. Oliguria
( ) d. Polyuria

a. X; b. X; c. —; d. X

■   ■   ■

13 The failure of cellular utilization of glucose causes potassium to leave the cells. The serum potassium level may therefore reflect normal or high serum values.

When serum potassium loss is the result of vomiting and renal excretion, the hemoconcentration can cause the serum potassium level to appear *_____ .

normal or high

■   ■   ■

ETIOLOGY

Between 20 and 25% of DKA clients are those who are newly diagnosed with DM, Type I. Table 14-1 lists the causes of DKA.

Table 14-1. CAUSES OF DKA	
Categories	**Causes**
Insulin deficiency	Undiagnosed DM, Type I Omission of prescribed insulin
Acute incidence	Infection Trauma Pancreatitis Major surgical interventions Gastroenteritis
Miscellaneous	Hyperthyroidism Steroids Adrenergic agonists

14 Most DKA reactions occur with *_____

_____ clients.

undiagnosed DM, Type I

    ■   ■   ■

15 Two common causes of DKA due to insulin deficiency are *_____ and

*_____ .

undiagnosed DM and omission of a prescribed insulin dose

    ■   ■   ■

16 Name three causes of an acute incidence of DKA. _____ ,

_____ , and _____ .

infection, trauma, and pancreatitis (others: major surgery, gastroenteritis)

    ■   ■   ■

CLINICAL MANIFESTATIONS

The most common symptoms of DKA are extreme thirst, polyuria, weakness, and fatigue. Hyperglycemia induces osmotic diuresis. Table 14-2 describes the signs and symptoms and laboratory results related to DKA. This table should be used as a guide for the assessment of clients with probable DKA.

Table 14-2. CLINICAL MANIFESTATIONS OF DKA

Signs and Symptoms	Rationale
Extreme thirst Polyuria	Elevated blood sugar and ketones increase the serum osmolality, causing thirst and osmotic diuresis.
Weakness, fatigue	Reduced cellular metabolism results in low energy levels.
Nausea, vomiting	Continuous vomiting causes a loss of body fluids and electrolytes. Dehydration results.
Vital Signs Temperature elevated or N	Infection causes an elevated temperature; dehydration can cause a slightly elevated temperature.
Pulse rapid	With a loss of body fluid, the heart beats faster to compensate in order to maintain circulation. Tachycardia of greater than 140 bpm denotes a severe fluid loss.
Blood pressure slightly to severely decreased	With early fluid loss from diuresis, the blood pressure decreases by 10–15 mm Hg.
Respiration rapid, vigorous breathing	Kussmaul breathing is a compensatory mechanism to decrease H_2CO_2 (acid) by blowing off CO_2
Poor skin turgor; dry, parched lips; disorientation, confusion	Dehydration frequently results in these symptoms; poor skin turgor; dry, parched lips; and confusion.
Abdominal pain with tenderness	Abdominal pain usually indicates severe ketoacidosis.
Laboratory Test Results Blood sugar 300–800 mg/dL	Blood sugar level is high; at times, it is not as high as HHNK. Sugar is not metabolized and utilized by the cells.
Electrolytes Potassium N, ↓, ↑	Potassium in the cells and plasma is low, but the serum potassium level may be high due to hemoconcentration. Normal or low levels can also occur.
Sodium N, ↓, ↑	Sodium is lost because of diuresis. Serum levels can be elevated due to dehydration.
Magnesium N, ↓, ↑ Chloride N, ↓ Phosphorus low N or ↓	Magnesium and phosphorus react the same as potassium. Chloride is excreted with sodium and water.
CO_2 ↓	The serum CO_2 is a bicarbonate determinant. With the loss of bicarbonate, the serum CO_2 is greatly decreased (<14 mEq/L).
Serum osmolality 300–350 mOsm/kg	Fluid loss (dehydration) increases the serum osmolality.

Table 14-2. (Continued)

Signs and Symptoms	Rationale
Hematology Hemoglobin, hematocrit ↑ WBC ↑	Because of fluid loss, hemoconcentration results, increasing the hemoglobin and hematocrit levels. Elevated white blood cells can indicate an infection.
Arterial Blood Gases (ABGs) pH ↓ $Paco_2$ ↓ HCO_3 ↓	The pH is low in the acidotic state. The $Paco_2$ is decreased because the lungs are expelling CO_2 (compensatory mechanism). The bicarbonate is lost through diuresis increase and in hydrogen and ketone (acid) levels.
Urine Glycosuria Ketonuria	Glucose and ketones spill into the urine.

Note: N = normal; ↑ = elevated; ↓ = decreased; bpm = beats per minute.

17 The four early clinical manifestations related to DKA are *_____ ,
_____ , _____ , and _____ .

extreme thirst, polyuria, fatigue, and weakness
■   ■   ■

18 Indicate which of the following vital signs is related to DKA:

( ) a. Elevated temperature
( ) b. Tachycardia
( ) c. Bradycardia
( ) d. Decreased blood pressure of 10–15 mm Hg
( ) e. High blood pressure
( ) f. Vigorous, rapid breathing
( ) g. apnea

a. X; b. X; c. —; d. X; e. —; f. X; g. —
■   ■   ■

19 Identify the changes that result in (a) the skin, (b) the lips and (c) the sensorium from dehydration associated with fluid loss and diuresis:

a. * _____

b. * _____

c. * _____

a. poor skin turgor; b. dry and/or parched lips; c. disorientation or confusion

■ ■ ■

20 The five electrolytes that frequently result in imbalance due to DKA are

_____ , _____ , _____ ,

_____ , and _____ .

potassium, sodium, magnesium, phosphorus (phosphate), and bicarbonate or serum CO_2 (also chloride)

■ ■ ■

21 With cellular breakdown, potassium is (lost/reabsorbed) _____ (from/into) _____ the cells.

When the acidotic state is corrected, potassium re-enters the cells and (hypokalemia/hyperkalemia) _____ may result.

lost; from; hypokalemia

■ ■ ■

22 With early fluid loss, the sodium level may be elevated because of increased aldosterone secretion (sodium-retaining hormone) response.

With continuous diuresis, the serum sodium level is _____ .

decreased

■ ■ ■

23 What causes the hemoglobin and hematocrit to be elevated? *_____ .

An elevated white blood cell (WBC) count is often due to an _____ .

hemoconcentration (due to fluid volume deficit); infection

■ ■ ■

24 A decrease in the pH and the arterial bicarbonate (HCO_3) indicates metabolic (acidosis/alkalosis) _____ resulting from DKA.

Why is the Pa_{CO_2} (arterial partial pressure carbon dioxide) decreased in DKA? *_____

_____ .

acidosis; it is a respiratory compensatory mechanism where the lungs blow off CO_2 to decrease the acidity in the blood

▪   ▪   ▪

CLINICAL MANAGEMENT

Treatment modalities for DKA include (1) vigorous fluid replacement, (2) insulin replacement, and (3) electrolyte correction. Osmotic diuresis can cause a fluid volume deficit of 4–8 liters of body fluid. In such a case immediate restoration of fluid loss is essential.

FLUID REPLACEMENT

25 In the first 24 hours, 80% of the total water and salt deficit should be replaced. There is less urgency for the other electrolytes since the rate of assimilation of the intracellular electrolytes is limited. Administration of potassium must be included, but *not in early treatment* (unless indicated) since an elevated serum potassium can be toxic.

With DKA, 80% of (salt and water/potassium and magnesium) *_____ should be replaced in the first 24 hours.

Cellular assimilation of electrolytes is (faster/slower) _____ than extracellular assimilation of electrolytes.

salt and water; slower

▪   ▪   ▪

26 For the first hour, 1–2 liters of a crystalloid (normal saline solution (0.9% NaCl) or lactated Ringer's solution) may be rapidly infused to reestablish the fluid volume balance. This may be followed by 1 liter every hour for the next 2 hours as indicated.

Rapid fluid replacement decreases the hyperglycemic state by causing a (hemoconcentration/hemodilution) _____ .

hemodilution

▪   ▪   ▪

27 Alternating normal saline solution with lactated Ringer's solution may be the IV therapy of choice of some physicians for improving fluid balance, renal perfusion, and blood pressure. ECF is restored directly from IV therapy. ICF replacement occurs in approximately 2 days.

When reestablishing fluid balance in the ECF space, the suggested amount of IV fluids for the first hour is *_____ . The purpose of rapid infusion of IV fluids is to improve *_____ , *_____ , and *_____ .

1–2 liters
fluid balance; renal perfusion; blood pressure

■   ■   ■

28 Restoration of ICF balance is somewhat (slower/faster) _____ than restoration of the ECF balance.

Indicate which solutions are used initially to correct the fluid imbalance:

( ) a. Dextrose in water (D_5W)
( ) b. Lactated Ringer's solution
( ) c. Normal saline solution (0.9% NaCl)

slower
a.—; b. X; c. X

■   ■   ■

29 A fluid overload in the ECF space should be avoided. What are four of the symptoms of overhydration or hypervolemia? *_____ , *_____ , *_____ , and *_____ .

constant, irritating cough, difficulty breathing (dyspnea), neck and hand vein engorgement, and chest rales

■   ■   ■

INSULIN REPLACEMENT

Ten to 15 years ago, massive doses of insulin were administered for the treatment of DKA. Today, less insulin is used when correcting DKA. Regular or crystalline insulin is given either intravenously and/or intramuscularly.

30 The parenteral routes used for correcting DKA include which of the following:

( ) a. Intravenous
( ) b. Subcutaneous
( ) c. Intramuscular

a. X; b. —; c. X

■   ■   ■

31 An initial bolus of 20–50 units of regular insulin is a practice of many physicians. The somewhat standard guideline for IV insulin replacement is an insulin bolus of 0.1–0.4 U/kg, followed by 0.1 U/kg per hour in IV fluids until the blood sugar level reaches 200–250 mg/dL.

Sample Problem: A client weighs 154 pounds or 70 kg. The physician's order reads regular insulin bolus of 0.4 U/kg and 0.1 U/kg per hour in normal saline solution. The amount of regular insulin to be administered as a bolus is _____ units, and the amount of regular insulin to be administered per hour in intravenous normal saline solution is _____ units. How much regular insulin is added to a 500-mL normal saline solution bag to run for 5 hours? _____ units.

28; 7; 35

　　　　　■　　　　　　　　■　　　　　　　　■

32 The blood sugar must be closely monitored during insulin replacement.

When the blood sugar level reaches _____ mg/dL, the IV fluids are usually switched to 5% dextrose in water. This prevents the possible occurrence of a (hypoglycemic/hyperglycemic) _____ reaction.

200–250; hypoglycemic

　　　　　■　　　　　　　　■　　　　　　　　■

33 The longer the acidosis persists, the more resistant the person is likely to be to insulin.

If acidosis persists, the person may require (more/less) _____ insulin.

Which of the following types of insulin can be administered intravenously?

( ) a. NPH
( ) b. Regular
( ) c. Protamine zinc insulin (PZI)
( ) d. Crystalline

more
a. —; b. X; c. —; d. X

　　　　　■　　　　　　　　■　　　　　　　　■

ELECTROLYTE CORRECTION

34   Potassium (K) replacement should start approximately 6–8 hours after the first dose of insulin has been administered (intravenously or intramuscularly) and as the acidotic state is being corrected. Serum potassium levels should be taken frequently. Potassium moves back into cells as fluid balance and the acidotic state are corrected.

If potassium is *not* given as acidosis is corrected, the serum potassium level would be (high/low) _____ . State the rationale for the reaction.

* _____ .

low
Potassium moves back into the cells leaving a serum potassium (K) deficit.
■   ■   ■

35   While fluid and insulin replacements are occurring, the serum potassium levels should be constantly monitored.

The serum potassium level (increases/decreases) _____ as fluids and insulin are being administered.

decreases
■   ■   ■

36   As acidosis is corrected, insulin is utilized more rapidly by the body for metabolizing sugar (glucose). (Hypoglycemia/hyperglycemia) _____ is most likely to result. Can you explain why?   *_____

_____

_____ .

hypoglycemia. When acidosis is corrected, there is less resistance to insulin. The insulin that had been previously administered (nonfunctional insulin due to acidosis) metabolizes the sugars for cellular use, causing a low blood sugar (hypoglycemia).
■   ■   ■

37 Magnesium, phosphate, and bicarbonate serum levels should be closely monitored. If the serum magnesium level is low, correcting hypokalemia does not fully result until the magnesium level is corrected.

There is controversy related to phosphate replacement when treating DKA. Phosphates are needed for neuromuscular function; thus serum phosphorus should be monitored along with the other electrolytes.

Another controversial issue is the use of bicarbonate therapy in the treatment of DKA. Usually, fluids and insulin replacement correct the acidotic state. If the pH falls below 7.1, bicarbonate replacement is usually prescribed.

The three electrolytes other than potassium and sodium that should be closely monitored are

_____ , _____ , and _____ .

magnesium, phosphate (phosphorus), and bicarbonate

■   ■   ■

38 Indicate when a bicarbonate infusion may be ordered:

( ) a. pH 7.15
( ) b. pH 7.05
( ) c. pH 6.95
( ) d. pH 7.21

a. —; b. X; c. X; d. —

■   ■   ■

CLINICAL APPLICATIONS

39 Dehydration is one of the major symptoms and concerns for persons in DKA.

When there is a marked intracellular and extracellular fluid depletion, the end result is which of the following:

( ) a. Decreased hemoconcentration
( ) b. Increased hemoconcentration
( ) c. Decreased blood volume
( ) d. Increased blood volume

a. —; b. X; c. X; d. —

■   ■   ■

40   While the client is receiving IV fluids and insulin, the nurse should observe for symptoms of hypoglycemia, also known as an insulin reaction, or a hypoglycemic reaction. These symptoms include cold, clammy skin; nervousness; weakness; dizziness; tachycardia; low blood pressure; and slurred speech. The blood sugar is frequently 50 mg/dL or lower.

How can the insulin reaction be corrected quickly?   *_____

_____ .

You may need to consult a nursing text; however, a glass or two of orange juice can raise the blood sugar rapidly.

■   ■   ■

41   When persons are treated for DKA with large doses of insulin, the nurse should observe for what type of reaction that might occur.   *_____ .

Too much insulin will cause symptoms similar to shock. Name three symptoms.

_____ ,   _____ , and   _____ .

insulin reaction; tachycardia, nervousness, and weakness (also low blood pressure, dizziness, and slurred speech)

■   ■   ■

42   Clients with diabetes who are ill are advised to go to bed because rest reduces metabolism. This decreases fat and protein catabolism.

These persons should also be protected from overheating and chilling. If they are in a state of vascular collapse, extra heat should *not* be applied since it can increase vasodilatation and intensify the failure of the circulation.

Rest reduces metabolism in an ill diabetic person; therefore, rest decreases the chance of

_____ and   _____ catabolism.

In the state of vascular collapse, extra heat may cause further (vasoconstriction/vasodilatation)   _____ .

fat and protein; vasodilatation

■   ■   ■

43 Jill Thompson arrived in the emergency room in a semicomatose state. Prior to admission, she had been vomiting and had complained of "feeling weak." The family stated she had a severe cold with a fever for weeks. They felt the vomiting was due to a viral infection.

The mucosa in her mouth was dry. Vomiting and dry mucosa would indicate

_____ .

Her respirations were rapid and deep, this can be an indication of which of the following:

( ) a. Kussmaul breathing
( ) b. Dyspnea

Her heart sinus rhythm was sinus tachycardia (pulse rate 120). Her breath had a very sweet smell. The family stated she did not have diabetes mellitus, but there was a familial history of it.

In the emergency room, a stat blood chemistry was done and a retention catheter was inserted. The blood sugar was 476 mg/dL, the normal range being 70–110 mg/dL. This indicates a (hypoglycemic/hyperglycemic) _____ state. The serum CO_2 combining power was very low, which indicates an _____ state.

dehydration
a. X; b. —
hyperglycemic; acidotic

■   ■   ■

Table 14-3 gives the laboratory studies of Jill Thompson, which show how her results deviated from the normal values at the time of her illness.

Table 14-3. LABORATORY STUDIES FOR MRS. THOMPSON

Laboratory Tests	On Admission	Day 1			Day 2	Day 3
Hematology						
Hemoglobin (12.9–17.0 g)	17.8					
Hematocrit (40–46%)	52					
Biochemistry						
BUN (blood urea nitrogen) (10–25 mg/dL)*	15					
Sugar feasting—postprandial (under 150 mg/dL)	476	825	458	382	60	144
Acetone	$\dfrac{+1}{1:10}$	$\dfrac{+1}{1:10}$	$\dfrac{\text{Trace}}{1:8}$			
Plasma/serum CO_2† $\dfrac{50\text{–}70 \text{ vol \%}}{22\text{–}32 \text{ mEq/L}}$	$\dfrac{7}{3}$	$\dfrac{10}{4}$	$\dfrac{14}{6}$	$\dfrac{18}{8}$	$\dfrac{34}{15}$	$\dfrac{44}{20}$
Plasma/serum chloride (95–108 mEq/L)	104		130	132	133	110
Plasma/serum sodium (135–146 mEq/L)	137		151	159	164	145
Plasma/serum potassium (3.5–5.3 mEq/L)	4.8		2.7	3.2	4.2	4.5

*mg/100 mL = mg/dL.

†*Plasma* and *serum* are used interchangeably.

44 Her urinalysis was as follows:

Color, dark yellow
Specific gravity, 1.024
Reaction, acid
Albumin, +3
Sugar, +4
WBC, many

Her specific gravity shows which of the following:

( ) a. A very high range
( ) b. A high average range
( ) c. A low range
( ) d. An indication of an increased amount of product in the urine

The +4 sugar in the urine indicates (hypoglycemia/hyperglycemia) _____ .

The +3 albumin in the urine indicates which of the following:

( ) a. Normal range
( ) b. Pathologic involvement, i.e., possible kidney cell injury

a. —; b. X; c. —; d. X
hyperglycemia
a. —; b. X

■   ■   ■

45 Jill's hemoglobin and hematocrit counts were which of the following:

( ) a. Normal
( ) b. Below normal
( ) c. Above normal
( ) d. An indication of mild edema
( ) e. An indication of mild dehydration

a. —; b. —; c. X; d. —; e. X

■   ■   ■

46 The feasting blood sugars (blood drawn after eating) on admission and the first day were which of the following:

( ) a. Normal
( ) b. Below normal
( ) c. Above normal
( ) d. An indication of hyperglycemia
( ) e. An indication of hypoglycemia

The second day her blood sugar was 60 mg/dL, which indicates a _____ reaction.

a. —; b. —; c. X; d. X; e —
hypoglycemic or insulin

■   ■   ■

47 Jill Thompson's serum CO_2 combining power was (normal/very low/very high)

_____ .

Her CO_2 combining power would indicate which of the following:

( ) a. Metabolic acidosis
( ) b. Metabolic alkalosis
( ) c. A bicarbonate loss
( ) d. A bicarbonate increase

very low
a. X; b. —; c. X; d. —

■   ■   ■

48 On admission, Jill Thompson's serum chloride, sodium, and potassium were in the (high/low/normal) _____ range.

On the first day, the laboratory studies indicated which of the following:

( ) a. Hyperchloremia
( ) b. Hypochloremia
( ) c. Hypernatremia
( ) d. Hyponatremia
( ) e. Hyperkalemia
( ) f. Hypokalemia

normal
a. X; b. —; c. X; d. —; e. —; f. X

■   ■   ■

49 In DKA there is frequently a serum sodium decrease before treatment due to which of the following:

( ) a. Fluid intake

( ) b. Vomiting

( ) c. Urine excretion

a. —; b. X; c. X

∎   ∎   ∎

CASE STUDY REVIEW

Jill Thompson, age 22, unknown diabetic, was admitted to the emergency room in a semicomatose state. Her respirations were deep and rapid, and her breath had a sweet smell. She had been urinating frequently. She had been vomiting for several days. Her laboratory results were Hgb 17.8 g, Hct 52, sugar feasting or postprandial 476 mg/dL, serum CO_2 3 mEq/L, serum sodium 137 mEq/L, serum chloride 104 mEq/L, and serum potassium 4.8 mEq/L.

1. According to Jill Thompson's history, identify three clinical symptoms of hyperglycemia.
   *_____ , *_____ , and *_____ .

2. Two clinical symptoms that indicated dehydration were *_____ and *_____ .

   What two laboratory results also indicated dehydration? _____ and _____ .

3. Her feasting sugar or postprandial blood sugar was _____ mg/dL. The normal range for a fasting blood sugar is _____ mg/dL and for feasting sugar is _____ mg/dL.

4. Jill Thompson's increased blood sugar causes the body fluids to be (hypomolar/hyperosmolar) _____ ; thus, osmotic diuresis results.

5. Polyuria can occur from ketonuria and _____ .

6. Her serum CO_2 was markedly _____ . What type of acid-base imbalance is present? *_____ .

7. Her acidosis is the result of fat catabolism, producing *_____ . This type of acidosis is referred to as *_____ .

In the emergency room, Jill Thompson received 2 liters of normal saline (0.9% NaCl), $NaHCO_3$, and insulin. The nurse checked her laboratory results and noted that her blood sugar remained high and her serum CO_2 remained low. Her electrolytes were Na 151 mEq/L, Cl 130 mEq/L, and K 2.7 mEq/L.

8. Her elevated serum sodium and chloride may be due to *_____ _____ .

9. The low serum potassium level may be due to *_____ _____ .

10. Potassium should be administered *_____ hours after correction of acidosis.

In the emergency room, Jill Thompson received 35 units of regular insulin. The first day of admission she received a total of 275 units of regular insulin and 2 liters of normal saline solution (1 liter contained 5% dextrose). Also, the first day she received KCl—100 mEq/L in 2 liters of IV fluids.

Her laboratory results the second day were blood sugar 60 mg/dL, serum CO_2 15 mEq/L and 20 mEq/L, serum Na 164 mEq/L, Cl 133 mEq/L, and K 4.2 mEq/L.

11. Blood sugars need to be monitored frequently. When the blood sugar level drops to *_____ , 5% dextrose in water should be given.

12. The nurse should observe for symptoms of hypoglycemia. Four of the symptoms are _____ , *_____ , _____ , and *_____ .

13. Her serum sodium and serum chloride levels were still elevated the second day. This may be due to *_____
_____ .

1. deep, rapid respirations (Kussmaul breathing), sweet smelling breath, and frequent urination
2. frequent urination and prolonged vomiting; hemoglobin and hematocrit
3. 476; 70–110; 150 or lower
4. hyperosmolar
5. glycosuria
6. decreased; metabolic acidosis
7. ketone bodies or ketosis (strong acid); diabetic ketoacidosis
8. The 2 liters of normal saline solutions. One liter of normal saline (0.9% NaCl) supplies 154 mEq/L of Na^+ and 154 mEq/L of Cl^-.
9. Rehydration causing dilution of potassium. Also, some of the potassium may be returning to the cells with the correction of DKA.
10. 6–8
11. 200–250 mg/dL or lower
12. nervousness, cold and clammy skin, tachycardia, and slurred speech (others: hunger, dizziness, low blood pressure)
13. 2 liters of normal saline solutions administered the first day

NURSING ASSESSMENT FACTORS

- Obtain a client's history of signs and symptoms related to fluid loss and incidences leading to the health problem. Record the vital signs and note abnormal findings such as tachycardia, slightly decreased blood pressure, vigorous-rapid breathing, and slightly elevated or high temperature. These can indicate dehydration and a possible acidotic state.
- Check for abnormal laboratory results that indicate DKA, such as elevated blood sugar (>300 mg/dL); elevated hemoglobin and hematocrit; decreased serum CO_2, normal or low serum potassium, sodium, magnesium, chloride, and/or phosphorus levels; decreased pH; decreased arterial HCO_3; and decreased $Paco_2$.
- Check urine for glycosuria and ketonuria. These are additional indicators of DKA.
- Assess urine output. Polyuria is an indicator of osmotic diuresis.

NURSING DIAGNOSIS 1

Fluid volume deficit, related to hyperglycemia and osmotic diuresis (polyuria).

NURSING INTERVENTIONS AND RATIONALE

1. Monitor vital signs (VSs). Vital signs that are indicative of fluid loss or dehydration include rapid, thready pulse rate; slightly decreased systolic blood pressure; rapid, vigorous breathing (Kussmaul breathing); and slightly elevated temperature.
2. Check for other signs and symptoms of fluid loss such as poor skin turgor; dry, parched lips; dry, warm skin; and dry mucous membranes.
3. Check the serum osmolality from laboratory results or from assessment of physical changes. Normal serum osmolality is 280–295 mOsm/kg. The serum osmolality level may also be obtained by doubling the serum sodium level or by using the formula given in Chapter 1.
4. Monitor blood sugar level. Levels greater than 200 mg/dL indicate hyperglycemia. Increased blood sugar levels can cause osmotic diuresis.
5. Observe for signs and symptoms of hypokalemia and hyperkalemia. Symptoms of hypokalemia are malaise, dizziness, arrhythmias, hypotension, muscular weakness, abdominal distention, and diminished peristalsis. Hypokalemia can occur as the acidotic state is corrected. Symptoms of hyperkalemia are tachycardia and then bradycardia, abdominal cramps, oliguria, numbness, and tingling in extremities.
6. Instruct the client to monitor his or her blood sugar level and/or urine to denote glycosuria. Clients can test their blood sugars with the use of a glucometer or some other approved testing device.
7. Administer normal saline solution and/or lactated Ringer's solution as prescribed to reestablish ECF. IV fluids for the first hour are usually given rapidly.

NURSING DIAGNOSIS 2

Nutrition: altered, less than body requirements, related to insufficient utilization of glucose and nutrients.

NURSING INTERVENTIONS AND RATIONALE

1. Administer regular (crystalline) insulin intravenously as prescribed in a bolus and in IV fluids to correct insulin deficiency. Recognize that 20–50 units or 0.1–0.4 U/kg of regular insulin may be given as a bolus. It is usually followed by administering 0.1 U/kg per hour in IV fluids.
2. Observe for signs and symptoms of a hypoglycemic reaction (insulin reaction) from possible overcorrection of hyperglycemia. The symptoms include cold, clammy skin, nervousness, weakness, dizziness, tachycardia, low blood pressure, and slurred speech.
3. Monitor IV fluids and adjust flow rate according to orders. If IV fluids are to run fast, observe for symptoms of overhydration.

NURSING DIAGNOSIS 3

Tissue perfusion: altered renal, cardiopulmonary, and peripheral, related to fluid volume deficit and lack of glucose utilization.

NURSING INTERVENTIONS AND RATIONALE

1. Monitor urine output, heart rate, blood pressure, and chest sounds for abnormalities. Fluid deficit limits tissue perfusion and decreases circulatory volume and nutrients available to the vital organs. Report abnormal findings.
2. Monitor arterial blood gases (ABGs), particularly the pH, $Paco_2$, Pao_2, and HCO_3. A decrease in pH and arterial HCO_3 determines the severity of the acidotic state. Tissue perfusion is decreased during acidosis.

OTHER NURSING DIAGNOSES

High risk for injury: cells and tissues, related to glucose intolerance and infection secondary to DKA. Fluid volume excess, related to excess administration of IV fluids.

CHAPTER 15

BURNS AND BURN SHOCK

LARRY PURNELL, R.N., PH.D.

Behavioral Objectives

Upon completion of this chapter, you will be prepared to:

- Explain the physiologic changes associated with fluid and electrolyte imbalances resulting from burns and burn shock.
- Describe the classifications of burned tissue involvement and degrees of burns.
- Explain one method used to determine the percentage of total body surface burns.
- State treatment priorities used in the clinical management of burns and burn shock.
- Apply selected principles of fluid balance in the assessment and care of burned patients in two clinical situations.
- Describe nursing assessment factors, nursing diagnoses, and nursing interventions related to burns and burn shock.

Introduction

Burns vary in severity depending upon the depth of tissue involvement and the percentage of burned surface area of the body. An extracellular fluid volume shift occurs soon after the burn and results in a fluid imbalance. A nursing assessment concerning the burn areas, tissue involvement, and signs and symptoms of fluid imbalance should be performed immediately. Monitoring vital signs, hourly urine output, and fluid replacement are a few of the prioritized nursing responsibilities required during the first 5–7 days after a moderate to severe burn.

This chapter discusses the pathophysiologic changes resulting from burns, classification systems used to assess tissue depth of the burns and the degrees of burns, methods used to determine percentage of total body surface burned, the three classifications of burns (mild, moderate, and critical), and important factors to consider in clinical management of burns. Two clinical situations of burned cases are presented. In the first situation, the focus is on fluid replacement during the first 48 hours. The focus in the second situation is on the assessment of burned areas by percent and laboratory studies as they relate to nursing assessment and the clinical management of fluid and electrolyte imbalances of burned clients. The nurse assesses the burn areas, the significance of the laboratory test results, and fluid replacement as it relates to nursing interventions. A case study review related to the second situation is provided. Nursing assessment factors, diagnoses, and interventions with rationales are listed following the second case study.

PATHOPHYSIOLOGY

1   Following a burn, there is an extracellular fluid volume shift in which fluid and electrolytes shift from the intravascular space (plasma) to the interstitial spaces of the burned area. (See Chapter 2 on ECF shift, if necessary.) This results in a(n) (increase/decrease) _____ of circulating plasma volume.

   decrease

   ■   ■   ■

2   With a decrease in circulating plasma volume, burn shock occurs. It is characterized by restlessness, confusion, tachycardia, decreased blood pressure, decreased urine output, metabolic acidosis, and a paralytic ileus.

   Burn shock results from   *_____.

   a decrease in circulating plasma volume

   ■   ■   ■

PHYSIOLOGIC CHANGES

Table 15-1 describes the physiologic changes associated with burns. There is an increased capillary permeability, increased serum osmolality, increased circulatory resistance, decreased cardiac output, decreased renal function, increased hemolysis, electrolyte imbalances, acidosis, increased hematocrit, and decreased protein level.

Table 15-1.   PHYSIOLOGIC CHANGES ASSOCIATED WITH BURNS AND BURN SHOCK

Physiologic Factors	Rationale
Capillary permeability: increased	There is a rapid shift of fluid and protein from the intravascular space (vessels) to the burned site. If more than 25% of the total body surface is burned, fluid (edema) accumulates in burned and unburned tissue spaces. Fluid shift to the burned site and tissue spaces is referred to as *fluid shift to the third space*. The fluid is nonfunctional, which causes vascular fluid deficit (hypovolemia). This is referred to as *burn shock*.
	Most of the fluid shift occurs during the first 18 hours but can persist for 48 hours postburn. Approximately 40–50% of vascular fluid can be lost to burned site and tissue spaces within the first 18 hours.
Serum osmolality: increased	Hemoconcentration results from loss of vascular fluid. The serum osmolality exceeds 295 mOsm/L since the proportion of solutes is greater than water.

Table 15-1. (Continued)

Physiologic Factors	Rationale
Electrolyte imbalances: decreased Serum Sodium (hyponatremia)	Sodium enters the edema fluid in the burned area, lowering the sodium content of the vascular fluid. Hyponatremia may continue for days to several weeks because of sodium loss to edema fluid, sodium shifting into cells, and later, diuresis. After 48 hours, fluid shifts from the burned and interstitial spaces to the vascular space. Sodium and excess fluid are excreted by the kidneys.
Cellular potassium: decreased	Potassium is lost from the cells.
Serum potassium: increased (hyperkalemia)	Potassium leaves the cells as sodium shifts into the cells. Hyperkalemia can occur if urine output is decreased. Serum potassium values may vary from normal to a deficit or an excess depending on the urine output and the length of time after the initial burn.
Serum calcium: decreased (hypocalcemia)	Hypocalcemia occurs because of calcium loss to edema fluid at the burned site (third-space fluid). Multiple infusions of citrated blood decreases the serum calcium level.
Serum protein: decreased	Protein is lost to the burned site due to increased capillary permeability. Serum protein levels remain low until healing occurs.
Hematocrit: increased	Hematocrit level is elevated due to hemoconcentration from hypovolemia. Anemia is present postburn due to blood loss at burned site and hemolysis, but it is not assessed until the client is adequately hydrated.
Hemolysis: increased (destruction of cells)	Hemolysis causes a liberation of hemoglobin (free hemoglobin) which can cause renal damage.
Cardiac output decreased	With more than 40% of the total body surface area burned, cardiac output can be decreased 50% or more due to hypovolemia. Cardiac output = stroke volume × heart rate. Tachycardia is a compensatory response. Beta receptors in the myocardium increase heart rate.
Circulatory resistance: increased	Hypovolemia and decreased blood pressure are sensed by pressoreceptors in the aorta and carotid bodies and in the sympathetic nervous system to cause vasoconstriction in order to increase blood flow to the vital organs, i.e., heart, brain, and lungs.
Renal function: decreased	Severe decreased blood volume (hypovolemia) causes a fall in blood pressure and oliguria or anuria. Systolic blood pressure below 60 mm Hg can cause renal insufficiency. Excess ADH (SIADH) is secreted during the first 48 hours, which causes water to be reabsorbed from the renal tubules and urine output to be decreased. Free hemoglobin from hemolysis is excreted by the kidneys as red-color urine and can cause renal damage.

Table 15-1. (Continued)	
Physiologic Factors	**Rationale**
Metabolic acidosis: increased	Burns cause cellular breakdown, and the cells release acid metabolites (lactic acid). Bicarbonate loss accompanies loss of sodium.

3   Capillary permeability is (increased/decreased) _____ during the first 48 hours postburn. If *less* than 25% of the total body surface is burned, fluid accumulates in which of the following:

( ) a. Burned site
( ) b. Unburned tissue spaces
( ) c. Both of the above

increased
a. X; b. —; c. —. If more than 25% of body surface area is burned, fluid shifts to the burned site and to unburned tissue spaces.

■   ■   ■

4   What is meant by fluid shift to the third space?   *_____

_____ .

Most of the fluid shift occurs during the first _____ hours, but may persist for _____ hours postburn. If 50% of the vascular fluid is lost to burned and unburned tissue spaces, severe (hypervolemia/hypovolemia) _____ occurs.

Fluid shifts from the vascular to the tissue (burned or unburned) spaces.
18; 48; hypovolemia

■   ■   ■

5   Hemoconcentration is present in early burns. Explain why.   *_____
_____ .

   When this occurs, the serum osmolality is (increased/decreased) _____
and the hematocrit is (increased/decreased) _____ .

Fluid leaves the vascular (intravascular) space, causing hypovolemia or dehydration.
increased; increased
   ■   ■   ■

6   Electrolyte imbalances occur postburn. Hyponatremia is common because of which of the
following:

(   ) a. Sodium is lost to edema fluid at the burned site.
(   ) b. Sodium shifts into cells.
(   ) c. Diuresis occurs 48 hours postburn.

a. X; b. X; c. X
   ■   ■   ■

7   Intracellular potassium is lost from the cells and is replaced by sodium. Decreased urine
output (oliguria) usually occurs in the early postburn period. With oliguria, the potassium level
(increases/decreases) _____ . Why?   *_____
_____ .

increases. Kidneys excrete 80–90% of potassium loss.
   ■   ■   ■

8   A serum calcium deficit may result from   *_____ .
Multiple infusions of citrated blood can cause (hypocalcemia/hypercalcemia)

_____ .

calcium loss to edema fluid at the burned site; hypocalcemia
   ■   ■   ■

9   Serum protein is (increased/decreased) _____ . Why?   *_____
_____ .

decreased. Protein leaks from the vascular system to the burned site because of increased
capillary permeability.
   ■   ■   ■

10 Erythrocytes or red blood cells are destroyed by hemolysis (destruction of red blood cells). The free hemoglobin released from the red blood cells may cause damage to the _____ system.

   Erythrocytes are destroyed as a result of which of the following:

( ) a. Increased plasma protein
( ) b. Hemolysis

renal
a. —; b. X

   ■   ■   ■

11 As a result of burned shock, there is (increased/decreased) _____ circulatory resistance and (increased/decreased) _____ cardiac output.

   increased; decreased

   ■   ■   ■

12 Once vascular fluid volume is reestablished, the diminished number of red blood cells (erythrocytes) becomes apparent; thus anemia results. Hemoconcentration is present (after/before) _____ rehydration.

   before

   ■   ■   ■

13 Renal function decreases as a result of which of the following:

( ) a. Hypervolemia
( ) b. Hypovolemia
( ) c. Systolic BP < 60 mm Hg
( ) d. SIADH (syndrome of inappropriate antidiuretic hormone secretion)

a. —; b. X; c. X; d. X

   ■   ■   ■

14 Metabolic acidosis can result from which of the following:

( ) a. Loss of serum bicarbonate
( ) b. Increase in acid metabolites
( ) c. Excess vascular fluid

a. X; b. X; c. —

   ■   ■   ■

15 Indicate which of the following may occur as the result of burns. Correct the wrong statements.

( ) a. Increased capillary permeability
( ) b. Elevated serum osmolality in early postburn
( ) c. Hypovolemia
( ) d. Hemolysis
( ) e. Hemoconcentration before hydration
( ) f. Metabolic alkalosis
( ) g. Increased serum protein
( ) h. Hyperkalemia with oliguria
( ) i. Hyponatremia
( ) j. Hypercalcemia

a. X; b. X; c. X; d. X; e. X; f. — (metabolic acidosis); g. — (decreased serum protein); h. X; i. X; j. — (hypocalcemia)

■   ■   ■

CLINICAL MANIFESTATIONS

DEGREE AND DEPTH OF BURNS

The degrees of burn are rated by two different classification methods. The older method, in which burns are classified as first-, second-, or third-degree burns, is still commonly used. The newer method classifies burns as (1) superficial, (2) partial thickness superficial, (3) partial thickness deep, and (4) full thickness. Because both classification methods are used in clinical practice, it is necessary to learn both methods. Burns involve three layers of skin: the *epidermis*, which is the outer layer of skin; the *dermis*, known as the true skin; and *subcutaneous tissues*, called the fatty tissues.

Depth of burn injury is described as superficial epidermal, partial thickness, and full thickness. These relate to first-, second-, and third-degree burns. Carefully study Table 15-2 and proceed to the frames that follow.

16 Define the following terms:

a. Epidermis *_____ .
b. Dermis *_____ .
c. Subcutaneous tissue *_____ .

a. the outer layer of skin; b. true skin; c. fatty tissue

■   ■   ■

17 Type and degree of burn injury is classified as *_____ ,
*_____ , and *_____ .

superficial epidermal; partial thickness; full thickness

or

first degree; second degree; third degree

■   ■   ■

Table 15-2.   DEGREE AND DEPTH OF BURNS AND THEIR CHARACTERISTICS

Type and Degree	Depth	Characteristics	Pain
Superficial epidermal (first degree)	Epidermis	Erythema, dry, blanches	Painful, hyperesthetic (very sensitive)
Partial thickness (first to second degree)	Epidermis Upper dermis	Pink to deep red blisters, moist blanches	Very painful
Deep (second degree)	Epidermis Deep dermis	Mottled, moist, or dry blisters	Extremely painful
Full thickness (third degree)	Epidermis Dermis Subcutaneous	Dry, pearly white to charred, inelastic and leathery	No pain or sensation

Note: From "Burn Trauma: The Emergent Phase of Care. Contemporary Perspectives in Trauma Nursing (An Independent Home Study Continuing Education Course)" by K. K. Bryant, Forum Medicum, Inc.: 4, 1991. Copyright 1991 by Forum Medicum. Adapted by permission.

---

18   Superficial epidermal burns involve which layer of skin? _____ .

epidermis

■   ■   ■

19   Superficial epidermal burns are characterized by   *_____ .
Superficial epidermal burns (are/are not) _____ painful.

erythema, dry and blanching; are

■   ■   ■

20   What two skin layers are involved in partial-thickness superficial burns?
_____ and   *_____ .

epidermis and upper dermis

■   ■   ■

21   Partial-thickness superficial burns are described as   *_____

_____ .

Partial-thickness superficial burns are (tender/very painful)   *_____ .

pink to deep red, blisters, and moist blanches; very painful

■   ■   ■

22 Which two skin layers are involved in partial-thickness deep burns? _____
and *_____ .

epidermis and deep dermis
■   ■   ■

23 Partial-thickness deep burns are described as *_____ .
Partial-thickness deep burns are (slightly painful/extremely painful) _____ .

mottled, moist, or dry blisters; extremely painful
■   ■   ■

24 Which three skin layers are involved in full-thickness burns? _____ ,
_____ , and *_____ .

epidermis, dermis, and subcutaneous tissue
■   ■   ■

25 Full-thickness burns are described as *_____ .
Full-thickness burns are (very painful/not painful) _____ .

dry, pearly white, inelastic, and leathery; not painful
■   ■   ■

26 Place SE for superficial epidermal, PT for partial thickness; and FT for full thickness according
to the depth, characteristics, and pain of burns.

____ a. Epidermis and upper dermis burned
____ b. Slightly painful
____ c. Epidermis, dermis, and subcutaneous tissues burned
____ d. Very painful
____ e. Epidermis only
____ f. Extremely painful
____ g. Dry and blanches
____ h. No pain
____ i. Epidermis and deep dermis burned
____ j. Moist or dry with blisters
____ k. Pearly white and leathery

a. PT; b. SE; c. FT; d. PT; e. SE; f. PT; g. PT; h. FT; i. PT; j. PT; k. FT
■   ■   ■

METHODS USED TO DETERMINE PERCENTAGE OF TOTAL BODY SURFACE BURNS

27   There are several methods used for determining the percentage of total body surface burns. The Berkow formula determines the percentage according to age and 19 predetermined surface body areas. Another method is the Lund and Browder chart, which estimates the body surface areas in small proportions, i.e., upper arm 2%, forearm 1½%, and hand 1½%. The rule of nines is frequently used as a quick method of estimation since it can be easily recalled. The three methods used to determine the percentage of total body surface area that has been burned are
*_____ , *_____ , and *_____ .

the Berkow formula, Lund and Browder chart, and rule of nines
■   ■   ■

Figure 15-1 explains the rule of nines used to estimate the amount and areas of body burns. The rule of nines uses 9% or multiples thereof in calculating the burned body surface. The five main regions in the estimation of burned surface are in italics. Be sure to know the five regions and the percentages of each.

Region	Percentage of Body Surface (%)
Head and neck	9
1. Anterior head and neck (4.5%)	
2. Posterior head and neck (4.5%)	
Upper extremities	18
3. Right arm—anterior (4.5%) and posterior (4.5%)	
4. Left arm—anterior (4.5%) and posterior (4.5%)	
Trunk and buttocks	36
5. Anterior surface (18%)	
6. Posterior surface (18%)	
Lower extremities	36
7. Right leg and thigh—anterior (9%) and posterior (9%)	
8. Left leg and thigh—anterior (9%) and posterior (9%)	
9. *Perineum and genitalia* (1%)	1

28   The rule of nines and the depth of burned tissue are used in planning parenteral therapy for burned persons.

What are the five main regions of the body used in the rule of nines?
*_____ , *_____ , *_____ ,
*_____ , and *_____ .

head and neck, upper extremities, trunk and buttocks, lower extremities, and perineum and genitalia
■   ■   ■

Figure 15-1. Rules of nines for estimation of body surface.

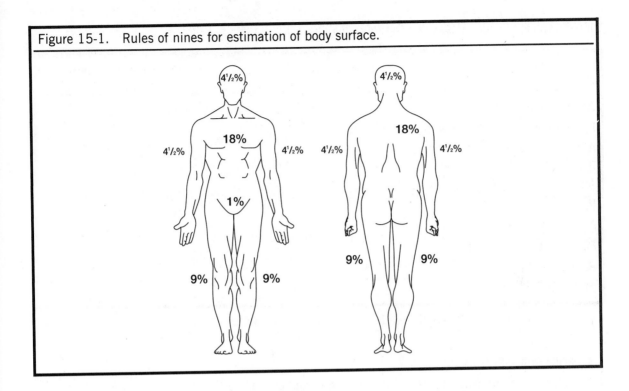

29 In planning parenteral therapy for burns, the *_____ and
*_____ are used.

    The estimated percentage used for the anterior and posterior surfaces of *each* arm is _____ %.

    The estimated percentage used for the anterior and posterior surfaces of the head and neck is _____ %.

rule of nines and depth of burned tissue (also burned surface area)
9; 9

           ■   ■   ■

30 The estimated percentage used for the anterior surface of the trunk is _____ %.

    The estimated percentage used for the anterior and posterior surfaces of *each* thigh and leg is _____ %.

18; 18

           ■   ■   ■

31 Complete the percentages on the following chart:

Region	Percentage of Body Surface (%)
Anterior head and neck	a. _____
Left anterior and posterior arm	b. _____
Anterior and posterior surfaces of trunk and buttocks	c. _____
Anterior surface of right thigh and leg	d. _____
Perineum and genitalia	e. _____
Anterior right arm	f. _____
Posterior trunk and buttocks	g. _____
Anterior and posterior surfaces of lower extremities	h. _____

a. 4½; b. 9; c. 36; d. 9; e. 1; f. 4½; g. 18; h. 36

■   ■   ■

CLASSIFICATIONS OF BURNS

Table 15-3 differentiates between minor, moderate, and critical burns according to the degrees and percentage of burns. Know the three classifications or burns, the degrees, and the percentages. It is important to note that this classification is for the adult person. Infants, children, the elderly, and individuals with chronic illnesses may need to be classified differently than the healthy adult.

Table 15-3. CLASSIFICATION OF BURNS

Minor Burns	Moderate Burns	Critical Burns
First degree	Second degree of 15–30% of body surface	Second degree of over 30% of body
Second degree of less than 15% of body surface	Third degree of less than 10% of body surface except hands, face, feet, or genitalia	Third degree of more than 10% of body surface or of hands, face, feet, or genitalia
Third degree of less than 2% of body surface		

32 The three classifications of burns are *_____ , *_____ , and
*_____ .

minor burns, moderate burns, and critical burns

■   ■   ■

33 To be classified as *minor burns,* the skin surface involved must be first degree or second degree of less than _____ % of body surface or third degree of less than _____ % of body surface.

15; 2

■   ■   ■

34 To be classified as *moderate burns,* the skin surface involved must be second degree of _____ to _____ % of body surface or third degree of less than _____ % of body surface, provided that the hands, face, feet, or genitalia are not burned.

15; 30; 10

■   ■   ■

35 To be classified as *critical burns,* the skin surface involved must be second degree of over _____ % of body surface or third degree of more than _____ % of body surface or the burn must be of the hands, face, _____ , or _____ .

30; 10
feet; genitalia

■   ■   ■

36 Place the word *minor* for minor burns, *moderate* for moderate burns, and *critical* for critical burns beside the following statements:

a. _____ Burns of the hands, face, feet, or genitalia
b. _____ Third-degree burns of less than 10% of body surface
c. _____ Third-degree burns of more than 10% of body surface
d. _____ Second-degree burns of 15–30% of body surface
e. _____ Second-degree burns of over 30% of body surface
f. _____ Second-degree burns of less than 15% of body surface
g. _____ Third-degree burns of less than 2% of body surface

a. critical; b. moderate; c. critical; d. moderate; e. critical; f. minor; g. minor

■   ■   ■

CLINICAL MANAGEMENT

37 Minor burns are generally treated in the physician's office or emergency room, and the person seldom needs hospitalization.

Moderate burns and burns (first and second degree) greater than 20% of total body area should receive intravenous fluids.

Minor burns and burns less than 20% of total body surface area frequently (do/do not) _____ need intravenous fluids unless the person is a child. Children with burns greater than 10% of total body surface area do need intravenous fluids.

do not

■   ■   ■

38 Persons with burns involving 20–40% of body surface require careful, planned intravenous replacement therapy for survival.

In those with over 50% of the body surface involved, the mortality rate is high regardless of careful, planned intravenous therapy.

Individuals with 20–40% of body surface burns, having received fluid replacement, have a (good/poor) _____ prognosis, whereas those with 50% or more have a (good/poor) _____ prognosis.

good; poor

■   ■   ■

39 Various formulas have been devised and used as a basis for initiating therapy in the treatment of burns.

Accurately measured hourly urine flow is an important index for the determination of adequate intravenous therapy. For all severely burned persons, an indwelling catheter is advisable to obtain   *_____ .

accurate hourly urine outputs

■   ■   ■

40   The desired rate of urine flow is 30–50 mL (cc) per hour. Less than 25 mL of urine output per hour for an adult indicates insufficient fluid intake or kidney dysfunction.

After 48–72 hours, the urine output can increase to 100 mL or more per hour from diuresis due to a fluid shift from the burned and unburned tissue areas into the intravascular space (vessels). For a burned person, the desired urine output per hour is *_____ . Less than 25 mL per hour indicates which of the following:

( ) a. Too much fluids
( ) b. Not enough fluids
( ) c. Kidney dysfunction

30–50 mL
a. —; b. X; c. X
■   ■   ■

41   During the first 48 hours fluid replacement should be at least three times the urine output because of the fluid shift to the burned and unburned tissue areas.

When the intravenous flow rate is increased to correct hypovolemia and to increase urine output, the nurse should observe for what type of fluid imbalance? _____ . Give three symptoms of overhydration. *_____ , _____ , and
*_____ .

overhydration; constant, irritating cough, dyspnea, and neck vein engorgement (also chest rales)
■   ■   ■

42   To determine whether poor urine output is due to renal damage or inadequate fluid intake, a Fluid Challenge Test can be used. This test consists of giving 500–1000 mL of fluid in $\frac{1}{2}$ hour.

A failure to increase urine output indicates *_____ .

renal damage
■   ■   ■

43 High protein liquids, between meals or at mealtime, are helpful for cell reconstruction. Which of the following liquids are high in protein?

( ) a. Eggnog
( ) b. Ginger ale
( ) c. Milkshake
( ) d. Coca-Cola

a. X; b. —; c. X; d. —

■   ■   ■

44 A very high hematocrit reading indicates *_____ .

Many physicians prefer to maintain the hematocrit (Hct) at 45 or above for the first 48 hours after the burn so that in rehydration, the hematocrit will do which of the following:

( ) a. Drop very low
( ) b. Return to a normal range
( ) c. Show a marked increase

a fluid volume deficit or hemoconcentration
a. —; b. X; c. —

■   ■   ■

45 The greatest fluid shift occurs during the first 18 hours after a burn and reaches its peak in 48 hours. Therefore, the critical period for fluid and electrolyte replacement is which of the following:

( ) a. The first 36 hours
( ) b. The first 48 hours
( ) c. The first 72 hours

a. —; b. X; c. —

■   ■   ■

46 A major hazard in burn cases is infection. This frequently delays the reabsorption of edema fluid from the site of the burn.

Surgical aseptic (sterile) techniques are employed to reduce the possibility of

_____ .

Infection causes the edematous fluid to be reabsorbed (more slowly/more quickly)
*_____ .

infection; more slowly

■   ■   ■

47 After 48 hours, capillary permeability lessens, fluid reabsorption begins, and edema starts to subside. This is considered to be the *stage of diuresis*. The stage of diuresis generally begins after 2 days; however, it may take as long as 2 weeks before the stage develops depending upon the severity of the burns. Explain what happens when the stage of diuresis begins:

  a. Capillary permeability (increases/decreases) _____ .
  b. Fluid (reabsorption/excretion) _____ begins.
  c. Edema starts to (increase/subside) _____ .

  a. decreases; b. reabsorption; c. subside

      ■   ■   ■

48 Extracellular fluid volume shift from the interstitial space to the intravascular space occurs during the stage of diuresis. This most likely occurs _____ hours after being burned. A delay in the stage of diuresis varies with *_____ .

  48; the severity of the burn

      ■   ■   ■

49 After 48 hours, IV therapy is frequently restricted or decreased, providing the serum sodium and potassium levels are near normal.

  Continuous IV therapy may result in overhydration. This can be hazardous since it can overload the circulation, causing pulmonary edema and cardiac failure.

  After 48 hours, IV fluid administration is (increased/decreased) _____ .

  Overloading the circulation can result in which of the following:

  ( ) a. Pulmonary edema
  ( ) b. Gastritis
  ( ) c. Cardiac failure
  ( ) d. Pancreatitis

  decreased
  a. X; b. —; c. X; d. —

      ■   ■   ■

FLUID CORRECTION FORMULAS

There are many formulas for calculating fluid replacement during the first 48 hours after burns. Table 15-4 gives three types of formulas. Brooke and Evans are similar except for the amount of colloid and electrolyte replacement. Parkland's formula does not call for colloid and free water during the first 24 hours. Parkland supporters believe that early colloid replacement shifts to the burned site, thus, by giving lactated Ringer's infusions, cardiac output increases and cell function is restored. Refer to Table 15-4 as needed.

Table 15-4.   FORMULAS FOR FLUID REPLACEMENT DURING FIRST 48 HOURS
FOR BURN SHOCK

Name	First 24 Hours	Second 24 Hours
Brooke Army Hospital	Colloid*: 0.5 mL/kg × % of burned area Electrolyte†: 1.5 mL/kg × % of burned area Water: 2000 mL D$_5$W	One-half (½) amount of colloid and electrolyte of the first 24 hours Water: 2000 mL D$_5$W
Evans	Colloid: 1 mL/kg × % of burned area Electrolyte: 1 mL/kg × % of burned area Water: 2000 mL D$_5$W	One-half (½) amount of colloid and electrolyte of the first 24 hours Water: 2000 mL D$_5$W
Parkland	Colloid: none Electrolyte: 4 mL/kg × % of burned area Water: none	Colloid: 20–60% of calculated plasma volume Water: 2000 mL D$_5$W

Note: Over 50% of body surface burns are calculated at 50% burns for fluid replacement purposes. 1 kg = 2.2 pounds.
*Colloid used: blood, dextran, plasma, albumin.
†Electrolyte used: lactated Ringer's or normal saline.

50   The three formulas used for fluid replacement during the first 48 hours postburn are

*_____ , _____ , and _____ .

the Brooke Army Hospital, Evans, and Parkland

 ■   ■   ■

51   Four solutions used for colloid replacement are   _____ ,

_____ , _____ , and _____ .

Two electrolyte solutions used are   *_____ and   *_____ .

blood, dextran, plasma, and albumin
lactated Ringer's and normal saline

 ■   ■   ■

CLINICAL APPLICATIONS

52 Mr. Greene, who weighed 154 pounds, or _____ kg, had 30% of his body surface burned.

   To estimate his fluid needs for the first 24 hours, calculate his fluid needs according to the Brooke's formula as:

   a. 0.5 mL colloid × 70 (kg of body weight) × 30 (% of burned body surface) = _____ mL of colloid to be given. [*Note:* When multiplying by 30, do not use the decimal point.]

   b. 1.5 mL electrolyte × 70 (kg of body weight) × 30 (% of burned body surface) = _____ mL of lactated Ringer's to be given.

   c. Plus 2000 mL of dextrose in water.

   The total amount of parenteral fluid that Mr. Greene should receive in the first 24 hours following his burns is _____ mL.

   70; a. 1050; b. 3150; c. 6200
   ■   ■   ■

53 For the second 24 hours, according to Brooke's formula, Mr. Greene should receive:

   a. _____ mL of colloid
   b. _____ mL of lactated Ringer's
   c. _____ mL of dextrose in water

   The total amount of parenteral fluid for the second 24 hours would be

   d. _____ mL.

   a. 525; b. 1575; c. 2000; d. 4100
   ■   ■   ■

54 After 48 hours of parenteral therapy, Mr. Greene should receive (more/less) _____ intravenous fluid.

   After 48 hours, fluid shifts from the burned and unburned tissue spaces to the vascular area, and if the same quantity of IV fluids is given, what type of fluid imbalance can occur? _____ .

   less; overhydration, hypervolemia, or fluid volume excess
   ■   ■   ■

55 Over 50% of body surface burns are calculated as _____ % burns for fluid replacement purposes.

   50
   ■   ■   ■

56 During the first 24 hours, one-half of the fluids is given in the first 8 hours and the other half is given in the remaining 16 hours.

Mr. Greene should receive _____ mL of intravenous fluids in the first 8 hours and _____ mL in the remaining 16 hours of the first day.

3100; 3100

■   ■   ■

Mrs. Silver, age 35, received 25% of second- and third-degree body surface burns when her farmhouse caught fire.
The following areas of her body were burned:

Face, 5%
Right arm and hand, 9%
Left arm, 5%
Back and upper chest, 6%

57 The total body surface area burned of Mrs. Silver is _____ %

25

■   ■   ■

58 Since the face, hand, and upper chest were burned, Mrs. Silver would be considered to have which of the following:

( ) a. Minor burns
( ) b. Moderate burns
( ) c. Critical burns

a. —; b. —; c. X

■   ■   ■

Mrs. Silver's laboratory studies were:

Hemoglobin	13.5 g
Hematocrit	44%
White blood count	20,300 cells/mm^3
Polymorphonuclear cells (polys)	65%

A venous section (cutdown) was performed. In the emergency room she received:

Two injections of morphine sulfate: 1. 10 mg (gr $\frac{1}{6}$) (IM)
                                                    2. later 10 mg (gr $\frac{1}{6}$) (IV)
1000 mL normal saline with 2 million units of aq. penicillin IV
1000 mL normal saline with 5 million units of aq. penicillin IV
Tetanus toxoid: 0.5 mL

Mrs. Silver received tetanus toxoid since she was subject to infection by anaerobic microbes, such as *Clostridium tetani.*

59 She received morphine sulfate for *_____ . She received aquious penicillin due to which of the following:

( ) a. Her hemoglobin was elevated.
( ) b. Her hematocrit was elevated.
( ) c. Her WBC was elevated.

relief of pain
a. —; b. —; c. X

∎   ∎   ∎

The laboratory studies of Mrs. Silver, given in Table 15-5, show how her results deviated from the normal values at the time of her illness.

60 Mrs. Silver's serum chloride, sodium, and potassium (are/are not) _____ in the normal range.

Due to her low serum CO_2 on admission, she is in a state of metabolic

_____ .

are; acidosis

∎   ∎   ∎

Laboratory Tests	On Admission	Day 1	Day 2	Day 3	Day 4	Day 5	Day 6	Day 7
Hematology Hemoglobin (12.9–17.0 g)	13.5	17.6						
Hematocrit (40–46%)	44	49 54	56 52 61 64	55	51	46	36	35
WBC (white blood count) (5000–10,000/mm³)	23,000		11,685					
Biochemistry BUN (blood urea nitrogen) (10–25 mg/dL)*	11	14						
Plasma/serum† CO_2 50–70 vol %	30	44	44		57		57	
22–32 mEq/L	14	20	20		26		26	
Plasma/serum chloride (95–108 mEq/L)	105	105	105		97		103	
Plasma/serum sodium (135–146 mEq/L)	141	137	137		134		141	
Plasma/serum potassium (3.5–5.3 mEq/L)	4.3	4.8	4.8		4.2		4.4	

Table 15-5. LABORATORY STUDIES FOR MRS. SILVER

*mg/100 mL = mg/dL.
†*Plasma* and *serum* are used interchangeably.

61 In the preceding frame you noted that Mrs. Silver's serum electrolytes were within normal range. Can you recall the normal range for the following electrolytes without referring to Table 15-5?

a. Plasma chloride. *_____

b. Plasma sodium. *_____

c. Plasma potassium. *_____

a. Cl, 95–108 mEq/L
b. Na, 135–146 mEq/L
c. K, 3.5–5.3 mEq/L

    ■   ■   ■

62 Her elevated hematocrit in relation to her hemoglobin during the first 48 hours following admission is *_____ ; and an indication of *_____ .

elevated; fluid volume deficit (You may have answered hemoconcentration. O.K.)

    ■   ■   ■

63 Her elevated WBC indicates which of the following:

( ) a. An increased number of white blood cells
( ) b. Infection
( ) c. Head cold
( ) d. Inflammatory stress response

a. X; b. X; c. —; d. X

    ■   ■   ■

64 Mrs. Silver weighed 65 kg and had a total of 25% body burns. Calculate the following fluid replacement needs using the Brooke Army Hospital formula:

a. $0.5 \times 65 \times 25 =$ _____ mL colloid

b. $1.5 \times 65 \times 25 =$ _____ mL electrolyte

plus _____2000_____ mL dextrose/water

c. Total _____ mL for first 24 hours

During the first 8 hours Mrs. Silver should receive one half of the intravenous fluid.

d. This amount is _____ mL. Intravenous fluids ordered for the first 8 hours are:

812.5 mL colloid

2437.5 mL electrolyte

__2000__ mL dextrose in water

5250 total for 24 hours

2625 mL for first 8 hours

Note: Lactated Ringer's is not ordered because her electrolytes are not low. You will notice in the clinical area that the figures are rounded off.

Orders for the second 8 hours include:

500 mL colloid

250 mL electrolyte

__400__ mL 5% dextrose in water

1150 mL for the second 8 hours

Later she received 1500 mL D_5W for the third 8 hours.

e. The total amount of colloid ordered is _____ mL.

f. The total amount of electrolyte ordered is _____ mL.

g. The total amount of dextrose in water ordered is _____ mL.

a. 812.5; b. 2437.5; c. 5250; d. 2600; e. 850; f. 2500; g. 1900

■   ■   ■

65 Calculate the amount of fluids that she should receive during the *second* 24 hours according to the Brooke formula.

a. _____ mL colloid

b. _____ mL electrolytes

c. _____ mL D_5W

a. 425; b. 1250; c. 950 or 1000

■   ■   ■

66 In Mrs. Silver's case, urine output was measured hourly and tested for specific gravity.

After the first 8 hours, Mrs. Silver's urine output was 250 mL per hour, so the IV fluid flow rate was decreased.

During the third 8 hours, her urine output had fallen to 5–10–15 mL per hour for three consecutive hours.

The fluid flow rate should be (increased/decreased) _____ .

Which of these intravenous fluids should be given to correct Mrs. Silver's decrease in urine output:

( ) a. Blood
( ) b. Normal saline
( ) c. 5% dextrose in water
( ) d. 10% dextrose in saline

increased
a. —; b. X; c. X; d. —

■   ■   ■

67 The specific gravity of Mrs. Silver's urine ranged from 1.005 to 1.017. The specific gravity of urine is the weight (waste products) in relationship to water, 1.000. The specific gravity norm for urine is (1.010–1.030).

Mrs. Silver's urine specific gravity of 1.005 and 1.008 indicates there are (more/less) _____ waste products in her urine than the norm. These waste products are more concentrated in her (urine/plasma) _____ .

less; plasma

■   ■   ■

CASE STUDY REVIEW

Mrs. Silver, age 35, received 25% second- and third-degree body surface burns. Using the rule of nines, her face received 5%, right arm and hand 9%, left arm 5%, and back and upper chest 6%. On admission, her hematocrit was 44%; on the first day it rose to 49 and 54%. By the second day, it was 56–64%. Her serum CO_2 on admission was 14 mEq/L, and on the second and third days it was 20 mEq/L. Her serum electrolytes were in normal range.

1. After a burn, there is an extracellular fluid volume shift from the _____ to the _____ space.
2. Mrs. Silver's hematocrit was _____ the first and second days following the burn. Explain why. *_____

_____ .

3. What type of acid-base imbalance did Mrs. Silver have the first three days?
   * _____ . Explain the reason for this imbalance.
   * _____
   _____ .

4. Besides fluid and electrolyte imbalance, another hazard in burn cases is
   _____ .

5. Name three methods used to estimate body burn surface. * _____ ,
   * _____ , and _____ .

6. Mrs. Silver's burns were classified as (minor/moderate/critical) _____ .
   Explain why. * _____
   _____ .

   Mrs. Silver's fluid replacement was based on the Brooke Army Hospital formula. Review the
   Brooke formula and Mrs. Silver's fluid replacement the first 24 hours.

7. In planning Mrs. Silver's parenteral therapy, the _____ formula was used
   based on the rule of nines. Name two other formulas for determining fluid needs.
   _____ and _____ .

8. An important index for the determination of adequate parenteral therapy is an accurate record
   of * _____ .

9. Urine output should be maintained between _____ and
   _____ mL per hour. Less than 25 mL of urine output can indicate
   * _____ or * _____ .

10. Mrs. Silver's colloid replacement solutions were _____ and
    _____ . What two other colloids can be used? _____ and
    _____ .

11. Name two types of electrolyte solutions used in parenteral therapy for burns.
    * _____ and * _____ .

12. Give the type of electrolyte solution that Mrs. Silver received and state why.
    * _____ . Why? _____
    _____ .

13. After 2 days or, at the longest, 2 weeks, the stage of diuresis occurs. This is when the
    extracellular fluid volume shifts from * _____ to * _____ .

14. Overhydration or hypervolemia is a hazard when large quantities of intravenous fluids are
    administered for fluid replacement and for increasing urinary output. Give four symptoms of
    overhydration. * _____ , _____ , * _____ , and
    * _____ .

1. *intravascular; interstitial*
2. *Elevated. Hemoconcentration was present due to ECF volume shift to the interstitial space
   (burned area), or you could answer dehydration due to ECF volume shift.*
3. *Metabolic acidosis. Due to a loss of serum bicarbonate and an increase in body acid
   metabolites (cellular breakdown).*
4. *infection*
5. *rule of nines, Lund and Browder's, and Berkow*
6. *Critical. Mrs. Silver had burns to the hand and face plus a total of 25% second- and
   third-degree burns.*

7. Brooke; Evans and Parkland
8. measured hourly urine output
9. 30; 50; insufficient fluid intake; kidney dysfunction
10. plasma and blood; albumin, and dextran
11. normal saline and lactated Ringer's solution
12. Normal saline. Mrs. Silver's serum electrolytes were in normal range, so saline was given. Also, saline (NaCl) replaces the sodium loss to the burn area and to diuresis.
13. interstitial spaces; the intravascular space
14. irritating cough, dyspnea, engorged neck and hand veins, and moist rales

NURSING ASSESSMENT FACTORS

- Assess vital signs: blood pressure, pulse, and respiration. An increase in pulse rate with a decrease in blood pressure (even slightly) and an increase in respiration can be indicative of shocklike symptoms due to hypovolemia resulting from the fluid shift to the burned site. A pulse pressure of less than 20 mm Hg can indicate severe hypovolemia.
- Assess burns, including the surface area and status of burned tissue. Burns are assessed according to the depth of tissue involvement, i.e., superficial, partial, partial-deep, and full thickness or by the degree of the burns (first, second, and third). The classification method used for burns, either by depth or degree, is determined by institutional preference.
- Record the skin surfaces involved indicating the color of the burn and the intensity of pain related to the burn site.
- A quick estimation of the percentage of total burned body surface areas can be accomplished using the rule of nines.
- Urine output is a key factor in fluid and electrolyte balance for burned clients. Insufficient urine output, <30 mL per hour or <250 mL per 8 hours, can indicate a change in body fluid loss resulting from a fluid shift to the burned areas and surrounding tissues (third-space fluid).

NURSING DIAGNOSIS 1

Fluid volume deficit, related to fluid shift to the burned site.

NURSING INTERVENTIONS AND RATIONALE

1. Monitor vital signs: every hour to every 4 hours depending on the severity of the burns and burn shock. A pulse rate greater than 100 may indicate impending or the presence of shock. Check strength of peripheral pulses. If systolic pressure is below 90 mm Hg, shock is probable.
2. Monitor urine output. Measure urine output and specific gravity at specified times such as ordered by the doctor or according to unit policy.
3. Check laboratory test results. Electrolytes, BUN, creatinine, protein, and CBC (hematocrit, hemoglobin, WBC) have implications for nursing care. Altered test results may be the result of hemodilution. Report significant changes to the physician.
4. Monitor fluid intake (oral and intravenous). The fluid intake can be as high as three times the amount of urine output depending upon the severity of the burns. IV therapy is usually not indicated if the percentage of burn is less than 20% of the body surface area for an adult and less than 10% of the body surface area for a child, elderly client, or a client with a debilitating preexisting illness.

5. Calculate the flow rate of IVs. During the first 24 hours, one half of the daily IV fluid order is usually administered in the first 8 hours and the second one half in the next 16 hours.
6. Monitor potassium replacement. When the client is receiving intravenous fluids with potassium and the serum potassium level is elevated due to hypovolemia in conjunction with a decreased urine output, notify the physician (a change in the IV order is indicated). Intravenous fluids without potassium should be run rapidly to improve renal function and to decrease the potassium level.

NURSING DIAGNOSIS 2

High risk for fluid volume excess, related to fluid shift from burned site to the vascular system and the administration of a large volume of IV fluids.

NURSING INTERVENTIONS AND RATIONALE

1. Monitor vital signs: blood pressure, pulse, respirations, and invasive hemodynamic parameters (e.g., CVP, PAP/PCWP) as appropriate.
2. Monitor fluid intake (oral and intravenous). Intravenous fluid is usually decreased after 3–5 days postburn as a result of the fluid shift back into the vascular system (blood vessels). If massive fluid replacement is continued as fluid shifts back into circulation, hypervolemia or overhydration results.
3. Observe the vascular system: vein engorgement, jugular vein distention, and hand vein engorgement can occur several days postburn and may indicate impending hypervolemia.
4. Monitor breath sounds. Report the presence of chest rales. Respiratory changes may occur due to hypervolemia (fluid overload).
5. Check laboratory test results: Electrolytes, BUN, creatinine, hematocrit, and hemoglobin have implications for care. The test results may be altered due to hemodilution. Report significant changes to the physician.
6. Weigh client daily or as indicated. Weight changes may indicate changes in fluid or nutritional status.
7. Monitor urine output. Urine output may be greatly increased (two to three times the normal volume) when the vascular system is overloaded. Insufficient urine output during the fluid shift to the vascular space may be indicative of renal impairment from burn shock or cardiac insufficiency.

NURSING DIAGNOSIS 3

Urinary elimination; decreased, related to hypovolemia.

NURSING INTERVENTIONS AND RATIONALE

1. Monitor fluid intake and urine output. Fluid intake requirements during the first several days following major burns is greatly increased due to fluid loss from the burns and the fluid shift to the burned site (third space). The administration of IV fluids must be decreased during the period in which body fluids shift back into circulation. If urine output remains low with the second phase of the fluid shift (back into circulation), renal insufficiency should be reported. Urine output should be closely monitored during the first postburn week.

2. Check laboratory test results. Elevated BUN and serum creatinine are usually indicative of renal dysfunction.
3. Monitor respiratory status. Auscultate lung fields for rales every 2–4 hours. Renal insufficiency resulting in hypervolemia frequently causes fluid congestion in the lungs.

NURSING DIAGNOSIS 4

High risk for ineffective airway clearance and high risk for ineffective breathing pattern, related to inhalation injury, tracheal edema, and/or hypervolemia.

NURSING INTERVENTIONS AND RATIONALE

1. Maintain client airway. Check for symptoms of inhalation injury: singed facial/nasal hairs, wheezing, stridor, hoarseness, and chest rales. Swelling and inflammation from inhalation injury obstruct air exchange.
2. Monitor respiratory status. Check respirations frequently, and assess chest sounds to evaluate quality of air exchange and respiratory status.
3. Administer oxygen per physician's order (usually by nonrebreather face mask) to reduce effects of reduced air exchange.
4. Maintain airway equipment at bedside (airway ambubag, tracheotomy tray) to be prepared for respiratory emergency.
5. Suction oropharyngeal and tracheal secretions prn to reduce the effects of obstruction of airway from increased burn secretions.
6. Turn position every 2 hours if not contraindicated to enhance full expansion of the lungs and movement of fluid and reduce respiratory complications.
7. Maintain head of bed 30°–45°, if permitted. This facilitates breathing by decreasing pressure on the diaphragm.

NURSING DIAGNOSIS 5

Tissue perfusion: altered, related to hypervolemia

NURSING INTERVENTIONS AND RATIONALE

1. Assess skin: color, temperature, quality, slow healing of lesions. Elevate edematous extremities. Keep warm and dry. Evaluate for signs of infection.
2. Mobilize. Turn every hour to prevent breakdown of pressure sites.
3. Monitor vital signs. Check peripheral pulses and assess chest sounds for pulmonary congestion.
4. Monitor laboratory test results: Hgb, Hct, electrolytes, BUN. Electrolytes, BUN, hematocrit, and hemoglobin may be elevated due to a decrease in vascular fluid.
5. Monitor weight. Weigh daily to determine loss or gain of fluid.
6. Monitor renal function. Observe fluid balances. Check amount of urine output and specific gravity to assess effectiveness of treatment regime.

NURSING DIAGNOSIS 6

High risk for body image disturbance, related to physical appearance from burn injury.

NURSING INTERVENTIONS AND RATIONALE

1. Assess causative factors. Have client describe self, encourage verbalization of feelings. Respond realistically, supporting positive perceptions and noting denial behaviors or overuse of defense mechanisms.
2. Assist client and significant others' acceptance of body changes. Establish therapeutic relationship, discuss fears and conflicts and encourage client to acknowledge and accept feelings. Provide accurate information. Encourage client to look at and touch affected body parts.
3. Promote wellness. Begin counseling as soon as possible. Provide positive feedback. Complete teaching exercises in small amounts at appropriate times. Refer to appropriate support groups.

Behavioral Objectives

Upon completion of this chapter, you will be prepared to:

- Explain the pathophysiologic changes associated with cirrhosis of the liver.
- Identify four etiologic factors associated with the development of cirrhosis of the liver.
- Describe the clinical manifestations related to cirrhosis of the liver.
- Identify abnormal laboratory results associated with cirrhosis of the liver.
- Discuss the clinical management for cirrhosis of the liver related to diuretic therapy, fluid restriction, dietary sodium restrictions, albumin infusions, and paracentesis.
- Identify important nursing assessment factors and nursing diagnoses related to cirrhosis of the liver.
- Discuss nursing interventions and rationale for nursing diagnoses associated with cirrhosis of the liver.

Introduction

Cirrhosis of the liver is characterized by an increase in inflammation and fibrous tissue in the liver tissue. Liver cell damage results in scar tissue, which inhibits liver function. Consequently, hepatic blood flow is obstructed and fluid and electrolyte imbalance occurs. Ascites is a common complication of cirrhosis.

PATHOPHYSIOLOGY

1   Liver (hepatic) disease is frequently associated with sodium and water retention caused by increased portal pressure and increased aldosterone secretion.

Water is retained in excess to sodium. In hepatic disease, the sodium and water retention is caused by *_____ ; *_____ .

increased portal pressure; increased aldosterone

■   ■   ■

2   Aldosterone, an adrenal cortical hormone, has a sodium retention effect that promotes water retention and encourages potassium excretion.

An increase in the aldosterone secretion results in a(n) (increase/decrease) _____ in the serum potassium level.

decrease

■   ■   ■

3   Although there is an excess in total body sodium, hyponatremia results because water is retained in excess of sodium.

Three other contributing causes of hyponatremia are:

1. Sodium moving into the intracellular space, replacing potassium, which leaves the cells because of dehydration, malnutrition, or diuresis
2. Prolonged use of potent diuretics
3. Low (or restricted) sodium diet

Hyponatremia frequently occurs with liver disorders because water is retained in (deficit/excess) _____ of sodium.

excess

■   ■   ■

4   Name three reasons wi₁ᵧ hyponatremia frequently occurs with cirrhosis of the liver.
*_____ , *_____ , and *_____ .

water is retained in excess of sodium, sodium moves into the cellular space and ascites, and prolonged use of potent diuretics results in salt and water losses

■   ■   ■

5   An increase in aldosterone secretions results in a(n) (increase/decrease) _____ in the serum potassium level. Name two other reasons hypokalemia results. _____ and _____ .

decrease; malnutrition and diuresis (potent potassium-wasting diuretics)

■   ■   ■

6   With cirrhosis of the liver, ascites may develop suddenly or insidiously. In Chapter 2, section on extracellular fluid volume excess (ECFVE), ascites was defined. Try to recall its definition.
*_____ .

an accumulation of fluid in the peritoneal cavity (abdomen)

■   ■   ■

One of the major complications of cirrhosis of the liver is the development of ascites. It occurs frequently with cellular liver damage and portal hypertension. The portal circulation, which is the liver's circulatory system, becomes affected when there is liver cell damage. The blood cannot circulate through the liver sufficiently; thus the portal pressure is significantly increased.

Ascites is a major problem in fluid and electrolyte imbalance which frequently accompanies severe cirrhosis of the liver. Thus emphasis is placed on ascites.

Study Table 16-1 carefully, noting where there is an increase or decrease in the pathophysiologic changes resulting in ascites. The rationale for these pathophysiologic changes is given. Refer to this table as needed.

Table 16-1.   PATHOPHYSIOLOGIC CHANGES ASSOCIATED WITH ASCITES

Physiologic Changes	Rationale
Portal obstruction hypertension increased	Portal obstruction resulting in portal vein hypertension alone does not cause ascites. When ascites accompanies portal hypertension, its presence can be explained because of liver damage. Surgical relief of portal hypertension relieves ascites without its fluid accumulating elsewhere in the body. Thus, portal hypertension influences fluid accumulation in the abdomen, but the fundamental cause of ascites lies in damage to the cellular structure of liver.
Capillary permeability increased	Capillary permeability is increased due to damage to the capillary endothelium, which contributes to transudation of fluid from the portal system into abdomen.
Plasma osmotic (oncotic) pressure decreased	With increased liver congestion and failure of the liver to synthesize albumin, protein-rich fluid leaves the capillaries and passes into the abdominal cavity, thus lowering the plasma osmotic pressure (hypoproteinemia and hypoalbuminemia result).
Retention of sodium and water increased	When plasma volume is reduced, an increased hormonal response (aldosterone) occurs, which decreases urinary output and causes retention of sodium and water.

7   Place I for increased and D for decreased beside the physiologic factors associated with ascites.

_____ a. Portal obstruction and hypertension
_____ b. Capillary permeability
_____ c. Plasma osmotic pressure
_____ d. Retention of sodium and water

a. I; b. I; c. D; d. I

■   ■   ■

8 Portal hypertension influences fluid accumulation in the abdomen, but the fundamental cause of ascites lies in   *_____ .

damage to the cellular structure of the liver

■   ■   ■

9 With ascites, there is a permeability defect of the capillary endothelium that contributes to
*_____ .

Capillary permeability (increases/decreases)   _____ .

the transudation of fluid; increases

■   ■   ■

10 Because of increased liver congestion and failure of the liver to synthesize albumin, the protein fluid leaves the _____ and passes into the   *_____
resulting in a(n) (increase/decrease) _____ in the plasma/serum osmotic pressure. The end result is (hypoproteinemia/hyperproteinemia) _____ .

capillaries; abdominal cavity; decrease; hypoproteinemia

■   ■   ■

11 The hormonal response of aldosterone secretions causes:

a. *_____ .
b. *_____ .

a. decrease in urinary output; b. retention of sodium and water

■   ■   ■

Place I for increased and D for decreased beside the physiologic changes as they occur with ascites. Give the rationale for each physiologic factor. After completing this review, refer to Table 16-1 for additional information.

____ Portal obstructions and hypertension
*_____

_____

_____ .

I. Portal hypertension influences ascites, but its presence is due to liver damage.

■   ■   ■

___ Capillary permeability

* ____

____

____.

I. A permeability defect of the capillary endothelium contributes to ascites.

■ ■ ■

___ Plasma osmotic pressure

* ____

____

____.

D. Due to liver congestion, protein fluid leaves the capillaries and passes into the abdomen decreasing the asmotic pressure.

■ ■ ■

___ Retention of sodium and water

* ____

____

____.

I. Increased hormonal response (aldosterone). This decreases urinary output and causes retention of Na and H_2O.

■ ■ ■

ETIOLOGY

Alcoholism with malnutrition is thought to be the primary cause of cirrhosis. Actually, hepatotoxins caused by chemicals and drugs are the leading cause of cirrhosis of the liver. Other causes include viral hepatitis and intrahepatic and extrahepatic cholestasis (obstruction or suppression of bile flow).

12 Name three causes of cirrhosis of the liver. ______________, * ______________, and * ______________.

hepatoxins (drugs and chemicals), alcoholism with malnutrition, and viral hepatitis (other: cholestasis)

■ ■ ■

CLINICAL MANIFESTATIONS

The signs and symptoms of cirrhosis of the liver are listed according to systems in Table 16-2.

Table 16-2. CLINICAL MANIFESTATIONS OF CIRRHOSIS OF THE LIVER

Body Areas	Signs and Symptoms
Gastrointestinal abnormalities	Anorexia, nausea, vomiting, indigestion, diarrhea, constipation, abdominal pain, ascites, esophageal varicies, weight loss
Renal abnormalities	Oliguria, hepatorenal syndrome (end-stage hepatic failure). BUN and serum creatinine are elevated.
Cardiovascular abnormalities	Ventricular dysrhythmias due to potassium deficit or excess
Neurologic abnormalities	Peripheral neuritis, paresthesias (abnormal sensation), sensory disturbances, sixth cranial nerve palsy
Respiratory abnormalities	Hyperventilation, respiratory alkalosis due to elevated serum ammonia levels
Integumentary abnormalities	Jaundice, vascular spiders, palmar erythema, pitting edema of the extremities, anasarca (late sign)
Laboratory Results	
Serum electrolytes ↓	Hypokalemia, hyponatremia, hypochloremia, hypomagnesemia, hypocalcemia
BUN, serum creatinine ↑	Blood urea nitrogen (BUN) > 25 mg/dL, serum creatinine > 1.5 mg/dL (late sign of hepatic failure)
Serum total bilirubin ↑	Serum bilirubin > 3.0 mg/dL. Jaundice is present.
Serum protein ↓ Serum albumin ↓	Serum protein and albumin deficit promote edema.
Prothrombin time (PT) ↑	Decrease in prothrombin time (PT). Bleeding occurs.
Serum ammonia ↑	Increased serum ammonia (end-stage hepatic failure)
Serum liver enzymes ↑	Elevated alkaline phosphatase, γ-glutamyl transferase, alanine aminotransferase (ALT/SGPT)

Note: ↑ = elevated; ↓ = decreased; > = greater than; < = less than

13 Cirrhosis causes many GI signs and symptoms. These are basically due to fluid and electrolyte imbalances.

Name four signs and symptoms of gastrointestinal disturbances. _____ , _____ , _____ , and _____ .

anorexia, nausea, vomiting, and indigestion (others: diarrhea, constipation, weight loss)

14 Ventricular dysrhythmias are often caused by potassium (deficit/excess/both)
_____ .

Because of an increased serum ammonia level, the client often hyperventilates, thus causing respiratory _____ .

both (potassium deficit occurs more frequently); alkalosis

■   ■   ■

15 Neurologic abnormalities are a common problem with cirrhosis. There is usually a vitamin B deficiency causing neurologic changes.

Two neurologic disturbances that are frequently observed are * _____ and
_____ .

peripheral neuritis and paresthesias [abnormal sensation (burning, prickling)]

■   ■   ■

16 Variations in skin disturbances are associated with cirrhosis. Jaundice usually occurs when the serum bilirubin exceeds 3.0 mg/dL. The liver is unable to conjugate bilirubin and excrete it as bile.

Vascular spiders (small dilated peripheral vessels) may be observed on the face and chest.

There may be redmottling of the palms of the hands (palmar erythema). However, this does not always mean liver disease.

Three integumentary abnormalities associated with cirrhosis are _____ ,
* _____ , and * _____ .

jaundice, vascular spiders, and palmar erythema

■   ■   ■

17 Pitting edema of the extremities is a common observation in progressive liver dysfunction. Edema in the extremities is likely due to a decreased serum albumin level (hypoalbuminemia) which causes a decrease in the serum/plasma colloid osmotic (oncotic) pressure. An extracellular fluid volume shift occurs from the _____ space to the
_____ space.

intravascular (vascular); interstitial (tissue)

■   ■   ■

18 Pitting edema ranges from +1 to +4. Which degree of pitting edema is the most severe (+2/+3)? _____ .

+3

■   ■   ■

19 With cirrhosis of the liver, there are many abnormal laboratory results occurring due to fluid and electrolyte imbalances and liver dysfunction.

Five serum electrolyte imbalances are _____ , _____ , _____ , _____ , and _____ .

hypokalemia, hyponatremia, hypomagnesemia, hypocalcemia, and hypochloremia

■   ■   ■

20 Hypokalemia occurs from cellular damage, potent potassium-wasting diuretics, inadequate nutrient intake and absorption, vomiting, and diarrhea.

The most likely cause of hypocalcemia is lack of vitamin D for calcium absorption from the GI tract and inadequate nutrient intake.

The three causes of hyponatremia (refer to Frame 3 if unknown) are *_____ , *_____ , and *_____ .

water is retained in excess of sodium, use of potent diuretics, and a low-sodium diet

■   ■   ■

21 Poor protein ingestion and protein synthesis results in (increased/decreased) _____ serum protein and serum albumin levels.

Decreased levels of blood protein results in edema formation in the extremities and ascites. In such cases the serum colloid osmotic pressure is (increased/decreased) _____ .

decreased; decreased

■   ■   ■

22 The decreased vitamin K uptake in the liver for prothrombin synthesis (prolongs/shortens) _____ the prothrombin time (PT).

The clotting time is (increased/decreased) _____ .

prolongs; decreased (bleeding tendency can result)

■   ■   ■

23 Hyperammoniemia is an indication of end-stage hepatic failure. When the liver is unable to convert ammonia to urea for excretion, serum ammonia levels increase. Ammonia is toxic to the cerebral cells.

With a buildup of ammonia levels, the client becomes drowsy, lethargic, and confused and a coma ensues.

The serum liver enzymes during liver dysfunction are (increased/decreased) _____ .

increased

■   ■   ■

CLINICAL MANAGEMENT

Clinical management for a client with advanced cirrhosis consists of decreasing the extent of ascites and peripheral edema. Treatment modalities include diuretic therapy, fluid restriction, dietary sodium restriction (500–1500 mg sodium), albumin infusion, and paracentesis if necessary. Eliminating the cause of cirrhosis, such as drugs or alcohol, may decrease the severity of the liver destruction.

24 Potent diuretic therapy is prescribed to promote fluid excretion by shifting fluid from the
*_____ and the *_____ .

Excessive use of diuretics can cause severe (hypovolemia/hypervolemia) _____ .

peritoneal cavity or ascites; interstitial (tissue) spaces or extremities; hypovolemia

■   ■   ■

25 A combination of potassium-wasting and potassium-sparing diuretics is frequently ordered.

Continuous use of potassium-wasting diuretics such as the thiazides or the loop (high-ceiling) diuretics can cause (hypokalemia/hyperkalemia) _____ .

hypokalemia

■   ■   ■

26 Fluid restrictions are often based on urine output and approximate amount of insensible fluid loss (skin and lungs). The fluid restriction may be 1000–1500 mL per day; however, the restriction varies per individual.

Sodium restriction also varies according to the situation and need. A low sodium diet consists of _____ mg per day.

Fluid intake may be restricted to _____ mL per day.

500–1500; 1000–1500

■   ■   ■

27 Administering albumin 25% solution reestablishes the vascular fluid volume. Albumin is a colloid and usually does not seep into the interstitial spaces. This solution increases the colloid osmotic (oncotic) pressure and pulls the fluid from the peritoneal cavity (ascites) and the extremities (peripheral edema).

Use of an albumin infusion (increases/decreases) _____ fluid loss from ascites and peripheral edema.

increases

∎   ∎   ∎

28 Paracentesis is prescribed mainly when there is respiratory distress and intra-abdominal pressure due to massive ascites.

Removing large quantities of fluid (>2000 mL) rapidly from the ascites area can result in a circulatory collapse.

When a large amount of ascites fluid is removed, fluid shifts occur to compensate for the fluid loss. Fluid shifts from the *_____ to the *_____ .

What type of fluid imbalance results? _____ .

intravascular (vascular) space; interstitial space (ascites); hypovolemia (a massive amount of fluid shifts from the vascular space to the ascites to maintain the ECF balance)

∎   ∎   ∎

CLINICAL APPLICATIONS

29 Persons with ascites eventually become refractory in regard to diuretic agents. Frequently, a paracentesis (surgical puncture of the abdominal cavity for relieving fluid) is required to relieve symptoms of pressure or respiratory distress or both.

With ascites, there is a tendency for the client to become refractory to

_____ .

diuretics

∎   ∎   ∎

30 *Paracentesis* means a *_____ .

surgical puncture of the abdominal cavity

∎   ∎   ∎

31 Paracentesis is generally required to relieve symptoms of _____ or
*
_____ .

pressure; respiratory distress
■   ■   ■

32 Repeated paracenteses result in a significant loss of protein, electrolytes, and water.
As a result of repeated paracenteses, what three substances may be lost?
_____ , _____ , and _____ .

protein, electrolytes, and water
■   ■   ■

33 The aftereffect of an abdominal paracentesis is an antidiuresis of water, with a hemodilution of sodium in the blood. Following this, there is a rapid outpouring of fluid into the abdominal cavity resulting in hemoconcentration of sodium and a drop in blood volume. This leads to a greater retention of sodium.

Abdominal paracentesis (is/is not) _____ a permanent cure for ascites.

After an abdominal paracentesis, antidiuresis of water results, causing hemodilution of
*
_____ .

is not; sodium in the blood
■   ■   ■

34 After hemodilution of serum sodium following a paracentesis, fluid pours into the
*
_____ . As a result, this blood volume is (increased/decreased)
_____ .

The nurse should observe for symptoms of serum sodium (excess/deficit)
_____ .

abdominal cavity; decreased; excess
■   ■   ■

35   Repeated paracenteses cause a significant loss in _____ ,
_____ , and _____ .

The removal of a large volume of fluid by a paracentesis causes a rapid shift of fluid from the plasma into the *_____ . Symptoms of circulatory collapse (shock symptoms) should be observed following the removal of a large volume of abdominal fluid.

Name at least five symptoms of shock.

a. *_____
b. *_____
c. *_____
d. *_____
e. *_____

water; protein; electrolytes; abdominal cavity (third-space fluid)
a. pallid, cold, clammy skin; b. fast pulse rate; c. apprehension and restlessness; d. fall in blood pressure; e. respirations are shallow and rapid (others: weakness, oliguria)

■   ■   ■

CASE STUDY

Mr. Moore, age 58, was admitted to the medical floor of the hospital complaining of shortness of breath with no chest pain. He had massive ascites with distended veins over the abdomen and +4 pitting leg edema. Mr. Moore's shortness of breath is most likely the result of ascites. His records show that his admissions in the past 8 years have been due to cirrhosis of the liver with ascites and peripheral edema. Congestive heart failure frequently accompanies severe liver damage with ascites; therefore, a cardiac glycoside is given. Mr. Moore is placed on diuretics and a cardiac glycoside drug (digoxin).

36   Diuretics are ordered to increase *_____ .

Digoxin is given to *_____ .

(Refer to section on CHF if necessary.)

fluid loss via urinary output
strengthen the heart beat and improve circulation of fluid

■   ■   ■

The laboratory studies of Mr. Moore in Table 16-3 show how his laboratory results deviate from the norms at the time of his illness.

Table 16-3. LABORATORY STUDIES OF MR. MOORE

Laboratory Tests	On Admission	2 Weeks Later	3 Weeks Later	4 Weeks Later
Hematology				
Hemoglobin (12.9–17.0 g)	10.4		12.6	
Hematocrit (40–46%)	34		41	
WBCs (white blood cells) (5000–10,000/mm^3)	8000			
Biochemistry				
BUN (blood urea nitrogen) (10–25 mg/dL)	47	55	132	190
Plasma/serum CO_2 $\frac{50-70 \text{ vol\%}}{22-32 \text{ mEq/L}}$	$\frac{44}{20}$	$\frac{48}{22}$		$\frac{29}{13}$
Plasma/serum chloride (95–108 mEq/L)	105	94	99	91
Plasma/serum sodium (135–146 mEq/L)	136	124	133	119
Plasma/serum potassium (3.5–5.3 mEq/L)	4.9	4.6	3.9	4.5
Plasma albumin (3.2–5.6 Gm/dL)	1.4			

Note: mg/100 mL = mg/dL. *Plasma* and *serum* are used interchangeably.

37 Mr. Moore's hemoglobin level on admission was 10.4 g, which can be indicative of secondary anemia or (hemodilution/hemoconcentration) _____ .

The BUN on his admission was 47 mg/dL, which can mean that *_____

_____ .

hemodilution;
he was dehydrated due to a lack of fluid, or renal insufficiency

38 Two weeks after admission, Mr. Moore's BUN became alarmingly elevated.

What does this mean in regard to his kidneys? _____

_____ .

the inability of the kidneys to excrete the waste product, e.g., uremia, or kidney failure, or
both

■   ■   ■

39 Mr. Moore's serum CO_2 on admission is 20 mEq/L, which can mean he is in a mild

_____ state.

acidotic

■   ■   ■

40 Mr. Moore's plasma albumin indicates (hyperalbuminemia/hypoalbuminemia)

_____ .

hypoalbuminemia

■   ■   ■

Mr. Moore's clinical management consists of:

1. Diuretics
   a. Lasix (furosemide) 160–200 mg (stat doses—immediate)
   b. Daily doses of Aldactone (spironolactone), an aldosterone antagonist and potassium-sparing diuretic

   Lasix (furosemide) is a potent diuretic that acts on the proximal and distal tubules and ascending limb of Henle's loop. If given in excessive amounts, furosemide can lead to a profound diuresis with water and electrolyte depletion.

   Aldactone (spironolactone) inhibits the production of aldosterone (the hormone that causes sodium and water retention and potassium excretion). Therefore, Aldactone promotes sodium and water excretion and inhibits potassium excretion.

   Hypokalemia can cause hepatic coma or liver failure. Low serum potassium has a tendency to increase ammonium accumulation, which precipitates hepatic toxicity.

2. Digoxin—0.25 mg daily
3. Low sodium diet—1.5 g
4. Limited fluid intake
5. Daily weights

41 Mr. Moore received furosemide (Lasix) by _____ doses. It is a potent diuretic that acts on what areas of the kidneys? *_____

_____ .

Large and continuous doses of Lasix can lead to profound diuresis, causing depletion of _____ and _____ .

Aldactone promotes excretion of _____ and _____ and inhibits excretion of _____ .

Digoxin is given daily to *_____ and *_____ .

A low-sodium diet and limited fluid intake can decrease the body's _____ and _____ .

stat; proximal and distal tubules and the loop of Henle
water; electrolytes
sodium; water; potassium
strengthen heart beat; improve circulation
sodium; water

■   ■   ■

42 Mr. Moore did not respond well to Lasix and Aldactone. Paracentesis is indicated when ascites becomes refractory to _____ .

A paracentesis is performed on the tenth day after admission and during the third week.

Following the removal of a large volume of fluid by paracentesis, the nurse should observe for symptoms of *_____ .

diuretics; circulatory collapse (shock)

■   ■   ■

43 On several occasions, Mr. Moore received albumin 25% intravenously. The purpose of an albumin solution is to draw the fluid from the *_____ into the *_____ to be excreted by the kidneys.

peritoneal cavity; intravascular (vascular) space

■   ■   ■

CASE STUDY REVIEW

Mr. Moore, age 58, is diagnosed as having cirrhosis of the liver with ascites and peripheral edema. He is in congestive heart failure, so he received digoxin and diuretics (Lasix and Aldactone). Diuretics promote the removal of fluids from the abdominal area, i.e., ascites. He is on a low-sodium diet (1 g). His serum sodium is low, 119–136 mEq/L.

1. Hyponatremia occurs in liver diseases in spite of the presence of an excess of total body sodium because water is *_____

   _____ .

2. Name three other conditions that contributed to Mr. Moore's hyponatremia.
   *_____ , *_____ , and *_____ .

3. Mr. Moore has ascites, which is *_____

   _____ .

4. Portal hypertension influences fluid accumulation in the abdomen, but the fundamental cause of ascites lies in *_____

   _____ .

5. With ascites, there is a capillary permeability (increase/decrease) _____ and a plasma osmotic pressure (increase/decrease) _____ .

6. Lasix (furosemide) is a (potassium-sparing/potassium-wasting) _____ diuretic. Aldactone (spironolactone) is a potassium- _____ diuretic. Why are these two types of diuretics frequently given together? *_____

   _____ .

   Mr. Moore was not responding to the diuretics. He was having difficulty in breathing due to his ascites. A paracentesis was performed.

7. Mr. Moore had a paracentesis done to alleviate which two symptoms? _____ , and *_____ .

8. A paracentesis was indicated, for he became refractory to which group of drugs?

   _____ .

9. Repeated paracenteses result in a great loss of _____ ,
   _____ , and _____ .

10. Following an abdominal paracentesis, antidiuresis of water results; there is an outpouring of fluid into *_____ , resulting in hemoconcentration and a drop in *_____ .

11. The nurse checked Mr. Moore's laboratory results. She noticed a low serum sodium. The nurse should observe for symptoms of _____ . Name four of the symptoms.
    *_____ , *_____ , _____ , and
    *_____ .

1. *retained in excess to sodium*
2. *sodium moves into the intracellular spaces, prolonged use of potent diuretics, and low-sodium diet*
3. *an accumulation of fluid in the peritoneal cavity*
4. *damage to the cellular structure of the liver*
5. *increase; decrease*

6. *potassium-wasting; sparing*
   Aldactone causes retention of potassium, thus preventing excessive potassium loss due to furosemide. Furosemide is a potent potassium-wasting diuretic.
7. *pressure and respiratory distress*
8. *diuretics*
9. *protein; electrolytes; water*
10. *the peritoneal cavity; blood volume or fluid volume*
11. *hyponatremia*
    abdominal cramps, muscular weakness, headaches, and nausea and vomiting

NURSING ASSESSMENT FACTORS

- Record vital signs (VSs) for baseline data to be compared with future VSs. Report abnormal findings. Tachycardia can indicate fluid volume deficit.
- Check urine output. If the urine output average is less than 25 mL per hour, notify the physician.
- Check lower extremities for pitting edema. Determine if the pitting edema is +1 to +4 (mild to severe fluid retention among the tissue spaces).
- Record body weight. The baseline weight can be compared with future daily weights; a loss or gain of weight indicates the amount of fluid discrepancy.
- Assess client's skin for signs of vascular spiders (angiomas) and the presence of jaundice, suggesting portal hypertension.
- Check the laboratory results and report abnormal findings. Serum potassium, sodium, magnesium, calcium, and chloride may be low. However, sodium and water are retained, so hyponatremia (sodium deficit) may occur due to a sodium shift into the cells and into the abdominal cavity, a low-sodium diet, and/or diuretics.

NURSING DIAGNOSIS 1

Fluid volume deficit: fluid shift to the third space (ascites), related to fluid and electrolyte imbalances secondary to cirrhosis of the liver.

NURSING INTERVENTIONS AND RATIONALE

1. Monitor vital signs. Compare with baseline vital signs. An increase in pulse rate, decrease in blood pressure, narrowing of pulse pressure (<20 mm Hg), and increase in breathing rate are indications of hypovolemia.
2. Check for signs and symptoms of hypokalemia since Mr. Moore is receiving a potent diuretic (Lasix) and digoxin. Symptoms include dizziness, cardiac dysrythmias, muscular weakness, abdominal distention, and diminished peristalsis (bowel sounds). Hypokalemia can enhance the action of digoxin and cause digitalis toxicity.
3. Monitor urine output. Urine output of less than 600 mL per 24 hours can indicate hypovolemia due to fluid shift into the abdominal cavity, kidney (renal) impairment, limited fluid intake, or excess aldosterone secretions.
4. Monitor daily body weight and compare with baseline weight. An increase of $4\frac{1}{2}$ pounds indicates approximately 2 liters of fluid retention (1 liter = 2.2 pounds). A loss of weight may indicate fluid loss from ascites and/or extremities (edema).
5. Measure abdominal girth daily. An increase in abdominal girth size indicates increased fluid in the peritoneal cavity (ascites).

6. Monitor fluid intake. Fluid restriction may be prescribed.
7. Continue to check all laboratory results. Report abnormal findings. Laboratory tests indicates client's progress, either toward recovery or nonresponsive to therapy.
8. Monitor skin for presence and decreasing evidence of jaundice. As the serum bilirubin decreases (<3.0 mg/dL), jaundice should be less apparent.
9. Observe for signs and symptoms of shock after paracentesis. Removal of large volumes of abdominal fluid can cause vascular fluid to shift into the abdomen. Symptoms of shock include cold, clammy skin; rapid pulse rate; apprehension and restlessness; rapid, shallow respirations; and a drop in blood pressure.

NURSING DIAGNOSIS 2

Nutrition: altered, less than body requirements, related to alcoholism and inadequate nutrient intake.

NURSING INTERVENTIONS AND RATIONALE

1. Monitor the client's nutrition intake. Encourage the client to eat a well-balanced diet.
2. Instruct the client to eat foods that are nutritionally high in protein. Increasing serum protein level increases the serum colloid osmotic pressure, which promotes abdominal fluid to shift to the vascular area.

OTHER NURSING DIAGNOSES

Skin integrity: impaired, related to fluid accumulation in the interstitial space (tissues) of the extremities and buttocks.

Ineffective breathing patterns, related to large volumes of fluid in the peritoneal cavity (ascites), which causes pressure on the diaphragm.

Activity intolerance, related to pressure in the diaphragm from ascites and edema in the extremities.

Health maintenance: altered, related to the chronicity of the disease process.

Coping: ineffective, related to impact on lifestyle and physical symptoms.

Behavioral Objectives

Upon completion of this chapter, you will be prepared to:

- Identify pathophysiologic changes associated with chronic obstructive pulmonary disease (COPD).
- Explain the clinical manifestations (early and late signs and symptoms) of emphysema and chronic bronchitis.
- Identify abnormal arterial blood gases (ABG) results by comparing the pH, $PaCO_2$, and HCO_3 results.
- Monitor the ABGs, hematology, breath sounds, lung expansion, and vital signs (VSs) of clients with COPD.
- Explain the clinical management for COPD.
- Identify appropriate nursing diagnoses with related nursing interventions and rationales to care for clients with COPD.

Introduction

Chronic obstructive pulmonary disease (COPD), also referred to as chronic obstructive lung disease (COLD), is a classification assigned to conditions associated with airway obstruction. The narrowing of the bronchioles increases the resistance to air flow.

Example of COPD are emphysema, chronic bronchitis, bronchiectasis, and asthma. Smoking is the leading cause of emphysema and chronic bronchitis. Other causes for COPD include alpha$_1$-antitrypsin deficiency (hereditary trait), chronic bacterial infection, air pollution, and inhalation of chemical irritants.

1   COPD is characterized by *_____ .

Another name for COPD is *_____ .

an airway obstruction; COLD or chronic obstructive lung disease

        ■   ■   ■

2   The leading cause of emphysema and chronic bronchitis is _____ .

Name two other causes for COPD.   *_____

and   *_____ .

smoking; alpha$_1$-antitrypsin deficiency and chronic bacterial infection (others: air pollution, inhalation of chemical irritants).

        ■   ■   ■

PATHOPHYSIOLOGY

Morphologic changes in emphysema are (1) thickening of bronchial walls caused by submucosal edema and excess mucous secretion; (2) loss of elastic recoil of lung tissue; and (3) destruction of the alveolar septa that promote overdistention and dead air space.

3   Name three morphologic changes in COPD.

a.   *_____

b.   *_____

c.   *_____

a. thickening of bronchial walls, b. loss of elastic recoil of lung tissue, c. destruction to alveolar septa or overdistended alveoli

■   ■   ■

Bronchitis and emphysema generally coexist. Table 17-1 lists the pathophysiologic changes associated with COPD conditions. The rationale for pathophysiologic changes is included.

Table 17-1.   PATHOPHYSIOLOGIC CHANGES IN CHRONIC OBSTRUCTIVE PULMONARY DISEASE (COPD)

Pathophysiologic Changes	Rationale
Decreased elasticity of bronchiolar walls (loss of elastic recoil)	Loss of elastic recoil causes a premature collapse of airways with expiration. Alveoli become overdistended when air is trapped in the affected lung tissue and dead air space is increased. Overdistention leads to rupture and coalescence of several alveoli.
Alveolar damage	Chronic air trapping and airway inflammation lead to weakened bronchiolar walls and alveolar disruption. Coalescence of adjacent alveoli results in bullae (parenchymal air-filled spaces > 1 cm in diameter). The total area of gas exchange is greatly reduced and pulmonary hypertension may develop.
Mucous gland hyperplasia and increased mucous production	Oversecretion of mucous is commonly found in bronchitis and advanced emphysema. Increased mucous production can cause mucous plugs which lead to airway obstruction.
Inflammation of bronchial mucosa	Inflammatory infiltration and edema of the bronchial mucosa commonly occur in bronchitis but are also found in advanced emphysema. Edema and infiltration cause thickening of bronchiolar walls.
Airway obstruction	This condition is caused primarily by narrowed bronchioles, edema and mucous plugs. Obstruction is greatest on expiration. During inspiration bronchial lumina widen to admit air; the lumina collapse during expiration.

Table 17-1.   (Continued)

Pathophysiologic Changes	Rationale

CO_2 retention
Increased Pa_{CO_2}
>45 mm Hg
(hypercapnia)
  Norms: 35–45 mm
      Hg
	Accumulation of carbon dioxide (CO_2) concentration in the arterial blood from inadequate gas exchange is the result of hypoventilation. CO_2 excess, >60 mm Hg, can lead to ventricular fibrillation.

Respiratory acidosis	CO_2 retention results from hypoventilation. Water combines with CO_2 to produce carbonic acid, and with increased CO_2 retention respiratory acidosis occurs ($H_2O + CO_2 = H_2CO_3$). The arterial blood gases reflect pH < 7.35; Pa_{CO_2} > 45 mm Hg.
Hypoxemia	Hypoxemia, or reduced oxygen (O_2) in the blood, is frequently caused by airway obstruction and alveolar hypoventilation. The thickened alveolar capillary membrane reduces O_2 diffusion.
Cor pulmonale (right-sided heart failure due to pulmonary hypertension)	Destruction of alveolar tissue leads to a reduction of the size of the pulmonary capillary bed. Pulmonary hypertension occurs when $\frac{2}{3}$ to $\frac{3}{4}$ of the vascular bed is destroyed. The workload of the right ventricle is then increased, thus causing right ventricular hypertrophy and eventually CHF.
Increased red blood cell (RBC) count	Secondary polcythemia occurs as a compensatory mechanism with prolonged hypoxemia. Hemoglobin and hematocrit are increased to enhance O_2 transport.
Alpha$_1$-antitrypsin deficiency	A genetic predisposition to alpha$_1$-antitrypsin deficiency is present. An antitrypsin or trypsin inhibitor is produced in the liver. A deficit of antitrypsin allows proteolytic enzymes (released in the lungs from bacteria or phagocytic cells) to damage lung tissue. The result is emphysema.

4   Airway obstruction is greatest on (inspiration/expiration) _____ .

  expiration

      ▪   ▪   ▪

5   The normal value of Pa_{CO_2} is _____ mm Hg.

     The term for CO_2 retention is _____ and the Pa_{CO_2} is
     _____ mm Hg.

     35–45; hypercapnia; >45

      ▪   ▪   ▪

6   A serious acid-base imbalance that occurs in advanced COPD is *_____ .

    Explain how this acid-base imbalance occurs. *_____

_____ .

    The pH is _____ and the Pa_{CO_2} is _____ .

respiratory acidosis
CO_2 combines with water to produce carbonic acid, thus causing acidosis.
<7.35; >45 mm Hg
      ■   ■   ■

7   The name for reduced oxygen (O_2) concentration in the blood is _____ .

    Decreased arterial O_2 causes the number of red blood cells to (increase/decrease)

_____ .

    The hemoglobin and hematocrit is (increased/decreased) _____ .

    Why? *_____ .

hypoxemia; increase; increased. More RBCs and hemoglobin are needed to carry oxygen.
      ■   ■   ■

8   Could a nonsmoker with an alpha$_1$-antitrypsin deficiency develop emphysema?

_____ .

    Explain the rationale for your answer. *_____

_____ .

Yes. Antitrypsin deficiency permits the proteolytic enzymes in the lungs to damage lung tissue.
      ■   ■   ■

9   Cor pulmonale is right-sided heart failure caused by *_____

_____ . It can result in COPD when alveolar tissue destruction leads to

*_____ .

pulmonary hypertension; a reduction in the size of the pulmonary capillary bed
      ■   ■   ■

CLINICAL MANIFESTATIONS

Early signs and symptoms of bronchitis and/or emphysema are fatigue and dyspnea after exertion. Table 17-2 lists the signs and symptoms of early to advanced COPD (chronic bronchitis and emphysema). Study the table carefully and refer to it as needed.

Table 17-2. CLINICAL MANIFESTATIONS OF COPD	
Signs and Symptoms	Rationale
Chronic fatigue	Fatigue, an early sign of COPD, is caused by hypoxia and the increased effort required to move air into and out of lungs.
Dyspnea	Difficulty in breathing and shortness of breath following exertion are early signs of COPD. In advanced COPD dyspnea occurs with little or no exertion.
Vital Signs	
BP increased	Increased blood pressure is due to increased sympathetic stimulation from stress.
Pulse rate increased	Increased pulse rate results from poor oxygenation. The body's attempts to compensate for hypoxemia (decreased oxygen in the blood) by increasing the heart rate to carry more oxygen.
Respirations labored and increased	Loss of elasticity of lung tissue causes the bronchioles to collapse during normal expiration, thus prolonging the expiratory phase of respiration. Accessory respiratory muscles are used to improve alveolar ventilation and gas exchange.
Barrel-shaped chest (AP diameter > lateral diameter)	This is the result of loss of lung elasticity, chronic air trapping, and chest wall expansion with chest rigidity. It may also be compounded by dorsal kyphosis which results from a bent-forward position used to facilitate breathing. Shoulders are elevated and the neck appears to shorten. Accessory muscles of respiration are used for breathing.
Cough (productive)	A cough is usually associated with bronchitis because of the excessive secretion of the mucous glands. In emphysema a cough is associated with respiratory infection or cardiac failure. Bacterial growth in retained mucous secretions leads to repeated infections and a chronic cough.
Cyanosis	In advanced COPD, marked cyanosis is due to poor tissue perfusion, which results from hypoxemia. Signs of cyanosis may also appear when the hemoglobin is below 5 g.

Table 17-2.   (Continued)

Signs and Symptoms	Rationale
Clubbing of nails	Clubbing of nails is commonly seen in association with hypoxemia and polycythemia. It may be due to capillary dilation in an attempt to draw more oxygen to the fingertips.
Laboratory Results	
Arterial blood gases (ABGs) pH < 7.35 $PaCO_2 > 45$ mm Hg $HCO_3 > 28$ mEq/L $PaO_2 < 70$ mm Hg BE $> +2$ (respiratory acidosis with metabolic compensation)	Increased CO_2 retention and water cause an excessive amount of carbonic acid. As a result of too much carbonic acid in the blood, acidosis develops and the pH is decreased. The $PaCO_2$ is the respiratory component of the ABGs. A decreased pH and an increased $PaCO_2$ indicate respiratory acidosis. The PaO_2 may be normal or greatly reduced, depending on the degree of distortion of ventilation/perfusion ratio. An increased bicarbonate (HCO_3) level indicates metabolic compensation to neutralize or decrease the acidotic state. A normal HCO_3 (24–28 mEq/L) indicates no compensation.
Hemoglobin (Hgb) and hematocrit (Hct) increased (hemoglobin may increase to 20 g)	Increased Hgb and Hct are due to hypoxemia. More hemoglobin can carry more oxygen. An elevated hemoglobin is a sign that cyanosis is more likely.

Electrolytes:
  Potassium, low to
  low normal
  Sodium, normal to
  slightly elevated
	The serum potassium level may be 3.0–3.7 mEq/L and can be the result of poor dietary intake related to breathlessness, potassium-wasting diuretics, or chronic use of steroid (e.g., cortisone). Usually the sodium level is normal but it can be elevated due to cardiac failure or excess IV saline infusions.

10   Two early signs and symptoms of COPD are _____ and
      *_____ .

      fatigue and dyspnea on exertion.

                              ■   ■   ■

11   Changes in VSs may include the following:
      1. Blood pressure. _____ .
      2. Pulse rate. _____ .
      3. Respiration. _____ .
      The expiratory phase of respiration is _____ .

      increased; increased; labored
      prolonged

                              ■   ■   ■

12   A common characteristic of COPD is a barrel-shaped chest. Explain.
      *_____

      _____ .

      loss of lung elasticity and chest wall expansion with chest rigidity or dorsal kyphosis from a
      bent position and using accessory respiratory muscles

                              ■   ■   ■

13   A cough is more common with what COPD problem? _____ .
      Respiratory infection is a complication of COPD. Explain why? *_____

      _____ .

      Bronchitis
      Bacteria grows in retained mucous secretions and respiratory infection results.

                              ■   ■   ■

14   What major type of acid-base imbalance occurs in COPD? *_____ .
      Indicate the arterial blood gases that occur with this acid-base imbalance:

      ( ) a. pH 7.46
      ( ) b. pH 7.32
      ( ) c. $Paco_2$ 55 mm Hg
      ( ) d. $Paco_2$ 32 mm Hg

      respiratory acidosis
      a. —; b. X; c. X; d. —

                              ■   ■   ■

15 Explain the significance of an elevated bicarbonate (HCO_3) level in respiratory acidosis.

*_____

_____ .

Elevated HCO_3 level indicates metabolic compensation. Conservation of bicarbonate helps to decrease the acidotic state.

      ■   ■   ■

16 Which of the following laboratory results frequently occur in chronic COPD? Correct the incorrect responses.

(   ) a. Hemoglobin decreased
(   ) b. Hematocrit decreased
(   ) c. Potassium low or low normal
(   ) d. Sodium loss

a. —, increased to carry more oxygen; b. —, increased; c. X; d. —; sodium normal or slightly elevated

      ■   ■   ■

CLINICAL APPLICATIONS

Joseph Hall, age 54, has smoked two packs of cigarettes for the last 35 years. He has repeatedly been admitted to the hospital over the last 7 years for COPD or emphysema. The nurse assessed Mr. Hall's physiologic status and noted dyspnea following exertion (breathlessness), barrel-shaped chest, and mild cyanosis. Joseph complained of constant fatigue. When checking his breath sounds, the nurse noted a prolonged expiration rate. Vital signs were BP 150/86, pulse rate 94, and respiration 26 and labored.

17 Which of Mr. Hall's clinical signs and symptoms taken on admission indicate COPD?

(   ) a. Breathlessness
(   ) b. Barrel-shaped chest
(   ) c. Mild cyanosis
(   ) d. Fatigue
(   ) e. Prolonged expiration

a. X; b. X; c. X; d. X; e. X

      ■   ■   ■

18 A risk factor of COPD which can be linked to Mr. Hall's problem is

_____ .

smoking

      ■   ■   ■

The results of the laboratory studies ordered for Mr. Hall are given in Table 17-3.

Table 17-3. LABORATORY STUDIES: MR. HALL			
Laboratory Tests	**On Admission**	**Day 1**	**Day 2**
Hematology			
Red blood cells (4.5–6 million)	6.6	6.5	6.2
Hemoglobin (Male: 13.5–18 g)	16.8	16.6	16.2
Hematocrit (Male: 40–54%)	57.8	57.2	55.6
White blood cells (5–10 mm³)	12.8	13.0	10.5
Biochemistry			
Potassium (K) (3.5–5.3 mEq/L)	3.5	3.6	3.7
Sodium (Na) (135–146 mEq/L)	140	138	139
Chloride (Cl) (95–108 mEq/L)	107	106	106
Carbon dioxide (CO_2)	30	36	38
Arterial blood gases (ABGs)			
pH (7.35–7.45)	7.24	7.32	7.34
$Paco_2$ (35–45 mm Hg)	73	68	60
Pao_2 (70–100 mm Hg)	45	70 (with O_2)	76 (with O_2)
HCO_3 (24–28 mEq/L)	28	34	37
BE (−2 to +2)	+2	+6	+9

19 Mr. Hall's RBC, hemoglobin, and hematocrit were elevated because of

*_____ .

poor oxygenation or hypoxemia

■   ■   ■

20 His potassium is low average. This can be the result of *_____

_____ .

*poor nutritional intake. He can be given a potassium-wasting diuretic for heart failure as a
result of prolonged respiratory distress.*

      ■   ■   ■

21 Sodium level may be normal or slightly elevated. His serum sodium value is in the
(high/normal/low) _____ range.

normal

      ■   ■   ■

22 The serum CO_2 is a bicarbonate determinant. An increased value (alkalosis) may be due to
base excess from bicarbonate intake or to metabolic (renal) compensation.

   In Mr. Hall's situation the cause is most likely *_____ .

metabolic (renal) compensation

      ■   ■   ■

23 On admission, his arterial blood gases (ABGs) indicate (respiratory alkalosis/respiratory
acidosis) *_____ (with/without) _____ metabolic
compensation.

   Explain his ABGs in response to your previous answer. *_____

_____ .

respiratory acidosis; without
*The pH is low, PaCO₂ is high, and HCO₃ and BE are normal values and thus there is no
compensation.*

      ■   ■   ■

24 On day 1 and day 2 his acid-base imbalance reflects *_____ .
   Is there metabolic compensation? _____ . Explain. *_____

_____ .

respiratory acidosis
*Yes. The HCO₃ and BE are elevated. This is a compensatory mechanism that brings the pH
close to normal value.*

      ■   ■   ■

25 Oxygen was administered to Mr. Hall at 2 liters per minute with a nasal O_2 cannula (nasal prongs). A ventimask delivered 24, 28, 35, and 40% of oxygen. A nonbreathing oxygen mask should *not* be used. Explain.   *_____

_____ .

The rate of O_2 flow with a nasal cannula should be no greater than _____ .

It delivers a high concentration of O_2, >90%. This decreases the hypoxic respiratory drive and can cause CO_2 narcosis.
2 liters per minute.

    ■   ■   ■

26 Mr. Hall's PaO_2 is (high/low) _____ . His PaO_2 indicates _____

_____ .

low; hypoxemia or low oxygen content in the blood

    ■   ■   ■

27 The nurse rechecked his breath sounds and noted rhonchi in the lower base of both lungs.

Mr. Hall's WBCs are elevated. Rhonchi and elevated WBCs could be indicative of

*_____ .

respiratory infection. This is the result of trapped mucous secretions and the presence of bacteria.

    ■   ■   ■

CLINICAL MANAGEMENT

Mr. Hall received bronchodilators and 2 liters per minute of oxygen. Breathing exercises were explained to him.

Table 17-4 lists methods of managing COPD.

28 Low-flow oxygen is frequently needed to decrease hypoxemia. When a nasal O_2 cannula is used, the flow should be _____ .

If a high concentration of oxygen is delivered, what might happen to the respiratory drive?

*_____ .

1–2 liters per minute
A high concentration of O_2 decreases hypoxic respiratory drive.

    ■   ■   ■

Table 17-4.   CLINICAL MANAGEMENT OF COPD

Management Methods	Rationale
Oxygen (O_2)	Low-flow oxygen: 1–2 liters per minute with a nasal O_2 cannula or ventimask with 24 or 28% is suggested. Mechanical ventilators may be needed to decrease CO_2 retention and to aid in ventilation. Care should be taken to avoid CO_2 narcosis; O_2 that is too high decreases the hypoxic respiratory drive.
Hydration	Fluid intake should be increased to 3–4 liters per day to liquify secretions and ease in expectoration *unless* cor pulmonale and/or CHF is present.
Bronchodilators: Isoproterenol (Isuprel) Metaproterenol (Alupent) Terbutaline (Brethine) Aminophylline Theophylline products	The purpose of these agents is to dilate bronchial tubes (bronchioles), to expectorate mucus, and to improve ventilation. Following use of a bronchodilator the client should deep breathe and cough. Bronchodilators can be administered through nebulizers (pressurized aerosols or IPPB with low-flow O_2 or compressed air), intravenously in IV fluids (aminophylline), or orally (theophylline products). Side effects of these drugs are tachycardia, cardiac dysrhythmias, and nausea/vomiting.
Antibiotics	When a respiratory infection is present, antibiotics are given intravenously (diluted in 100 mL of solution) or orally.
Chest physiotherapy	Chest clapping loosens the thick, tenacious mucous secretions that must be "coughed up." Deep breathing and coughing should follow. Diaphragmatic breathing improves tidal volume and increases alveolar ventilation. Pursed-lip breathing prevents airway collapse so that trapped air in the alveoli can be expelled.
Exercise	Walking and stationary bicycling improve respiratory status and state of well being.
Relaxation techniques	Practicing relaxation techniques decreases anxiety, fear, and panic. Decreased dyspnea can result from relaxation.

29 Why is hydration important in the management of COPD? *_____

_____ .

Increased fluid intake should be contraindicated when _____

and/or _____ are present.

to liquify secretions and ease in expectoration
cor pulmonale; CHF

■   ■   ■

30 Bronchodilators are used for the following purposes:

a. * _____

b. * _____

c. * _____

a. to dilate the bronchial tubes/bronchioles; b. to expectorate mucous;
c. to improve ventilation

■   ■   ■

31 Indicate which of the following side effects may result from constant use or overuse of bronchodilators:

( ) a. Bradycardia
( ) b. Tachycardia
( ) c. Nausea, vomiting
( ) d. Cardiac dysrhythmias
( ) e. Hypotension
( ) f. Skin rash

a. —; b. X; c. X; d. X; e. —; f. —

■   ■   ■

32 Identify three examples of chest physiotherapy and explain their purposes:

a. * _____ .
    Purpose * _____ .

b. * _____ .
    Purpose * _____ .

c. * _____ .
    Purpose * _____ .

a. chest clapping; to loosen thick, tenacious mucous secretions
b. diaphragmatic breathing; to increase alveolar ventilation
c. pursed-lip breathing; to prevent airway collapse

■   ■   ■

33 Use of a relaxation technique performed daily can improve ventilation. Explain how.
* _____ .

It decreases anxiety, fear, and panic related to breathlessness.

■   ■   ■

CASE STUDY REVIEW

Mr. Joseph Hall, age 54, has had numerous admissions for severe dyspnea related to emphysema. His clinical signs, symptoms, and findings are stated under clinical applications.

1. Emphysema is classified as a *_____
_____ . Two other lung disorders under this classification are _____
and _____ .

2. Name three physiologic changes that occur in COPD.
*_____ , *_____
_____ , and *_____
_____

3. What is the major risk factor in COPD? _____ .

4. Name the protein produced in the liver that inhibits proteolytic enzymes in the lung.
_____ . A deficit of this protein causes *_____ and the
disease _____ .

5. Four signs and symptoms of COPD are _____ ,
_____ , *_____ ,
and _____ .

6. Mr. Hall's RBC, hemoglobin, and hematocrit values are elevated. Give the reason.
*_____

Mr. Hall's ABG on admission are pH 7.35, $Paco_2$ 73 mm Hg, and HCO_3 28 mEq/L. On day 2 his ABG were pH 7.34, $Paco_2$ 60 mm Hg, HCO_3 37 mEq/L, BE +9.

7. Mr. Hall's acid-base imbalance on admission is *_____
_____ . Is there metabolic compensation? _____ .

8. On day 2 his ABGs indicate *_____ .
Is there metabolic compensation? _____ . Explain. *_____
_____

Mr. Hall received 2 liters per minute of oxygen and ampicillin in IV fluids.

9. Clients with emphysema should not be given a high concentration of oxygen.
Why? *_____

10. Why was Mr. Hall given ampicillin? *_____
_____ .

11. Name three nursing actions to assist Mr. Hall with his breathing.
*_____
*_____
*_____ .

1. *chronic obstructive lung disease (COPD); bronchitis and asthma*
2. *decreased elasticity of lung tissue or loss of elastic recoil, alveoli overdistention and damage, and excess mucous production (others: edema of the bronchial mucosa, hypoxemia)*
3. *smoking*
4. *antitrypsin; damage to lung tissue; emphysema or COPD*
5. *fatigue, dyspnea, barrel-shaped chest, and coughing (others: cyanosis, abnormal ABGs)*
6. *poor oxygenation or hypoxemia*

7. *respiratory acidosis; no*
8. *respiratory acidosis*
   Yes. HCO$_3$ and BE are elevated to decrease acidotic state.
9. *Delivery of a high concentration of oxygen decreases hypoxic respiratory drive.*
10. *His WBC is elevated, indicating a possible infection (respiratory).*
11. *chest clapping, teaching diaphragmatic breathing, and teaching pursed-lip breathing [others: explaining relaxation technique, mild exercise, increase fluids (hydration)]*

NURSING ASSESSMENT FACTORS

- Obtain a client history of respiratory-related problems such as dyspnea at rest and on exertion, increasing shortness of breath, wheezing, fatigue, and activity intolerance.
- Auscultate and percuss the lung areas noting diminished breath sounds, decreased lung expansion, wheezing, crackles, and hyperresonance (hollow sound).
- Check vital signs (VSs) for baseline reading to compare with future VS readings.
- Check the arterial blood gas (ABGs) report. Compare results with the norms: pH 7.35–7.45, Paco$_2$ 35–45 mm Hg, HCO$_3$ 24–28 mEq/L, BE −2 to +2.

NURSING DIAGNOSIS 1

Gas exchange: impaired, related to alveoli damage and the collapse of the bronchial tubes (bronchioles).

NURSING INTERVENTIONS AND RATIONALE

1. Monitor ABGs. Notify the physician when report is returned and abnormal changes are noted. A marked decrease in pH and a marked increase in Paco$_2$ (respiratory acidosis) should be reported immediately.
2. Check the electrolytes and hematology findings when returned and report abnormal results. Elevated hemoglobin and hematocrit indicate hypoxemia.
3. Monitor breath sounds and lung expansion by auscultating and percussing lung area.
4. Assist with the use of aerosol bronchodilators. Check breath sounds after use of aerosol treatments. If breath sounds are not clear or improved, the physician should be notified.

NURSING DIAGNOSIS 2

Airway clearance: ineffective, related to excess mucous secretions and the collapse of the bronchial tubes secondary to COPD.

NURSING INTERVENTIONS AND RATIONALE

1. Check breath sounds for rhonchi and rales. Provide chest physiotherapy (chest clapping) for rhonchi and have client deep breathe and cough to clear bronchial secretions.
2. Instruct the client how to do breathing exercises; i.e., pursed-lip breathing (to prevent airway collapse) and diaphragmatic breathing (to increase alveolar ventilation).

3. Instruct the client not to get overfatigued and to avoid smoking, carefully use chemical irritants (bleaches, paints, and aerosol hair spray), avoid people with respiratory infections, air pollution, excess dust, pollen, and extreme heat or cold weather, all of which increase breathlessness.
4. Instruct the client to use bronchodilators as directed. Overuse of pressurized bronchodilator aerosol can cause a rebound effect.
5. Monitor fluid and food intake. Hydration is important to liquify tenacious mucous secretions. Frequent small feedings may be necessary.
6. Instruct the client to recognize early signs of respiratory infections, i.e., change in sputum color, elevated temperature, and coughing.

NURSING DIAGNOSIS 3

Cardiac output: decreased, related to breathlessness and hypoxemia secondary to COPD.

NURSING INTERVENTIONS AND RATIONALE

1. Monitor vital signs. Report increase in pulse rate and changes in the rate of respiration. Labored breathing is a common sign of a respiratory problem.
2. Encourage the client to limit activities that increase the body's need for oxygen.

NURSING DIAGNOSIS 4

Anxiety, related to breathlessness, dependence on others, and the treatment regime.

NURSING INTERVENTIONS AND RATIONALE

1. Encourage the client to select and engage in a relaxation technique; help in the selection. Relaxation helps to decrease oxygen need by body tissues.
2. Explain the treatment and nursing care to the client and family members and answer questions or refer them to the physician.
3. Be supportive of client and family members.
4. Refer to support groups, community agencies, and/or assistance programs.

NURSING DIAGNOSIS 5

Activity intolerance, related to breathlessness and fatigue.

NURSING INTERVENTIONS AND RATIONALE

1. Assist the client with the activities of daily living (ADLs) as needed.
2. Encourage the client to try mild exercises in the afternoon or when breathlessness is not severe. Avoid early mornings when mucous secretions are increased and after meals when energy is needed for digestion.
3. Observe for signs and symptoms for COPD, i.e., changes in vital signs, dyspnea, fatigue, barrel-shaped chest and cyanosis. Barrel-shaped chest results from dilated alveoli, inability to expel trapped air in the alveoli, and long-term effect of COPD.

OTHER POTENTIAL NURSING DIAGNOSES

1. Breathing patterns: ineffective, related to CO_2 retention and poor gas exchange secondary to COPD.
2. Tissue perfusion altered: related to hypoxemia.
3. Nutrition: altered, less than body requirements, related to breathlessness.
4. Comfort: altered, related to breathlessness and muscle pain (diaphragm, intercostal).
5. Coping: ineffective, related to breathlessness and life style changes.
6. High risk for injury: lungs, related to smoking and respiratory infections.
7. Physical mobility: impaired, related to breathlessness.
8. Self-care deficit, related to the inability to take part in ADLs because of dyspnea or breathlessness.

abdomen   the portion of the body lying between the chest and the pelvis.

acid   any substance that is sour in taste and that neutralizes a basic substance.

acid metabolites   see metabolites.

ACTH   abbreviation for adrenocorticotropic hormone. A hormone secreted by the hypophysis or pituitary gland. It stimulates the adrenal cortex to secrete cortisone.

afterload   resistance in the vessels against which the ventricle ejects blood during systole.

aged   age of 65 years or older.

albumin   simple protein. It is the main protein from the blood.

   serum   Primary function is to maintain the colloid osmotic pressure of the blood.

alimentary   pertaining to nutrition; the alimentary tract is a digestive tube from the mouth to the anus.

alkaline   any substance that can neutralize an acid and that, when combined with an acid, forms a salt.

alveolus   air sac or cell of the lung.

amphoteric   ability to bind or release excess H^+.

anesthetic   an agent causing an insensibility to pain or touch.

anion   a negatively charged ion.

anorexia   a loss of appetite.

anoxia   oxygen deficiency.

antipyretic   a medication that reduces body core temperature.

anuria   a complete urinary suppression.

aortic arch   the arch of the aorta soon after it leaves the heart.

aphasia   a loss of the power of speech.

arrhythmia   irregular heart rhythm.

arterioles   minute arteries leading into a capillary.

arteriosclerosis   pertaining to thickening, hardening, and loss of elasticity of the walls of the blood vessels.

artery   a vessel carrying blood from the heart to the tissue.

ascites   an accumulation of serous fluid in the peritoneal cavity.

atrium   a chamber. In the heart it is the upper chamber of each half of the heart.

atrophy   decrease in size of structure.

autoregulation   control of blood flow to tissue by a change in the tissue.

azotemia   an excessive quantity of nitrogenous waste products in the blood increased BUN and creatinine.

biliary   pertaining to or conveying bile.

blood   intravascular fluid composed of red and white blood cells and platelets.

bradycardia   pulse rate less than 50 beats per minute.

brain interstitium   spaces between the brain tissues.

brain parenchyma   functional tissue of the brain.

brain stem herniation   protrusion of the medulla, pons, and midbrain into the spinal canal.

bronchiectasis   dilatation of a bronchus.

BUN   abbreviation for blood urea nitrogen. Urea is a by-product of protein metabolism.

butterfly (winged tip)   an infusion device designed for short-term parenteral therapy. Each set consists of a wing-tip needle with a metal cannula, plastic or rubber wings and plastic catheter or hub. The needle is $\frac{1}{2}$–$1\frac{1}{2}$ inches long with needle gauges of 15–26. The infusion needle and clear tubing are bonded into a single unit. It is commonly used for children and elderly who may have small or fragile veins.

capillary   a minute blood vessel connecting the smallest arteries (arterioles) with the smallest veins (venules).

capillary permeability   diffusion of substances from capillary walls into tissue spaces.

carbonic anhydrase inhibitor   an agent used as a diuretic that inhibits the enzyme carbonic anhydrase.

cardiac output   amount of blood ejected by the heart each minute.

cardiac reserve   capacity of the heart to respond to increased burden.

carotid sinus   a dilated area at the bifurcation of the carotid artery that is richly supplied with sensory nerve endings of the sinus branch of the vagus nerve.

cation   a positively charged ion.

cerebral hemorrhage   bleeding into brain tissue from rupture in a blood vessel.

cerebral spinal fluid   fluid contained within the ventricles of the brain and spinal cord.

cerebrospinal fluid   fluid found and circulating through the brain and spinal cord.

cirrhosis   a chronic disease of the liver characterized by degenerative changes in the liver cells.

colloid   gelatinlike substance, e.g., protein.

colloid osmotic pressure   pressure exerted by nondiffusible substances.

congestive heart failure (CHF)   circulatory congestion related to pump failure.

contraindication   nonindicated form of therapy.

conversion table:
> 1 kilogram (kg) = 2.2 pounds (lb)
> 1 gram = 1000 milligrams (mg) or 15 grains (gr)
> 1 liter (L) = 1 quart or 1000 milliliters (mL)
> 1 cubic centimeter (cc) = 1 milliliter (mL); 100 mL = dL
> 1 deciliter (dL) = 100 mL
> 1 drop (gtt) = 1 minim (m)
> qh = every hour
> × = times

cortisone   a hormone secreted by the adrenal cortex.

creatinine   end product of creatine (amino acid).

crystalloids   diffusible substances dissolved in solution that pass through a selectively permeable membrane.

CVP   abbreviation for central venous pressure. It is the venous pressure in the vena cava or the heart's right atrium.

cyanosis   a bluish or grayish discoloration of the skin due to a lack of oxygen in the hemoglobin of the blood.

cytogenic   originating within the cell.

decerebrate   condition wherein the brain cells are affected, causing the extremities to be in rigid extension.

decompensation   failure to compensate.

decorticate   condition wherein the cortex of the brain is affected, causing the extremities to be in rigid flexion.

deficit   lack of.

dependent edema   see edema.

dermis   the true skin layer.

dextran   colloid hyperosmolar solution.

dextrose   a simple sugar, also known as glucose.

diabetes mellitus   a disorder of carbohydrate metabolism due to an inadequate production or utilization of insulin.

diabetic acidosis   an excessive production of ketone bodies (acid) due to a lack of insulin and inability to utilize carbohydrates, also called diabetic ketoacidosis.

dialysate   an isotonic solution used in dialysis that has similar electrolyte content to plasma or Ringer's solution, with the exception of potassium.

diaphoresis   excessive perspiration.

diffusion   the movement of each molecule along its own pathway irrespective of all other molecules; going in various directions, mostly from greater to lesser concentration.

diplopia   double vision.

630

disequilibrium syndrome   rapid shift of fluids and electrolytes during hemodialysis which causes CNS disturbances.

dissociation   a separation.

diuresis   an abnormal increase in urine excretion.

diuretic   a drug used to increase the secretion of urine.

   potassium-sparing diuretic   retains potassium and excretes other electrolytes.

   potassium-wasting diuretic   excretes potassium and other electrolytes.

diverticulum   a sac or pouch in the wall of an organ.

dry weight   normal body weight without excess water.

duodenal   pertaining to the duodenum, which is the first part of the small intestine.

dyspnea   a labored or difficult breathing.

edema   an abnormal retention of fluid in the interstitial spaces.

   dependent edema   fluid present in the interstitial spaces due to gravity (frequency found in extremities after being in standing or sitting position).

   nondependent edema   fluid present in the interstitial spaces, but not necessarily due to gravity along, e.g., cardiac, liver, or kidney dysfunction.

   pitting edema   depression in the edematous tissue.

   pulmonary edema   fluid throughout the lung tissue.

   refractory edema   fluid in the interstitial spaces that does not respond to diuretics.

e.g.   for example.

electrolyte   a substance that, when in solution, conducts an electric current.

endothelium   flat cells that line the blood and lymphatic vessels.

enzyme   a catalyst, capable of inducting chemical changes in other substances.

epidermis   an outer layer of the skin.

erythrocytes   red blood cells.

erythropoietin   factor secreted by the kidneys that stimulates bone marrow to produce red blood cells.

excess   too much.

excretion   an elimination of waste products from the body.

excretory   pertaining to excretion.

extract   outside of.

extracellular fluid volume shift (ECF shift)   shift of fluid within the ECF compartment from intravascular to interstitial spaces or from the interstitial to the intravascular spaces.

febrile   pertaining to a fever.

flatus   gas in the alimentary tract.

generic name   reflects the chemical family to which a drug belongs. The name never changes.

globulin   a group of simple proteins.

glomerulus   a capillary loop enclosed within the Bowman's capsule of the kidney.

glucose   formed from carbohydrates during digestion and frequently called dextrose.

glycogen   a stored form of sugar in the liver or muscle that can be converted to glucose.

glycosuria   sugar in the urine.

gt   abbreviation for drop.

gtt   abbreviation for drops.

hematocrit   the volume of red blood cells or erythrocytes in a given volume of blood.

hemoconcentration   increase in number of red blood cells and solutes, and a decrease in plasma volume.

hemodilution   an increase in the volume of blood plasma due to a lack of red blood cells and solutes or an excess of intravascular fluid.

hemoglobin   conjugated protein consisting of iron-containing pigment in the erythrocyte.

hemolysis   destruction of red blood cells and causing release of hemoglobin into the serum.

heparin   anticoagulant.

hepatic coma   liver failure.

hernia   a protrusion of an organ through the wall of a cavity.

   inguinal   protrusion of the intestine at the inguinal opening.

homeostasis   uniformity or stability. State of equilibrium of the internal environment.

hormone   a chemical substance originating in an organ or gland, which travels through the blood and is capable of increasing body activity or secretion.

   ADH   abbreviation for antidiuretic hormone; a hormone to lessen urine secretion.

hydrocephalus   increased fluid retention in the ventricles of the brain.

hydrostatic pressure   pressure of fluids at equilibrium.

hyperalimentation   intravenous administration of a hyperosmolar solution of glucose, protein, vitamins, and electrolytes to promote tissue synthesis.

hyperbaric oxygenation   oxygen under pressure carried in the plasma.

hypercalcemia   a high serum calcium.

hypercapnia   increased carbon dioxide in the blood.

hyperchloremia   a high serum chloride.

hyperglycemia   condition where blood glucose levels are elevated above normal.

hyperkalemia   a high serum potassium.

hypernatremia   a high serum sodium.

hyperosmolar   increased number of osmols per solution. Increased solute concentration as compared to plasma.

hypertension   high blood pressure.

   essential   a high blood pressure that develops in the absence of kidney disease. It is also called primary hypertension.

hypertonic   a higher solute concentration than plasma.

hypertrophy   increased thickening of a structure.

hyperventilation   breathing at a rate greater than needed for body requirements.

hypervolemia   an increase in blood volume.

hypocalcemia   a low-serum calcium.

hypochloremia   a low-serum chloride.

hypoglycemia   low blood sugar.

hypokalemia   a low-serum potassium.

hyponatremia   a low-serum sodium.

hypo-osmolality   condition where number for formed particles in the serum is decreased.

hypo-osmolar   decreased number of osmols per solution. Decreased solute concentration as compared to plasma.

hypophysis   the pituitary gland.

hypotension   a low blood pressure.

hypotonic   a lower solute concentration than plasma.

hypoventilation   breathing at a rate lower than required to meet metabolic demands.

hypovolemia   a decrease in blood volume.

hypoxia   decreased oxygen content in body tissue.

hypoxemia   reduced oxygen content in the blood.

i.e.   that is.

incarcerated   constricted, as an irreducible hernia.

infusion   an injection of a solution directly into a vein.

in-needle catheter (INC)   an infusion device designed for short-term parenteral therapy (opposite of the over needle catheter—ONC) which is constructed exactly opposite the ONC. Needle length is 1½–3 inches with a catheter length of 8–36 inches. The catheter is available in gauges of 8–22. The INC set comes with a catheter sleeve guard which must be secured over the needle bevel to prevent severing the catheter. It is commonly used for more prolonged infusions. Catheters used in INCs and ONCs are constructed of silicone, Teflon, polyvinyl chloride, or polyethylene.

insensible perspiration   water loss by diffusion through the skin.

insulin   a hormone secreted by the beta cells of the islets of Langerhans found in the pancreas. It is important in the oxidation and utilization of blood sugar (glucose).

inter   between.

interstitial edema   accumulation of excess fluid between cells; this is extracellular fluid.

632

intervention   action.

intra   within.

intracerebral edema   accumulation of excess fluid within the brain tissue and structures.

intracerebral hypertension   increased pressure within the brain structures.

intracranial pressure   pressure exerted by fluid within the brain structures.

ion   a particle carrying either a positive or negative charge.

ionization   separation into ions.

ionizing   separating into ions.

iso-osmolar   same number of osmols per solution as compared to plasma.

isotonic   same solute concentration as plasma.

ketone bodies   oxidation of fatty acids.

ketonuria   excess ketones in urine.

Kussmaul breathing   hyperactive, abnormally vigorous breathing.

lassitude   weariness.

lidocaine   also known as xylocaine. A drug used as a surface anesthetic. It also can be used to treat ventricular arrhythmias.

lymph   an alkaline fluid. It is similar to plasma except that its protein content is lower.

lymphatic system   the conveyance of lymph from the tissues to the blood.

malaise   uneasiness, ill feeling.

medulla   the central portion of an organ, e.g., adrenal gland.

membrane   a layer of tissue that covers a surface or organ or separates a space.

mercurial diuretic   a drug that affects the proximal tubules of the kidneys by inhibiting reabsorption of sodium.

midbrain   connects the pons and cerebellum with the cerebral hemispheres.

metabolism   the physical and chemical changes involved in the utilization of particular substances.

metabolites   the by-products of cellular metabolism or catabolism.

milliequivalent   the chemical activity of elements.

milligram   measures the weight of ions.

milliosmol   1/1000th of an osmol. It involves the osmotic activity of a solution.

molar   1 gram molecular weight of a substance.

myocardium   the muscle of the heart.

narcotic   a drug that depresses the central nervous system, relieves pain, and can induce sleep.

necrosis   destroyed tissue.

nephritis   inflammation of the kidney.

nephrosis   degenerative changes in the kidney.

neuromuscular   pertaining to the nerve and muscle.

neuromuscular junction   the innervation of the nerve with a muscle.

nondependent edema   see edema.

nonvolatile acid   fixed acid resulting from metabolic processes, excreted by the kidneys.

oliguria   a diminished amount of urine.

oral rehydration fluid   oral fluids designed to replace fluid and electrolyte losses in clients (usually children) who are able to tolerate liquids. These fluids are made up of similar concentrations of glucose, sodium, potassium, chloride, and bicarbonate of soda. Examples include WHO, Hydra-lyte, Rehydra-lyte, Lytren, ReSol, and Infalyte.

osmol   a unit of osmotic pressure.

osmolality   osmols or milliosmols per kilogram of water.

osmolarity   osmols or milliosmols per liter of solution.

osmosis   the passage of a solvent through a partition from a solution of lesser solute concentration to one of greater solute concentration.

osmotic pressure   the pressure or force that develops when two solutions are of different concentrations and are separated by a selectively permeable membrane.

otorrhea   drainage from the ear.

over-needle catheter   an infusion device designed for short-term parenteral therapy (opposite of the INC). The bevel of the needle extends beyond the catheter, which is 1¼–8 inches in length. The needle is available in gauges of 8–22. It is more comfortable for the client. See also in-needle catheter.

oxygenation   the combination of oxygen in tissues and blood.

oxyhemoglobin   hemoglobin carrying oxygen.

packed cells   red blood cells (RBCs).

pallor or pallid   pale.

PAP   abbreviation for pulmonary artery pressure. It measures the pressure in the pulmonary artery.

paracentesis   the surgical puncture of a cavity, e.g., abdomen.

parathyroid   an endocrine gland secreting the hormone parathormone, which regulates calcium and phosphorus metabolism.

parenteral therapy   introduction of fluids into the body by means other than the alimentary tract.

parietal lobe   lobe on the side of the brain lying under the parietal bone.

patency   the state of being opened.

PCWP   abbreviation for pulmonary capillary wedge pressure. Its reading indicates the pumping ability of the left ventricle. Left ventricular end-diastolic pressure (LVEDP) is the best indicator of ventricular function. PCWP reflects LVEDP.

perfusion   passing of fluid through body space.

pericardial sac   fibroserous sac enclosing the heart.

pericarditis   inflammation of the pericardium or the membrane that encloses the heart.

peristalsis   wavelike movement occurring with hollow tubes such as the intestine for the movement of contents.

peritoneal cavity   a lining covering the abdominal organs with the exclusion of the kidneys.

permeability   capability of fluids and/or other substances, e.g., ions, to diffuse through a human membrane.

  selectively permeable membrane   refers to the human membrane.

  semipermeable membrane   refers to artificial membranes.

phlebitis   inflammation of the vein.

physiologic   pertaining to body function.

pitting edema   see edema.

plasma   intravascular fluid composed of water, ions, and colloid. Plasma is frequently referred to as serum.

plasmanate   commercially prepared protein product used in place of plasma.

pleural cavity   the space between the two pleuras.

pleurisy   inflammation of the pleura or the membranes that enclose the lung.

polyionic   many ions or ionic changes.

polyuria   an excessive amount or discharge of urine.

pons   that part of the brain that connects the cerebral hemispheres.

porosity   the state of being porous.

portal circulation   circulation of the blood through the liver.

postoperative   following an operation.

potassium-sparing diuretics   see diuretics.

potassium-wasting diuretics   see diuretics.

prednisone   synthetic hormonal drug resembling cortisone.

preload   pressure of the blood that fills the left ventricle during diastole.

pressoreceptor   sensory nerve ending in the aorta and carotid sinus, which when stimulated causes a change in the blood pressure.

pressure gradient   the difference in pressure which makes the fluid flow.

proprioception   awareness of one's movement and position in space.

protein   nitrogenous compounds essential to all living organisms.

  plasma   relates to albumin, globulin, and fibrinogen.

  serum   relates to albumin and globulin.

pruritis   itching

psychogenic polydipsia   psychologic effect of drinking excessive amounts of water.

pulmonary artery pressure   see PAP.
pulmonary capillary wedge pressure   see PCWP.
pulmonary edema   see edema.
pulse pressure   the arithmetic difference between the systolic and diastolic blood pressure.

rales   pertaining to rattle. It is the sound heard in the chest due to the passage of air through the bronchi which contain secretions or fluid.
rationale   the reason.
reabsorption   the act of absorbing again an excreted substance.
refractory edema   see edema.
retention   retaining or holding back in the body.
reticular activating system   alert awareness system of the brain formed from the thalamus, hypothalamus, and cortex.
rhinorrhea   drainage from the nose.

sclerosis   hardening of an organ or tissue.
selectively permeable membrane   see permeability.
semi-Fowler's position   45° elevation.
semipermeable membrane   see permeability.
sensible perspiration   the loss of water on the skin due to sweat gland activity.
serous cavity   a cavity lined by a serous membrane.
serum   consists of plasma minus the fibrinogen. It is the same as plasma except that after coagulation of blood, the fibrinogen is removed. Serum is frequently referred to as plasma.
sign   an objective indication of disease.
solute   a substance dissolved in a solution.
solvent   a liquid with a substance in solution.
specific gravity   a weight of a substance, e.g., urine. Water has a specific gravity of 1.000. The specific gravity of urine is higher.
steroid   an organic compound. It is frequently referred to as an adrenal cortex hormone.
stress   effect of a harmful condition or disease(s) affecting the body.
stroke volume   amount of blood ejected by the left ventricle with each contraction.
sympathetic nervous system   a part of the autonomic nervous system. It can act in an emergency.
symptom   subjective indication.

tachycardia   a fast heart beat.
tetany   a nervous affection characterized by tonic spasms of muscles.
thrombophlebitis   inflammation of a vein with a thrombus or a blood clot.
total parenteral nutrition (TPN)   also known as hyperalimentation.
trade name   the name given to a drug by its manufacturer.
transudation   the passage of fluid through the pores of a membrane.
trauma   an injury.

urea   the final product of protein metabolism that is normally excreted by the kidneys.
uremia   a toxic condition due to the retention of nitrogenous substances (protein by-products), such as urea, which cannot be excreted by the kidneys.

Valsalva maneuver   procedure in which individual takes deep breath and bears down to increase intrathoracic pressure for prevention of air injection. Forced exhalation closes the glottis.
vasoconstriction   decrease in size of a blood vessel.
vasodilation   increase in size of a blood vessel.
vasogenic   originating within the blood vessels.
vasomotor   pertaining to the nerves having a muscular contraction or relaxation control of the blood vessel walls.
vasopressors   drugs given to contract muscles of the blood vessel walls to increase the blood pressure.
vein   a vessel carrying unoxygenated blood to the heart.

ventilation   the circulation of air.

   pulmonary   the inspiration and expiration of air from the lungs.

ventricles   the lower chambers of the heart.

venules   minute veins moving from capillaries.

vertigo   dizziness.

volatile acid   acid excreted as a gas by the lungs.

winged-tip infusion device   see butterfly.

American Nurses Association (1991). *Standards of clinical nursing practice.* Kansas City: American Nurses Association.

Baird, S. B., McConkle, R., & Grant, M. (1991). *Cancer nursing: A comprehensive textbook.* Philadelphia: Saunders.

Baker, W. L. (1985). Hypophosphatemia. *American Journal of Nursing, 85*(9), 998–1003.

Barrows, J. J. (1982). Shock demands drugs. *Nursing 1982, 12*(2), 34–41.

Baxter, C. R., & Waeckerle, J. F. (1988). Emergency treatment of burn trauma. *Journal of Trauma, 17,* 1305–1315.

Beckwith, N. (1987). Fundamentals of fluid resuscitation. *Nursing Life, 2*(3), 51–55.

Bidani, A. (1991). Electrolyte and acid-base disorders, 1013–1035.

Birney, M. H., & Penney, D. G. (1990). Atrial natriuretic peptide: A hormone with implications for clinical practice. *Heart and Lung, 19*(2), 174–182.

Bloch, A. S. (1990). *Nutrition management of the cancer patient.* Rockville, MD: Aspen.

Borgen, L. (1978). Total parenteral nutrition. *American Journal of Nursing, 78*(2), 224–228.

Bouchard-Kurtz R., & Speese-Owens, N. (1981). *Nursing care of the cancer patient* (4th ed.). St. Louis: Mosby.

Bryant, K. K. (1991). Burn trauma: The emergent phase of care. *Contemporary perspectives in trauma nursing.* An independent home study course for individual continuing education. Chicago: Forum Medicum.

Brunner, L. S., & Suddarth, D. S. (1988). *Textbook of medical-surgical nursing* (6th ed.). Philadelphia: Lippincott.

Burnside, I. (1988). *Nursing and the aged: A self care approach* (3rd ed.). New York: McGraw-Hill.

Butts, E. E. (1987). Fluid and electrolyte disorders associated with diabetic ketoacidosis and hyperglycemic hyperosmolar nonketotic coma. *Nursing Clinics of North America, 22*(4), 827–836.

Cannon, P. J. (1989). Sodium retention in heart failure. *Cardiology Clinics, 7*(1), 49–59.

Carpenito, L. J. (1992). *Nursing diagnosis: Application to clinical practice* (4th ed.). Philadelphia: Lippincott.

Cefalu, W. T. (1991). Diabetic ketoacidosis. *Critical Care Clinics, 7*(1), 89–107.

Chambers, J. K. (1987). Fluid and electrolyte problems in renal and urologic disorders. *Nursing Clinics of North America, 22*(4), 815–825.

Chernecky, C. C., & Ramsey, P. W. (1984). *Critical nursing care of the client with cancer.* E. Norwalk, CT: Appleton-Century-Crofts.

Chernow, B., Bamberger, E., & Stoiko, M. (1989). Hypomagnesemia in patients in postoperative intensive care. *Chest, 95*(2), 391–396.

Christopher, K. L. (1980). The use of a model for hemodynamic balance to describe burn shock. *Nursing Clinics of North America, 15*(3), 617–627.

Clark, J. C., & McGee, R. N. (1992). *Core curriculum for oncology nursing.* Philadelphia: Saunders.

Coroenwald, S., Frogge, M. H., Goodman, M., & Yarbro, C. H. (1992). *Comprehensive cancer nursing review.* Boston: Jones & Bartlett.

Cunningham, S. G. (1982). Fluid and electrolyte disturbances associated with cancer and its treatment. *Nursing Clinics of North America, 17*(4), 579–591.

Davis, K. D., & Attie, M. F. (1991). Management of severe hypercalcemia. *Critical Care Clinics, 7*(1), 175–189.

Doran, A. (1992). S.I.A.D.D.: Is your patient at risk? *Nursing 92, 22*(6), 60–63.

Elbaum, N. (1977). Detecting and correcting magnesium imbalance. *Nursing 1977, 7*(8), 34–35.

Felver, L., & Pendarvis, J. H. (1989). Electrolyte imbalances. *AORN Journal, 49*(4), 992–1005.

Freeman, B. I., & Burkart, J. M. (1991). Hypokalemia. *Critical Care Clinics, 7*(1), 143–153.

Fundamentals of body water and electrolytes. (1981). Travenol Laboratories, Parenteral Products, Deerfield, IL.

Fundamentals of fluid and electrolyte imbalances. (1982). Travenol Laboratories, Parenteral Products, Deerfield, IL.

German, K. (1987). Fluid and electrolyte problems associated with diabetes insipidus and syndrome of inappropriate antidiuretic hormone. *Nursing Clinics of North America, 22*(4), 785–795.

Gershan, J. A., Freeman, C. M., Ross, M. C., & members of the Research committee, Greater Milwaukee area chapter of the American Association of Critical Care Nurses (1990). *Heart and Lung, 19*(2), 152–156.

Giesecke, A. H., Grande, C. M., & Whitten, C. W. (1990). Fluid therapy and the resuscitation of traumatic shock. *Critical Care Clinics, 6*(1), 61–71.

Green, M. G. (1991). *Harriet Lane handbook* (12th ed.). St. Louis: Mosby Yearbook.

Groer, M. W., & Shekleton, M. E. (1983). *Basic pathophysiology* (2nd ed.). St. Louis: Mosby.

Guyton, A. C. (1981). *Textbook of medical physiology* (5th ed.). Philadelphia: Saunders.

Hayter, J. (1978). Emergency nursing care of the burned patient. *Nursing Clinics of North America, 13*(2), 223–243.

Hecker, J. (1988). Improve techniques in IV therapy. *Nursing Times, 84*(34), 28–33.

Heitkemper, M. M., & Bond, E. (1988). Fluid and electrolytes: Assessment and interventions. *Journal of Enterostomal Therapy, 15*(1), 18–23.

Hikey, J. V. (1986). *The clinical practice of neurological and neurosurgical nursing* (2nd ed.). Philadelphia: Lippincott.

Hollifield, J. W. (1989). Electrolyte disarray and cardiovascular disease. *American Journal of Cardiology, 63,* 21B–26B.

Intravenous Nurses's Society (1990). *Intravenous nursing standards of practice.* Belmont, ME: Intravenous Nurses's Society.

Jones, A. M., Moseley, M. J., Halfmann, S. J., Heath, A. H., & Henkelman, N. J. (1991). Fluid volume dynamics. *Critical Care Nurse, 11*(4), 74–76.

Jones, D. H. (1991). Fluid therapy in the PACU. *Critical Care Nursing Clinics of North America, 3*(1), 109–130.

Kamel, K. S., Ethier, J. H., & Richardson, M. A. (1990). Urine electrolytes and osmolality: When and how to use them. *American Journal of Nephrology, 10*(2), 89–102.

Kamel, K. S., Magner, P. O. C., Ethier, J. H., & Halperin, M. L. (1989). Urine electrolytes in the assessment of extracellular fluid volume contraction. *American Journal of Nephrology, 9*(4), 344–347.

Karb, V. B. (1989). Electrolyte abnormalities and drugs which commonly cause them. *Journal of Neuroscience Nursing, 21*(2), 125–128.

Kee, J. L. (1987). Potassium imbalance. *Nursing 1987, 17*(9), 32 K, M, P.

Kee, J. L. (1991). *Laboratory and diagnostic tests with nursing implications* (3rd ed.). E. Norwalk, CT: Appleton & Lange.

Kee, J. L., & Gregory, A. P. (1974). The ABC's (and mEq's) of fluid balance in children. *Nursing 1974, 4*(6), 28–36.

Kehoe, C. (1991). Malignant ascites: Etiology, diagnosis, and treatment. *Oncology Nursing Forum, 18,* 523–530.

Keyes, J. L. (1974). Blood-gas and blood-gas transport. *Heart and Lung, 3*(6), 945–954.

Keyes, J. L. (1976). Blood-gas analysis and the assessment of acid-base status. *Heart and Lung, 5*(2), 247–255.

King, C. R., Hoffart, N., & Murray, M. E. (1992). Acute renal failure in bone marrow transplantation. *Oncology Nursing Forum, 19,* 1327–1335.

Kiss, S., & Kaiser, J. (1990). *Emergency nursing: A physiologic and clinical perspective.* Philadelphia: Saunders.

Kleihenz, T. J. (1985). Preload and afterload. *Nursing 1985, 15*(5), 50–55.

Klemm, P. (1992). *Total nutritional admixture (TNA): Programmed instruction.* Baltimore: Johns Hopkins Hospital Department of Nursing.

Kokko, J. P., & Tanner, R. L. (1990). *Fluids and electrolytes* (2nd ed.). Philadelphia: Saunders.

Kositzke, J. A. (1990). A question of balance, dehydration in the elderly. *Journal of Gerontologic Nursing, 16*(5), 4–11, 40–41.

Krieger, J. N., & Sherrard, D. J. (1991). *Practical fluids and electrolytes.* E. Norwalk, CT: Appleton & Lange.

Lancaster, L. E. (1987a). *Core curriculum for nephrology nursing.* Pitman, NJ: Jannetti, Anthony J.

Lancaster, L. E. (1987b). Renal and endocrine regulation of water and electrolyte balance. *Nursing Clinics of North America, 22*(4), 761–772.

Lancour, J. (1978). ADH and aldosterone: How to recognize their effects. *Nursing 1978, 8*(9), 36–41.

Leaf, A., & Cotran, R. (1985). *Renal pathophysiology* (3rd ed.). New York: Oxford University Press.

Levy, D. B., & Peppers, M. P. (1991). IV fluids used in shock. *Emergency, 23*(4), 22–26.

Luckmann, J., & Sorensen, D. C. (1987). *Medical-surgical nursing* (3rd ed.). Philadelphia: Saunders.

MacLeod, S. (1975). The rational use of potassium supplements. *Postgraduate Medicine, 57*(2), 123–127.

Matheson, M. (1989). Intravenous therapy. *Critical Care Nurse, 9*(2), 21–34.

McCance, K., & Huether, S. (1990). *Pathophysiology: The biologic basis for disease in adults and children.* St. Louis: Mosby.

McConnell, E. A. (1987). Fluid and electrolyte concerns in intestinal surgical procedures. *Nursing Clinics of North America, 22*(4), 853–859.

McDermott, K. C., Almadrones, L. A., & Bajorunas, D. R. (1991). The diagnosis and management of hypomagnesemia: A unique treatment approach and case report. *Oncology Nursing Forum, 18,* 1145–1152.

McFadden, M. E., & Gatoricos, S. E. (1992). Multiple systems organ failure in the patient with cancer, Part I: Pathophysiologic perspectives. *Oncology Nursing Forum, 19,* 719–727.

Meador, B. (1982). Cardiogenic shock. *RN, 45*(4), 38–42.

Medical Center of Delaware (1992). *Calculating infusion rate.* Newark, DE: Medical Center Orientation Materials.

Menzel, L. (1980). Clinical problems of fluid balance. *Nursing Clinics of North America, 15*(3), 549–576.

Metheny, N. M. (1990). Why worry about IV fluids? *American Journal of Nursing, 90*(6), 50–57.

Metheny, N. M. (1992). *Fluid and electrolyte balance* (2nd ed.). Philadelphia: Lippincott.

Metheny, N. M., & Snively, W. D. (1983). *Nurses' handbook of fluid balance* (4th ed.). Philadelphia: Lippincott.

Meyers, K. A., & Hickey, M. K. (1988). Nursing management of hypovolemic shock. *Critical Care Nursing Quarterly, 11*(1), 57–67.

Millam, D. (1991). Myths and facts . . . About IV therapy. *Nursing 91, 21*(6), 75–76.

Miller, C. A. (1990). *Nursing care of older adults: Theory and practice.* Glenview, IL: Scott Foresman/Little, Brown.

Moiser, L. C. (1991). Anaphylaxis: A preventable complication of home infusion therapy. *Journal of Intravenous Nursing, 14*(2), 108–112.

Mueller, K. D., & Boisen, A. M. (1989). Keeping your patient's water level up. *RN, 52*(7), 65–68.

Nanji, A. (1983). Drug-induced electrolyte disorder. *Drug Intelligence and Clinical Pharmacy, 17,* 175–185.

Narins, R. G. (1982). Diagnostic strategies in disorders of fluid, electrolyte and acid-base homeostasis. *American Journal of Medicine, 72,* 496–518.

Norris, M. K. (1989). Dialysis disequilibrium syndrome. Action stat! *Nursing 1989, 19*(4), 33.

O'Donnell, T. F., & Belkin, S. C. (1978). The pathophysiology, monitoring, and treatment of shock. *Orthopedic Clinics of North America, 9*(3), 589–610.

Olinger, M. L. (1989). Disorders of calcium and magnesium metabolism. *Emergency Medicine Clinics of North America, 7*(4), 795–819.

Otto, S. (1991). *Oncology nursing.* St. Louis: Mosby Year Book.

Peppers, M. P., Geheb, M., & Desai, T. (1991). Hypophosphatemia and hyperphosphatemia. *Critical Care Clinics, 7*(1), 201–213.

Perkin, R., & Levin, D. L. (1980). Common fluid and electrolyte problems in the pediatric intensive care unit. *Pediatric Clinics of North America, 27*(3), 567–586.

Perry, A., & Potter, P. (1983). *Shock.* St. Louis: Mosby.

Phipps, W. J., Long, B. C., & Woods, N. F. (1987). *Medical surgical nursing* (3rd ed.). St. Louis: Mosby.

Plumer, A. L. (1987a). Parenteral fluids and related fluid and electrolyte abnormalities (chap. 9). In *Principles and practice of intravenous therapy* (4th ed.). Boston: Little, Brown.

Plumer, A. L. (1987b). Rationale of fluid and electrolyte therapy (chap. 8). In *Principles and practice of intravenous therapy (4th ed.).* Boston: Little, Brown.

Poe, C. M., & Radford, A. L. (1985). The challenge of hypercalcemia in cancer. *Oncology Nursing Forum, 12*(6), 29–34.

Porth, C. M. (1990). *Pathophysiology* (3rd ed.). Philadelphia: Lippincott.

Price, C. (1989). Continuous renal replacement therapy, from a professional nursing perspective. *Nephrology News and Issues, 3*(7), 31–34.

Ragland, G. (1990). Electrolyte abnormalities in the alcoholic patient. *Emergency Medicine Clinics of North America, 8*(4), 761–771.

Rice, V. (1981). Shock, a clinical syndrome. *Critical Care Nurse, 1*(5), 34–43.

Rice, V. (1985). Shock management, Part II. Pharmacologic interventions. *Critical Care Nurse, 5*(1), 42–56.

Rose, B. D. (1989). *Clinical physiology of acid-base and electrolyte disorders* (3rd ed.). New York: McGraw-Hill.

Ross Roundtable Report, 12th. (1992). Enteral nutrition support for the 1990's: Innovations in nutrition, technology and techniques. Columbus, OH: Ross Laboratories (Division of Abbott Laboratories).

Rutherford, C. (1989). Fluid and electrolyte therapy: Considerations for patient care. *Journal of Intravenous Nursing, 12*(3), 175–183.

Salem, M., Munoz, R., & Chernow, B. (1991). Hypomagnesemia in critical illness. *Critical Care Clinics, 7*(1), 225–247.

Schrier, R. W. (1986). *Renal and electrolyte disorders* (3rd ed.). Boston: Little, Brown.

Shakir, K. M. M., & Amin, R. M. (1991). Hypoglycemia. *Critical Care Clinics, 7*(1), 75–87.

Smith, Z. H., & VanGeilick, A. J. (1992). Management of neutropenic enterocolitis in the patient with cancer. *Oncology Nursing Forum, 19,* 1337–1342.

Snider, M. A. (1974). Helpful hints on IV's. *American Journal of Nursing, 74,* 1978–1981.

Sommers, M. (1990). Rapid fluid resuscitation: How to correct dangerous deficits. *Nursing 1990, 20*(1), 52–60.

Statland, H. (1963). *Fluid and electrolyte in practice* (3rd ed). Philadelphia: Lippincott.

Stein, J. H. (1988). Hypokalemia: Common and uncommon causes. *Hospital Practice,* March 30, 1988.

Sterns, R. H. (1991). The management of hyponatremic emegencies. *Critical Care Clinics, 7*(1), 127–141.

Swonger, A. K., & Matejski, M. P. (1991). *Nursing pharmacology* (2nd ed.). Philadelphia: Lippincott.

Teaming up to send the end-stage COPD patients home. *Nursing 1984, 14*(1), 65–76.

Tripp, A. (1976). Hyper and hypocalcemia. *American Journal of Nursing, 76,* 1142–1145.

Twombly, M. (1983). Shift to third space. *Monitoring fluid and electrolytes precisely: Nursing skillbook.* Horsham, PA: Intermed Communications.

Valle, G. A., & Lemberg, L. (1988). Electrolyte imbalances in cardiovascular disease: The forgotten factor. *Heart and Lung, 17*(3), 324–329.

Vanatta, J. C., & Fogelman, M. J. (1988). *Moyer's fluid balance* (4th ed.). Chicago: Yearbook Medical.

VanHook, J. W. (1991). Hypermagnesemia. *Critical Care Clinics, 7*(1), 215–223.

Votey, S. R., Peters, A. L., & Hoffman, J. R. (1989). Disorders of water metabolism: Hyponatremia and hypernatremia. *Emergency Medicine Clinics of North America, 7*(4), 749–765.

Waltman, N. L., Bergstrom, N., Armstrong, N., Norrell, K., & Braden, B. (1991). Nutritional status, pressure sores, and mortality in elderly patients with cancer. *Oncology Nursing Forum, 18,* 867–873.

Watson, J. E. (1987). Fluid and electrolyte disorders in cardiovascular patients. *Nursing Clinics of North America, 22*(4), 797–803.

Whaley, L., & Wong, D. (1991). *Pediatric quick reference* (4th ed). Philadelphia: Mosby Yearbook.

Wilhelm, L. (1985). Helping your patient settle in with TPN. *Nursing 1985, 15*(4), 60.

Wittaker, A. (1985). Acute renal dysfunction. *Focus on Critical Care, 12*(3), 12–17.

Wong, D. (1993). *Essentials of pediatric nursing* (4th ed.). Philadelphia: Mosby Year Book.

Young, M. E., & Flynn, K. T. (1988). Third-spacing. When the body conceals fluid loss. *RN, 51*(8), 46–48.

Yurick, A. G., Spier, B. E., Robb, S. S., & Ebert, N. J. (1989). *The aged person and the nursing process* (3rd ed.). E. Norwalk, CT: Appleton & Lange.

Zalaga, G. P. (1991). Hypocalcemic crisis. *Critical Care Clinics, 7*(1), 191–199.

Zull, D. N. (1989). Disorders of potassium metabolism. *Emergency Medicine Clinics of North America, 7*(1), 771–793.